D1574475

1997
YEAR BOOK OF
HAND SURGERY®

Statement of Purpose

The YEAR BOOK Service

The YEAR BOOK series was devised in 1901 by practicing health professionals who observed that the literature of medicine and related disciplines had become so voluminous that no one individual could read and place in perspective every potential advance in a major specialty. In the final decade of the 20th century, this recognition is more acutely true than it was in 1901.

More than merely a series of books, YEAR BOOK volumes are the tangible results of a unique service designed to accomplish the following:

- to *survey* a wide range of journals of proven value
- to *select* from those journals papers representing significant advances and statements of important clinical principles
- to provide *abstracts* of those articles that are readable, convenient summaries of their key points
- to provide *commentary* about those articles to place them in perspective.

These publications grow out of a unique process that calls on the talents of outstanding authorities in clinical and fundamental disciplines, trained literature specialists, and professional writers, all supported by the resources of Mosby, the world's preeminent publisher for the health professions.

The Literature Base

Mosby and its editors survey more than 1,000 journals published worldwide, covering the full range of the health professions. On an annual basis, the publisher examines usage patterns and polls its expert authorities to add new journals to the literature base and to delete journals that are no longer useful as potential YEAR BOOK sources.

The Literature Survey

The publisher's team of literature specialists, all of whom are trained and experienced health professionals, examines every original, peer-reviewed article in each journal issue. More than 250,000 articles per year are scanned systematically, including title, text, illustrations, tables, and references. Each scan is compared, article by article, to the search strategies that the publisher has developed in consultation with the 270 outside experts who form the pool of YEAR BOOK editors. A given article may be reviewed by any number of editors, from one to a dozen or more, regardless of the discipline for which the paper was originally published. In turn, each editor who receives the article reviews it to determine whether or not the article should be included in the YEAR BOOK. This decision is based on the article's inherent quality, its probable usefulness to readers of that YEAR BOOK, and the editor's goal to represent a balanced picture of a given field in each volume of the YEAR BOOK. In addition, the editor indicates when to include figures and tables from the article to help the YEAR BOOK reader better understand the information.

Of the quarter million articles scanned each year, only 5% are selected for detailed analysis within the YEAR BOOK series, thereby assuring readers of the high value of every selection.

The Abstract

The publisher's abstracting staff is headed by a seasoned medical professional and includes individuals with training in the life sciences, medicine, and other areas, plus extensive experience in writing for the health professions and related industries. Each selected article is assigned to a specific writer on this abstracting staff. The abstracter, guided in many cases by notations supplied by the expert editor, writes a structured, condensed summary designed so that the reader can rapidly acquire the essential information contained in the article.

The Commentary

The YEAR BOOK editorial boards, sometimes assisted by guest commentators, write comments that place each article in perspective for the reader. This provides the reader with the equivalent of a personal consultation with a leading international authority—an opportunity to better understand the value of the article and to benefit from the authority's thought processes in assessing the article.

Additional Editorial Features

The editorial boards of each YEAR BOOK organize the abstracts and comments to provide a logical and satisfying sequence of information. To enhance the organization, editors also provide introductions to sections or individual chapters, comments linking a number of abstracts, citations to additional literature, and other features.

The published YEAR BOOK contains enhanced bibliographic citations for each selected article, including extended listings of multiple authors and identification of author affiliations. Each YEAR BOOK contains a Table of Contents specific to that year's volume. From year to year, the Table of Contents for a given YEAR BOOK will vary depending on developments within the field.

Every YEAR BOOK contains a list of the journals from which papers have been selected. This list represents a subset of the more than 1,000 journals surveyed by the publisher and occasionally reflects a particularly pertinent article from a journal that is not surveyed on a routine basis.

Finally, each volume contains a comprehensive subject index and an index to authors of each selected paper.

The 1997 Year Book Series

Year Book of Allergy, Asthma, and Clinical Immunology: Drs. Rosenwasser, Borish, Gelfand, Leung, Nelson, and Szefler

Year Book of Anesthesiology and Pain Management®: Drs. Tinker, Abram, Chestnut, Roizen, Rothenberg, and Wood

Year Book of Cardiology®: Drs. Schlant, Collins, Gersh, Graham, Kaplan, and Waldo

Year Book of Chiropractic®: Dr. Lawrence

Year Book of Critical Care Medicine®: Drs. Parrillo, Balk, Calvin, Franklin, and Shapiro

Year Book of Dentistry®: Drs. Meskin, Berry, Kennedy, Leinfelder, Roser, Summitt, and Zakariasen

Year Book of Dermatologic Surgery®: Drs. Greenway, Papadopoulos, and Whitaker

Year Book of Dermatology®: Drs. Sober and Fitzpatrick

Year Book of Diagnostic Radiology®: Drs. Federle, Gross, Dalinka, Maynard, Rebner, Smirniotopolous, and Young

Year Book of Digestive Diseases®: Drs. Greenberger and Moody

Year Book of Drug Therapy®: Drs. Lasagna and Weintraub

Year Book of Emergency Medicine®: Drs. Wagner, Dronen, Davidson, King, Niemann, and Roberts

Year Book of Endocrinology®: Drs. Bagdade, Braverman, Horton, Kannan, Landsberg, Molitch, Morley, Nathan, Odell, Poehlman, Rogol, and Ryan

Year Book of Family Practice®: Drs. Berg, Bowman, Davidson, Dexter, and Scherger

Year Book of Geriatrics and Gerontology®: Drs. Beck, Burton, Ostwald, Rabins, Reuben, Roth, Shapiro, and Whitehouse

Year Book of Hand Surgery®: Drs. Amadio and Hentz

Year Book of Hematology®: Drs. Spivak, Bell, Ness, Quesenberry, Wiernik, and Blume

Year Book of Infectious Diseases®: Drs. Keusch, Barza, Bennish, Poutsiaka, Skolnik, and Snydman

Year Book of Medicine®: Drs. Klahr, Cline, Petty, Frishman, Greenberger, Malawista, Mandell, and O'Rourke

Year Book of Neonatal and Perinatal Medicine®: Drs. Fanaroff, Maisels, Stevenson

Year Book of Nephrology, Hypertension, and Mineral Metabolism: Drs. Schwab, Bennett, Emmett, Hostetter, Kumar, and Toto

Year Book of Neurology and Neurosurgery®: Drs. Bradley and Wilkins

Year Book of Neurology and Neurosurgery®: Drs. Bradley and Wilkins

Year Book of Nuclear Medicine®: Drs. Gottschalk, Blaufox, Neumann, Strauss, and Zubal

Year Book of Obstetrics, Gynecology, and Women's Health: Drs. Mishell, Herbst, and Kirschbaum

Year Book of Occupational and Environmental Medicine®: Drs. Emmett, Frank, Gochfeld, and Hessl

Year Book of Oncology®: Drs. Ozols, Cohen, Glatstein, Loehrer, Tallman, and Wiersma

Year Book of Ophthalmology®: Drs. Wilson, Augsburger, Cohen, Eagle, Flanagan, Grossman, Laibson, Maguire, Nelson, Penne, Rapuano, Sergott, Spaeth, Tipperman, and Ms. Salmon

Year Book of Orthopedics®: Drs. Sledge, Poss, Cofield, Dobyns, Griffin, Springfield, Swiontkowski, Wiesel, and Wilson

Year Book of Otolaryngology–Head and Neck Surgery®: Drs. Paparella and Holt

Year Book of Pathology and Laboratory Medicine: Drs. Mills, Bruns, Gaffey, and Stoler

Year Book of Pediatrics®: Dr. Stockman

Year Book of Plastic, Reconstructive, and Aesthetic Surgery®: Drs. Miller, Cohen, McKinney, Robson, Ruberg, Smith, and Whitaker

Year Book of Podiatric Medicine and Surgery®: Dr. Kominsky

Year Book of Psychiatry and Applied Mental Health®: Drs. Talbott, Ballenger, Breier, Frances, Meltzer, Schowalter, and Tasman

Year Book of Pulmonary Disease®: Dr. Petty

Year Book of Rheumatology®: Drs. Sergent, LeRoy, Meenan, Panush, and Reichlin

Year Book of Sports Medicine®: Drs. Shephard, Alexander, Drinkwater, Eichner, George, and Torg

Year Book of Surgery®: Drs. Copeland, Bland, Deitch, Eberlein, Howard, Luce, Seeger, Souba, and Sugarbaker

Year Book of Thoracic and Cardiovascular Surgery®: Drs. Ginsberg, Wechsler, and Williams

Year Book of Urology®: Drs. Andriole and Coplin

Year Book of Vascular Surgery®: Dr. Porter

1997

The Year Book of HAND SURGERY®

Editors
Peter C. Amadio, M.D.
Vincent R. Hentz, M.D.

Editors Emeritus
Robert A. Chase, M.D.
James H. Dobyns, M.D.

International Assistant Editors
Guy Foucher, M.D.
Seiichi Ishii, M.D.
Priv. Dr. Med. C.L. Jantea
Antonio Landi, M.D.
Caroline LeClercq, M.D.
Alberto Lluch, M.D., Ph.D.
Yasuo Ueba, M.D.

Mosby

St. Louis Baltimore Boston Carlsbad Chicago Naples New York Philadelphia Portland
London Madrid Mexico City Singapore Sydney Tokyo Toronto Wiesbaden

Mosby
Dedicated to Publishing Excellence

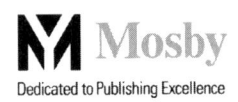

A Times Mirror
Company

Vice President and Publisher, Continuity Publishing: Kenneth H. Killion
Director, Editorial Development: Gretchen C. Murphy
Developmental Editor: Catherine Flanagan
Acquisitions Editor: Linda M. Sheehan
Associate Production Editor: Andrea Field
Freelance Staff Supervisor: Barbara M. Kelly
Illustrations and Permissions Coordinator: Nancy Dunne
Director, Editorial Services: Edith M. Podrazik, B.S.N, R.N.
Information Specialist: Kathleen Moss, R.N.
Information Specialist: Terri Santo, R.N.
Circulation Manager: Lynn D. Stevenson

1997 EDITION
Copyright © April 1997 by Mosby–Year Book, Inc.

All rights reserved. No part of this publication may be reproduced, stored in a retrieval system, or transmitted, in any form or by any means, electronic, mechanical, photocopying, recording, or otherwise, without prior written permission from the publisher.

Permission to photocopy or reproduce solely for internal or personal use is permitted for libraries or other users registered with the Copyright Clearance Center, provided that the base fee of $4.00 per chapter plus $.10 per page is paid directly to the Copyright Clearance Center, 21 Congress Street, Salem, MA 01970. This consent does not extend to other kinds of copying, such as copying for general distribution, for advertising or promotional purposes, for creating new collected works, or for resale.

Printed in the United States of America
Composition by Reed Technology and Information Services, Inc.
Printing/binding by Maple-Vail

Mosby–Year Book, Inc.
11830 Westline Industrial Drive
St. Louis, MO 63146
Customer Service: customer.support@mosby.com
                www.mosby.com/Mosby/CustomerSupport/index.html

Editorial Office:
Mosby–Year Book, Inc.
161 North Clark Street
Chicago, IL 60601
series.editorial@mosby.com

International Standard Serial Number: 0739-5949
International Standard Book Number: 0-8151-0162-7

Editors

Peter C. Amadio, M.D.
Professor of Orthopedic Surgery, Mayo Medical School; Consultant, Department of Orthopedics and Surgery of the Hand, Mayo Clinic, Rochester, Minnesota

Vincent R. Hentz, M.D.
Professor of Surgery and Chief, Division of Hand Surgery, Stanford University School of Medicine, Stanford, California

Editors Emeritus
Robert A. Chase, M.D.
Emile Holman Professor of Surgery and Anatomy, Emeritus, Stanford University School of Medicine, Stanford, California

James H. Dobyns, M.D.
Emeritus Professor of Orthopedic Surgery, Mayo Foundation, Rochester, Minnesota; Clinical Professor, University of Texas Health Science Center, San Antonio, Texas

International Assistant Editors
Guy Foucher, M.D.
Chirurgien, Strasbourg, France

Seiichi Ishii, M.D.
Professor of Orthopedic Surgery, Sapporo Medical University, Sapporo, Japan

Priv. Dr. Med. C.L. Jantea
Upper Limb Service, Orthopaedic Department, Heinrich-Heine-University Dusseldorf, Dusseldorf, Germany

Antonio Landi, M.D.
Facoltà di Medicina e Chirurgia, Università degli Studi di Modena, Modena, Italy

Caroline LeClercq, M.D.
Ancien Chef de Clinique, Assistante des Hospitaux de Paris, Institut de la Main, Paris, France

Alberto Lluch, M.D., Ph.D.
Assistant Professor of Orthopedic Surgery, University of Barcelona, Institut Kaplan for Surgery of the Hand and Upper Extremity, Barcelona, Spain

Yasuo Ueba, M.D.
Professor, Division of Occupational Therapy, College of Medical Technology, Kyoto University, Kyoto, Japan

Contributing Editors

Edward Akelman, M.D.
Associate Professor of Orthopaedic Surgery, Brown University, Providence, Rhode Island

Kai-Nan An, Ph.D.
Professor of Bioengineering, Mayo Medical School; Chairman, Division of Orthopedic Research, Mayo Clinic, Rochester, Minnesota

Marie A. Badalamente, Ph.D.
State University of New York, Stonybrook, New York

Robert D. Beckenbaugh, M.D.
Professor of Orthopedic Surgery, Mayo Medical School; Consultant, Department of Orthopedics and Surgery of the Hand, Mayo Clinic, Rochester, Minnesota

Keith Bengstson, M.D.
Consultant in the Department of Physical Medicine and Rehabilitation, Mayo Medical Center, Rochester, Minnesota

Richard A. Berger, M.D., Ph.D.
Associate Professor of Orthopedic Surgery and Anatomy, Mayo Medical School; Consultant, Departments of Orthopedics, Surgery of the Hand, and Anatomy, Mayo Clinic, Rochester, Minnesota

Gabrielle Bergman, M.D.
Assistant Professor of Radiology, Stanford University Hospital, Stanford, California

Thomas H. Berquist, M.D.
Professor of Radiology, Mayo Medical School; Chair, Department of Diagnostic Radiology, Mayo Clinic, Jacksonville, Florida

Charles Burgar, M.D.
Assistant Professor of Functional Restoration, Stanford University Hospital, Stanford, California

William P. Cooney, III, M.D.
Professor of Surgery, Mayo Medical School; Chair, Division of Hand Surgery, Department of Orthopedic Surgery, Mayo Clinic, Rochester, Minnesota

Paul Dell, M.D.
Professor and Chief of Hand and Microsurgery, University of Florida, Gainesville, Florida

William Engberger, M.D.
Associate Professor of Orthopedic Surgery, University of Wisconsin, Madison, Wisconsin

Roslyn B. Evans, O.T.R./L., C.H.T.
Indian River Hand Rehabilitation, Inc., Vero Beach, Florida

Marybeth Ezaki, M.D.
Assistant Professor, Department of Orthopedic Surgery, University of Texas Southwestern Medical School, Dallas, Texas

Joseph M. Failla, M.D.
Senior Staff, Department of Orthopedic Surgery, Head of Section of Hand Surgery, Henry Ford Hospital, Detroit, Michigan

Thomas Feeley, M.D.
Professor of Anesthesiology, Stanford Health Systems, Stanford, California

Earl Fleegler, M.D.
Director, Hand Program, Albert Einstein Medical Center, Philadelphia, Pennsylvania

Robert L. Horner, M.D.
Retired Assistant Professor of Orthopedic Surgery, Division of Hand Surgery, Mayo Medical Center, Rochester, Minnesota; Voluntary Staff, US Veterans Medical Center, Long Beach, California

James House, M.D.
Professor of Orthopedic Surgery, University of Minnesota, Minneapolis, Minnesota

Lawrence C. Hurst, M.D.
Department of Orthopedics, SUNY at Stonybrook, Stonybrook, New York

Craig H. Johnson, M.D.
Senior Associate Consultant, Division of Plastic and Reconstructive Surgery, Department of Surgery and Division of Hand Surgery, Department of Orthopedic Surgery, Mayo Clinic, Rochester, Minnesota

Jesse B. Jupiter, M.D.
Associate Professor of Orthopedic Surgery; Director, Orthopedic Hand Service, Massachusetts General Hospital, Boston, Massachusetts

Morton L. Kasdan, M.D.
Clinical Professor of Plastic and Reconstructive Surgery, University of Louisville, Louisville, Kentucky

J.A. Katarincic, M.D.
Instructor in Orthopedics, Mayo Medical Center, Rochester, Minnesota

Michael Keith, M.D.
Professor of Orthopedic Surgery, Case Western Reserve University, Cleveland, Ohio

T. Kiefhaber, M.D.
Assistant Clinical Professor of Orthopaedic Surgery, University of Cincinnati, Cincinnati, Ohio

L. Andrew Koman, M.D.
Professor, Surgical Sciences, Department of Orthopaedic Surgery, Bowman Gray School of Medicine, Wake Forest University, Winston-Salem, North Carolina

Amy L. Ladd, M.D.
Assistant Professor of Functional Restoration–Hand Surgery, Stanford University School of Medicine, Stanford, California

Maurice LeBlanc, Ph.D.
Visiting Scholar–School of Medicine; Visiting Lecturer–School of Engineering, Stanford University, Stanford, California

William L. Lineaweaver, M.D.
Associate Professor of Functional Restoration–Hand Surgery, Stanford University School of Medicine, Stanford, California

Ronald L. Linscheid, M.D.
Professor of Orthopedic Surgery, Mayo Medical School; Consultant Emeritus, Department of Orthopedics and Surgery of the Hand, Mayo Clinic, Rochester, Minnesota

Graham D. Lister, M.D.
Professor of Surgery, Division of Plastic and Reconstructive Surgery, Washington University School of Medicine, St. Louis, Missouri

Susan E. Mackinnon, M.D.
Professor of Surgery, Chief Division of Plastic and Reconstructive Surgery, Washington University School of Medicine, St. Louis, Missouri

N. Bradley Meland, M.D.
Associate Professor of Plastic Surgery, Mayo Medical School; Head, Section of Hand Surgery, Mayo Clinic, Scottsdale, Arizona

Bernard F. Morrey, M.D.
Professor of Orthopedic Surgery, Mayo Medical School; Chair, Department of Orthopedics, Mayo Clinic, Rochester, Minnesota

Owen J. Moy, M.D.
Hand Center of Western New York, Millard Fillmore Hospital, Buffalo, New York

Peter A. Nathan, M.D.
Portland Hand Surgery and Rehabilitation Center, Portland, Oregon

Tom Norris, M.D.
Pacific Medical Center, San Francisco, California

Edward R. North, M.D.
Washington Hand Surgery, Kirkland, Washington

Shawn W. O'Driscoll, M.D.
Associate Professor of Orthopedic Surgery, Mayo Medical School; Consultant, Department of Orthopedics, Mayo Clinic, Rochester, Minnesota

A. Lee Osterman, M.D.
Professor of Orthopedic and Hand Surgery, Thomas Jefferson University Hospital, Philadelphia Hand Center, Philadelphia, Pennsylvania

Clayton A. Peimer, M.D.
Professor, Department of Orthopedics, State University of New York at Buffalo School of Medicine; Chief of Hand Surgery, Department of Orthopedics, Millard Fillmore Hospital, Buffalo, New York

Vincent D. Pellegrini, Jr., M.D.
Department of Orthopedics and Rehabilitation, The Pennsylvania State University/The Milton S. Hershey Medical Center, Hershey, Pennsylvania

John Rayhack, M.D.
Director, Wrist and Hand Center, Tampa, Florida

R.K. Roenigk, M.D.
Professor of Dermatology, Mayo Medical Center, Rochester, Minnesota

Leonard K. Ruby, M.D.
Professor of Orthopedic Surgery, Tufts University School of Medicine, Boston, Massachusetts

William J. Shaughnessy, M.D.
Assistant Professor of Orthopedics, Mayo Medical School; Consultant, Department of Orthopedics, Mayo Clinic, Rochester, Minnesota

Peter J. Stern, M.D.
Professor and Chairman, Department of Orthopedic Surgery, University of Cincinnati College of Medicine, Cincinnati, Ohio

Robert M. Szabo, M.D.
Professor of Hand, Microvascular, and Orthopedic Surgery, University of California, Davis, California

Julio Taleisnik, M.D.
Clinical Professor of Surgery (Orthopedics), University of California, Irvine, California

Francisco Valero-Cuevas, Ph.D
Stanford University, School of Engineering (Mechanical Engineering), Stanford, California

Steven F. Viegas, M.D.
Professor and Chief, Division of Hand Surgery, Department of Orthopaedic Surgery and Rehabilitation; Professor of Anatomy and Neuroscience, The University of Texas Medical Branch, Galveston, Texas

Peter Wu, M.D.
Assistant Professor of Physical Medicine and Rehabilitation, Stanford Health System, Stanford, California

Felix M. Zajac, Ph.D.
Director, Rehabilitation R&D Center, VA Palo Alto Health Care System; Professor, Departments of Medical Engineering and Functional Restoration, Stanford University, Stanford, California

Table of Contents

JOURNALS REPRESENTED	xvii
INTRODUCTION	xix
1. Anatomy and Biomechanics	1
2. Diagnosis, Evaluation, and Anesthesia	21
3. Skeletal Trauma and Reconstruction	39
4. Soft-tissue Trauma and Reconstruction	67
5. Tendon Trauma and Reconstruction	89
6. Nerve Trauma and Reconstruction	103
7. Compression Neuropathy	113
8. Wrist	149
General	149
Carpus	158
Distal Radius	193
Distal Radioulnar Joint	214
9. Elbow	229
10. Neuromuscular Disorders	245
11. Cumulative Trauma Disorders	255
12. Arthritis	275
13. Tumors	297
14. Congenital Problems	315
15. Rehabilitation, Occupation, and Sports	327
16. Microsurgery	343
17. Vascular and Dystrophic Disorders	353
18. Research	361
SUBJECT INDEX	379
AUTHOR INDEX	465

Journals Represented

Mosby and its editors survey more than 1,000 journals for its abstract and commentary publications. From these journals, the editors select the articles to be abstracted. Journals represented in this YEAR BOOK are listed below.

Acta Radiologica
American Journal of Industrial Medicine
American Journal of Nephrology
American Journal of Orthopedics
American Journal of Public Health
American Journal of Roentgenology
American Journal of Sports Medicine
Annales de Chirurgie Plastique et Esthetique
Annales de Chirurgie de la Main
Annals of Emergency Medicine
Annals of Neurology
Annals of Plastic Surgery
Archives of Dermatology
Archives of Orthopaedic and Trauma Surgery
Arthritis and Rheumatism
Arthroscopy
Arthroskopie
British Journal of Anaesthesia
British Journal of Plastic Surgery
Canadian Journal of Surgery
Clinical Anatomy
Clinical Orthopaedics and Related Research
Contact Dermatitis
Ergonomics
Hand Surgery
International Orthopaedics
Journal of Biomechanics
Journal of Bone and Joint Surgery (American Volume)
Journal of Bone and Joint Surgery (British Volume)
Journal of Clinical Epidemiology
Journal of Environmental Medicine
Journal of Hand Surgery (American)
Journal of Hand Surgery (British)
Journal of Hand Therapy
Journal of Occupational and Environmental Medicine
Journal of Orthopaedic Research
Journal of Orthopaedic Science
Journal of Orthopaedic Trauma
Journal of Pediatric Orthopedics
Journal of Reconstructive Microsurgery
Journal of Rheumatology
Journal of Shoulder and Elbow Surgery
Journal of Trauma: Injury, Infection, and Critical Care
Journal of Workers Compensation
Journal of the Japanese Society for Surgery of the Hand
La Main
Medical Problems of Performing Artists

Microsurgery
Neurology
Neurosurgery
Nouvelles Dermatologiques les
Occupational and Environmental Medicine
Orthopedics
Paraplegia
Plastic and Reconstructive Surgery
Radiology
Revista Espanola de Cirugia de la Mano
Revista de Ortopedia y Traumatologia
Scandinavian Journal of Plastic and Reconstructive Hand Surgery
Scandinavian Journal of Rheumatology
Skeletal Radiology
The 1995 Jefferson Orthopaedic Journal

STANDARD ABBREVIATIONS

The following terms are abbreviated in this edition: acquired immunodeficiency syndrome (AIDS), cardiopulmonary resuscitation (CPR), central nervous system (CNS), cerebrospinal fluid (CSF), computed tomography (CT), deoxyribonucleic acid (DNA), electrocardiography (ECG), health maintenance organization (HMO), human immunodeficiency virus (HIV), intensive care unit (ICU), intramuscular (IM), intravenous (IV), magnetic resonance (MR) imaging (MRI), and ribonucleic acid (RNA).

NOTE

The YEAR BOOK OF HAND SURGERY® is a literature survey service providing abstracts of articles published in the professional literature. Every effort is made to assure the accuracy of the information presented in these pages. Neither the editors nor the publisher of the YEAR BOOK OF HAND SURGERY® can be responsible for errors in the original materials. The editors' comments are their own opinions. Mention of specific products within this publication does not constitute endorsement.

To facilitate the use of the YEAR BOOK OF HAND SURGERY® as a reference tool, all illustrations and tables included in this publication are now identified as they appear in the original article. This change is meant to help the reader recognize that any illustration or table appearing in the YEAR BOOK OF HAND SURGERY® may be only one of many in the original article. For this reason, figure and table numbers will often appear to be out of sequence within the YEAR BOOK OF HAND SURGERY®.

Introduction

This 1997 edition of the YEAR BOOK OF HAND SURGERY continues our tradition of searching the world literature for the very best articles in hand surgery. This year we welcome two new journals: *La Main*, which has replaced *Annales de Chirurgie de la Main* as the official journal of the French Society for Surgery of the Hand (GEM), and *Hand Surgery*, official journal of the Asia Pacific Federation of Societies for Surgery of the Hand. We continue to depend on our International editors for papers published in languages other than English, and would like to again thank Drs. LeClercq, Foucher, Lluch, Landi, Jantea, Ishii, and Ueba. This will be Dr. Antonio Landi's last YEAR BOOK as international editor for Italy. We are grateful for his contributions over the past few years. We are currently searching for a successor.

As always, we thank our families for their forbearance, our secretaries for their support, and the staff at Mosby–Year Book, particularly our developmental editor, Catherine Flanagan, for making all this possible.

Peter C. Amadio, M.D.
Vincent R. Hentz, M.D.

1 Anatomy and Biomechanics

Special Issue: Biomechanics
Bell-Krotoski JA, Riordan DC, Giurintano DJ, et al (Gillis W Long Hansen's Disease Ctr, Carville, La; Tulane Univ, New Orleans, La; Univ of New Mexico, Albuquerque; et al)
J Hand Ther 8:63–174, 1995   1–1

▶ The April/June 1995 issue of the *Journal of Hand Therapy* is a special issue entitled "Biomechanics: The Forces of Change and the Basis for All That We Do." The editors invited a number of authors from various fields including engineers, surgeons, and therapists to address significant contributions to the field of hand rehabilitation through the introduction and application of engineering concepts to clinical theory and practice. The articles are grouped according to content with basic anatomy and biomechanics discussed initially, followed by articles devoted to biomechanical research regarding specific joints, such as the thumb. The issue concludes with treatment-related articles and articles addressing specific measurement issues including instruments and objectivity. All of these articles have direct relevance to the field of hand rehabilitation. Because the entire issue is deemed outstanding, we have asked one of our contributing editors, Roslyn B. Evans, O.T.R./L., C.H.T., to comment on this special issue on biomechanics.

P.C. Amadio, M.D.

▶ This special issue on biomechanics may well be the most outstanding issue produced by the *Journal of Hand Therapy* since its inception in 1987. The disciplines of biomechanical engineering, hand surgery, and hand therapy have collaborated to address 2 critical issues in upper extremity management: assessment and the application of force to healing tissues.

Biomechanical terms and principles are defined in language common to both the engineer and the hand clinician and are used consistently throughout the issue in articles that discuss objective measures, instrumentation, assessment, the relationship of soft tissues to externally applied forces through exercise and splinting, and the performance properties of splinting materials. Quantification of forces and complication of inaccurately applied clinical forces are emphasized. Torque range of motion is described as a means of quantifying the amount of tension applied for objective measurement of joint angle. The use of the Haldex and other strain gauge instruments is described as these instruments relate to hand treatment. The new concept of total end range time and its relationship to joint end range is defined.[1] The contributors encourage the clinician to think in terms of force and time and how these 2 variables can be manipulated to stimulate tissue remodeling and homeostasis.

Never before has objective measurement been more important. We are now asked to justify the efficacy of every procedure or treatment with outcome studies. We are asked to quantify loss and clinical improvement with treatment and relate both to function. Reliable functional outcomes are dependent on reliable and valid assessment; reliable assessment is dependent on reliable and valid instrumentation and testing. As the authors point out, few clinical assessment instruments in hand rehabilitation meet even the most basic measurement criteria. Aside from a few hand function tests, only 4 hand assessment instruments meet the basic requirements of instrument reliability.[2] These include the volumeter, the goniometer, Jamar dynamometer, and Semmes Weinstein monofilaments.

As hand therapists and hand surgeons, we stand to learn much from the engineer regarding instrumentation concepts, an area in which we receive little training. A number of examples are offered throughout this issue, and one of the best concerns evaluation of sensibility. It is the engineer who has helped us to define the importance of controlled force with any sensory testing instrument. Two-point discrimination and the hand-held vibrometer are not reliable and valid testing instruments because the forces applied with the human hand are widely variable; even so, these tests are often used to evaluate clinical results. Inaccurate measurements and untested beliefs result in errors that find their way into the literature and complicate treatment by being relied on as fact by other clinicians.[3]

Defining the application of force to healing tissues is simplified, not complicated, by the application of biomechanical principals. Simple biomechanics teaches us why a high outrigger is more effective than a low outrigger with dynamic splinting; why the metacarpophalangeal joint placed in modest flexion, instead of full flexion, decreases internal flexor tendon forces with active motion; and why low-load and prolonged stress with serial casting is more effective in elongations connective tissue than dynamic splinting and exercise. The point is clearly made in this issue that the engineer should be included as an essential part of the research or rehabilitation team in the practice of hand surgery and hand therapy. Dr. Paul Brand envisioned this concept over 30 years ago and, together with David Thompson, Ph.D., produced much of the work that has contributed to critical thinking in our discipline. The Carville influence is present in almost every article in this special issue. As clinicians, we have much to gain by its review.

R.B. Evans, O.T.R./L., C.H.T.

References

1. Flowers KR, LaStayo P: Effect of total end range time on improving passive range of motion. *J Hand Ther* 7:150–157, 1994.
2. Fess EE: Guidelines for evaluating assessment instruments. *J Hand Ther* 8:145, 1995.
3. Bell-Krotoski JA, Fess EE: Biomechanics: The forces of change and the basis for all that we do. *J Hand Ther* 8:66, 1995.

Contact Areas in the Thumb Carpometacarpal Joint
Ateshian GA, Ark JW, Rosenwasser MP, et al (Columbia Univ, New York; Raleigh Orthopaedic Clinic, NC; Univ of Michigan, Ann Arbor)
J Orthop Res 13:450–458, 1995   1–2

Background.—Osteoarthritis of the thumb carpometacarpal joint is less common than osteoarthritis of the distal interphalangeal joints of the fingers; however, it is more disabling because advanced osteoarthritis of the thumb can result in a 50% loss of hand function. The articular surfaces of the thumb carpometacarpal joint are saddle-shaped, and incongruity has been suggested as a major factor in the development of arthritis. Instability of the joint has also been implicated. To understand the mechanics and origin of osteoarthritis in this joint, precise determination of contact areas as a function of joint position is important. Direct in situ testing and stereophotogrammetry were used to study thumb carpometacarpal articular contact.

Methods.—Thirteen fresh-frozen cadaver hands were studied. Contact areas in the joint were determined under the functional position of lateral (key) pinch and in extremes of the joint's range of motion. Contact areas were compared with known sites of cartilage erosion. Data were collected in vitro with the thumb in the lateral pinch position under a 25 N load and with the thumb in flexion, extension, abduction, adduction, and neutral positions under muscle loads of 0 to 5 N. Stereophotogrammetry was used to determine the contact areas of the articular surfaces of the thumb carpometacarpal joint when in these positions.

Results.—Contact areas associated with the lateral pinch position were located primarily on the central, volar, and volar-ulnar regions of the trapezium and the metacarpal (Fig 6). Contact areas were distinctly separated between the dorsoradial and volar-ulnar regions in 3 specimens. Contact occurred exclusively on the dorsoradial region of the trapezium in another. For 9 specimens, maps of cartilage thickness were also generated. The most common sites of thin cartilage were the volar-ulnar, ulnar, and dorsoradial regions of the trapezium. Thinning in these sites may be the result of cartilage wear.

Discussion.—The lateral pinch position produced stresses in the same regions in which cartilage thinning occurred. High states of stress in these regions may initiate the process of cartilage degeneration. This optical

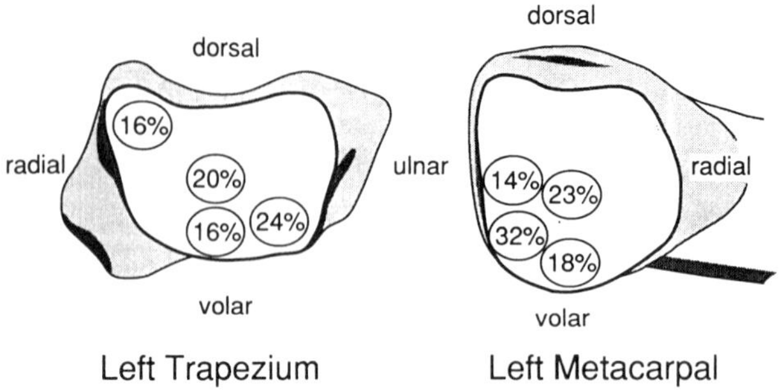

FIGURE 6.—The contact areas for all specimens, in lateral pinch with a 25-N load. All results from the right hand are transposed onto this schema of a carpometacarpal joint from the left thumb (Courtesy of Ateshian GA, Ark JW, Rosenwasser MP, et al: Contact areas in the thumb carpometacarpal joint. *J Orthop Res* 13:450–458, 1995.)

technique is advantageous in that it obviates the need to insert devices or substances into the joint space (which might affect contact mechanics).

▶ The authors use a sophisticated optical technique of stereophotogrammetric analysis to study the contact areas of the thumb trapeziometacarpal joint. Such a technique avoids any artifact secondary to introduction of materials between joint surfaces. The results agree with previous reports using pressure sensitive Fuji film; during the principal functional position of lateral pinch, joint contact areas were concentrated in the volar and ulnar aspects of the facing surfaces of the trapezium and metacarpal (Fig 6). In 3 specimens, dorsoradial contact regions were also noted. Although areas of cartilage thinning coincided with identified areas of joint surface contact, the method did not allow distinction between cartilage thinning resulting from degenerative disease and that present in the setting of a normal articular cartilage surface. Taken in the context of previously published data regarding pathoanatomy of disease in trapeziometacarpal joints, this work confirms the primary volar contact during lateral pinch and also identifies an area of dorsoradial contact, perhaps secondary to rotational malalignment of joint surfaces.

Alternatively, dorsoradial contact and cartilage thinning may well be secondary to physiologic aging, as previous researchers have hypothesized, rather than secondary to pathologic articular surface disease. Broader application of this sophisticated technique of optical analysis on additional specimens, in the context of gross anatomical disease as distinguished from changes of physiologic aging, will certainly contribute to our understanding of the pathophysiology of trapeziometacarpal osteoarthritis.

V.D. Pellegrini, Jr., M.D.

An Anatomical Study for Innervation and Vascular Supply of the Nail Bed and Matrix and a Histological Study of their Nerve Endings

Hayashi H, et al (Jikei Univ, Tokyo, Japan)
J Jpn Soc Surg Hand 12:515–520, 1995
1–3

Methods.—The distribution of innervation and vascular supply of the nail bed and matrix was investigated. Four fresh cadaver hands with 20 fingers were dissected using microscopic magnification. Colored latex was injected from the arteries of the wrist. From anatomical findings, the nerve and vascular distributions of the nail bed and matrix were provided from the finger pulp.

Results.—All branches of the nail bed entered into the rima ungualum, which is surrounded by the medial edge of the interosseous ligament and the distal phalanx. This indicates that the branches of the nail bed are protected by the lateral interosseous ligament.

Methods.—A histologic study of the innervation of the nail bed and matrix was also performed, using 3 fresh cadaver fingers. Transverse sections were made and dyed by Bodian staining. Vertical cross sections were made using an amputated finger and dyed by Masson and Bodian staining. The nerve endings and sensory receptors were observed under the microscope. Quantitative analysis of Meissner's corpuscles in the distal one third of the nail bed and in the soft tissue under the nail bed were performed using the vertical cross-sections.

Results.—Few free nerve endings were recognized in the collagen tissues of the nail bed, and Meissner's corpuscles were observed in the superficial layer of the nail bed and in the soft tissues under the nail matrix. The numbers of Meissner's corpuscles were $13.3/mm^2$ in the distal one third of nail bed and $6.6/mm^2$ in the soft tissue under nail matrix.

▶ This histologic study on the innervation and vascular supply to the nail bed and matrix provides interesting information regarding the origin, divisions, and distribution of the nerves and vessels under the nail. The most interesting information for me regards the sensory receptors in the nail matrix and bed.

According to this study, only free nerve endings and Meissner's corpuscles are present, and neither Merkel's disks nor pacinian's corpuscles are observed there. Nail removal causes severe pain, presumably by free nerve endings, and the nail is sensitive to slow vibration owing to Meissner's corpuscles. It is deemed that the nail is less sensitive to constant pressure and quick vibrations because of the lack of Merkel's disks and pacinian corpuscles under the nail. Electrophysiologic study is necessary to further confirm these aspects of sensitivity of the nail.

Y. Ueba, M.D.

The Axes of Rotation of the Thumb Interphalangeal and Metacarpophalangeal Joints

Hollister A, Giurintano DJ, Buford WL, et al (Rancho Los Amigos Med Ctr, Downey, Calif; Gillis W Long Hansen's Disease Ctr, Carville, Calif; Univ of Texas, Galveston; et al)
Clin Orthop 320:188–193, 1995

Introduction.—The normal function and pathology of the thumb can be best understood with an accurate model of its kinematics. Although the carpometacarpal joint of the thumb has been studied in detail, less is known about the metacarpophalangeal and interphalangeal joints of the thumb. In this study, a mechanical device called an axis finder was used to determine the axes of rotation of the metacarpophalangeal and interphalangeal joints of the thumb.

Methods.—The axis of rotation from 5 thumb metacarpophalangeal and 7 interphalangeal cadaveric joints were located using an axis finder. To determine the axis of the interphalangeal joint, the axis finder was pinned to the distal phalanx bone. The interphalangeal joint was then moved through a normal range of motion with flexion and extension of the distal phalanx; the axis finder was adjusted to locate the axis. After the axis was located, a 1.6-mm K-wire was positioned along the axis through the distal phalanx. To locate the axis of the metacarpophalangeal joint, the axis finder was pinned to the thumb proximal phalanx. The metacarpophalangeal joint was also moved through a normal range of motion until the axis was located. Another 1.6-mm K-wire was positioned along the located axis through the metacarpal. The K-wire was later removed and the abduction-adduction axis of the joint was located using the axis finder. The interphalangeal and metacarpophalangeal joints were dissected and angles and locations of the wires in relationship to bone were measured.

Results.—For the interphalangeal joint, one fixed axis of rotation was identified. The axis of rotation was found to be parallel to the flexion creases, passing between the dorsal and volar creases. The axis of rotation also passed through the Cleland's ligaments and was distal and volar to the epicondyles. For the metacarpophalangeal joint, 2 axes of rotation were found: a flexion-extension axis and an abduction-adduction axis. The flexion-extension axis was found to be fixed for all positions through flexion and extension. This axis was volar and distal to the metacarpal epicondyles. The abduction-adduction axis passed through the metacarpal and was between the 2 sesamoids of the volar plate. This axis was fixed in relation to the proximal phalanx.

Conclusion.—The interphalangeal joint was found to have one fixed axis of rotation, parallel to the flexion crease of the joint and offset to the phalanx. Two fixed axes were found for the metacarpophalangeal joint, neither of which was perpendicular to the phalanges. Improved knowledge about the location and function of the mechanical axes of the thumb will help in the construction of prosthetic joints and in reconstructive surgery.

▶ By use of a mechanical method, the axis of rotation of the interphalangeal joint of the thumb was determined to parallel the interphalangeal joint flexion crease and is thus offset with respect to the phalanx. This explains the pronation that occurs with flexion, another of evolution's little refinements that permits the thumb pulp to face the digital pulps in grasp. Although the authors describe metacarpophalangeal motion as occurring about 2 fixed axes, the joint's motion seems better described by the addition of a third axis about which pronation and supination occur.

V.R. Hentz, M.D.

A Graphic Analysis of the Biomechanics of the Massless Bi-articular Chain: Application to the Proximal Bi-articular Chain of the Human Finger
Leijnse JNAL (Erasmus Univ, Rotterdam, The Netherlands)
J Biomech 29:355–366, 1996

Objective.—This report introduces a model that visualizes the relationship between morphologic characteristics and function in the bi-articular chain, and permits graphic analysis of motor force in the unloaded and loaded chain, the load range of the motors, the range of preferential loading (loads that can be sustained with little force), the feasibility of equilibrium, and the condition of control.

Observations.—Results were applied to the proximal three-motor bi-articular chain of the human finger when controlled by the superficial flexor, interosseous, and extensor only. It was noted that the anatomical position of the superficial flexor and extensor is an essential factor in the optimal function of this chain, that the proximal bi-articular chain of the human finger can sustain certain flexion loads very well, but is structurally weak when extension loads are applied, and that the chain is not optimally controllable. These findings suggest that the third joint and the other finger motors (deep flexor and lumbrical) have an important part in improvement of finger control.

Conclusions.—In terms of the proximal 3-tendon bi-articular chain of the human finger, it is concluded that the loadability and controllability of the chain of the proximal finger is essentially determined by the marked antagonism of the extensor and superficial flexor. The other motor pairs are not antagonistic at all. The chain is structurally weak in the extensor-flexor load range. It also is not well conditioned for optimal control, and fairly small alterations in the moment arms of the extensor and/or flexor may lead to an uncontrollable chain.

▶ This work concentrates on the worthwhile task of expanding on work done by others in their group (Leijnse and Kalker, 1995[1]; Leijnse, et al., 1992[2]; Leijnse, et al., 1993[3]), thoroughly addresses previously raised questions such as feasibility of solutions (Spoor, 1983[4]) and introduces "moment arm vectors" to find optimality of control. However, I do not consider it a significant contribution to the field of finger biomechanics for the following reasons:

(1) The simplified model of the finger (2 segments and 3 muscles) used in this paper permits the development of interesting and important interactions among finger geometry and musculotendons (such as extensor-flexor interactions necessary to produce an extension force at the second phalanx, or the sensitivity of solutions to anatomical parameters). Unfortunately, this very simplification also precludes the meaningful theoretical and clinical extrapolation of their methodology and concepts to anatomically correct fingers.

(2) It omits mention of other important work, which is not only graphic in nature (Chao and An, 1978[5]), but also considers a more anatomically correct model of the fingers (i.e., 3 segments and 6 muscles) to thoroughly address the clinically important issues of finger equilibrium, muscle redundancy and optimality, and uniqueness and feasibility of muscle force combinations.

F. Valero-Cuevas, Ph.D.

References

1. Leijnse J, Kalker J: A two-dimensional kinematic model of the lumbrical in the human finger. *J Biomech* 28:237–249, 1995.
2. Leijnse JN, Bonte JE, Landsmeer JM, et al: Biomechanics of the finger with anatomical restrictions: The significance for the exercising hand of the musician. *J Biomechanics* 25:1253–1264, 1992.
3. Leijnse JN, Snijders CJ, Bonte JE, et al: The hand of the musician: Kinematics of the bidigital finger system with anatomical restrictions. *J Biomechanics* 26:1169–1179, 1993.
4. Spoor CW: Balancing a force on the fingertip of a two dimensional finger model without intrinsic muscles. *J Biomechanics* 16:497–504, 1983.
5. Chao EY, An, KN: Graphical interpretation of the solution to the redundant problem in biomechanics. *J Biomech Eng* 100:159–167, 1978.

Human Wrist Motors: Biomechanical Design and Application to Tendon Transfers
Loren GJ, Shoemaker SD, Burkholder TJ, et al (Univ of California, San Diego; Göteborg Univ, Sweden)
J Biomech 29:331–342, 1996

1–6

Background.—Strength is commonly used to determine neuromuscular function. Accurate interpretation of strength necessitates an understanding of joint kinematics, muscle tension, tendon compliance, and interactions among these factors. Moment arm, muscle architecture, and tendon compliance were determined in human cadaver forearms and used to model the wrist torque-joint angle relation.

Methods.—Five cadaver arms were studied. Instantaneous moment arms were determined by differentiating tendon excursion in joint rotation. Predictions of maximum isometric tension of each wrist muscle-tendon unit were based on muscle physiologic cross-sectional area. Muscle forces were subsequently adjusted for sarcomere length changes from joint rotation and tendon strain. Torque profiles were established for each prime wrist motor, and the effects of moment arm, muscle force, and tendon compliance on the torque profile of each motor were quantified.

Findings.—Considerable variation in wrist extensor motor torque was noted throughout range of motion. Moment arm-joint angle relations primarily determined the contours of the extensor torque profiles. By contrast, near-maximal torque over the entire range of motion resulted from wrist flexor motors. Flexor torque profiles were less affected by moment arm and relied more on muscle force variations with wrist rotation and tendon strain.

Conclusions.—Interactions among the joint, muscle, and tendon produce a unique torque profile for each wrist motor. These findings have significant implications for biomechanical modeling and operative tendon transfer.

▶ This report emphasizes the role of torque in determining muscle performance and provides some useful advice regarding applications for tendon transfer surgery. To me, all this underlines the complexity of tendon transfer surgery. There seems to be no substitute for a conscientious analysis of strength, excursion, angle of pull, and moment arm, among other factors, when analyzing alternatives.

P.C. Amadio, M.D.

Tendon Biomechanical Properties Enhance Human Wrist Muscle Specialization
Loren GJ, Lieber RL (Univ of California, San Diego; VA Med Ctr, San Diego)
J Biomech 28:791–799, 1995   1–7

Introduction.—The various skeletal muscles are highly specialized with respect to how much force they generate. Muscles of differing architectural conformation generate different peak tensions through a particular range. The degree to which tendon compliance influences the contractile properties of skeletal muscles is uncertain.

Objective and Methods.—The biomechanical properties of the tendons of the prime wrist movers were studied in 5 cadavers by subjecting them to loads predicted to be physiologic. The muscles studied were the extensor carpi radialis brevis (ECRB) and longus (L), the extensor carpi ulnaris, the flexor carpi radialis, and the flexor carpi ulnaris (FCU). Tendon area was estimated by manual digital micrometry, saline displacement, and computed microscopic analysis after tensile failure testing. Peak tension was predicted using a specific tension value of 22.5 N/cm^2. Collagen was assayed, and a model was used to predict the extent of sarcomeric shortening taking place at the expense of tendon lengthening for a maximal contraction.

Findings.—Loading to peak tension resulted in significantly different strain values for the different tendons. Strain was greatest in the FCU and least in the ECRL. It averaged about 2.5% for the various tendons, but final deformation corresponded to a strain of approximately 14%. The amount of strain correlated positively with the ratio of tendon length to fiber length ratio of the muscle-tendon unit—a measure of intrinsic compliance. The maximum expected decrease in sarcomere length was approximately 0.6 μm for the FCU, and the minimum was about 0.2 μm for the ECRB at peak tension. Analysis of elongation to failure—the conventional method—failed to reveal significant biomechanical differences among the various tendon-muscle units. The wrist flexor tendons contained significantly less collagen than the extensors, but there was no substantial difference among the radial and ulnar deviators.

Implications.—The biomechanical properties of wrist tendons do not merely reflect the architectural properties of the corresponding muscles. Instead, they add to overall specialization of the muscle-tendon unit. It may not be valid to infer functional properties from the results of traditional deformation-to-failure studies.

▶ Tendons not only act like a link to transfer muscle force to the skeleton; because they have compliance, they also affect the force-length relation of the muscle-tendon unit. This study on flexor and extensor tendons of human wrist cadavers shows that these muscle-tendon units differ in how much their tendons elongate per unit length per maximum force developed by the muscle (i.e., tendon strain at maximum force differs among the wrist muscle-tendon units). The implications of this finding on function are that the effect of tendon on the overall force-length properties of the muscle-tendon unit is determined not only by the relative length of tendon to the length of the muscle fibers but also by the intrinsic properties of the tendon (e.g., tendon strain at maximum force). On the basis of well-known force-length properties of muscle fibers, the authors calculate that tendon strain could affect muscle force generation among wrist tendons by as little as 10% (ECRL) or as much as 50% (FCU). As important as these data and calculations are to understanding the intrinsic properties of muscle-tendon units, I believe the ultimate challenge lies in developing methods to find their properties in situ. This will be no easy task.

F.M. Zajac, Ph.D.

Efficiency of the Flexor Tendon Pulley System in Human Cadaver Hands
Rispler D, Greenwald D, Shumway S, et al (Univ of Chicago; Massachusetts Gen Hosp, Boston)
J Hand Surg [Am] 21A:444–450, 1996   1–8

Objective.—The flexor tendon pulley system was examined in 4 cadaver hands.

Methods.—The transverse carpal ligament was exposed in 12 fingers. Individual flexor tendons were sutured together, as were extensor tendons. Tensile testing was accomplished by attaching a 200-g weight to the extensors and a 50-g weight to the flexors. Digits were flexed at 4 cm/min. Viscoelastic changes were measured using an analogue-digital converter system at 10 samples/sec for triplicate runs. Pull was measured until 0.1 kg of force was measured. Load and distance pulled were measured by a force transducer and a linear variable differential transformer. Excursion efficiency was calculated as the ratio of control excursion to experimental excursion. Work efficiency was calculated as the ratio of experimental work to control work. Combinations of annular pulleys measured were A1, A1 + A5, A3 + A5, A1 + A3 + A5, A2, A4, and A2 + A4.

Results.—Excising A5 or A3 and A5 did not affect work or excursion efficiency. Excising A1 significantly improved work efficiency by 118% but did not change excursion efficiency. Excising A1 and A5 significantly improved work efficiency by 116% but did not change excursion efficiency. Excising A1, A3, and A5 and excising A2 increased work efficiency by 106% and 102%, respectively, but significantly decreased excursion efficiency to 96% and 95%, respectively. Excision of A4 and of A2 and A4 significantly decreased work efficiency by 85% and 92%, respectively and significantly decreased excursion efficiency to 83% and 82%, respectively. With skin and pulleys intact, work efficiency decreased significantly to 92%, whereas excursion efficiency was essentially unchanged.

Conclusion.—Excision of A4 resulted in the largest biomechanical work and excursion efficiency losses. Preservation of the A2, A3, and A4 pulley combination was necessary to maintain work and excursion efficiency.

▶ This interesting paper looks at the excursion and work of tendons after pulley excision. The work function studied was fingertip pressure. The authors seemed surprised to find that A4 excision had a greater effect on this variable than did A2 excision. However, because tip pressure is primarily a function of the flexor digitorum profundus, I think the finding is readily understandable. Grip force, which brings the flexor digitorum sublimis into play, would probably show a stronger role for A2. Clearly, both A2 and A4 are important when one considers the gamut of finger–hand function.

P.C. Amadio, M.D.

Mechanical Analysis of the Palmar Aponeurosis Pulley in Human Cadavers
Phillips C, Mass D (Univ of Chicago)
J Hand Surg [Am] 21A:240–244, 1996   1–9

Introduction.—The anatomy of the palmar aponeurosis (PA) pulley has previously been described, but less is known about its biomechanical function. The functional importance of the PA pulley was anatomically studied.

Materials.—Six freshly frozen upper extremities obtained at autopsy were dissected. The index, long, and ring fingers of each hand were used, for a total of 18 fingers tested. The parameters measured included tendon load, tendon excursion, and tendon work. Data were obtained in the intact pulley system and after the sequential division of the PA pulley alone and in combination with the proximal annular pulleys.

Results.—Sectioning the PA pulley alone did not significantly affect any of the efficiency parameters. Excursion efficiency was significantly decreased, however, when the PA pulley was sectioned in combination with either or both of its proximal annular pulleys. After all 3 proximal pulleys had been sectioned, there was a significant increase in load efficiency and a significant decrease in work efficiency. The data suggest that the PA pulley in combination with the proximal annular pulleys acts to decrease the tendency to bow-stringing around the metacarpophalangeal joint. Thus the apparent role of the PA pulley as part of the flexor tendon pulley system is not only to ensure efficient finger range of motion, but also to influence the gliding capability of the tendons themselves.

Conclusion.—The PA pulley has a major biomechanical role in the flexor tendon pulley system. Although damage to the PA pulley alone would not cause a functional deficit, damage to the PA pulley and certain annular pulleys could leave some functional deficit.

▶ This useful article provides details on the mechanical effects of the PA pulley, originally described by Manske and Lesker.[1] The pulley seems to have its major role as a backup, particularly to A1. It is probably advisable to preserve PA when doing, for example, a trigger finger release.

P.C. Amadio, M.D.

Reference

1. Manske PR, Lesker PA: Palmar aponeurosis pulley. *J Hand Surg* 8:259–263, 1983.

In-vitro Strength of Flexor-Tendon Repairs
Sanders DW, Bain GI, Johnson JA, et al (Univ of Western Ontario, London; St Joseph's Health Centre, London, Ontario)
Can J Surg 38:528–532, 1995   1–10

Background.—Although many advances have been made in surgical technique for flexor-tendon repair in the hand, clinical failures still occur. New suture methods that withstand early active motion have been developed. The initial static strength, technical ease, and repair site bulk associated with the conventional Tajima repair and with these newer techniques were compared.

Methods.—Thirty-nine fresh-frozen cadaveric flexor digitorum superficialis tendons from index, long, and ring fingers were harvested and divided transversely. The tendons were randomly assigned to the Tajima method or to 1 of 3 new methods—the Halsted, Savage, or Silfverskiold techniques (Fig 1).

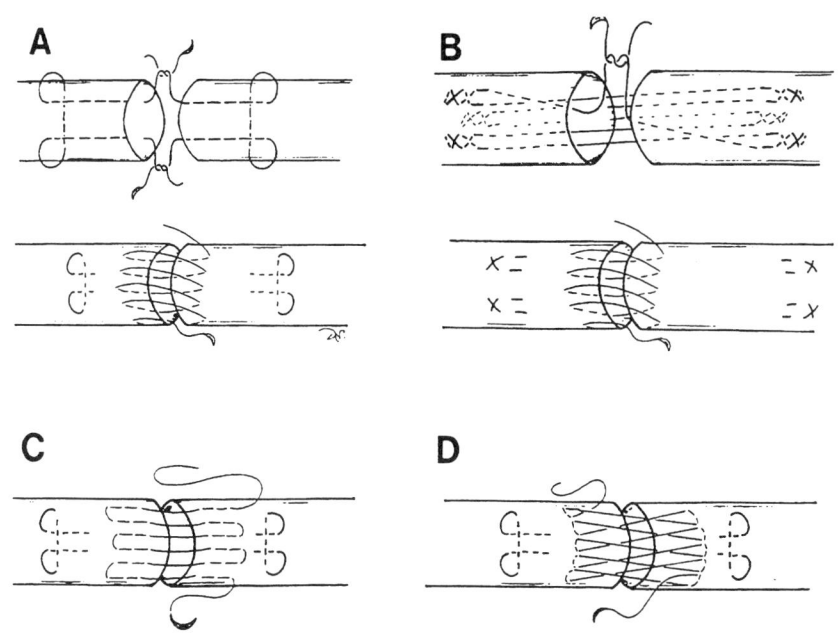

FIGURE 1.—Suture techniques. A, Tajima technique with 2-strand 4-0 Ethibond (Ethicon Sutures Ltd., Peterborough, Ontario) core suture and 6-0 Ethilon epitendinous running suture. B, Halsted technique with 4-0 Ethibond Kessler core suture (single knot) and 6-0 Ethibond horizontal mattress epitendinous stitch. C, Savage technique with 4-0 Ethibond core suture and 6-0 Ethilon running epitendinous suture. D, Silfverskiold technique with 4-0 Ethibond Kessler core suture and 6-0 Ethilon epitendinous cross-stitch. (Reprinted from Sanders DW, Bain GI, Johnson JA, et al: In-vitro strength of flexor-tendon repairs, by permission of the publisher, *Can J Surg*, 38:528–532, 1995.)

Findings.—The greatest loads were tolerated by the Savage repair, followed by the Halsted, Silfverskiold, and Tajima techniques. The least time-consuming was the Silfverskiold, followed by the Tajima, Halsted, and Savage. All methods increased the cross-sectional dimensions of the tendon. The Silfverskiold technique increased the dimensions by 50% or more and the Savage, by more than 100%. All the new techniques provided better static strength than did the Tajima, but none performed ideally.

Conclusions.—None of the suture methods tested in this study performed perfectly. Ideally, such repair would resist gap formation and rupture at physiologic cyclic loads without adversely affecting tendon gliding or healing. Additional in vitro and in vivo research is needed.

▶ For many years, almost all hand surgeons used similar suture techniques in repairing lacerated flexor tendons. The Bunnell "criss-cross" technique became a relic of past days. We are probably witnessing the same relegation of the long-favored Kessler or Tajima technique in favor of techniques that provide much higher resistance to gap formation at the repair site, in order to begin active motion at the earliest possible moment. Additional core strands and different surface weaving techniques are being touted as necessary to permit safe early active motion. However, we must accept a wider cross-section at the repair site in exchange. This evolution is ongoing.

V.R. Hentz, M.D.

Biomechanical Alterations in the Carpal Arch and Hand Muscles After Carpal Tunnel Release: A Further Approach Toward Understanding the Function of the Flexor Retinaculum and the Cause of Postoperative Grip Weakness
Fuss FK, Wagner TF (Univ of Vienna; Gen Hosp of Wiener, Neustadt, Austria)
Clin Anat 9:100–108, 1996   1–11

Background.—One of the most serious problems after carpal arch surgery is grip weakness, which can severely impair patients during the first 3 months after surgery. Grip weakness is caused by bowstringing of the flexor tendons because of loss of the carpal ligament pulley and widening of the carpal arch, resulting in biomechanical changes. In one study, reconstruction of the flexor retinaculum by z-plasty did not result in significant loss of grip strength. Another study measured increased distance between the palmar tips of the trapezium ridge and the hamate hook and found a mean increase of 10.4% or 2.7 mm at follow-up. It was also reported that this increase was associated with the degree of loss of grip strength. There is a general lack of knowledge in 4 areas of the function of the flexor retinaculum and postoperative grip weakness.

Study.—Carpal arch widening under stress situations was studied. Changes in thenar and hypothenar muscle mechanics after transverse carpal arch transection and z-plasty were analyzed along with grip weakness and the role of the thenar and finger muscles.

Methods.—Five fresh forearms with hands were dissected on the palmar side to expose the muscle attachments to the flexor retinaculum. The fiber arrangements and attachment of the flexor retinaculum and ligaments were examined. Details of examination of joint mechanics and muscle mechanics are given. Twenty patients with carpal tunnel syndrome and 20 controls were clinically evaluated. Hands were examined before and 4 months after carpal tunnel release. Patients with postoperative grip weakness were questioned about when grip weakness was most noticeable. Force measurements were obtained in controls and in patients before and after surgery and were used to determine whether grip weakness resulted from the thenar or finger muscles.

Results.—Differences between the maximal and minimal distance covered by an intact flexor retinaculum and the increase in maximal distance on carpal tunnel release were significant. The distance between the attachments of the trapezopisiform band increased after carpal tunnel release under external supination. The distance between attachments of the scaphoideohamate band increased after carpal tunnel release under external pronation. Carpal tunnel release also caused an anatomical attachment loss for these muscles: the superficial head of the flexor pollicis brevis, the

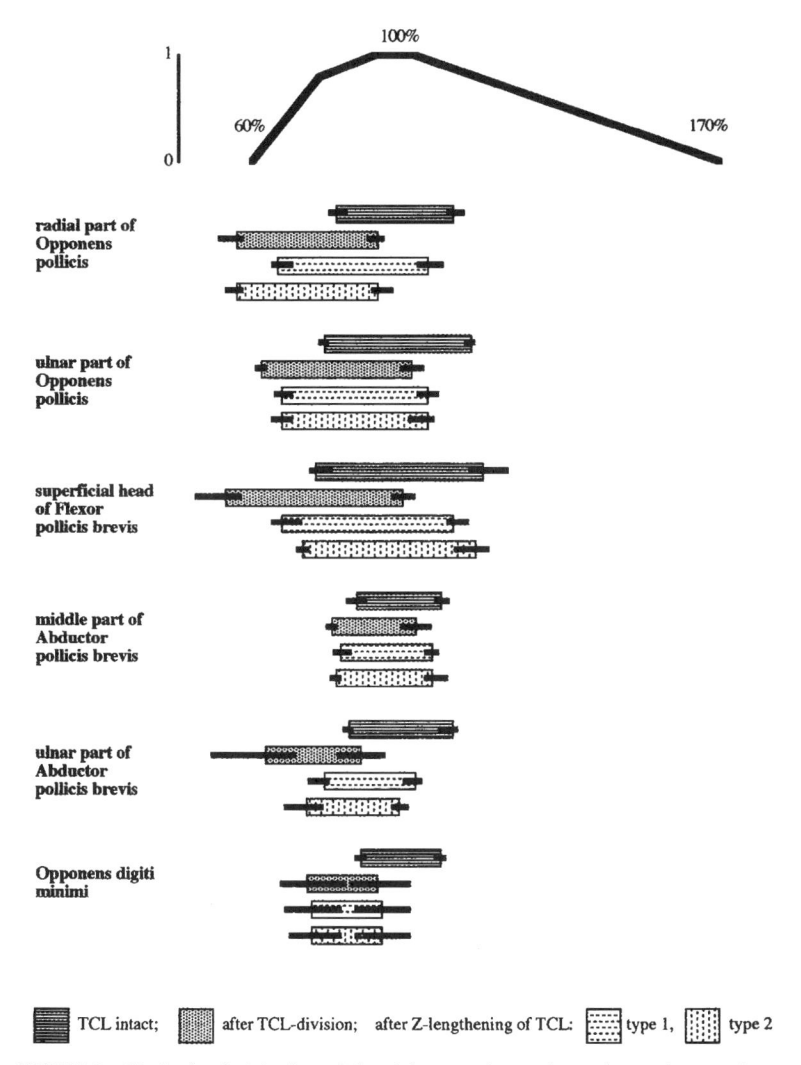

FIGURE 6.—Maximal and minimal muscle length between the muscle attachments (mean and extreme values) before and after z-plasty. These values are shown in relation to the muscle force-relative muscle length curve. *Note*: 1 = maximal muscle force; 100% = rest length. *Abbreviations*: TCL, transverse carpal ligament (flexor retinaculum). (Courtesy of Fuss FK, Wagner TF: Biomechanical alterations in the carpal arch and hand muscles after carpal tunnel release: A further approach toward understanding the function of the flexor retinaculum and the cause of postoperative grip weakness. *Clin Anat* 9:100–108, Copyright 1996. Reprinted by permission of Wiley-Liss, Inc., a subsidiary of John Wiley & Sons.)

ulnar part of the abductor pollicis brevis, the opponens pollicis, and the opponens digiti minimi (Fig 6). Preoperative and postoperative evaluation of the reaction force of the distal phalanx resulted in 3 groups of patients: 1) patients with significant loss of strength who had problems with grasping, lifting, twisting off lids, screwing, pulling ropes, and pinching; 2) those whose force values remained relatively constant; and 3) those whose strength significantly increased.

Conclusions.—These findings show that decreased postoperative thenar strength is related to muscle shortening when the thenar musculature is not atrophied. When there is thenar atrophy, muscle shortening affects the situation less than muscle recovery after carpal tunnel release. Increased muscle strength is to be expected. The cause of decreased and increased finger strength is unclear.

▶ Many authors have commented on the weakness that may occur after carpal tunnel surgery. These authors relate it not to the loss of pulley function of the flexor tendons. Rather, they ascribe it to shortening of the resting length of the thenar muscles, particularly the opponens pollicis, and to some extent also the abductor pollicis brevis. This is logical because bowstringing would increase moment arms and thus increase force of the long flexors for grip. The effect should be seen more in pinching, and forms of opposition grasp involving the thumb (unscrewing a jar lid, for example).

P.C. Amadio, M.D.

Suggested Reading

Olsen BS, Vœsel MT, Søjbjerg JO, et al: Lateral collateral ligament of the elbow joint: Anatomy and kinematics. *J Should Elbow Surg* 5:103–112, 1996.

▶ Olsen and co-workers, in Aarhus, Denmark, have performed an anatomical and biomechanical study of the lateral collateral ligament (LCL) complex of the elbow. They confirmed the importance of the LCL in varus and rotational stability of the elbow. Their investigation has the advantages of reproducibility by mechanically simulating external rotation and varus moments about the elbow by monitoring displacement of the radius and ulna in 3 dimensions. They confirmed that releasing the LCL causes varus and external rotational instability of the elbow.

They also confirmed the ligamentous insertion on the ulna at and distal to the annular ligament, having originated on the humerus at the origin of the LCL. This structure, which has been described to be an integral part of the LCL complex of the elbow that is distinct only at its insertion, is the ulnar part of LCL also called the lateral ulnar collateral ligament (LUCL). Its structure and function is homologous with that of the anterior bundle of the medial collateral ligament. Collectively the LCL and LUCL are the primary varus and valgus stabilizers of the elbow; the ulnar part of the LCL is also the primary constraint against posterolateral rotatory instability elbow.

This excellent study adds scientific documentation to recent papers regarding elbow stability and the ligamentous anatomy, clarifying some issues in this area. Three points could perhaps be clarified further. First, posterolateral rotatory instability of the elbow is a complex, 3-dimensional displacement, not simply a uniplanar displacement. Therefore, one has to be careful when extrapolating from this more simplistic experimental design to the more complex kinematic pattern of instability in the clinical situation. A previous study of our own,[1] in which we performed the lateral pivot shift test for posterolateral rotatory instability and measured displacements, confirmed that we were unable to mimic the complex 3-dimensional motion of this instability pattern with a mechanical apparatus.

Second, the authors refer to the LUCL as being the posterior part of the LCL complex. Although the additional anterior fibers give the impression that the LUCL is a posterior component, one must recognize the homology between the anterior bundle on the medial side and the ulnar part of the LCL on the lateral side. These 2 structures assume similar locations from anterior to posterior, and because the medial one is already termed the anterior bundle, it potentially confuses one's understanding of function to refer to the lateral structure as the posterior part. There is, indeed, a posterior part of the LCL that is analogous to the posterior part of the medial collateral ligament that is quite different from the LUCL.

Third, the authors conclude that rotation of the forearm has no influence on humeroulnar stability. This may have been true in their experimental setup but is not at all the case in the treatment of patients with unstable elbows. A patient who has posterolateral rotatory instability of the elbow will be unstable in supination and, perhaps, even in midrotation but will be stable in full (gently forced) pronation provided that the medial soft tissues are intact. This has significant implications for treating patients after elbow and fracture dislocations for example.

S.W. O'Driscoll, M.D.

Reference

1. O'Driscoll SW, Morrey BF, Korinek S, et al: The pathoanatomy and kinematics of posterolateral rotatory instability of the elbow. *Orthop Trans* 14:306, 1990.

Saint-Cast Y, Dagregorio G: Bases anatomique du greffon vasularisé de Carlos Zaidemberg (artère du processus styloïde radial) (Anatomical basis of Carlos Zaidemberg's vascularized graft [radial styloid process artery]). *La Main* 1:113–118, 1996.

▶ This brilliant anatomical work, which was awarded the Raoul Tubiana's prize for the best paper at the last GEM meeting, proves the constancy of the artery of the radial styloid process described by Carlos Zaidemberg, et al., in the *American Journal of Hand Surgery* 4 years ago.[1] Moreover, it describes at length the course and anatomical variations of this artery, which the authors classified into 4 types.

A short technical note published in the same issue[2] gives all the details on the operative procedure, with step-by-step illustrations and variations according to the anatomical type of artery.

Nonunion and avascular necrosis after scaphoid fractures remain frequent problems in our practice. Inlay bone grafting remains the treatment of choice, with a successful outcome in most cases. However, in difficult cases, including failed prior surgery, vascularized bone grafts may be a better option. Several such types of grafts have already been described, such as the pronator quadratus bone graft (Kawai[3]) and the second metacarpal vascularized bone graft (Brunelli[4]).

According to the authors, this new option provides a single approach and a fairly straightforward dissection of the pedicled graft, provided one raises enough soft tissue around the artery, which is rather thin (0.3–0.8 mm at its origin, 0.2–0.4 mm at the point at which it reaches the radial styloid). The main problem lies with the length of the pedicle (14–23 mm), which does not allow the graft to reach the most lateral part of the volar defect. The graft is inserted transversally, and the scaphoid height must be maintained with two volar K-wires, according to the authors.

Zaidemberg used this technique on 11 patients with an average immobilization of 6.2 weeks and a bony union in all cases. The authors add a further 15 cases in this article but do not provide the results. In light of these 2 articles, Zaidemberg's technique should be regarded as one of the few sources of vascularized bone graft when treating difficult cases of scaphoid nonunion.

C. LeClercq, M.D.

References

1. Zaidemberg C, Siebert JW, Angrigiani C: A new vascularized bone graft for scaphoid nonunion *J Hand Surg (Am)* 16:474–478, 1991.
2. Saint-Cast Y, Dagregorio G: Le greffon vascularisé de Carlos Zaidemberg—Artère du processus styloïde radiale—dans le traitment des pseudarthroses du scaphoïde. *La Main* 1:119–123, 1996.
3. Kawai H, Yamamoto K: Pronato quadratus pedicled bone graft for old scaphoid fractures. *J Bone Joint Surg Br* 70:829–831, 1988.
4. Brunelli F, Mathoulin CH, Saffar PH: Description d'un greffon osseux vascularisé au niveau de la tête du deuxième métacarpien. *Ann Chir Main* 11:40–45, 1992.

▶ This article stresses the anatomical data relevant to surgical technique. Zaidemberg's work stimulated other useful studies, and Bishop[1] has recently described new possibilities of vascularized bone graft harvested on the distal radius, providing a clarification according to the situation of the artery relative to the extensor compartments.

G. Foucher, M.D.

Reference

1. Sheetz KK, Bishop AT, Berger RA: The arterial blood supply of the distal radius and ulna and its potential use in vascularized pedicled bone grafts. *J Hand Surg [Am]* 20:902–914, 1995.

Prevel CD, McCarty M, Katona T, et al: Comparative biomechanical stability of titanium bone fixation systems in metacarpal fractures. *Ann Plast Surg* 35:6–14, 1995.

▶ The authors used a transverse metacarpal osteotomy model to study the rigidity of various plate and screw constructs. The hardware tested included Synthes, 5-hole plates (1.5 mm and 2.0 mm); Leibinger 4-hole plates (from 1.2 mm to 2.3 mm); Leibinger 3-dimensional, 4-hole and 8-hole plates (from 1.2 mm to 2.3 mm). Apex dorsal, apex volar, and torsional loading modes were tested. It is not surprising that the "3-dimensional" design, with its joined parallel plates and twice the number of screws produced the highest rigidity of all 3 bending modes. Although their overall data showed that rigidity increased with plate thickness, it was interesting to note that no statistical increase in rigidity was obtained by moving from the Synthes 1.5 mm plate to the thicker and wider 2.0 mm design.

T. Kiefhaber, M.D.

Wang X, Merzenich MM, Sameshima K, et al: Remodeling of hand representation in adult cortex determined by timing of tactile stimulation. *Nature* 378:71–75, 1995.

▶ This is an interesting continuation of long-term experiments whose goal is to determine, in part, how the brain processes afferent stimuli. The study determined that coincident stimulation of areas that are remote from each other resulted in these fingers being integrated in their cortical representation. However, fingers stimulated asynchronously were segregated in their cortical representation. The contact surfaces of the digits, therefore, develop very large areas of cortical representation on the basis of the constant synchronous stimulation.

V.R. Hentz, M.D.

Weiler PJ, Bogoch ER: Kinematics of the distal radioulnar joint in rheumatoid arthritis: An *in vivo* study using centrode analysis. *J Hand Surg* 20A:937–943, 1995.
▶ The authors studied 4 normal and 6 rheumatoid wrists with CT scans of the distal radioulnar joint in 5 positions: full pronation, midpronation, neutral, midsupination, and full supination. Using centrode analysis, they found that in normal wrists, the centrode lies in a relatively small area within the head of the ulna and is consistent with previous studies showing that there is both rotation of the radius around the ulna and translation in the dorsal-palmar plane. In the patients with rheumatoid wrists with severe involvement, the centrode was erratic in location and was often outside the head of the ulna, suggesting that rheumatoid arthritis disturbs the normal distal radioulnar joint kinematics. This is not new information, but it is nice to see the data quantified; moreover, they noted that with mild degrees of involvement, centrode disruption was not as severe and was more nearly normal. This method may have greater application for detecting subtle instabilities in a traumatic situation.

L.K. Ruby, M.D.

Phillips CS, Falender R, Mass DP: The flexor synovial sheath anatomy of the little finger: A macroscopic study. *J Hand Surg* 20A: 636–641, 1995.
▶ This paper on the anatomy of the synovial sheath of the little finger is interesting and worth reviewing for hand surgeons who treat synovial sheath infections.

R.A. Chase, M.D.

2 Diagnosis, Evaluation, and Anesthesia

The Value of Wrist Arthroscopy: An Evaluation of 129 Cases
de Smet L, Dauwe D, Fortems Y, et al (Univ Hosp Pellenberg, Leuven, Belgium)
J Hand Surg [Br] 21B:210–212, 1996   2–1

Background.—Wrist arthroscopy has become routine and is indicated by soft-tissue and bone abnormalities. The value of diagnostic and therapeutic arthroscopy of the wrist was reviewed.

Patients and Findings.—The results of 129 arthroscopies were analyzed. Patients were followed up for at least 6 months. Seventy-seven arthroscopies were therapeutic, and 52 were diagnostic. Diagnostic benefits were documented in 42.5% of the procedures and therapeutic benefits, in 22.5%. Combined diagnostic and therapeutic benefits were evident in 30%. In 5%, arthroscopy was not useful. Two patients had arthroscopy-related complications. One tendon incision occurred over a Kirschner wire in a patient in the treatment group, and 1 superficial infection occurred in a patient in the diagnostic group.

Conclusion.—Although arthroscopy is a valuable tool, it should not be thought of as the universal solution in the diagnosis and treatment of all wrist problems. The current data do not indicate clearly which clinical problem is suitable for wrist arthroscopy.

▶ This large retrospective study confirms the diagnostic power of wrist arthroscopy when used after adequate history and expert clinical examination. As stated, these retrospective data are biased by a cooperative setting that determines the procedure's success rate and does not delineate the clinical problems best suited for arthroscopy. However, this article and the body of existing peer-reviewed literature demonstrates the diagnostic accuracy and interventional potential of arthroscopy. It is important to remember that arthroscopy is an adjunct to managing wrist problems and should not be used as an alternative to obtaining a history, performing a clinical examination, or ordering less invasive diagnostic modalities. Controlled, randomized trials are necessary to define the specific indications for the use of arthroscopy over traditional procedures.

L.A. Koman, M.D.

Left-hand Dominance and Hand Trauma
Taras JS, Behrman MJ, Degnan GG (Philadelphia Hand Ctr, Pa)
J Hand Surg (Am) 20A:1043–1046, 1995   2–2

Objective.—Some evidence suggests that hand dominance may have a bearing on the risk for injury; left-handed individuals appear to be more accident prone. The relation between hand dominance and the relative risk for sustaining amputating hand injuries or minor trauma was studied retrospectively.

Methods.—The records of 15 women and 110 men, aged 16–74 years, who had been treated for digital amputation during a 3-year period were reviewed. For comparison, the records of 116 patients with minor hand trauma were also reviewed.

Findings.—The prevalence of left-hand dominance was 35% in patients with amputating hand injury and 11% in patients with minor hand trauma. Although more amputating injuries occurred on the left side, left-handed patients were more likely to have an amputating injury of their dominant hand (70%) than right-handed patients (51%). The most common mechanism of amputating injuries was by power saw; the risk for sustaining a significant injury to the dominant hands with a power saw was 10.8 times higher in left-handed individuals than in right-handed individuals.

Conclusion.—Left-handed individuals have a relative risk for sustaining an amputating injury that is 4.9 times greater than that of right-handed individuals. In general, tools, assembly lines, and work stations are designed for right-handed individuals, which means that left-handed individuals must use their nondominant, less-skilled hand in a controlling position. Additional safety measures and redesign of tools, assembly lines, and workshops are needed to reduce the prevalence of serious hand injuries among left-handed individuals.

▶ These very interesting findings show once again that it is a right-handed world and that most tools and devices are built primarily for right-handed individuals. The left-handed individual has always been "left out" of making decisions regarding the design of nearly everything. Left-handers arise! Apparently you have nothing to lose but your fingers.

V.R. Hentz, M.D.

Identification of Low-effort Patients Through Dynamometry
Stokes HM, Landrieu KW, Domangue B, et al (Univ of New Orleans, La)
J Hand Surg (Am) 20A:1047–1056, 1995   2–3

Introduction.—The Jamar dynamometer is the most reliable, valid instrument for measuring grip strength as an indicator of recovery from injury. The accuracy of this tool depends on the patient's willingness to exert maximal effort during assessment. It is difficult to separate patients

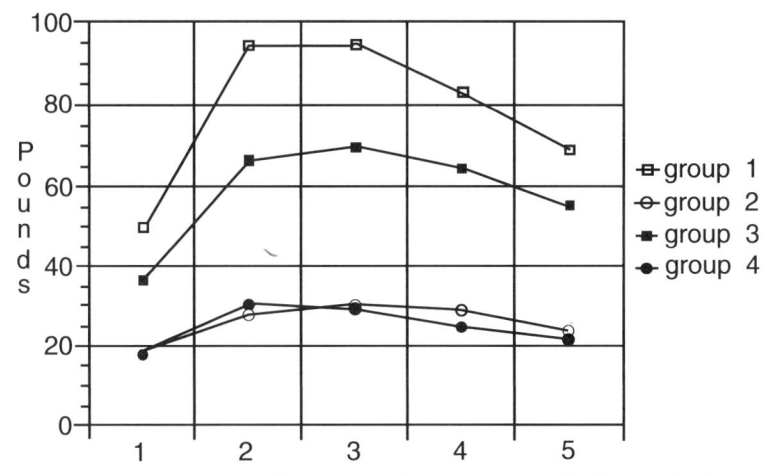

FIGURE 1.—Five-rung test plotted by group. The feigning groups (2 and 4) have similar, flatter curves than the sincere groups (1 and 3), who produced normal bell-shaped curves. (Courtesy of Stokes HM, Landrieu KW, Domangue B, et al: Identification of low-effort patients through dynamometry. *J Hand Surg (Am)* 20A:1047–1056, 1995.)

who will not exert themselves on these tests from those who have not recovered from injury. The 5-rung grip test and the rapid exchange grip (REG) test have been used to evaluate patients suspected of low effort. Objective criteria were developed that can be used to accurately assess patients suspected of low effort on grip evaluations.

Study Group.—The study group was composed of 4 types of participants: 40 healthy volunteers, 30 healthy volunteers who were instructed to feign a weak grip in 1 hand, 32 patients with hand injury whose recovery times were consistent with their injuries, and 27 patients with hand injury who were suspected by clinicians of exerting low effort on grip evaluation. All participants were administered the 5-rung dynamometer test followed by the REG, with a switch rate of 1.5 seconds.

Results.—After the 5-rung dynamometer test, significantly less variability across trials was seen in the low-effort group and in patients instructed to feign low effort than in either of the other 2 groups (Fig 1). Peak rapid exchange and peak 5-ring grip strength were reliably different only in patients suspected of low effort and in those asked to feign low effort (Fig 2). A model was derived to identify patients who exerted low effort on grip strength tests: $Y' = 3.6 + .01624(RE) - .023282(T3)$, where $T3$ is trial 3 on the 5-rung dynamometer test and RE is peak rapid exchange. This model permitted accurate identification of patients suspected of exerting low effort in more than 96% of cases in this series.

Conclusions.—The tests and model presented in this paper can be used to evaluate the motivation of patients with hand injury at any time during the course of therapy. This model permits an objective assessment of such subjective issues as motivation and sincerity of effort.

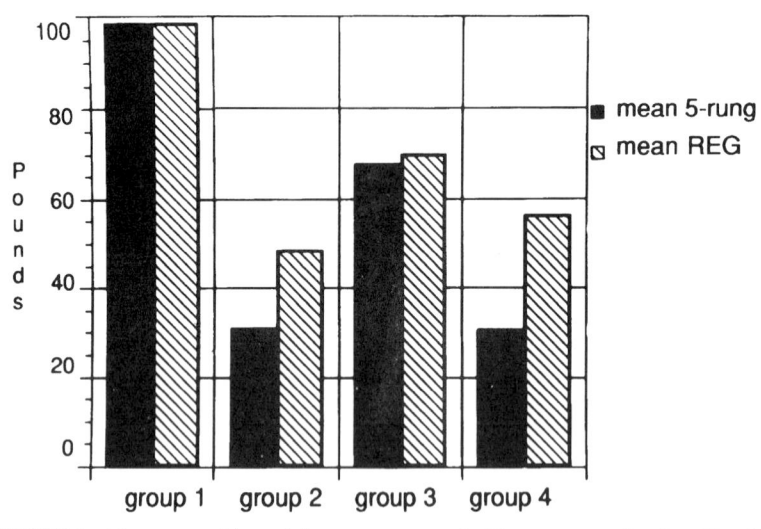

FIGURE 2.—Mean scores of the peak 5-rung test compared with mean scores of peak rapid exchange grip (*REG*) test. Sincere groups (1 and 3) had no significant difference in peak scores of the 2 tests. Differences in the feigning groups (2 and 4) were significant. (Courtesy of Stokes HM, Landrieu KW, Domangue B, et al: Identification of low-effort patients through dynamometry. *J Hand Surg (Am)* 20A:1047–1056, 1995.)

▶ The potential role of subjectivity in the interpretation of the presumably objectively derived Jamar dynamometer grip readings can't be stressed enough. Stokes and coauthors remind us that we should be using this tool if we suspect less than sincere effort.

V.R. Hentz, M.D.

A Gap Detection Tactility Test for Sensory Deficits Associated With Carpal Tunnel Syndrome
Jeng O-J, Radwin RG (Univ of Madison, Wis)
Ergonomics 38:2588–2601, 1995   2–4

Background.—Quantitative, noninvasive tools are needed to evaluate symptoms of carpal tunnel syndrome (CTS) and other peripheral neuropathies. In most cases of CTS, sensory symptoms are the earliest and primary deficit. Electrophysiologic testing does not measure symptoms or functional deficits, and patients with sensory symptoms of median nerve compression do not always show measurable changes in sensory or nerve conduction. Two-point discrimination tests are not sensitive to gradual decrease in nerve function created by external compression. Alternative sensory testing methods are time consuming, expensive, and not readily available; results may depend on the experience of the examiner.

Study.—Population normative data were obtained using a new aesthesiometer for gap detection tactility testing for sensory deficits associated with CTS. The reliability of the test and the factors that affect the sensory threshold were also studied.

Methods.—Gap detection thresholds were measured with the converging staircase method of limits model. Important factors that affect gap detection thresholds were studied in 16 normal persons 21 to 66 years of age. The test evolved sensing a tiny gap in a smooth surface by probing with the finger.

Results.—The threshold of actively probing with the index finger had a threshold almost more sensitive than passive touch, similar to two-point discrimination. As contact force increased from 25 g to 75 g, the average threshold decreased by 24%. Performance in this tactility test quickly stabilized and showed few learning effects; results were highly repeatable. No significant threshold differences were seen between testing on different days or between dominant and nondominant hands. A contact force of 50 g was recommended because it required moderate force, but it resulted in a smaller threshold than did 25 g or 75 g. A second study was conducted using 8 normal persons and 10 patients with CTS. The average gap detection threshold was 0.20 mm for normal persons and 0.40 mm in patients. The average gap detection threshold without finger probing was 1.71 mm for normal persons and 2.53 mm in patients, an increase of 48%. For static thresholds for normal persons and patients, age had a small but significant effect.

Discussion.—Patients with CTS may not detect surface scratches in a tactile inspection test unless the scratches are twice as large as those detected by persons without the syndrome. The gap test was easily administered, determined tactile sensitivity rapidly, was learned quickly, and had highly repeatable results. A contact force of 50 g was recommended. The dynamic test had low intersubject variability.

▶ The authors introduce a new test for quantifying sensory deficit. The test involves evaluating the patient's ability to detect a tiny gap in an otherwise smooth surface by probing with the finger. When active probing with the index finger was allowed, the threshold was much lower (0.19 mm) than when only passive touch was allowed (1.63 mm). The authors have evaluated this device in patients with CTS. Although there was a statistical difference between the patients with the syndrome and normal persons in this study, the scatter of the data reminds us that "to make a difference, there must be a difference," and emphasizes the importance of clinical judgment in determining needs for surgical intervention. There is a definite need for noninvasive, inexpensive tests that can be administered in a practical amount of time. However, although this instrument and similar ones may be useful for screening patients and confirming clinical suspicions, indications for surgery for CTS remain a clinical decision.

S.E. Mackinnon, M.D.

Sensitivity and Specificity of Ultrasound in the Diagnosis of Foreign Bodies in the Hand

Bray PW, Mahoney JL, Campbell JP, et al (Univ of Toronto)
J Hand Surg (Am) 20A:661–666, 1995

Purpose.—Previous studies have demonstrated the clinical value of high-resolution ultrasonography (US) for detecting and evaluating retained foreign bodies (FBs) in the hand, particularly those that are typically invisible on standard radiographs. The sensitivity and specificity of US for the diagnosis of FBs in the hand were assessed.

Methods.—The study material consisted of 15 fresh-frozen cadaver hands that were each divided into 21 standardized locations for FB insertion, for a total of 315 potential insertion sites. Cylindrical wood, metal, and glass objects made in 2 sizes were used as FBs. The smaller objects measured 1 × 4 mm and the larger ones, 2 × 5 mm (Fig 2). A computer program was used to determine where the 166 FBs were to be inserted. The remaining 149 empty sites served as controls. After insertion of the FBs, anteroposterior and lateral radiographs of each hand were obtained. A single radiologist who was blinded to the FB locations read all the films. The hands were then scanned by high-resolution US at a frequency of 10 MHz. A single radiologist, experienced in US examination of the extremities, performed and interpreted all US scans.

Results.—Foreign bodies occupied 104 (49.5%) of the 210 potential insertion sites in the phalanges and 62 (59%) of the 105 potential palmar

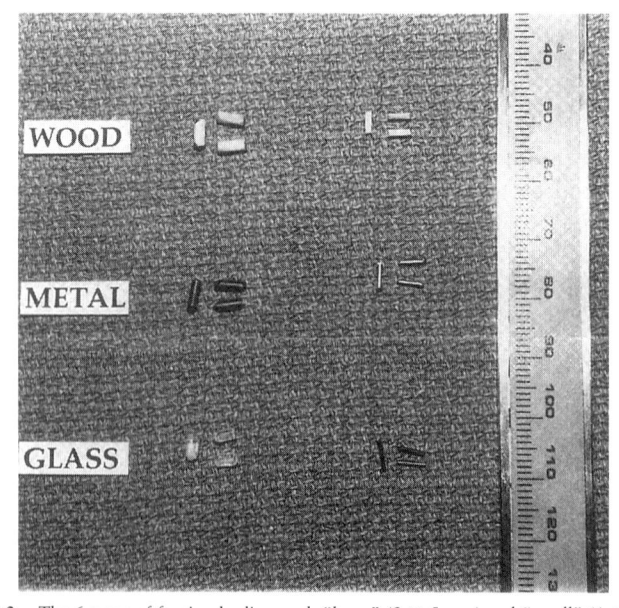

FIGURE 2.—The 6 types of foreign bodies used: "large" (2 × 5 mm) and "small" (1 × 4 mm) sizes of wood, metal, and glass. (Courtesy of Bray PW, Mahoney JL, Campbell JP, et al: Sensitivity and specificity of ultrasound in the diagnosis of foreign bodies in the hand. *J Hand Surg* 20A:661–666, 1995.)

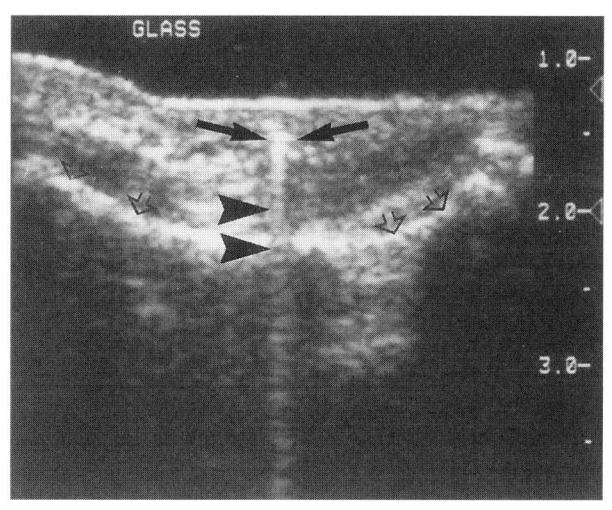

FIGURE 4.—Longitudinal sonogram of soft tissue anterior to metacarpal (*open arrows*) demonstrates echogenic foreign body (*arrows*) with strong reverberation artifact (*arrowheads*). The foreign body is a piece of glass measuring 1 × 4 mm. (Courtesy of Bray PW, Mahoney JL, Campbell JP, et al: Sensitivity and specificity of ultrasound in the diagnosis of foreign bodies in the hand. *J Hand Surg* 20A:661–666, 1995.)

insertion sites. All metal FBs, 50 glass FBs (92.6%), and no wooden FBs were detected on standard radiographs. On US examination, 156 of the 166 FBs were detected and 10 were falsely analyzed as negative, for a sensitivity of 94%. There was 1 false positive result and 148 true negative results, for a specificity of 99%. The FB dimensions could be accurately measured by US to within ± 1 mm. Both glass and wooden FBs were

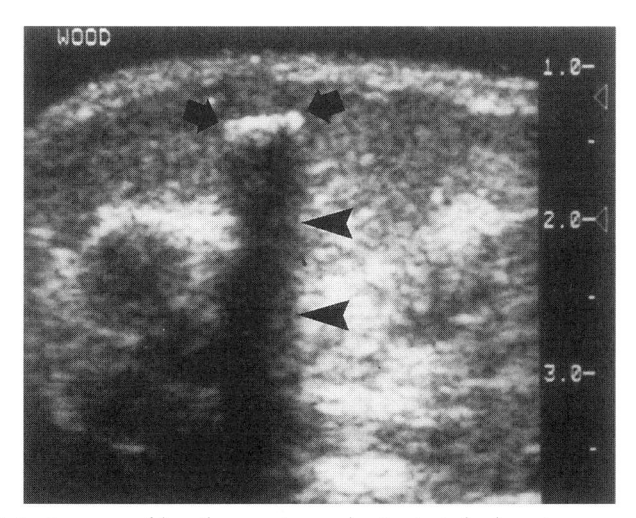

FIGURE 5.—Sonogram of hypothenar eminence showing typical echogenic appearance of wood fragment (*arrows*) with strong acoustic shadowing (*arrowheads*). The foreign body measured 1 × 4 mm. (Courtesy of Bray PW, Mahoney JL, Campbell JP, et al: Sensitivity and specificity of ultrasound in the diagnosis of foreign bodies in the hand. *J Hand Surg* 20A:661–666, 1995.)

readily detected on US (Figs 4 and 5); the appearance of metal objects varied.

Conclusion.—The selectively combined use of standard radiography and high-resolution US should enable the experienced radiologist to detect almost all FBs embedded in the soft tissues of the hands with a minimal use of resources.

▶ Although plain radiography remains the initial examination in the algorithm for imaging detection of FBs, US can be used to detect nonradiodense FBs larger than 1 × 3 to 4 mm, as is well shown in this experimental, cadaveric study.

G. Bergman, M.D.

Diagnosis by Ultrasound of Dislocated Ulnar Collateral Ligament of the Thumb
Höglund M, Tordai P, Muren C (Södersjukhuset, Stockholm)
Acta Radiol 36:620–625, 1995
2–6

Background.—Forced abduction and extension of the thumb can cause a rupture of the ulnar collateral ligament. After complete rupture, the ligament may be displaced and folded back proximally to the aponeurosis. Treatment decisions are based on the severity of this displacement. Clinical estimation of the extent of such injury, however, can be difficult. The value of ultrasound in demonstrating whether the ulnar collateral ligament was

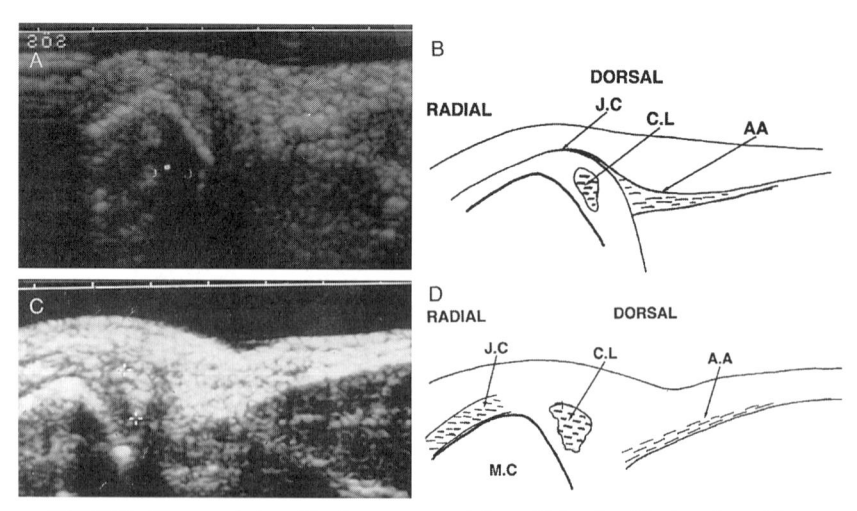

FIGURE 6.—Transversal view of the first metacarpophalangeal joint. **A and B**, the collateral ligament (C.L) is located under the adductor aponeurosis (A.A) and the joint capsule (J.C). **C and D**, the CL is located outside and proximally to the AA. Joint capsule as it inserts to the metacarpal bone. (Courtesy of Höglund M, Tordai P, Muren C: Diagnosis by ultrasound of dislocated ulnar collateral ligament of the thumb. *Acta Radiol* 36:620–625, 1995.)

folded back proximally to the adductor aponeurosis in 1 group of patients was investigated.

Methods.—Sixty-four patients, aged 10–81 years, were examined. Ligaments were assessed in the longitudinal and transverse planes (Fig 6). Ultrasonographic findings were correlated with surgical findings in 39 patients.

Findings.—Surgical and ultrasonographic findings were in agreement in 82% of patients. The extent of the injury suggested was overestimated by ultrasound in 10% of patients and underestimated in 8%. Ultrasound predictions were highly significantly correlated with operative findings.

Conclusions.—Diagnostic efforts should focus on ligament displacement in patients who have injury to the ulnar collateral ligament of the metacarpophalangeal joint of the thumb. Although conventional radiography demonstrates skeletal involvement, it does not show the position of the ligament. Ultrasound should be done when clinical assessment does not clearly indicate the extent of the ligament injury. The decision to operate is greatly influenced by the outcome of the ultrasound examination.

▶ Clinical evaluation of suspected ulnar collateral ligament injury will, as usual, dictate the need for specific imaging techniques in a given clinical setting. The presence of a significant hematoma or ecchymosis reduces the utility of ultrasound and MRI. In this setting, conventional arthrography with anesthetic injection allows improved stress testing and diagnosis of ulnar collateral ligament injury along with osseous injury. Although invasive, this technique is still useful and cost-effective.

Ultrasound is effective in experienced hands but can be limited by hematoma and local hemorrhage. It is most accurate, as the authors state, when the ruptured ligament is displaced proximal to the adductor aponeurosis. This technique should therefore be kept in mind for certain selected patients who have a palpable defect (tumor) or in those who do not have significant hemorrhage or hematoma.

T.H. Berquist, M.D.

Magnetic Resonance Imaging of Acute Tendon Injury in the Finger
Scott JR, Cobby M, Taggart I (Frenchay Hosp, Bristol, England)
J Hand Surg (Br) 20B:286–288, 1995

Introduction.—Accurate clinical assessment of flexor tendon function in a finger after acute nonpenetrating trauma is difficult. Magnetic resonance imaging (MRI) is widely used for assessing tendons in the shoulder and ankle. An experience with MRI for the assessment of flexor tendon function in patients with acute finger injuries is reported.

Case Report 1.—Man, 33, right-handed, sustained a nonpenetrating hyperextension injury when he closed a car door on his left index finger. Results of neurologic and plain radiographic examinations were normal, but clinical examination could not exclude closed rupture of the flexor digitorum profundus (FDP) tendon. Sagittal and axial MRI of the finger confirmed the integrity of the FDP tendon and its insertion.

Case Report 2.—Man, 35, ambidextrous, sustained a nonpenetrating hyperextension injury to the right ring finger. Conventional radiographs were negative for fracture or dislocation. Sagittal and axial MRI of the injured finger confirmed the integrity of the FDP tendon.

Case Report 3.—Man, 23, right-handed, sustained a nonpenetrating hyperextension injury to the left ring finger. The FDP tendon function could not be accurately assessed because of localized posttraumatic soft-tissue edema of the distal part of the finger. Sagittal and axial MRI of the injured finger clearly showed an avulsed FDP tendon that had retracted to the level of the proximal interphalangeal joint. The patient underwent FDP tendon repair and was undergoing hand rehabilitation at the time of this report.

Comment.—Because MRI can differentiate tendons from surrounding inflammatory changes and hemorrhage, the morbidity and extra cost associated with surgical exploration was avoided in 2 of 3 patients with nonpenetrating hyperextension injuries. Both of these patients were able to start hand therapy immediately, thus shortening the period of disability.

▶ Magnetic resonance imaging is widely used for detecting abnormalities of the tendons in the ankle and foot. This article illustrates that MRI is also useful in detecting tendon injuries in the fingers.

G. Bergman, M.D.

Evaluation of the Arthroscopic Valgus Instability Test of the Elbow
Field LD, Altchek DW (Mississippi Sports Medicine and Orthopaedic Ctr, Jackson; Hosp for Special Surgery, New York)
Am J Sports Med 24:177–181, 1996   2–8

Objective.—Although medial collateral ligament (MCL) injury can result in instability of the elbow, the condition is difficult to diagnose. By using 7 cadaveric elbows, the extent to which the MCL must be injured before there is arthroscopic evidence of valgus instability, the amount of ulnohumeral joint opening required before evidence of injury can be observed, and the elbow position at which this opening can best be viewed were studied.

Methods.—The MCL was exposed, the elbows were placed in a vise, and a valgus stress was applied with the forearm in neutral rotation. The joint opening was visualized and measured at 15-degree increments from 15 degrees to 120 degrees of flexion. The MCL was sequentially sectioned from the anterior bundle to the posterior bundle, and valgus testing and joint opening measurements were repeated each time.

Results.—The ulnohumeral joint was not visible until the posterior bundle was cut. Under valgal stress, the joint then opened 4 to 10 mm. Maximal opening and maximal visualization occurred in all elbows at 60 degrees and 75 degrees of flexion. Forearm pronation enlarged the joint opening, and forearm supination reduced the joint opening.

Conclusion.—The anterior bundle must be sectioned completely before arthroscopic valgus instability of the elbow can be observed.

▶ This is a very interesting article about a relatively new area, arthroscopic assessment of elbow instability. The diagnosis of partial tears of the MCL, especially in athletes, who frequently perform movements with their arms overhead, can be difficult. Traditionally diagnosis has been primarily based on history and physical examination with confirmation by surgical exploration of the ligament. Magnetic resonance imaging and CT arthrography have been investigated. Arthroscopic assessment of valgus opening of the elbow has also been discussed in the literature. This is the first scientific investigation of the normal vs. abnormal amounts of medial opening during valgus stress when the elbow is viewed arthroscopically. My colleagues and I and several other investigators have found this test to be helpful in a clinical setting. The authors have demonstrated that the normal elbow really does not open at all on an arthroscopic stress test. This finding is in slight disagreement with what has been found with basic science studies, which have shown 2-degree to 4-degree laxity of the normal elbow. The finding by Field and colleagues might be related to the difficulty in performing the test, which my experience has confirmed. Certainly, any observable degree of opening in the experimental study was consistent with at least a partial disruption, and, of course, complete disruption of the MCL was associated with reproducible medial joint opening with valgus stress. One should remember that partial tears are usually accompanied by attenuation of the ligament; thus, the extent of opening may be greater than seen in this experimental study of acute injuries.

S.W. O'Driscoll, M.D.

Comparison of Continuous Brachial Plexus Infusion of Butorphanol, Mepivacaine and Mepivacaine–Butorphanol Mixtures for Postoperative Analgesia
Wajima Z, Shitara T, Nakajima Y, et al (Kitamurayama Kohritsu Hosp, Japan)
Br J Anaesth 75:548–551, 1995
2–9

Introduction.—For surgery of the upper extremity, the continuous brachial plexus block provides constant postoperative analgesia, sympathectomy, and increased blood flow to the arm. This method has been shown to be superior to continuous IV infusion for the delivery of butorphanol. The effects of continuous infusion of 3 types of solutions into the axillary sheath were compared for their effectiveness on postoperative pain relief.

TABLE 2.—Mean Visual Analogue Scale Scores After Surgery

	Time (h) 3	6	9	12	18	24	36	60
Group B ($n = 14$)	2.5 (2.1) [0–6.2]	2.3 (2.5) [0–8.3]	1.5 (1.8) [0–5.1]	1.0 (1.6) [0–5.2]	1.5 (2.3) [0–7.5]	0.7 (1.2) [0–3.6]	1.0 (1.8) [0–5.2]	1.2 (2.5) [0–9.1]
Group M ($n = 9$)	5.0 (2.4) [0–8.1]	4.1 (2.0) [0–7.1]	3.6 (1.8) [0–6.5]	3.2 (1.8) [0–6.1]	2.9 (1.2) [0–4.0]	3.1 (1.5) [0–5.5]	2.7 (2.5) [0–8.2]	1.6 (1.6) [0–4.0]
Group MB ($n = 10$)	0.3 (0.6) [0–1.9]	1.6 (2.1) [0–6.4]	1.1 (1.5) [0–4.4]	1.0 (1.2) [0–3.0]	1.1 (1.2) [0–2.5]	1.0 (1.1) [0–2.9]	1.5 (1.9) [0–4.9]	0.2 (0.6) [0–1.8]
Kruskal-Wallis test	$H = 15.5$ ($P < 0.0005$)	$H = 6.3$ ($P < 0.05$)	$H = 7.8$ ($P < 0.05$)	$H = 9.6$ ($P < 0.01$)	$H = 7.8$ ($P < 0.05$)	$H = 11.5$ ($P < 0.005$)	$H = 5.8$ (ns)	$H = 4.0$ (ns)
Post hoc comparison	M > MB ($P < 0.01$) B > MB ($P < 0.05$)	ns	M > MB ($P < 0.05$)	M > B ($P < 0.05$)	M > MB ($P < 0.05$)	M > MB ($P < 0.05$) M > B ($P < 0.05$)		

Note: Values in parentheses are the standard deviation; values in brackets are the range. Data were analyzed by Kruskal–Wallis' and Dunn's procedures.
Abbreviations: B, patients receiving butorphanol; M, patients receiving mepivacaine; MB, patients received both butorphanol and mepivacaine.
(Courtesy of Wajima Z, Shitara T, Nakajima Y, et al: Comparison of continuous brachial plexus infusion of butorphanol, mepivacaine, and mepivacaine–butorphanol mixtures for postoperative analgesia. Br J Anaesth 75:548–551, 1995.)

TABLE 4.—Number of Patients Who Required Supplementary Analgesia and Who Developed Side Effects After Surgery

	Group B ($n = 14$)	Group M ($n = 9$)	Group MB ($n = 10$)
Required supplementary analgesia	5	6	2
Nausea	7*	0	3
Vomiting	4	0	1
Slight drowsiness	3	0	1
Dizziness	2	0	1

Note: The incidence of nausea differed significantly among the 3 groups ($P < .05$); the incidence in group B (butorphanol) was higher than that in group M (mepivacaine).
Abbreviations: B, patients receiving butorphanol; M, patients receiving mepivacaine; MB, patients received both butorphanol and mepivacaine.
*$P = .05$ compared with group M.
(Courtesy of Wajima Z, Shitara T, Nakajima Y, et al: Comparison of continuous brachial plexus infusion of butorphanol, mepivacaine, and mepivacaine-butorphanol mixtures for postoperative analgesia. Br J Anaesth 75:548–551, 1995.)

Methods.—Thirty-three patients undergoing arm surgery were studied. Operations ranged from open reductions to tendon transfers. The axillary block was established with 30 mL of 1.5% mepivacaine. Ten mL of mepivacaine was injected every 90 minutes. Sedation with IV medazolam was given at the discretion of the anesthesiologist. After surgery, 10 mL of mepivacaine was given to the plexus sheath and the patients were randomly assigned to 1 of 3 groups: 9 patients to butorphanol (83.3 µg/h), 14 patients to .5% mepivacaine (50 mL/24 h), and 10 patients to both drugs. Diclofenac was available as needed for comfort. Pain was rated on a visual analogue scale 3, 6, 9, 12, 18, 24, 36, and 60 hours after surgery. Symptoms, arterial pressure, heart rate, and ventilation frequency were monitored.

Results.—At 3 hours after surgery, patients receiving both drugs had significantly less pain (Table 2). Over time, patients receiving both drugs had consistently less pain than the other 2 groups. At 4 hours after surgery, the total diclofenac use was greater in the mepivacaine group than in the group receiving both drugs. Respiratory depression did not occur. Patients receiving butorphanol only had more nausea than did patients receiving mepivacaine only (Table 4).

Conclusion.—The best analgesia was obtained in the group receiving both butorphenol and mepivacaine, followed by the group receiving butorphanol only. The differences were most significant 3 hours after surgery; few differences were seen during the remainder of the study. Further pain relief may occur with an increased concentration of anesthetic and increased rate of administration of or dose of the opiod.

▶ A continuous brachial plexus block is being used with increased frequency to manage pain after hand surgery. The combination of local anesthetic and narcotics in postoperative continuous epidural analgesia has an additive effect, thereby permitting lower doses of each. The current study demonstrates that the best postoperative analgesia was achieved using a combination of local anesthetic and narcotic for infusion in the brachial plexus sheath within the first 3 hours; after that point, addition of local anesthetic provided no better analgesia than did narcotic alone. In view of the success of combined therapy in epidural analgesia, it may be possible that equally good results can be obtained by using a higher concentration of local anesthetic later in the infusion period.

T. Feeley, M.D.

Bier's Block: A Change of Injection Site
Blyth MJG, Kinninmonth AWG, Asante DK (Glasgow Royal Infirmary Univ, Scotland)
J Trauma: Injury Infect Crit Care 39:726–728, 1995   2–10

Introduction.—Bier's block, or IV regional anesthesia, is the anesthetic method of choice for the closed manipulation of simple, distal radial metaphyseal fractures. The traditional injection site in the dorsum of the hand can present difficulties with subsequent plaster application and with venous access close to the fracture site that is often swollen and painful. Proximal injection in the antecubital fossa is an alternative technique that offers several practical advantages.

Study Design.—During a 3-month period, 100 patients hospitalized with distal radial metaphyseal fractures requiring manipulation under Bier's block were randomly allocated to 2 groups of 50 patients. On the injured side, anesthesia was injected into the dorsum of the hand in the first group and into the antecubital fossa in the second group. The proximal cuff was inflated to a pressure of 300 mm Hg, and 40 mL of .5% prilocaine was injected over a 90-second period. Pain at the fracture site and at the cuff was graded on a visual analogue scale.

Outcome.—The 2 groups were well matched for age, morphologic characteristics, fracture type, associated swelling, tourniquet pressure, and time. Pain experienced at the fracture site or at the cuff did significantly differ between the 2 groups (Table 1). However, fewer technical problems

TABLE 1.—Pain Experienced

Injection Site	Dorsum of Hand	Antecubital Fossa
Pain at fracture site		
Mean	2.66	3.46
Number in sample	50	50
p is greater than 0.05		
Pain at cuff		
Mean	3.16	3.30
Number in sample	50	50
p is greater than 0.05		

(Courtesy of Blyth MJG, Kinninmonth AWG, Asante DK: Bier's block: a change of injection site. *J Trauma (Injury Infect Crit Care)* 394:726–728, 1995.)

TABLE 2.—Problems at Injection Site

Injection Site	Dorsum of Hand	Antecubital Fossa
Number in sample	50	50
Number of failed cannulations	12	3
Injection site bleeding	5	0
Injection site hematoma	5	0

(Courtesy of Blyth MJG, Kinninmonth AWG, Asante DK: Bier's block: a change of injection site. *J Trauma (Injury Infect Crit Care)* 394:726–728, 1995.)

associated with venous access and subsequent plaster application occurred in the antecubital fossa group (Table 2). No major complications developed, particularly those relating to signs of systemic toxicity.

Conclusion.—For closed manipulation of simple forearm fractures, proximal injection of the anesthetic agent in the antecubital fossa is a safe and practical alternative to the traditional distal injection sites. Proximal injection in the antecubital fossa at a slow speed and cuff pressures of 300 mm Hg reduces the incidence of local injection site complications while maintaining adequate levels of anesthesia at both the fracture and cuff sites.

▶ This study of distal radius fracture reduction under a Bier's block demonstrates that the effectiveness of the techniques does not depend on the site of injection. Although most clinicians acknowledge that the antecubital fossa vein is easier to cannulate, fear of systemic injection and decreased efficacy results in the infrequent use of this vein for procedures on the wrist and hand. In this study, the antecubital fossa vein provided anesthesia equivalent to that of the dorsum of the hand without evidence of systemic injection from either site. It must be noted that the authors used cuff pressures of at least 300 mm Hg and a slow injection technique (infusion over 90 seconds) to minimize systemic absorption.

T. Feeley, M.D.

Anesthesia for Hand Surgery in Patients with Epidermolysis Bullosa [in French]
Chevaleraud E, Ragot JM, Glicenstein J (Clinique Oudinot, Paris)
Ann Chir Main 14:296–303, 1995   2–11

Introduction.—Epidermolysis bullosa (EB) is a rare, genetic, mechanobullous dermatosis characterized by the formation of cutaneous bullae in the skin and squamous epithelium. The recessive dystrophic form of the disease (RDEB) has a cicatricial course, causing retraction and pseudosyndactylization of the fingers, often leading to complete destruction of the hand. The anesthetic management during hand surgery in a series of young patients with RDEB was reported.

Patients.—Since January 1988, 23 patients aged 3–35 years required anesthesia for 185 operations on 62 hands. Eleven patients were children younger than 8 years who weighed less than 20 kg. Only 28 operations were done under general anesthesia; the other 157 were performed with locoregional blocks of the upper extremities. Of 157 first-line local anesthesias, 148 were brachial plexus blocks administered via the axillary route, 7 were axillary blocks performed after halothane inhalation induction, and 2 were interscalene blocks because severe blistering in the axillary region precluded using the axillary access route. Children were premedicated with oral midazolam 1 hour before induction with the regional block. One parent was asked to stay with the child for the duration of the procedure. Local anesthesia was induced with lidocaine 2% and bupivacaine 0.5%.

Outcome.—Postoperative pain was controlled with oral acetaminophen with codeine preparations. There were no major complications associated with the use of local anesthesia. Operations were performed 1 week apart without complications. Because anemic children cannot be transfused because their illness precludes the use of a pneumatic cuff, oral iron and vitamin supplements and high-protein drinks were given between operations, but the children did not like the protein drinks and their use for this purpose proved unsatisfactory. Antibiotics were not administered.

Conclusions.—Locoregional plexus blocks of the upper extremity can be used with good results during hand reconstruction in children with RDEB who weigh at least 10 kg, thus eliminating the need for general anesthesia.

▶ The use of regional anesthesia is becoming increasingly common in pediatric hand surgery, and this study, in patients as young as 3 years. For delicate surgery on small hands, a field in which not fidgeting is as important as a pain-free experience for the patient. Especially in younger patients, the anesthesiologist must be expert in titrating the sedation which is used; both too little and too much (just short of general anesthesia) can result in a patient who won't (or can't) lie still.

P.C. Amadio, M.D.

Suggested Reading

González VM, Stewart A, Ritter PL, et al: Translation and validation of arthritis outcome measures into Spanish. *Arthritis Rheum* 38(10):1429–1446, 1995.
▶ For those who need it, here is the reference for the Spanish version of the HSQ/SF-36 questionnaire. The appendix includes all the questions in Spanish.

P.C. Amadio, M.D.

Castellini-Modena PL: Prime considerazioni sul Coordinamento Nazionale diModena Soccorso (Analysis of National Coordination by Modena Assistance). *Riv Chir Riab Mano Arto Sup* 31(1S):63–67, 1994.

▶ The supplement of *Rivista di Chirurgia e Riabitazione della Mano e dell'arto Superiore* (Italian Journal of Hand Surgery) has been entirely devoted to the work of a combined Commitee of the Italian Society for Surgery of the Hand (SICM) and the Italian Society of Microsurgery (SIM). The Commitee has been named CUMI and has been assigned to address "il Coordinamento Urgenze microvascolari in Italia" (the coordination of microvascular emergencies in Italy).

The analysis of the overall work produced by this committee might be useful for similar projects arising in other continents. This specific paper might be useful when considering the organizing aspects regarding the coordination of the microvascular emergencies in a wide area, region, or entire national territory.

A. Landi, M.D.

Haramati N, Hiller N, Dowdle J, et al: MRI of the Stener lesion. *Skeletal Radiol* 24:515–518, 1995.
▶ The investigators doubt whether MRI is sufficiently accurate to diagnose a so-called Stener lesion.

V.R. Hentz, M.D.

Hahn P, Heindl E: Does an ulnar nerve lesion influence the motion of the index finger? *J Hand Surg* 21B(2):252–254, 1996.
▶ A little.

P.C. Amadio, M.D.

Bain GI, Bennett JD, Richards RS, et al: Longitudinal computed tomography of the scaphoid: A new technique. *Skeletal Radiol* 24:271–273, 1995.
▶ This is a good description of the optimal method for CT scanning of scaphoid fractures. The degree of healing and deformity is better shown with longitudinal CT scanning with conventional CT scanning in axial, sagittal, and coronal planes, and plain radiography.

G. Bergman, M.D.

Yin Y, Wilson AJ, Gilula LA: Three-compartment wrist arthrography: Direct comparison of digital subtraction with nonsubtraction images. *Radiology* 197:287–290, 1995.
▶ According to this article, the digital subtraction technique for wrist arthrography improves identification of the site of communication between joint compartments, as compared with conventional spot-film technique. The conventional technique was better for detection of all communication sites, however, because it often requires wrist motion whereas digital subtraction technique requires the wrist to be immobilized during the examination. When the two techniques were used in combination, the value added by the subtraction technique was small.

G. Bergman, M.D.

3 Skeletal Trauma and Reconstruction

Surgical Treatment of Severe Fracture Dislocations of the Proximal Interphalangeal Joint
Büchler U (Univ of Bern, Switzerland)
Hand Surg 1:31–35, 1996

Introduction.—Unstable impacted fracture-dislocations of the proximal interphalangeal joint of the finger that involve more than 40% of the surface of the joint plateau usually have poor response to conservative treatment. Surgery is difficult in these cases, however, and carries the risk for technical failure. The technique presented here is based on the author's experience with 27 such fracture-dislocations.

Fracture Components.—The fracture involves impaction of 1 or more major fragments and numerous smaller fragments, an outward bursting of the walls of the metaphysis, fragmentation and collapse of a segment of the metaphyseal wall, and joint subluxation. Linear or trispiral tomograms in 2 planes can reveal details of the impaction frature if roentgenograms are inadequate.

Technique.—Adequate optical exposure is necessary for a successful outcome. The joint inspection portal is created on the side showing the greatest effect of impaction, and the joint is entered between the central slip and the dorsal edge of the proper collateral ligament. If this does not provide an adequate overview, the proper collateral ligament is detached close to its origin and deflected distally.

The reduction–internal fixation technique begins with disimpaction of the depressed fragments. After the fragments are freed (a process that may require considerable force), they are levered into the correct position. To facilitate anatomical reduction, coaxial alignment of the joint should be assured, dorsal to palmar pressure should be applied to the base of the middle phalanx, and the head of the proximal phalanx should be used as a template for reduction. Cancellous bone grafts taken from the distal radius are used to fill the void resulting from disimpaction. Circular coherence of the outer shell can usually be restored using 1 or 3 cortical 1.5-mm compression screws. Simple external pressure is usually adequate for reducing secondary zigzag fractures of the metaphyseal wall. After closure, a unilateral dynamic external fixator is applied when there is a residual tendency toward dorsal subluxation in full extension.

Closure.—Mobilization is usually started before postoperative day 4 depending on the condition of the outer soft tissue. Consolidation can be confirmed by tomograms after 6 weeks, and the external fixation device can then be removed. More aggressive therapy is then started, and increased loading is permitted at 8 weeks.

▶ The intra-articular fracture of the base of the middle phalanx has to be considered a severe injury when the fracture is associated with an impaction and involvement of more than 40% of its surface. In these situations, surgical reconstruction of the joint is the therapy of choice.

The author demonstrates the surgical approach to the joint from the lateral aspect by dissecting the check rein ligament, the palmar plate, and the collateral ligament. Bone grafting is performed after disimpaction of the fragments and reconstruction of the articular surface. A minimal osteosynthesis may be performed if there is no intrinsic stability.

The major problem in this type of fracture occurs in cases in which the fragments are too small and cannot be realigned to reconstruct the joint surface of the base of the proximal phalanx. In these cases, I recommend using fibrin glue, perichondrium, or periosteum to avoid extrusion of the cancellous bone in the joint. Further opening of the tendon sheath of the flexor tendon should be avoided because this structure has a so-called ligamentotaxis effect on the stability of the middle phalanx.

Priv. Dr. Med. C.L. Jantea

Dynamic Digital Traction for Unstable Comminuted Intra-articular Fracture-Dislocations of the Proximal Interphalangeal Joint
Morgan JP, Gordon DA, Klug MS, et al (Wright State Univ, Dayton, Ohio)
J Hand Surg (Am) 20A:565–573, 1995   3–2

Introduction.—Comminuted fracture dislocations about the proximal interphalangeal (PIP) joint with significant articular surface disruption are extremely difficult to treat. Consensus does not exist on a therapeutic procedure of choice; any can result in contracture, loss of motion, functional decline, and post-traumatic arthritis. Recently, R.R. Schenck described a treatment that combines use of traction with early motion. The efficacy of this treatment was evaluated.

Methods.—Fourteen patients with comminuted, unstable intra-articular PIP joint fracture dislocations were available for an average 24-month follow-up after treatment with digital traction and immediate motion. The

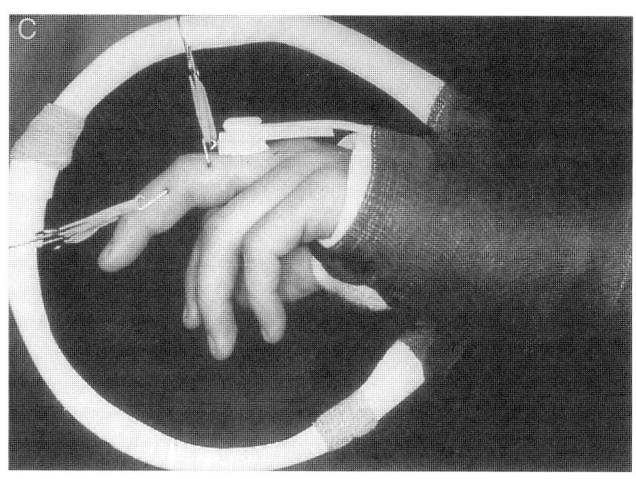

FIGURE 2C.—Completed assembly of device. Pins are bent into a hook shape for attachment of rubber bands. Metacarpophalangeal extension block may be added to encourage full proximal interphalangeal extension without outside help. (Courtesy of Morgan JP, Gordon DA, Klug MS, et al: Dynamic digital traction for unstable comminuted intra-articular fracture-dislocations of the proximal interphalangeal joint. *J Hand Surg (Am)* 20A:565–573, 1995.)

technique used involves institution of early motion; the traction device is applied in the physician's office (Fig 2C). The metacarpophalangeal joint is not immobilized, but a dorsal extension block is added to prevent hyperextension. Patients are instructed to perform passive range-of-motion exercises at least 8 times a day; motion begins on the day of application and continues throughout the duration of traction. Radiography and reevaluation of tension are indicated after 2–5 days and then weekly until the device is removed after 4–6 weeks. More traditional hand therapy is then instituted. Dynamic PIP extension and flexion splinting, as needed, are begun at 6 weeks; strengthening with putty is begun at 8 weeks. Patients are discharged from therapy 10–12 weeks after injury.

Results.—Most patients showed dorsal fracture dislocation and pilon-type injuries. Average involvement of the articular surface of the joint was 80%. At the time of final follow-up examination, patients who had isolated injuries averaged a 95-degree active arc of motion at the PIP joint; for all patients, the average active arc of motion was 89 degrees. Fracture union, joint remodeling, and preservation of joint space were evident on radiographs. Functional joint restoration was excellent; patients were very satisfied and returned to previous levels of activity. Residual pain in 7 patients was mild and associated primarily with cold weather and heavy activity. No patient experienced pain at rest or during usual activity. No patient required secondary surgical intervention to improve results.

Discussion.—This technique is based on the tenets that joint and fracture alignment can be restored by ligamentotaxis through traction and that joint healing and restoration of function are promoted by early motion. Risk for iatrogenic injury and further trauma to the joint (with resultant stiffness) are minimized by this closed technique. Use of local anesthesia and readily available materials makes this technique highly cost-effective and convenient, but patients must be tolerant and compliant. Dynamic digital traction is thus recommended for treatment of unstable comminuted PIP joint fractures, even those involving subluxation or dislocation.

▶ This article is a thorough, detailed analysis of a minimally invasive technique to treat severe fractures and fracture dislocations of the PIP joint. The overall results, particularly with respect to PIP joint mobility, are outstanding considering the magnitude of these injuries. Interestingly, most patients did lose some terminal joint flexion. The primary advantage of traction in combination with early mobilization is that it largely avoids proximal interphalangeal joint stiffness, an all too frequent sequela to more invasive fixation techniques. The proximal interphalangeal joint seems to be somewhat forgiving in terms of anatomical restoration of the articular surface. In the pilon injury, for example, there is central depression of the articular surface of the middle phalanx. Ligamentotaxis cannot be counted on to elevate depressed articular fragments. However, if the reduction can restore colinearity between the proximal and middle phalanges and is combined with early mobilization, considerable articular remodeling results; this remodeling allows satisfactory restoration of joint motion.

On the basis of personal experience, as well as of this article, I can only conclude that this is a very reasonable treatment option for compliant patients with severe PIP joint injuries.

P.J. Stern, M.D.

Cerclage Fixation for Fracture Dislocation of the Proximal Interphalangeal Joint
Weiss A-PC (Brown Univ, Providence, RI)
Clin Orthop 327:21–28, 1996

3–3

Background.—Achieving excellent functional outcomes is difficult in the treatment of dorsal fracture dislocations of the proximal interphalangeal joint. In recent years, minimally invasive internal fixation methods have gained popularity, as they result in better biological healing responses while providing fracture fragment stabilization. A technique of cerclage wiring for severe simple and multifragmented volar margin fractures of the middle phalanx in patients with a dorsal fracture dislocation of the proximal interphalangeal joint was developed.

Technique.—The technique involves making a volar zigzag incision and flexor sheath incision between the A-2 and A-4 pulleys. The flexor digitorum profundus and flexor digitorum sublimis tendons are then retracted to the side, exposing the volar plate. Cancellous bone grafting under 1 or more fragments helps stabilize the fragment reduction. This grafting is accomplished by direct application or through the cortical window. Sharp dissection is performed to free 1–2 mm of the periosteum circumferentially around the bony fragments of the middle phalanx.

Results.—Twelve patients underwent volar cerclage wiring. Mean follow-up was 2.1 years. Eleven patients had no degenerative joint changes. Only 1 showed evidence of early volar articular surface beaking. The mean final active arc of motion at the proximal interphalangeal joint was 89 degrees. The mean degree of extension loss at the proximal interphalangeal joint was 8 degrees. There were no implant failures, irritations, or infections.

Conclusions.—Cerclage fixation for fracture dislocation of the proximal interphalangeal joint has several advantages. The articular surface is restored, postoperative stability to the fracture fragments is excellent, and early active and passive range of motion is possible. In addition, there is no implant protrusion.

▶ Dorsal fracture dislocation of the proximal interphalangeal joint is a very common injury and most injuries can be treated by closed means. There are a few instances when the joint is irreducible or unable to be held reduced by a closed procedure. If maintaining reduction is the problem, a dorsal blocking K-wire, an Agee force couple, or a hinged external fixator may be helpful. Failing this, open reduction may be necessary. The author describes a fixation technique requiring extensive soft-tissue dissection followed by fixation with a No. 24-gauge cerclage wire. Exactly how soon the patients are mobilized postoperatively and other details of the postoperative rehabilitation program are not described and would make the article more helpful. The results of an average range of motion of 89 degrees are quite good, however, for any patient sustaining this injury despite the treatment.

J.A. Katarincic, M.D.

Corrective Osteotomy for Post-traumatic Malunion of the Phalanges in the Hand
Büchler U, Gupta A, Ruf S (Univ of Bern, Switzerland)
J Hand Surg (Br) 21B:33–42, 1996   3–4

Background.—Phalangeal malunion can result in rotation, angulation, deviation, shortening, or a combination of deformities, thereby impairing hand function. The results of corrective osteotomy for post-traumatic malunion of the phalanges in 1 series of patients were reported.

Patients.—Fifty-seven patients, aged 5–61 years, who underwent phalangeal corrective osteotomies for post-traumatic malunion between 1978 and 1990 were included. A total of 59 rotational, radial-ulnar deviation, flexion-extension, length adjustment procedures, and combinations were done. Rigid internal fixation was used. Half the patients underwent concurrent tenocapsulolysis.

Outcomes.—Surgical correction was satisfactory in 76% of patients. Bony union was achieved in all patients. Eighty-nine percent of patients had a net gain in active range of motion. Surgical outcomes were excellent or good in 96% of patients who underwent corrective osteotomies for malunion involving the bone only and in 64% of those who underwent corrections for malunion with multiple structure involvement.

Conclusions.—With comprehensive planning, meticulous technique, and intensive aftercare, corrective osteotomy of the phalanges can yield satisfactory results. In patients who have complex, multistructural involvement, capsulotomy, tenolysis, nerve grafting, and skin flap applications are important and may be performed safely in 1 stage when rigid internal fixation is used. The best functional outcomes are unassociated with type and degree of bony deformity or procedure complexity but are associated with the nature of the initial injury.

▶ The phalangeal skeleton serves as a foundation for a most unique architecture in nature—the human digit. The mere fact that the ratio of the lengths of the 3 phalanges in the digits represents that of Fibonacci's series of logarithmic spirals adds more to this premise. Failure to maintain correct digital alignment and length will, by itself, lead to an imbalance of the extrinsic, as well as intrinsic, tendons and subsequently the digital articulations. It is also evident that trauma associated with these gliding structures can manifest itself in an adverse outcome, regardless of the overall alignment of the skeleton.

Büchler et al. have laid out for the reader a comprehensive understanding of the nature of malunions of the phalanges and associated tendon and joint dysfunction and a rational plan for approaching these problems operatively. This enormous study represents the senior author's experience in dealing with a host of complex problems involving the digits. I must emphasize the authors' conclusion that "comprehensive planning, meticulous technique, and intensive aftercare" will yield satisfactory results.

Two major contributions can be found in this study. First, the authors identify the types of skeletal deformity by virtue of location, the vector of the deformity, and the relationship to associated articulations. This identification is the most clearly defined in the literature.

Perhaps just as important is the authors' identification of the relationship of capsular contracture, tendon adhesion, and other soft tissue deficiencies that are so often associated with these problems. Just as in the acute injury, the authors have defined the problems by virtue of isolated injuries as compared with combined injuries, being both skeletal as well as soft tissue. Further, they have identified the need for both length correction and stable internal fixation, particularly when associated with soft tissue reconstruction.

The authors have compared their results with those in the literature. It is quite evident from reading this paper, however, that the cases identified in the authors' experience were substantially more defined, the outcome more carefully scrutinized, and the overall results more accurately defined.

This paper is absolutely a must for anyone involved in surgery of the hand. It serves as a landmark for this particular problem.

J.B. Jupiter, M.D.

Flexible Intramedullary Nailing for Metacarpal Fractures
Gonzalez MH, Igram CM, Hall RF Jr (Univ of Illinois, Chicago)
J Hand Surg (Am) 20A:382–387, 1995   3–5

Introduction.—Flexible intramedullary nailing is a technique used for several types of long-bone fractures. A .8-mm prebent, blunted nail (Smith and Nephew, Memphis, Tenn.) has been designed specifically for metacarpal fractures. Image control is used to guide insertion of the nails without opening the fracture site. The records of 83 patients undergoing nonthumb metacarpal fixation between 1983 and 1988 were retrospectively reviewed.

Methods.—The patients had a total of 98 metacarpal fractures. Closed metacarpal fractures ($n = 96$) were reduced in a closed procedure and underwent flexible intramedullary fixation with multiple 0.8-mm prebent rods. Two open metacarpal fractures were similarly fixed. Insertion of rods was antegrade in 73 fractures and retrograde in 25. Average duration of follow-up was 9 months.

Technique Summary.—The portal site is located with an image intensifier. Four holes are drilled into the bone tilted 45 degrees toward the fracture site, and a single, flexible blunt-tip rod is inserted into 1 of them (Fig 1A and 1B). With image intensifier guidance and traction, an assistant then reduces the fracture, after which the rod is advanced until it engages the opposite cortex (Fig 1C). Once satisfactory reduction is confirmed, the canal is "stacked" with 3 or 4 more rods and all the rods are cut flush with the cortex. The hand is placed in a clam-digger splint for 4 weeks.

Results.—Short oblique and transverse fractures are amenable to flexible intramedullary fixation; long oblique and bicortical comminuted fractures are a contraindication for this procedure. All fractures healed. Complications included bending of the rods after repeat trauma (2 instances) and the backing out of rods (1 instance). All but 2 patients gained 90 degrees of flexion at the metacarpophalangeal joint; all gained full extension. One patient required reoperation because of rotation deformity.

Conclusions.—Flexible intramedullary nails offer the advantages of use of closed reduction, lack of wire protruding from skin or bone, absence of need for rod removal, opportunity for early motion, and rotational control. Flexible intramedullary pinning of carefully selected metacarpal fractures provides excellent results with few complications.

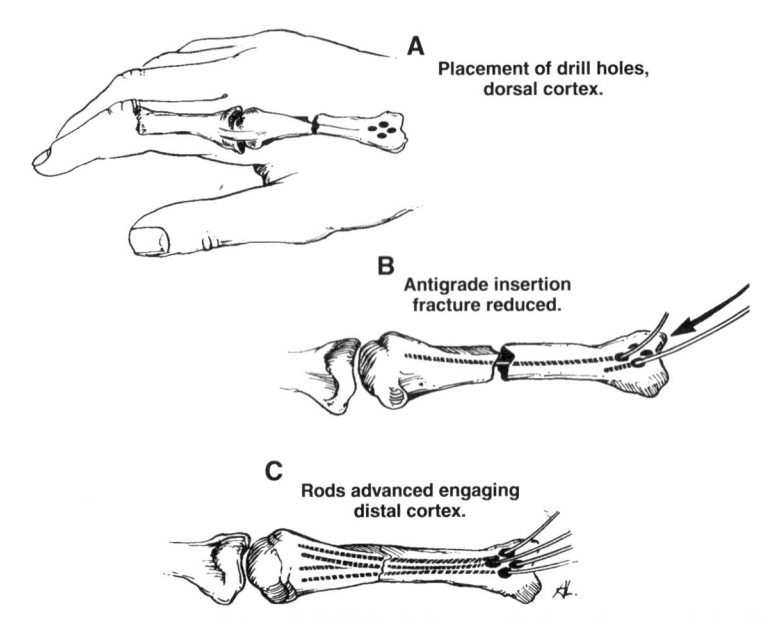

FIGURE 1.—Operative technique. A, drill holes. B, fracture reduction and passage of wire. C, rods advanced "stacking canal." (Courtesy of Gonzalez MH, Igram CM, Hall RF Jr: Flexible intramedullary nailing for metacarpal fractures. *J Hand Surg (Am)* 20A:382–387, 1995. Medical illustration by Allen Levenson, C.M.I., Los Angeles, CA, (310) 540-5424.)

▶ Intramedullary fixation of metacarpal shaft fractures with multiple pins is not new. In this series, the authors obtained excellent results with a technique for inserting flexible, prebent pins. The advantages to this technique are the following[1]: (1) indirect reduction that prevents exposure or devascularization of the fracture site; (2) 3-point fixation that prevents fracture rotation; and (3) the pins are buried and, unlike external implants, do not need to be removed.

The surgeon should keep in mind several caveats: (1) indications are limited to diaphyseal fractures, which are transverse or short oblique; (2) pins can migrate into an adjacent joint and can back out if not well seated within the medullary canal; and (3) care must be taken during insertion to ensure that rotational alignment is proper and that the fracture is not distracted.

On a personal note, I have found intramedullary fixation (using a Steinman pin) particularly effective for replantation in severe open fractures in which conservation of time is critical.

P.J. Stern, M.D.

Reference

1. Foucher G: "Bouquet" osteosynthesis in metacarpal neck fractures: A series of 66 patients. *J Hand Surg (Am)*, 20A:586–590, 1995.

Internal Fixation of Oblique Metacarpal Fractures

Firoozbakhsh K, Moneim MS, Doherty W, et al (Sharif Univ of Technology, Tehran, Iran)
Clin Orthop 325:296–301, 1996
3–6

Introduction.—Although several biomechanical studies have evaluated different fixation methods for the bones of the hand, most have used only simple quasistatic loadings applied with an Instron testing machine. However, static loading tests may not provide adequate information on impact injuries, such as those experienced in falls or in sports. This information might be useful in choosing the best fixation technique for patients at risk of impact loading. A series of impact loading studies was performed to assess the internal fixation of oblique metacarpal fractures.

Methods.—Oblique osteotomy and internal fixation were performed in 120 fresh-frozen human metacarpal bones. Various internal fixation techniques were used: dorsal plating with lag screws, 2 dorsal lag screws, crossed Kirschner wire tension band, 5 stacked intramedullary Kirschner wires, and paired intramedullary Kirschner wires. Compressive impact and bending impact tests were then applied. The impact forces were selected to mimic the sudden blows associated with sports injuries and other impact-type injuries.

Results.—The compressive impact tests produced failure within 6 msec, whereas the bending impact test produced almost immediate failure. The strongest internal fixation techniques were the dorsal plate and the intramedullary rod—they were about as strong as intact specimens on compressive impact testing, although 19% weaker in bending impact tests. The weakest of all the fixation techniques evaluated was 2 dorsal lag screw fixation. It was 59% weaker than dorsal plating on compressive impact testing and 47% weaker in bending impact tests.

Conclusions.—A biomechanical study of metacarpal internal fixation using impact loading demonstrated that dorsal plate and intramedullary rod fixation are best able to resist impact loading. The weakest technique in this regard is 2 dorsal lag screw fixation. The authors use plates and screws for transverse and short oblique fractures, with screws alone for long oblique fractures.

▶ This biomechanical study tested the strength of oblique metacarpal fracture fixation constructs preferred by the authors in compression and bending. As expected, the combination of dorsal plate and intrafragmentary lag screw fixation was the strongest, and 2-screw fixation the weakest. These data, however, would not lead me to routinely use a plate and screws for a metacarpal fracture. Fixation such as multiple K-wires, either crossed, intramedullary, or to an adjacent intact metacarpal, could in many cases be accomplished closed, and although unable to sustain the forces applied in this study, they could withstand the forces of gentle active motion, or be temporarily protected by splinting. Also, multiple lag screw fixation without plating may be weak to the authors' testing, but is preferred in a patient who needs to gently use the hand early.

J.M Failla, M.D.

Arthroscopic Treatment of Acute Complete Thumb Metacarpophalangeal Ulnar Collateral Ligament Tears
Ryu J, Fagan R (West Virginia Univ, Morgantown; Texas Tech Univ, El Paso)
J Hand Surg (Am) 20A:1037–1042, 1995   3–7

Introduction.—Ulnar collateral ligament (UCL) injuries of the thumb metacarpophalangeal (MP) joint are common. Acute partial ruptures are usually treated by MP joint immobilization, but the treatment of acute complete UCL ruptures remains controversial. An arthroscopic technique for the reduction of Stener lesions that permits healing without open surgical repair is described.

Patient Group.—Arthroscopy was performed on 9 patients with acute UCL rupture between July 1985 and December 1989. One patient did not continue with follow-up. Of the 8 remaining patients, 7 had injuries in their dominant thumb. Six of the 8 patients were men (mean age, 30 years).

Technique.—An arthrobot and a Chinese finger trap on the thumb were used to vertically suspend the hand, with its own weight providing traction. A 20-gauge needle was inserted into the MP joint, followed by a #11 blade, blunt trocar, and arthroscope. A second portal, just palmar to the radial collateral ligament, the radiopalmar portal, was established and used for irrigation and

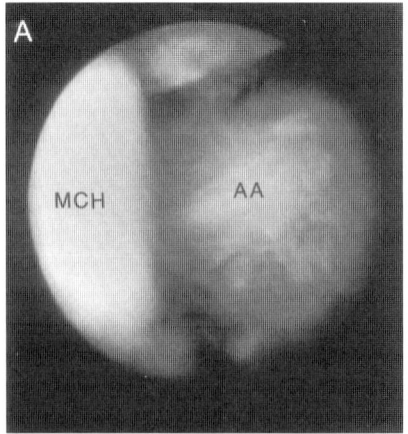

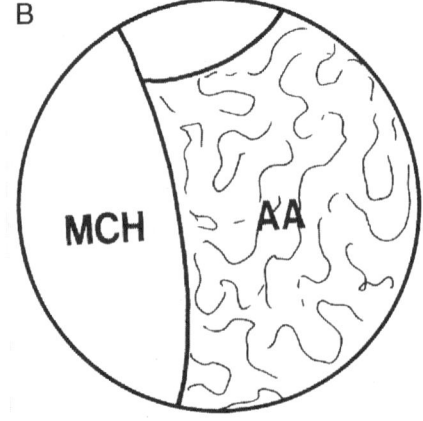

FIGURE 2.—**A,** thumb metacarpophalangeal joint with Stener lesion. **B,** the metacarpal head (*MCH*) is shown on the left. The adductor aponeurosis (*AA*) is shown on the right. (Courtesy of Ryu J, Fagan R: Arthroscopic treatment of acute complete thumb metacarpophalangeal ulnar collateral ligament tears. *J Hand Surg (Am)* 20A:1037–1042, 1995.)

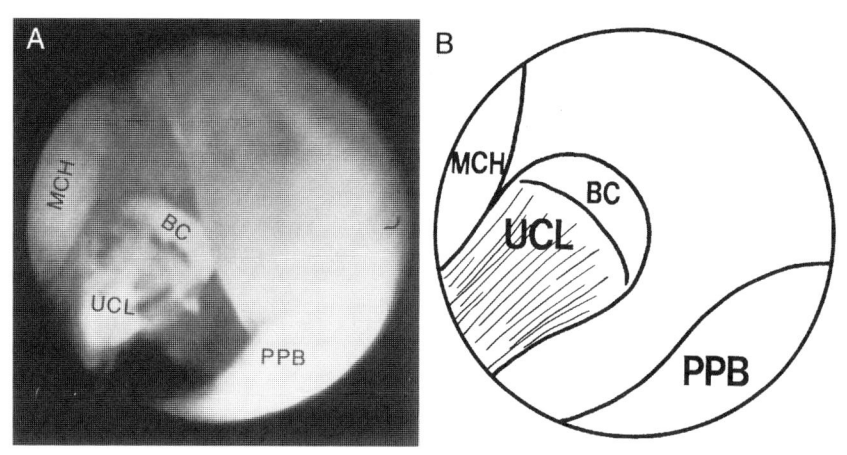

FIGURE 3.—**A,** after Stener lesion reduction, the ulnar ligament (*UCL*) is shown with a small bony fragment (*BC*) at the end. **B,** a portion of the metacarpal head (*MCH*) is shown in the left. *Abbreviation: PPB,* proximal phalangeal base. (Courtesy of Ryu J, Fagan R: Arthroscopic treatment of acute complete thumb metacarpophalangeal ulnar collateral ligament tears. *J Hand Surg (Am)* 20A:1037–1042, 1995.)

drainage. The surgery was performed after inflation of a pneumatic tourniquet. A small probe was introduced through the radiopalmar portal, along the metatarpal head; passed through the proximal edge of the apneurosis around the anticipated origin site of the UCL; and pulled toward the joint. This brought the distal UCL end within the joint. A Kirschner wire was used to immobilize the MP joint in a 20- to 30-degree flexed position. A thumb spica short arm cast was applied. The wire was removed after 4 weeks and the cast, after 6 weeks. Daily active and passive range of motion exercises were then initiated under the care of a therapist.

Results.—The average initial follow-up lasted 21 months. Tip pinch, key pinch, and grip strength were all equal to or greater than those on the contralateral side. Laxity of the MP joint was not increased. Joint motion was within 99% of that on the contralateral side. No pain or functional limitation was reported. At 30- to 48-month follow-up, no changes were reported by patients. The only complication in ths series was a pin track infection in 1 patient. The wire was removed 2 weeks early, and the patient was given oral antibiotics. The infection resolved without further probems.

Case Report.—Boy, 13 years, sustained a complete UCL tear of his dominant thumb MP joint while playing football. His initial stress radiograph demonstrated a 50-degree radial deviation with a small avulsion fracture. Arthroscopy of the MP joint confirmed the presence of a Stener lesion (Fig 2). The UCL was brought back into the joint (Fig 3). The end of the UCL was placed at the base of the proximal phalanx (Fig 4). A Kirschner wire was used to immobilize

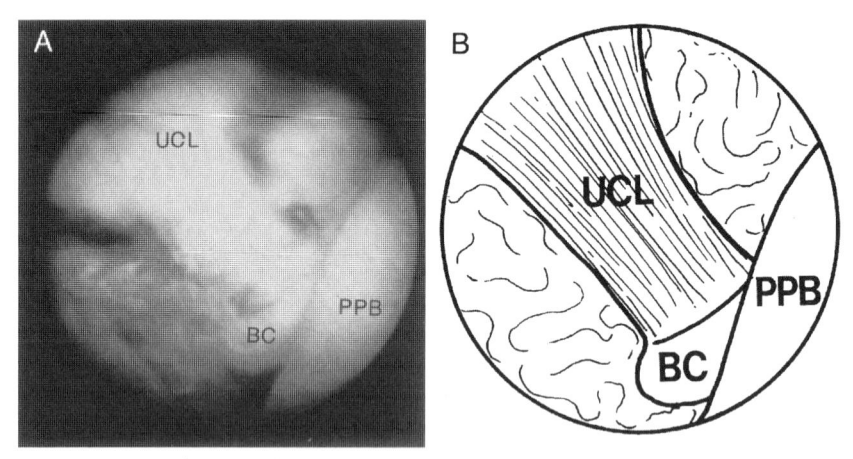

FIGURE 4.—**A,** the ulnar collateral ligament (*UCL*) is placed where it anatomically belongs. **B,** the proximal phalangeal base (*PPB*) is shown in the lower right corner. *Abbreviation: BC,* bony fragment. (Courtesy of Ryu J, Fagan R: Arthroscopic treatment of acute complete thumb metacarpophalangeal ulnar collateral ligament tears. *J Hand Surg (Am)* 20A:1037–1042, 1995.)

the joint in 20-degree flexion. The wire was removed after 4 weeks. The patient returned to playing football without problems 3 months after surgery.

Conclusions.—In this series of 8 patients with acute complete tears of the UCL of the thumb MP joints, treatment done with arthroscopic reduction of the Stener lesion provided excellent results. Additional experience and longer follow-up periods are required before this technique can be recommended.

▶ The author used a very small (1.7-mm) arthroscope that was originally designed for temporomandibular joint arthroscopy to identify and reposition a displaced and torn UCL. The results in this small series equal or succeed the functional results seen after open repair. These 9 patients had clinical examination results that strongly indicated the existence of a so-called Stener lesion. The slope of the learning curve, however, cannot be established by reading the article. Some practice on cadavers seems advisable for the uninitiated surgeon.

V.R. Hentz, M.D.

Treatment of Thumb Ulnar Collateral Ligament Ruptures With the Mitek Bone Anchor
Kozin SH (Temple Univ, Philadelphia)
Ann Plast Surg 35:1–5, 1995   3–8

Background.—Thumb ulnar collateral ligament (UCL) injuries are common. Although several techniques have been described for UCL reattachment, they tend to be difficult, time-consuming, frustrating, or ineffective. One experience with the Mitek bone anchor technique in the open reduction and primary repair of acute UCL injuries was reported.

Patients and Outcomes.—Seven patients were treated for complete ulnar collateral ligament disruptions. They were 4 men and 3 women, aged 20 to 89 years. Four patients were found to have a Stener lesion. Within the mean 1-year follow-up, all patients had regained a stable metacarpophalangeal joint to valgus stress. Radiographs showed accurate placement of the bone anchor with protraction of the metallic wings in cancellous bone. On range of motion assessment, patients had a 7% loss of metacarpophalangeal flexion-extension and a 21% loss of interphalangeal motion. Mean pinch strength was 98% in apposition and 97% in opposition of the uninvolved hand. Compared with the uninjured extremity, grip strength was 96%.

Conclusions.—The Mitek bone anchor facilitates UCL repair by obviating the need for connecting drill holes, pull-out sutures, and external buttons. The clinical outcomes associated with the use of the Mitek bone anchor have been favorable. Thus, this technique is recommended for the fixation of complete UCL ruptures at the thumb metacarpophalangeal joint.

▶ The use of anchor bolts to attach soft tissues such as tendon or ligament to bone has gained in popularity. The systems are reasonably easy to learn and use. In my view, their principal disadvantage is that their design does not allow firm anchoring over a wide area. If only 1 bolt is used, the 2 filaments of the attached suture arise from a very small hole in the bone. If they are then passed upward through the tissue to be anchored in close proximity to one another, the suture grasps only a small amount of tissue. On the other hand, if the 2 sutures are passed widely apart, thereby "grasping" a large volume of tissue, as the knot is tied under tension, the 2 parts of the suture between bone and soft tissue tend to come together. This in turn distracts the soft tissues away from the proposed anchor point. The use of 2 anchors with cross ties seems preferable when there is concern about the stability of the attachment.

V.R. Hentz, M.D.

Isolated Injuries to the Dorsoradial Capsule of the Thumb Metacarpophalangeal Joint
Krause JO, Manske PR, Mirly HL, et al (Washington Univ, St Louis, Mo)
J Hand Surg (Am) 21A:428–433, 1996   3–9

Background.—The most common injury to the metacarpophalangeal (MP) joint of the thumb involves the ulnar collateral ligament. Radial collateral ligament (RCL) injuries are less common. Little attention has been given to isolated dorsal capsular injuries. A series of patients with dorsoradial capsular injuries of the thumb MP joint without clinical RCL or ulnar collateral ligament laxity was described.

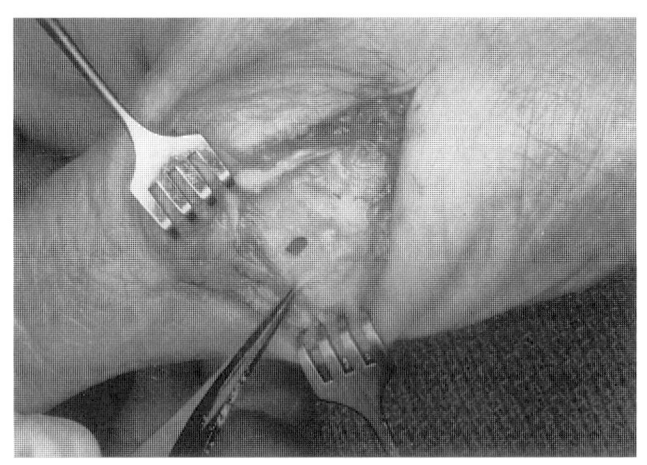

FIGURE 2.—Intraoperative photograph demonstrating defect in dorsoradial capsule of the metacarpophalangeal joint of the thumb. (Courtesy of Krause JO, Manske PR, Mirly HL, et al: Isolated injuries to the dorsoradial capsule of the thumb metacarpophalangeal joint. *J Hand Surg [Am]* 21A:428–433, 1996.)

Methods and Findings.—Eleven patients aged 10–45 years who had injuries to the dorsoradial capsule of the thumb MP joints were seen between 1989 and 1993. The mechanism of injury was breaking a fall (5 patients), a direct blow (3), and a sports-related injury (3). Seven injuries were confirmed at operative exploration and repaired by imbrication or a direct technique (Fig 2). No complications resulted from surgery. Six of the 7 patients later returned to unrestricted activity with no need for analgesics. One patient continued to report tenderness over the dorsoradial capsule and minor pain.

Conclusion.—Although much less common than collateral ligament injuries, isolated injuries to the dorsoradial capsule of the thumb MP joint do occur. Patients with palmar subluxation of the proximal phalanx will probably need surgical exploration and repair. Nonoperative treatment was ineffective in the patients in this series with palmar subluxation and extensor lag.

▶ This important paper includes the thumb in the concept that a dorsal capsular tear of the MP joint of a finger can lead to chronic pain, which can be relieved by immobilization or surgery. One difference between the thumb MP joint and a finger MP joint is that in the finger, one usually has to deal with a saggital band injury as well. This paper also makes evident the difference that the dorsal capsular tear in the thumb can cause palmar MP joint subluxation and loss of some extension, even without RCL injury. This could be caused by the extensor pollicis brevis (EPB) in some patients attaching directly into the dorsoradial capsule rather than into the proximal phalanx; its function is, thus, decreased when the capsule is torn. I have noted this during surgery for RCL injury with palmar subluxation, as well as during cadaver dissection, with the EPB inserted into the capsule in 10% of cases and into the proximal phalanx, or distally with the extensor pollicis longus, in the rest. It would be interesting to supplement this clinical data with a biomechanical cadaver study by creating a dorsoradial capsular injury and checking for palmar MP joint subluxation.

J.M. Failla, M.D.

Splint Immobilization of Gamekeeper's Thumb
Landsman JC, Seitz WH Jr, Froimson AI, et al (Case Western Reserve Univ, Cleveland, Ohio)
Orthopedics 18:1161–1165, 1995   3–10

Introduction.—Instability of the metacarpophalangeal joint of the thumb resulting from chronic and acute insults to the ulnar collateral ligament is often referred to as "gamekeeper's thumb." Closed management of complete ruptures has resulted in failure rates as high as 50%. It has also been reported that early reconstruction, within 2 weeks of injury, as opposed to delayed reconstruction will achieve better results. The treatment protocol for acute, complete ruptures of the ulnar collateral ligament of the thumb metaphalangeal joint has been reexamined. Results of nonoperative splinting developed for patients who refused surgical repair of acute rupture of the ulnar collateral ligament were retrospectively reviewed in 40 thumbs for 6 years.

Methods.—Thumb spica splint immobilization was used for 39 patients with 40 gamekeeper's thumbs. Treatment began within 1 week of injury. Splinting ranged from 8–12 weeks, with patients wearing a thumb spica custom-made splint 24 hours a day—a hand-based splint worn during the day and a more rigid forearm-based splint at night. Patients were observed every 2 weeks during the healing phase, and at the end of 8 weeks, they were reexamined. Follow-up continued up to 5 years, with an average of 2.4 years.

Results.—No complications were seen. Fifteen of 39 patients continued normal work activities, and these included 34 surgeons and an anesthesiologist. In the follow-up, 34 of 39 (or 85%) of these injuries healed without arthrosis, stiffness (range of motion within 80% of the contralateral hand), significant instability, or pain. Splint immobilization resulted in healing for all bony avulsion lesions. Persistent instability and pain were seen in 6 ruptures (15%) at 12 weeks and they were treated with surgical reconstruction.

Conclusion.—Revision may be necessary for currently accepted guidelines for surgical intervention as primary treatment for ligamentous disruption at the thumb metacarpophalangeal joint. An effective primary treatment modality may be splint immobilization. Surgery may be used for the minority of patients who demonstrate persistent laxity.

▶ The conclusions from this article are contrary to the mainstream recommendations for the management of acute thumb metacarpophalangeal

(MCP) ulnar collateral injury: As the authors note, the literature states that 15% to 60% of patients will have a Stener lesion. If this is true, I believe operative intervention for unstable injuries is warranted to ensure that the ligament is positioned where it can heal. Current teaching states that failure to address the Stener lesion operatively will usually result in symptomatic chronic MCP instability. Although nonoperative management is appealing, chronic instability in my experience is a significant problem. The goal now becomes reestablishment of pain-free stability, either by MCP fusion or ligament reconstruction, usually with a tendon graft. Both of these procedures have their own set of problems.

In their discussion, the authors state that ligament disruptions in other areas (such as the medial collateral ligament of the knee) can heal uneventfully with immobilization. Such an analogy is inappropriate, as in the case of the knee, the ligament is nondisplaced. Ryu, et al.[1] have shown that acute Stener lesions can be successfully managed arthroscopically by positioning the ligament adjacent to the proximal phalangeal base without suture reattachment. This makes sense to me and is analogous to successful nonoperative management of medial collateral ligaments of the knee. It is interesting to note that all of the bony avulsions healed. Because bony avulsion rarely results in a Stener lesion, it seems appropriate to manage most of these injuries nonoperatively.

Finally, this article does not detail the nonoperative results and surgical management of the failures. I am unconvinced that splint management of unstable nonbony ligamentous avulsions is superior and I hope the authors will design a prospective comparative study addressing this issue.

P.J. Stern, M.D.

Reference

1. Ryu J, Fagan R: Arthroscopic treatment of acute complete thumb metacarpophalangeal ulnar collateral ligament tears. *J Hand Surg* 20-A: 1037-1042, 1995.

Treatment of Infected Clench-fist Human Bite Wounds in the Area of Metacarpophalangeal Joints
Chadaev AP, Jukhtin VI, Butkevich AT, et al (Russian State Med Univ, Moscow)
J Hand Surg [Am] 21A:299–303, 1996   3–11

Background.—Treating infected clench-fist human bite wounds in the metacarpophalangeal joints can be difficult, especially when pyarthrosis or osteomyelitis develop. Generally, patients do not seek medical attention for this injury until significant inflammation is present. One series of patients with infected clench-fist human bite wounds in the area of the metacarpophalangeal joints was reviewed.

Patients and Findings.—Two hundred twenty-one patients were included. The joint capsule was not violated in 79 patients; the wounds of these patients were debrided and irrigated with an antiseptic solution. The wounds were then drained with microirrigators and closed primarily. In 53 patients, the joint had been violated but with no osseous or articular involvement. For these patients, treatment consisted of débridement, irrigation, drainage, and skin closure. In 89 patients with articular or bond destruction, treatment was the same as in the second group, but a distraction device was added to fix and unload the joint. Seventy-three of the 79 patients in the first group were available for follow-up assessment. Outcomes were excellent in 71 and satisfactory in 2. Forty-seven of the 53 patients in group 2 were available for follow-up, 38 of whom had excellent results; 7, satisfactory; and 2, unsatisfactory. Among the 73 patients followed in the third group, 39 had excellent results; 24, satisfactory; and 10, unsatisfactory.

Conclusion.—Treatment outcomes in patients with pyarthrosis associated with clenched-fist injury depends on the degree of joint involvement. The application of a distraction device, which prevents joint fusion and preserves joint mobility, is recommended for such patients.

▶ This Russian article is one of the largest series of metacarpophalangeal human bite wounds and, although retrospective, offers some important concepts. The authors note some differences between their series and similar series from the United States. For example, in their series, 79% of the injuries involved the long or index finger, whereas in the United States, most injuries affect the ring and small finger. The predominant organism isolated was *Staphylococcus aureous* (86%). No mention was made of *Eikenella corrodens;* this may reflect culturing techniques.

The authors classify infection as injuries involving soft tissue only rather than bone and joints. All patients had appropriate incision and drainage. The postoperative regimen included microcatheters and local antibiotic infusion. To date, no data show that such antibiotic administration is effective, and the response seen may just as likely reflect the importance of adequate irrigation and drainage. Parental administration of antibiotics of appropriate sensitivity was also used, reflecting the necessary use of antibiotic medication.

The legacy of this article lies in its treatment of the destroyed septic metacarpophalangeal joint. Rather than simple resection or fusion, the authors salvaged joint motion by the use of a hinged distractor. By this technique, 77% had had good to excellent results compared with only 33% in a control group that had simple resection. By experience, the stable fibrous pseudo-joint that was obtained here is clearly preferable to metacarpophalangeal joint fusion; I would therefore recommend such a distraction technique in those faced with salvaging an infected metacarpophalangeal joint.

A.L. Osterman, M.D.

Oblique Ulnar Shortening Osteotomy by a Single Saw Cut
Labosky DA, Waggy CA (West Virginia Univ, Morgantown)
J Hand Surg (Am) 21A:48–59, 1996

Background.—Considerable precision in ulnar shortening osteotomy is needed to obtain accurate apposition of the cut bone ends and to produce the correct amount of shortening. In the Milch cuff resection, or double-cut method, the amount of shortening is equal to the amount of bone removed, which makes the procedure straightforward. The width of the bone removed is equal to the cuff of bone resected plus twice the width of the saw kerf (the amount of material removed by a saw blade) of the blade used to make the cuts (Fig 2). The 2 cuts, however, must be very close to parallel to achieve accurate alignment of the bony fragments after the osteotomy. In the single-cut method, the saw kerf of the blade cuts away material, thereby resulting in a bony defect with parallel walls. Rigid osteosynthesis eliminates the need for parallel cuts, as bone ends appose exactly. Varying the angle of the cut alters the amount of shortening, thereby resulting from a specific saw blade kerf. This single-cut technique is simpler and more accurate when the kerf diameter of the specific blade used in the shortening osteotomy is known. Three experiments were performed to investigate the usefulness of the single-cut technique.

Methods and Findings.—The first experiment was done to determine the diameter of the saw kerfs of as many bone saw blades and blade combi-

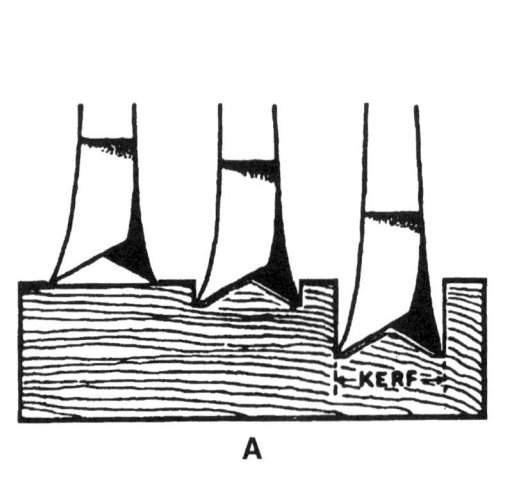

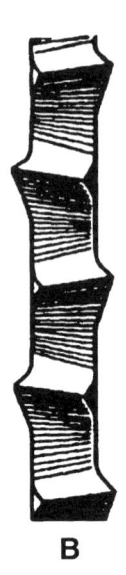

FIGURE 2.—**A**, the saw kerf defines the thickness of material removed by a saw blade. **B**, the kerf of material removed by a saw blade is shown to be a function of the thickness of the blade itself and the amount of offset of the teeth. The offset of the teeth, called the set of teeth, causes the blade to cut a kerf wider than the thickness of the blade, thus helping prevent binding of the blade in the saw kerf. (Courtesy of Labosky DA, Waggy CA: Oblique ulnar shortening osteotomy by a single saw cut. *J Hand Surg (Am)* 21A:48–59, 1996.)

nations as possible. Most of the blades tested produced kerfs substantially larger than the thickness defined by the manufacturer because of saw tooth set. The kerfs of some of the thinnest blades were equal to blade thickness because there was no saw tooth set. The range of single-blade kerfs was 0.4–1.4 mm. Stacks of 2 or 3 blades produced saw kerfs unequal to the sum of the individual blade kerfs (Fig 6). The thickest kerf—4.45 mm—resulted from 3 DePuy 5606–18 or 5606–31 blades stacked in a Magaforce oscillating saw.

In experiments 2 and 3, the actual shortening produced by the single-cut technique was measured and compared with the osteotomies performed by the double-cut method. At 0, 45, and 60 degrees, the 6 experimental osteotomies that used a single-cut kerf produced shortenings very close to the predicted values. When the single- and double-cut methods were compared, all 3 single-kerf experimental groups were significantly more

NESTED BLADES **TWO INDIVIDUAL BLADES**

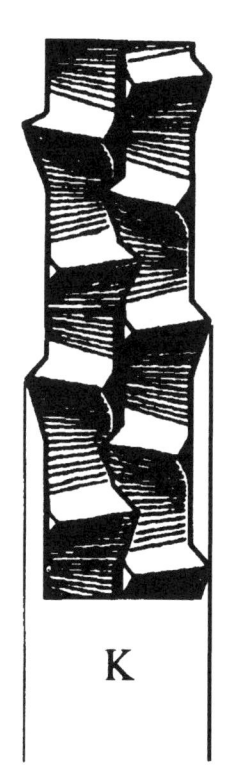

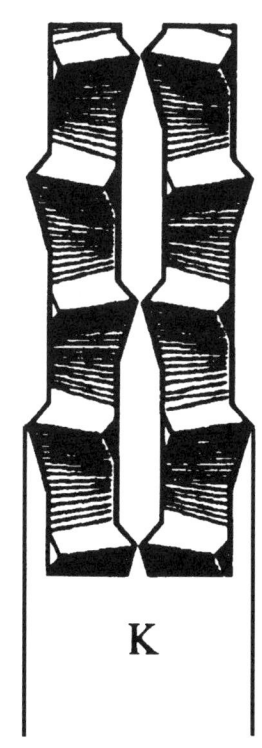

FIGURE 6.—Two saw blades are stacked as they would be on a bone saw (**left**). The teeth of blades with large saw tooth set nest together when the blades are stacked. The kerf cut by these 2 nested blades is, therefore, smaller than twice the kerf cut by a single blade as demonstrated on the **right**. (Courtesy of Labosky DA, Waggy CA: Oblique ulnar shortening osteotomy by a single saw cut. *J Hand Surg (Am)* 21A:48–59, 1996.)

accurate than the double-cut technique in approximating the desired shortening.

Conclusions.—In these experiments, the single-cut technique resulted in a more predictable amount of shortening than did the double-cut technique in the removal of bone cuff. The single-cut method can be used to shorten any long bone.

▶ The authors have provided us with information regarding a useful technique for accurately aligning opposing surfaces of shortening osteotomies of long bones, specifically the ulna. The actual precision of the technique seems to exceed the precision capabilities predicted clinically but most certainly seems to be an improvement over the standard techniques other than the precision oblique osteotomy system (Rayhack).

R.D. Beckenbaugh, M.D.

Clinical Results of the One-bone Forearm
Peterson CA II, Maki S, Wood MB (Mayo Clinic, Rochester, Minn; Kagoshina City, Japan)
J Hand Surg (Am) 20A:609–618, 1995   3–13

Introduction.—Reconstruction is challenging in patients with forearm instability associated with structural bone defects caused by trauma, congenital deformity, or previous surgery. Although some patients may be adequately treated with simple internal fixation and bone grafting, structural bone grafting or prosthetic segmental-spacer interposition, or osteotomy, other patients may be most effectively treated by surgical creation of a 1-bone forearm with radioulnar synostosis. An 18-year experience with 1-bone forearm construction in patients who were ineligible for other reconstructive procedures is reported.

Methods.—The clinical records, operative reports, radiographs, and follow-up questionnaire for 19 patients who underwent radioulnar synostosis between 1973 and 1991 were reviewed. The instability was secondary to trauma in 13 patients and secondary to congenital deformity or previous tumor resection in 6 patients. Thirteen had undergone previous failed reconstruction procedures. The surgical technique varied, depending on the preoperative bone status and results of soft-tissue evaluation. The fusion was located in the proximal third of the forearm in 3 patients, the middle third in 7, and the distal third in 9. Three patients without the distal radius and portions of the carpus required wrist fusion, with free, vascularized fibula transfer used in 2. Autologous bone grafting was used at the fusion site in 14 patients. The forearms were fused in neutral rotation in 10 patients and in varying degrees of pronation (range, 5 to 40½ degrees) in 9 patients. Clinical outcome was assessed on the basis of function, pain, and radiographic union.

Results.—The results were excellent in 7 patients, good in 6, fair in 5, and poor in 1. Factors that predicted an unsatisfactory outcome included traumatic cause, 2 or more previous failed reconstructive procedures, history of severe nerve injury, and previous infection. Major complications occurred in 10 patients and included nonunion, infection, hardware failure, and fracture. Of the 6 patients with nonunion, only 1 required a revisional procedure. The others were treated with bracing and activity restriction.

Conclusions.—Radioulnar synostosis may be an effective technique for salvaging angular, axial, or rotatory radioulnar instability in patients with osseous defects. The complication rate can be high, however, especially in patients whose injury was caused by trauma.

▶ Several surgeons at the Mayo Clinic describe the salvage technique of the 1-bone forearm procedure for radioulnar instability. Although the patients had multiple diagnoses, they all shared the major indication for this procedure: radioulnar instability. Unfortunately, there were many other variables in this retrospective study, not the least of which was inconsistency in technique. Nonetheless, this is an honest report that supports my personal experience: Radioulnar synostosis is a useful, sometimes the only, salvage procedure, but it is fraught with a high rate of complications, including nonunion.

L.K. Ruby, M.D.

Distal Anterior Radius Bone Graft in Surgery of the Hand and Wrist
Mirly HL, Manske PR, Szerzinski JM (Washington Univ, St Louis)
J Hand Surg (Am) 20A:623–627, 1995
3–14

Background.—The traditional donor site for autogenous bone grafting of the hand and wrist has been the iliac crest. More recently, use of local upper-extremity sites has been reported. Use of the distal anterior radius, however, has been infrequently mentioned. Over a 10-year period, this donor site was used for bone grafting in 131 surgeries of the hand and wrist performed by the senior author. Surgeries included curettage and bone grafting of 9 cysts, arthrodesis of 75 joints, and 47 scaphoid nonunions.

Technique.—The distal anterior radius is exposed with careful dissection. A 1 × 1-cm window is cut in the anterior cortex using a small, 4.5-mm oscillating saw blade. This window is then removed with a narrow osteotome (Fig 1D). Curettes are used to obtain cancellous bone from the distal radius. If necessary, osteotomes may be used to remove the graft material as a block. Gelfoam is placed in the donor site before soft-tissue repair and closure.

Results.—All of the cysts, 63 of the 75 arthrodeses, and 35 of the 47 scaphoid nonunions healed, yielding an overall healing rate of 82%. Time

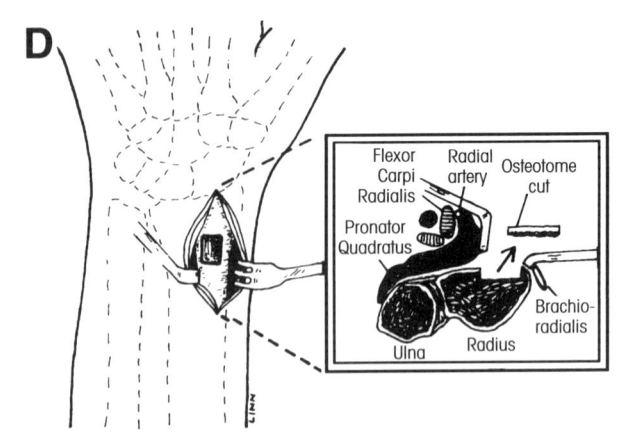

FIGURE 1D.—Osteotomy completed in frontal and transverse planes. (Courtesy of Mirly HL, Manske PR, Szerinski JM: Distal anterior radius bone graft in surgery of the hand and wrist. *J Hand Surg (Am)* 20A:623–627, 1995.)

until union averaged 15 weeks and was slightly longer for scaphoid nonunions than for the other surgeries. This longer time may reflect the learning curve associated with the internal fixation technique used. One complication involved fracture through the donor site after minimal trauma 46 months after surgery. This fracture healed with casting; no other complications occurred.

Conclusion.—The distal anterior radius is an excellent source of bone graft for surgery of the hand and yields little morbidity. This site should not be used for surgical procedures involving the distal radius.

▶ The authors provide an additional source of bone graft for small procedures. Its utility in small joints is well documented by the senior author.

A.L. Ladd, M.D.

Distal Interphalangeal Joint Arthrodesis Comparing Tension-band Wire and Herbert Screw: A Biomechanical and Dimensional Analysis
Wyrsch B, Dawson J, Aufranc S, et al (Vanderbilt Univ, Nashville, Tenn)
J Hand Surg (Am) 21A:438–443, 1996   3–15

Background.—Arthrodesis of the distal interphalangeal (DIP) joint is indicated to relieve various painful conditions as well as for joint stabilization. Several different fixation techniques have been used, including interosseous or tension band wires (TBW) and, more recently, Herbert compression screws. Although Herbert screws are widely used, there are few data on their effectiveness in the DIP joint. A cadaver study was performed to evaluate the use of Herbert screws for DIP joint fusion.

Methods.—In the first part of the study, measurements were made to determine whether the distal phalanx of adult fingers is large enough to accommodate the large-threaded Herbert screw. Simulated arthrodeses were then prepared in 15 male and 15 female cadaver DIP joints. These constructs were compared for 3-point anteroposterior and lateral bending and for axial torsion.

Results.—The initial measurements showed that the mean height of the distal phalanx was 3.555 mm, smaller than the 3.90 mm diameter of the screw. In 25 of 30 specimens—including all 15 female specimens—the tip of the distal phalanx was either fractured or penetrated during screw placement. In many of these cases, the nail bed was stretched or otherwise violated. On biomechanical analysis, the Herbert screw fusions showed significantly greater anteroposterior bending strength and torsional rigidity than the TBW fusions. There was no difference in lateral bending strength.

Conclusions.—Herbert screw arthrodesis of the DIP joint appears to be biomechanically stronger than TBW arthrodesis. The thread diameter of the Herbert screw is larger than the height of the distal phalanx in most specimens, but the size problem can be overcome by use of the Herbert mini screw. Controlled trials comparing various fixation techniques are needed; past studies have shown that compression arthrodesis gives better results than the Kirschner wire technique.

▶ In this study, Wyrsch and co-workers biomechanically compare 2 fixation techniques for DIP joint fusion: tension band arthrodesis and Herbert screw. They conclude that the Herbert screw is superior, and this may be of clinical importance. From a practical viewpoint, tension band arthrodesis is rarely employed for DIP fusions. Today, if pins are chosen, most surgeons recommend Kirschner pins with or without supplemental interosseous wiring.

I agree with the authors that the primary problem with DIP joint fusion is nonunion. I am not convinced that the particular technique of fusion correlates with nonunion.[1] Rather, nonunion results when there has been inadequate preparation of the bone surfaces, poor coaptation, or a technical error.

The finding that the diameter of the lagging threads is usually greater than the anterorposterior height of the distal phalanx is a significant one. Nail deformity and/or hypersensitivity of the fingertip secondary to a "proud" screw head are clinical problems that can lead to patient dissatisfaction. As the authors suggest, the Herbert mini-screw (the maximum length of which is currently 18 mm) is an excellent solution, assuming there is adequate length to achieve solid fixation in the middle phalanx.

P.J. Stern, M.D.

Reference

1. Stern PJ, Fulton DB: Distal interphalangeal joint arthrodesis: An analysis of complications. *J Hand Surg* 17A:1139–1145, 1992.

Osseointegrated Thumb Prostheses: A Concept for Fixation of Digit Prosthetic Devices

Lundborg G, Brånemark P-I, Rosén B, et al (Lund Univ, Malmö, Sweden; Inst for Applied Biotechnology, Göteborg, Sweden)
J Hand Surg [Am] 21A:216–221, 1996   3–16

Background.—Several techniques have been developed for reconstructing the thumb after traumatic amputation. Osseointegration is the anchorage of an implant in bony tissue without fibrous tissue. The technique has been used for dental prostheses and fixed bone-conducting hearing aids. The principle was used in an alternative technique for fixating a thumb prosthesis to the first metacarpal bone in 3 patients.

Technique.—A local skin flap was raised on top of the thumb stump. The most distal cortical layer was drilled, and cancellous bone from the iliac crest was packed around a self-taping titanium fixture inserted longitudinally into the medullary canal. Approxi-

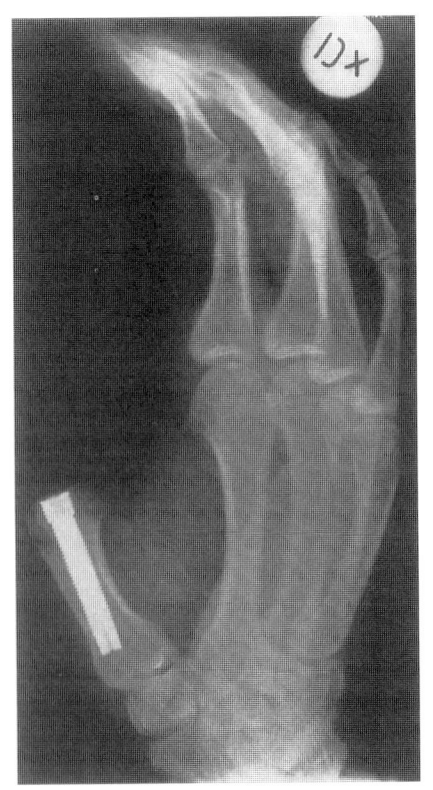

FIGURE 1.—X-ray film appearance of an osseointegrated titanium fixture 3 months after surgery (case 1). (Courtesy of Lundborg G, Brånemark P-I, Rosén B, et al: Osseointegrated thumb prostheses: A concept for fixation of digit prosthetic devices. *J Hand Surg [Am]* 21A:216–221, 1996.)

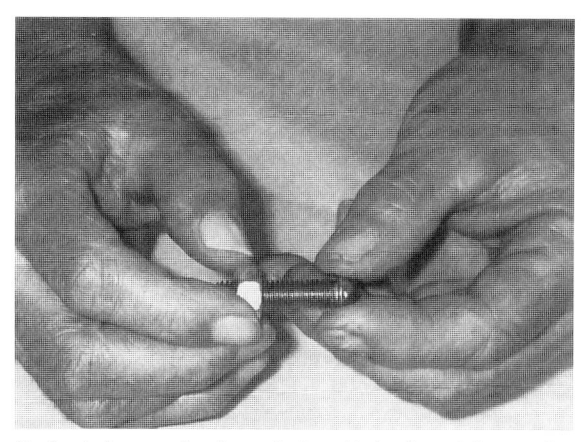

FIGURE 4.—Pinch grip between thumb prosthesis and index finger 2.5 years after surgery (case 2). (Courtesy of Lundborg G, Brånemark P-I, Rosén B, et al: Osseointegrated thumb prostheses: A concept for fixation of digit prosthetic devices. *J Hand Surg [Am]* 21A:216–221, 1996.)

mately 3 months later, the stage 2 surgery involved repeated raising of the skin flap, followed by trimming the distal part of the metacarpal bone to the level of the fixture head. The special abutment was attached to the fixture, and the skin around the abutment was trimmed to the thickness of a split graft. After 2–4 weeks, a silicone thumb prosthesis was anchored to the abutment and locked in place with a small screw device that the patient could handle.

Methods.—Three patients with traumatic amputation of the thumb at the metacarpophalangeal joint level underwent the procedure. Hand function and tactile capacities were assessed at regular follow-up examinations.

Results.—No complications or skin problems occurred during healing. The osseointegration of the implant was perfect and was maintained during the 18 months to 3 years of follow-up (Fig 1). The patients learned to use the thumb prosthesis quickly and achieved good fine manipulation function (Fig 4). Each patient also had some tactile discrimination.

Conclusions.—When other techniques for thumb reconstruction are not possible, an osseointegrated thumb prosthesis presents an appropriate alternative. The observed tactile perception is probably due to the transfer of tactile stimuli to intraosseous nerves through the osseointegrated implant.

▶ This novel approach for thumb reconstruction uses principles of osseointegration established by Brånemark. Possibly unanticipated was the sensory feedback and tactile discrimination achieved through the bone prosthesis interface and the lack of reactive changes between the stem and titanium implant. This technique seems to have achieved long-term success. Will the titanium implant within the thumb metacarpal have permanency over time, or will loosening occur as a consequence of repetitive loads from pinch and grasp? We await the commercial release of this prosthesis to determine whether similar success can be achieved by others.

W.P. Cooney, III, M.D.

Suggested Reading

Krakauer JD, Stern PJ: Hinged device for fractures involving the proximal interphalangeal joint. *Clin Orthop Rel Res* 327:29–37, 1996.
▶ The authors present 20 patients (12 treated within 2 weeks of injury and 8 treated more than 4 weeks after injury), in which the Compass PIP hinged device (Smith & Nephew Richards, Inc., Memphis, Tenn.) is used as a dynamic external fixator. As with other devices, precise placement of the hinge in alignment with the center rotation of the PIP joint is required. A major limitation of this compass hinge is the need to have precise joint alignment. I am somewhat surprised to note in this series that operative intervention of the fracture itself was required in 11 of the 12 patients treated within 2 weeks of injury. I have been able to gain realignment of the joint articular surfaces and initiate early motion without resorting to open reduction of either the comminuted fragments or the central depression fracture. The somewhat restricted range of motion postoperatively in this series may be related in part to the open fracture treatment involved.

In the group of patients who were seen late, I agree that open reduction is required to accurately align fracture fragments and to remove postfracture hematoma and scar tissue. The authors' success in these late cases is relatively good when considering that the majority of patients had previous surgery, including volar plate arthroplasty. The authors recommend a volar approach to surgical exposure; many hand surgeons would disagree with this. In this approach, exposure can be difficult. In addition it is necessary to release the collateral ligaments from the ulnar insertion on the middle phalanx. In my opinion, this has the risk of devascularizing the fracture components. A volar approach should only be used if one is considering volar plate arthroplasty. I also disagree with the recommendation that the joint must be reduced to 60 degrees of flexion or less to warrant extension-block splinting. My experience demonstrates that extension block splinting can be used up to a position of 80 degrees of flexion provided there is gradual, careful extension of the joint over time, with alignment maintained. I do agree that pinning a joint to maintain a reduction position is undesirable and can lead to stiffness and occasionally to recurrent dislocation. Although the authors do not report any mechanical problems with the compass device, I have noted fractures through the plastic hinge in 2 patients in my care.

W.P. Cooney, III, M.D.

Allison DM: Fractures of the base of the middle phalanx treated by a dynamic external fixation device. *J Hand Surg (Br)* 21B:305–310, 1996.
▶ Allison presents a technique for treatment of comminuted, intra-articular fractures at the base of the middle phalanx with the use of a dynamic traction spring device. Others use a stainless steel spring wire with double loops providing between 6 and 1,000 g of tension. A greater force can be provided, thus making the spring smaller or larger. As with the Agee and the Hastings devices, the proximal K-wire is placed through the center of the joint of rotation. These devices therefore allow for distraction with early motion using the force coupled principle. Considering the nature of the injury, the authors have excellent results—they gained an average of 80 to 85 degrees of flexion with a loss of

approximately 10 degrees of extension. I agree that this Agee technique and the dynamic fixator of Hotchkiss are preferable to external frame devices such as those described by Shenk and Fahmy. I agree that these fractures are not amenable to open reduction and internal fixation and that more predictable results can occur with a distraction and early motion program. I congratulate the authors on this novel approach to comminuted fractures at the base of the middle phalanx.

W.P. Cooney, III M.D.

Starker I, Eaton RG: Kirschner wire placement in the emergency room; Is there a risk? *J Hand Surg (Br)* 20B:535–538, 1995.
▶ The authors' prospective study demonstrates that closed reduction and internal fixation for finger and hand fractures can be performed successfully in an outpatient emergency department with few complications *if* certain conditions are met. Sterile technique must be observed at all times. Adequate equipment must be available, including wire drivers, clamps, pin cutters, and radiographic control. A portable mini-C arm is ideal. Finally, the authors used immobilization after pin fixation with pin removal at 3–4 weeks. Not all closed fractures are amenable to treatment in this manner, and considerable judgment is required to select and obtain proper pin fixation. This is not a procedure for the novice, but it can be a safe and successful treatment method without the costs associated with a trip to the operating room.

E.R. North, M.D.

Ip WY, Ng KH, Chow SP: A prospective study of 924 digital fractures of the hand. *Injury* 27:279–285, 1996.
▶ A good reference.

P.C. Amadio, M.D.

Trousdale RT, Linscheid RL: Operative treatment of malunited fractures of the forearm. *J Bone Joint Surg* 77A:894–902, 1995.
▶ Surgical treatment for malunion of the forearm is predictably complicated and technically difficult. The greatest correction of rotational deformity and instability at the distal radioulnar joint is attained if surgery is performed within the first year.

A.L. Ladd, M.D.

Ouellette EA, Freeland AE: Use of the minicondylar plate in metacarpal and phalangeal fractures. *Clin Orthop Rel Res* 327:38–46, 1996.
▶ As these authors point out, minicondylar plates may be helpful, particularly in the metacarpals, but are not without their problems: there were more complications than patients, and only a third of patients retained 220 degrees or more of total active motion. These implants need to be used with caution, especially in the phalanges. The advantage of enabling early motion may be outweighed by the risk of disastrous failure. In many cases, less complex fixation will suffice. Less stable fixation, requiring secondary tenolysis or capsulotomy, may be preferable to an attempt at aggressive fixation that results in an infected nonunion.

P.C. Amadio, M.D.

Brazier J, Moughabghab M, Migud H, et al: Les fractures articulaires de la base du premier mé tacarpien: Etude comparative del'ostéosynthèse directe et de l'embrochage extra-focal (Articular fractures of the base of the first metacarpal: comparative study of direct osteosynthesis and closed pinning). *Ann Chir Main* 15:91–99, 1996.

▶ As in most contemporary series of Bennett's fracture cases, the results in terms of alignment, pain, motion, and grip all marginally favor open reduction, but with such variability (perhaps aggravated by including Rolando type fractures in the mix, and a total population of just 35 cases) that the results barely reach statistical significance.

P.C. Amadio, M.D.

Dong PR, Seeger LL: Fractures of the sesamoid bones of the thumb. *Am J Sports Med* 23:336–339, 1995.

▶ The authors revisit the problem of fracture of the sesamoid bones of the thumb secondary to hyperextension injuries of the metacarpophalangeal point, They suggest the utility of oblique radiographs in this setting, because a sesamoid fracture is often not apparent in true lateral radiographs of the thumb. In fact, if we define a true lateral radiograph of the thumb as one in which the sesamoid bones are overlapping, the majority of thumb radiographs do not qualify as "true lateral" radiographs. As such, most sesamoid fractures may be visible on the "standard" radiographs often obtained in the emergency department; the true lateral radiograph provided by the authors is actually an oblique projection with the sesamoid bones not overlapping, and does indeed demonstrate a proximal pole fracture.

V.D. Pellegrini, Jr., M.D.

4 Soft-tissue Trauma and Reconstruction

Temporary Ectopic Implantation for Salvage of Amputated Digits
Graf P, Gröner R, Höri W, et al (Technical Univ, Munich)
Br J Plast Surg 49:174–177, 1996   4–1

Background.—In certain types of amputation associated with extensive soft-tissue damage, although the amputated extremity is in good condition, a débridement of the crushed tissue is needed, resulting in a segmental defect that makes replantation impossible. In such patients, temporary ectopic implantation may be used to salvage the amputated part. Successful temporary ectopic implantation of digits was reported for the first time.

Case Report.—Man, 24, was injured when a train ran over his left hand. He sustained no other serious injuries. He had a subtotal oblique amputation of all the fingers and severe crushing of the whole integument of the midhand and the intrinsic musculature, except for a skin bridge on the radial side of the thumb. The amputated ring and little fingers were intact distal to the metacarpophalangeal joints. The extensor tendons were lacerated at the metacarpal level, and the flexor tendons were partly avulsed from the muscles or were lacerated at the wrist. The motor branch of the median nerve was avulsed from the thenar muscles, and the ulnar neurovascular bundle was crushed to the wrist. The fingers were completely amputated at the first débridement, and the fourth and fifth digits were implanted into the right forearm. The radial artery was anastomosed end-to-end to the common digital artery. The 2 radial artery venae comitantes were anastomosed to superficial digit veins. The extensor tendons of the amputated fingers were fixed to the tendon of the brachioradialis muscle and the flexor tendons to the tendon of the flexor carpi radialis muscle. Four months after injury, the fingers were replanted onto the left hand. Despite vigorous physiotherapy during ectopic implantation, the mobility of the interphalangeal joints declined. The extensor and flexor tendons of the digits became detached from the respective tendons and markedly shrunk. The tendon sheaths contained extensive adhesions of the flexor tendons. Thus tendon reconstructions were not done. Sensibility was restored using 4 sural nerve grafts coapted to the ulnar and digital nerves. After 6 operations, the replanted digits were stiff but useful, with an ever-improving sensibility and temperature perception.

Conclusions.—Temporary ectopic implantation is recommended very rarely in patients with amputation injuries associated with extensive soft tissue damage in whom immediate replantation with adequate shortening or preservation of length is not possible. All other options should be excluded before ectopic implantation is attempted. The recipient site should allow easy revascularization and provide a long vascular pedicle to obviate the need for vascular grafts at the second stage. The final mobility of replanted fingers relies on the length of time between the ectopic implantation and the second-stage replantation. The second stage of reconstruction should be done early.

▶ The authors have reported on an uncommonly used technique for treating amputations combined with severe soft-tissue injuries of the recipient tissues. They nicely outline their indications for the procedure in the treatment of total and subtotal amputations. The procedure is a last resort after primary closure without replantation, primary replantation after shortening, or primary replantation with reconstruction to maintain length have all been considered and rejected. The results of the reported case may have been compromised by the time until replantation, and the authors encourage a shorter implantation time. Advantages of different temporary implantation sites are also discussed. The procedure adds to the reconstructive microsurgeon's armamentarium, but, as with many procedures, serious consideration should be given to the risk–benefit ratio.

J.A. Katarincic, M.D.

Efficacy and Tolerability of Lamisil® (Terbinafine): Multicenter Study in the Treatment of Cutaneous and Ungual Mycoses
Sayag J, Badillet G, Zagula M (CHU La Timone, Paris)
Nouv Dermatol 14:547–552, 1995   4–2

Introduction.—Numerous studies have demonstrated the efficacy of oral and topical terbinafine (Lamisil) preparations in treating cutaneous and ungual mycoses. Even for ungual mycoses of the big toe, which are the most difficult to treat, a cure rate of 92% has been reported. This open, multicenter trial evaluated the feasibility of using terbinafine in the dermatology office setting.

Patients.—Between December 1992 and June 1993, 1,400 patients were entered into the study by 524 French dermatologists with urban practices. Only patients with culture-positive onychomycoses of the feet or cutaneous mycoses that had been refractory to treatment were eligible. Pregnant or lactating women, as well as patients younger than 18 years of age were excluded. Oral terbinafine therapy was initiated after a wash-out period of 1 month for systemic antifungal agents and 15 days for topical antifungal products.

Results.—Of the 914 patients who met the study's inclusion criteria and were given oral terbinafine tablets, 465 (average age, 45 years) were treated for onychomycoses of the big toe, and 449 (average age, 42.2 years) were treated for refractory cutaneous mycoses. Clinical and mycologic cure was obtained in 95.2% of patients with onychomycoses of less than 1 year's duration and in 89.3% of those who had had onychomycoses for more than 1 year at the start of terbinafine therapy. Global cure was also obtained in 88.9% of patients with refractory cutaneous mycoses of less than 1 year's duration and in 84.4% of those with a longer history. *Trichophyton, Microsporum,* and *Epidermophyton* infections were cured in 88% of the affected patients. All 6 patients with cutaneous *Candida* infections were also completely cured. Terbinafine was well tolerated by approximately 90% of the patients. Only 6.5% of patients withdrew from the study because of side effects. No major side effects occurred.

Conclusions.—Oral terbinafine is effective and safe for treating onychomycoses and cutaneous mycoses that are refractory to topical treatment and require systemic therapy. The drug is well tolerated and is safe for use in the dermatology office setting.

▶ This French multicenter study of 1,400 patients, conducted by 524 dermatologists, established the benefit of using terbinafine (Lamisil) in 465 patients with onychomycosis of the feet and 449 patients with difficult-to-treat cutaneous mycoses. The response rates were 89.8% and 89.4%, respectively.

Terbinafine is a valuable addition to the armamentarium of antifungal drugs. It is effective in vitro against a broad spectrum of pathogenic fungi, including dermatophytes. Terbinafine is a highly dermatophilic and lipophilic drug that easily penetrates the stratum corneum and nail plate and achieves levels exceeding the minimum inhibitory concentration for most dermatophytes in a short period. Drug levels decline slowly in the nail over weeks after discontinuation of therapy. The drug is generally well tolerated; most side effects are transient and mildly to moderately severe. The pharmacokinetics of terbinafine and its primarily fungicidal action against dermatophytes in vitro form the basis for its increased efficacy, shorter treatment times, lower relapse rates, better compliance, and cost-effectiveness compared with the conventional antifungal agent, griseofluvin.

Another relevant article is one by Shear and Gupta.[1] In addition, itraconazole is also a highly effective and popular new oral medication for the same conditions.[2]

R.K. Roenigk, M.D.

References

1. Shear N, Gupta A: Terbinafine for the treatment of pedal onychomycosis: A foot closer to the promised land of cured nails? *Arch Dermatol* 131:937, 1995.

2. Cawenbergh G, DeGreef H, Heykants J, et al: Pharmacokinetic profile of orally administered itraconazole in human skin. *J Am Acad Dermatol* 18:263–268, 1988.

Antifungal Pulse Therapy for Onychomycosis: A Pharmacokinetic and Pharmacodynamic Investigation of Monthly Cycles of 1-Week Pulse Therapy With Itraconazole

de Doncker P, Decroix J, Piérard GE, et al (Univ of Antwerp, Wilrijk, Belgium; Free Univ of Brussels, Belgium; Janssen Research Found, Beerse, Belgium; et al)
Arch Dermatol 132:34–41, 1996   4–3

Background.—Continuous-dosing regimens of oral therapies are generally used in the treatment of onychomycosis. The suggested dose of itraconazole in patients with this condition is 200 mg/day for 3 months. The efficacy and nail kinetics of intermittent pulse-dosing treatment with oral itraconazole in patients with onychomycosis were investigated.

Methods.—Fifty patients with confirmed onychomycosis of the toenails, mostly *Trichophyton rubrum*, were enrolled in the randomized trial. Twenty-five patients were assigned to 3 pulses and 25 to 4 pulses of 1-week itraconazole treatment. Toenails were examined clinically and mycologically and drug levels in the distal ends of the fingernails and toenails were determined once a month for 6 months, then every 2 months for up to 1 year.

Findings.—In patients undergoing 3-pulse treatment, the mean itraconazole concentration in the distal ends of the toenails ranged from 67 ng/g at 1 month to 471 ng/g at 6 months. In the distal ends of the fingernails, it ranged from 103 ng/g at 1 month to 424 ng/g at 6 months. After 11 months, the drug was still evident in the distal end of the toenails in a mean concentration of 186 ng/g. The greatest individual concentrations, reached at 6 months, were 1,064 ng/g for toenails and 1,166 ng/g for fingernails. At the final follow-up, toenails in 84% of the patients were cured clinically as determined by a negative potassium hydroxide preparation in 72% and by culture in 80%.

In patients undergoing 4-pulse treatment, the mean itraconazole concentration in the distal ends of the toenails ranged from 32 ng/g at 1 month to 623 ng/g at 8 months. In the distal ends of the fingernails, it ranged from 42 ng/g at 1 month to 380 ng/g at 6 months. The greatest individual concentrations, reached at 7 months for toenails and 9 months for fingernails, were 1,449 and 946 ng/g, respectively. The drug was still evident in the distal ends of the toenails at a mean level of 196 ng/g after 12 months. At the last follow-up, toenails were clinically cured in 76% of the patients as determined by a negative potassium hydroxide preparation in 72% and by culture in 80%. The primary efficacy parameters did not differ significantly between the treatment groups. Patients in both groups tolerated the drug well, showing no significant side effects.

Conclusions.—Three- or four-pulse therapy with itraconazole is safe and effective in the treatment of onychomycosis. Three pulses may be effective in most affected toenails.

▶ Itraconazole is a broad-spectrum triazole derivative that is highly effective against yeast and dermatophytes for the treatment of onychomycosis. This drug is highly lipophilic and keratophilic with good oral absorption when it is taken with meals and has extensive tissue distribution. Itraconazole readily penetrates into the nail via the matrix and bed. Initial therapy for itraconazole consists of 100 mg orally per day for 3 months, although clinical resolution does not occur until the nail has completely regrown. This study shows the efficacy of pulse therapy (400 mg orally per day for 1 week each month for 3 or 4 months). Clinical cure rates were between 76% and 84% and negative mycological examination results were between 72% and 80%. The data suggest that pulsed therapy is an effective and safe treatment option for onychomycosis.

R.K. Roenigk, M.D.

Short-pedicle Vascularized Nail Flap
Endo T, Nakayama Y (Univ of Tsukuba, Ibaraki, Japan)
Plast Reconstr Surg 97:656–661, 1996

Purpose.—Reconstruction of a missing or deficient fingernail is a challenging surgical problem. Long-pedicle flaps for this purpose have been described, but these procedures take a long time and leave long, unsightly scars. A short-pedicle vascularized flap for fingernail reconstruction was described.

Technique.—The flap uses the second or third toenail as a donor because it is similar in size and shape to the fingernails. The pedicle is dissected over the periosteum to define the dorsal digital artery and dorsal cutaneous vein (Fig 1). When the recipient finger has a congenital nail defect, the recipient artery is the digital artery of the same finger. In injured fingers, the digital artery of the neighboring finger is used to ensure a safe anastomosis. After the pedicle is transferred, the toe defect is closed with the use of a split-thickness skin graft. The surgeon uses an operating microscope to perform the arterial and venous anastomoses at the level of the proximal interphalangeal joint; nerve anastomoses are not usually done.

Findings.—Three patients who underwent nail flap transfer to the index and little fingers were described. The procedure took an average of 3.5 hours, with only 50 minutes needed to harvest the vascularized nail flap. The short pedicle required only a small incision, so there were no large scars of the hand or foot. The cosmetic results were excellent, and the transferred nails grew well.

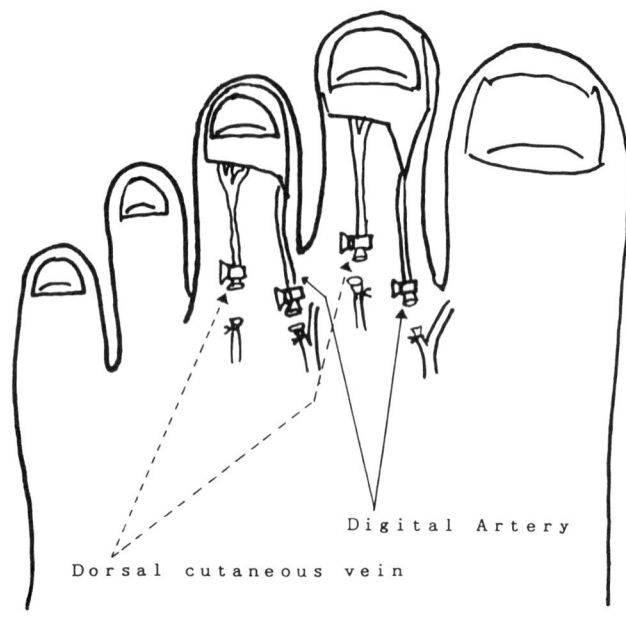

FIGURE 1.—Schematic drawing of the vascularized nail flap with short pedicle. The second or third toe is usually selected as the donor site. (Courtesy of Endo T, Nakayama Y: Short-pedicle vascularized nail flap. *Plast Reconstr Surg* 97:656–661, 1996.)

Discussion.—The short-pedicle vascularized nail flap gives excellent cosmetic results in patients who have traumatic or congenital defects of the fingernails. It can be used to reconstruct nail defects of any finger, except the thumb. The use of a short pedicle minimizes scarring at the donor and recipient sites and avoids the need to sacrifice a major artery.

▶ Endo and Nakayama, from Ibaraki, Japan, have published a very nice report on vascularized nail transfer for congenital onychodysplasia and post-traumatic nail deformities. The donor site, periosteum and joint capsule to the toe, is treated with a split-thickness skin graft, and the authors stated that they have had no problems with this approach. The entire nail complex, with a small dart of dorsal toe skin, is transferred with a single digital artery and a single subcutaneous dorsal vein. The pedicle length is limited to 2.5 cm to the web space of the toe to cause less scarring at the donor site. The authors prefer to use the digital artery on the recipient finger in congenital malformation cases but state that they sacrificed the digital artery from the adjoining finger in traumatic cases. Interestingly, in the case they present in their article, they used a digital artery on the traumatized finger; I would agree with this approach. I do not think it would be necessary in most cases to sacrifice a digital artery in the donor finger for microsurgical reconstruction of the nail bed.

Although in most practices I believe that this technique would have rare indications, all of us who practice hand surgery occasionally see a young patient who is very concerned about a post-traumatic nail bed defect. This technique certainly seems to be one that we could offer the patient. The results are good as long as the patient's expectations are realistic.

N.B. Meland, M.D.

A Neurovascular Island Flap for Volar-Oblique Fingertip Amputations: Analysis of Long-term Results
Tsai T-M, Yuen JC (Christine M Kleinert Inst for Hand and Micro Surgery, Louisville, Ky)
J Hand Surg (Br) 21B:94–98, 1996   4–5

Objective.—Although many different flaps and techniques have been used, the management of volar-oblique fingertip amputations continues to pose challenging problems. A variation of the homodigital neurovascular flap has been used in this situation. The long-term results of neurovascular island flap repair of volar-oblique fingertip amputations were reported.

Methods.—Sixteen patients, whose status was followed for more than 2 years after primary reconstruction, were included. All patients had partial amputation of the fingertip or volar skin defects measuring less than 1.5 cm in length. The flap, based on a single neurovascular pedicle, consisted of a sickle-shaped island of volar-lateral-dorsal skin (Fig 1). The patients were re-examined after a mean follow-up of 5 years. The evaluation included objective assessments of active and passive range of motion and 2-point discrimination and subjective assessments of patient satisfaction.

Results.—Active-passive range of motion averaged 54–55 degrees at the distal interphalangeal joint, 96–98 degrees at the proximal interphalangeal joint, and 83–83 degrees at the metaphalangeal joint. Seventy-five percent of repairs demonstrated 2-point discrimination better than 10 mm. All patients returned to work within 1 month. Eighty-eight percent of patients expressed satisfaction with their results. Six had moderate to severe problems with cold intolerance, 3 each had hypersensitivity and stiffness, and 2 had numbness.

Conclusions.—The neurovascular island flap technique described gives good long-term results in patients with volar-oblique fingertip amputations. The technique has several key advantages, including the need for only a single operation, the use of a local donor site for sensory cover, and minimal immobilization. The functional results are good, and the patient satisfaction rate is high.

▶ This is an excellent article with a novel idea for fingertip reconstruction. The technique is well described in Figure 1. Although for defects greater than 1 cm in a volar-oblique fashion injury my preference has been a reverse neurovascular island flap, in smaller defects the technique the authors describe has many benefits over the latter. It does not sacrifice the digital artery and it maintains intact innervation to the fingertip, with 75% of patients maintaining 2-point discrimination of better than 10 mm at 2 years.

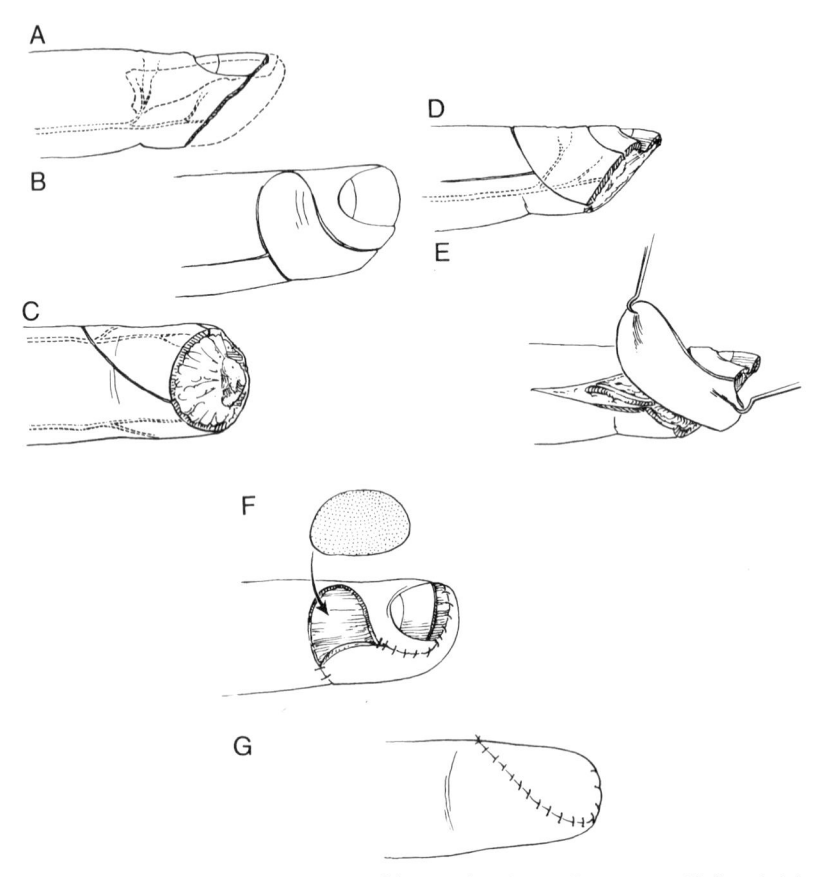

FIGURE 1.—Diagrammatic representation of the procedure. **A**, vascular anatomy with fingertip injury. **B and C**, dorsal and lateral view of flap design. Flap is located 5 mm lateral and proximal to the nail bed. **D**, the volar flap is designed to be as wide as the distal nail bed. **E**, the flap is ready to advance. **F**, the donor defect is covered with a split thickness skin graft or a full thickness skin graft from the wrist or amputated part. **G**, the finished appearance. (Reproduced with the kind permission of the Christine M. Kleinert Institute for Hand and Micro Surgery, Louisville, USA. Courtesy of Tsai T-M, Yuen JC: A neurovascular island flap for volar-oblique fingertip amputations: Analysis of long-term results. *J Hand Surg (Br)* 21B:94–98, 1996.)

I do not believe that this rate can be achieved by a reverse artery island flap. I am somewhat surprised by the amount of flexion maintained in these patients at the distal interphalangeal (DIP) joint with the large skin graft over the DIP joint that is required in all cases. Although the authors do not state which type of a skin graft they use over the DIP joint to close the donor site, it appears that split-thickness grafts were used. If I were to use this technique in my clinical practice, I would use a full-thickness skin graft for that defect.

The authors also state that they use a bulky immobilizing dressing for 10–14 days. I think it would be safe to start motion, even with a full-thickness skin graft, at 10 days.

The article is well written, with 24 months of follow up. It should be recommended reading for all hand surgeons who manage fingertip injuries.

N.B. Meland, M.D.

Utilizing the Osseointegration Principle for Fixation of Nail Prostheses
Baruchin AM, Nahlieli O, Vizethum F, et al (Ben-Gurion Univ of the Negev, Ashkelon, Israel; Hadassah Hebrew Univ, Jerusalem, Israel)
Plast Reconstr Surg 96:1665–1671, 1995   4–6

Background.—In patients who have injuries to the fingertips, it can be very difficult to restore a normal-looking fingernail. For most deformities, artificial nails are less expensive and offer a better final appearance than surgical reconstruction. Although an acceptable prosthetic fingernail has been available for many years, there have been problems in attaching the prosthetic nails to the fingers. An experience with an osseointegrated anchorage device for the fixation of fingernail prostheses is reported.

Technique.—Proximally based skin flaps are used to achieve good surgical bone exposure and to provide a thick, protective soft-tissue cover during healing. The bone is drilled, and a titanium implant is placed through the phalangeal cortex. The fixture is matched to the prepared bone to achieve the very close fit needed for osseointegration. The implant is installed, the cover screw is inserted, and the site is covered with a skin flap for at least 4 months. At that time, the site is re-entered, the cover screw is removed, and the fixture is tightened. An impression is then made for creation of an acrylic translucent nail by a maxillofacial prosthodontist. The nail is connected to the fixture with either a screw-type fixture or an attachment.

Experience.—The experience included 5 men and 8 women, aged 14 to 50 years. The patients had lost a total of 9 fingernails as a result of trauma. They received 2 types of IMZ titanium plasma-sprayed implant systems: a 3.3-mm diameter and 8-mm long dental implant and a 3.3-mm diameter and 6-mm long craniofacial implant. One early failure occurred in a patient who was noncompliant with hygiene requirements. At an average follow-up of 18 months, the results were good in all other cases. Early in the series, a minor technical problem with loosening of the abutment screws was addressed by replacing them with lateral new abutment screws.
Conclusions.—Preliminary experience suggests that the principle of osseointegration can be successfully applied to the fixed anchorage of fingernail prostheses. Titanium alloy fixtures appear to provide the most inert and biocompatible material. The results have been good, and no problems

with titanium allergy or toxicity, tumor growth, or other adverse reactions have occurred.

▶ This is the first prospective study of a system for rigid anchoring of a nail prosthesis. Although the long-term reliability of transmucosal implants has been well established, there has been some doubt regarding the ability of transcutaneous systems to stand up to long-term wear. The average duration of follow-up in this study was only 18 months, too short a time to adequately judge long-term stability. Nonetheless, the technique has real merit, given the relatively limited appeal of surgical reconstruction of the entire nail mechanism after traumatic loss. The cemented-on prosthetic nails used today serve only a cosmetic role. They are too unstable to be used in the manner of a true nail. The osseointegrated nail not only is stable enough to be used to assist in picking up small objects, but it can also serve another of the nail's important functions, proprioception, by transmitting stimulus through the bony attachment.

V.R. Hentz, M.D.

Treatment of Amputated Fingertip
Yoshimura M (Yoshimura Orthopedic Clinic, Japan)
J Jpn Soc Surg Hand 12:555–558, 1995   4–7

Background.—To prevent functional and cosmetic disturbance of the nail during amputation through the nail, both the soft tissue and the bone must be repaired. For these cases, plastic surgery of the nail has been used to keep the nail intact.

Procedure.—Midlateral incisions are made on both sides of the finger from the finger stump to the middle phalanx. The dorsal flap and palmar flap are elevated. The distal phalanx is shortened by several millimeters. This procedure was used to treat 35 amputated fingers in 32 cases. The fingers involved were 1 thumb, 14 index fingers, 16 middle fingers, 9 ring fingers, and 1 little finger.

Findings.—The average length of finger shortening was 10.9 mm; the minimum was 4 mm, and the maximum was 17 mm. When the regenerated nail was compared with the opposite healthy nail, no problem was observed in the width of the nail; however, the average shortening of the nail was 2.4 mm (range, 0 mm to 5 mm). Sensation of the fingertip was normal in 26 fingers. Numbness was seen in 8 fingers and paresthesia was seen in 1 finger.

Conclusion.—Most patients were satisfied with the cosmetic and functional results of the procedure. The disadvantage of this procedure is shortening of the finger.

▶ Many operative techniques are available for treating amputated fingertip. Claw nail deformity results when only soft tissue is repaired. The plastic procedure involving bone grafting is complicated and results in sustained sensory disturbance. The author developed a new plastic surgical technique to keep the nail intact. He has treated 35 fingers of 32 patients with his procedure and has prevented nail deformity.

The advantages of this procedure are as follows: (1) the technique is simple and safe; (2) the fingertip is covered by normal skin that has normal sensation; (3) no microvascular technique is needed; (4) the nail regenerates without deformity. The disadvantage of the procedure is that further shortening of phalanx is needed to close the wound of the fingertip. This procedure is recommended for treating the amputated fingertip through the nail.

S. Ishii, M.D.

Pulp Plasty After Toe-to-Hand Transplantation
Wei F-C, Yim KK (Chang Gung Mem Hosp, Taipei, Taiwan, Republic of China; Stanford Univ, Calif)
Plast Reconstr Surg 96:661–666, 1995   4–8

Background.—After toe-to-hand transplantation, the bulbous-appearing pulp of the transplanted digit can be debulked using pulp plasty. Although this procedure is simple, its effects have not been well documented. The effects of pulp plasty on the function and appearance of the operated digit were retrospectively reviewed.

Technique.—The procedure is done on an outpatient basis with local anesthesia and tourniquet control. The surgeon makes a longitudinal elliptical incision in the middle of the pulp, corresponding to the most bulbous part of it. The incision is usually extended from the distal end of the paronychium to the interphalangeal crease. The surgeon removes a wedge of subcutaneous tissue down to the bone and tendon insertion with its overlying skin. To prevent injury to the neurovascular bundle and formation of depressed scar, the surgeon must be careful to avoid dissecting and removing excess soft tissue laterally on both sides. The skin is closed with 5-0 nylon suture before tourniquet release, and hemostasis is achieved by compression.

Patients.—Of 107 patients undergoing pulp plasty between January 1990 and June 1993, 51 were available for detailed follow-up assessment at 1 month or more after the procedure. These patients were 35 men and 16 women, aged 13 to 56 years. A total of 82 transplanted toes were debulked by pulp plasty at a mean of 14 months after toe-to-hand transplantation. Average duration of follow-up was 20 months.

Findings.—According to subjective criteria, appearance was improved in 67.1% of the debulked digits and function was improved in 63.4%. Painful scarring was rare. No patient reported hypersensitivity. The procedure did not adversely affect sensation. For 87.8% of the digits, pulp plasty was judged to be worthwhile.

Conclusions.—Pulp plasty is a simple, effective procedure for debulking digits after toe-to-hand transplantation. Patient satisfaction with the functional and cosmetic outcomes of this adjunctive treatment is high.

▶ This article provides a useful description of a secondary procedure that follows toe transplantation. The procedure itself appears to significantly improve the shape of the toe with minimal effort. The availability and efficacy of the operation should become part of "informed consent" when toe transplantation is discussed with a patient.

W.L. Lineaweaver, M.D.

Ulnar Parametacarpal Flap: Anatomical Study and Clinical Application [in French]
Bakhach J, Saint Cast Y, Gazarian A, et al (Hôpital du Tondu-Pellegrin, Bordeaux)
Ann Chir Plast Esthét 40:136–147, 1995   4–9

Introduction.—A new island skin flap, harvested on the ulnar border of the hand, allows surgeons to cover the palm and the dorsum of the hand with antegrade flow and to reach the distal interphalangeal joint of the fifth finger when based on its distal anastomosis with retrograde flow.

Anatomy.—The cubitodorsal artery, a branch of the ulnar artery, was studied in 43 cadavers (Fig 3). This artery originates at a mean of 3.5 cm proximal to the pisiform; the length varies from 1–2.5 cm and the mean diameter is 1 mm. The artery bifurcates in an upward branch (Becker's flap) and in a downward carpal branch that passes between the ulnar styloid and the pisiform; thus, 3 cutaneous branches are seen. The medial branch is

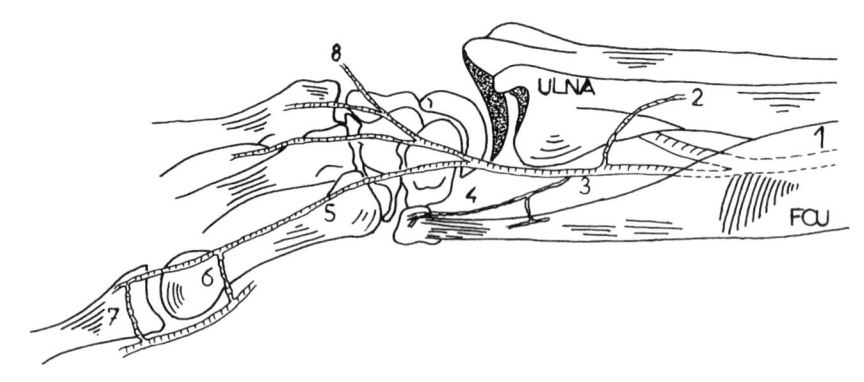

FIGURE 3.—Dorsal carpal branch of the ulnar artery. Shown are the ulnar artery (*1*), proximal branch (*2*), distal branch (*3*), pisiform bone artery (*4*), medial branch of the distal artery (*5*), anastomotic network with the ulnar collateral artery of the little finger (*6* and *7*), and anastomosis with the dorsal carpal network (*8*). *Abbreviation:* FCU, flexor carpi ulnaris. (Courtesy of Bakhach J, Saint Cast Y, Gazarian A, et al: Ulnar parametacarpal flap: anatomical study and clinical application. *Ann Chir Plast Esthét* 40:136–147, 1995.)

constant, running on the abductor minimi muscle and anastomosing constantly with the ulnar palmar collateral artery of the auricular at the neck of the fifth metacarpal joint. A second, more distal anastomosis with the collateral proper digital artery was found in 20% of the dissections. The skin territory extends from the ulnar border of the hand to the third metacarpal.

> *Technique.*—The dissection begins on the medial border, and the incision includes the abductor aponeurosis. The pedicle is not individualized, and the aponeurosis is lifted and separated from the metacarpal bone. It is important to include a 1-cm piece of skin on the radial border of the fifth metacarpal joint. The available proximal length of the pedicle is 5 centimeters. When distally based, the pivot point is the neck of the fifth metacarpal joint, and the proximal limit is the dorsal carpal crease.

Conclusion.—This new island, or free flap, can include a piece of vascularized bone from the fifth metacarpal joint or a nerve branch from the dorsal cutaneous ulnar branch.

▶ This new flap will have a definite place in the armamentarium of the hand surgeon. It has a more constant pedicle than the reverse metacarpal flap of the fourth space. In my limited experience, the most useful indication is the flap with retrograde flow, which allows covering of the dorsum of the metacarpophalangeal joints after dorsal tenoarthrolysis for stiffness in extension. It is also a versatile flap that can be used to cover extensive skin loss of the fifth finger and the proximal phalanx of the ring finger.

G. Foucher, M.D.

▶ A flap based only on the dorsal branch of the ulnar artery was first described by *Becker and Gilbert in 1988*.[1] The current authors extend this work and describe several different adaptations of this flap both as a proximally and distally based pedicle flap and as a small free flap for specific defects. Although the article is written in French, it is well illustrated, and the legends are in English. Given the renewed interest in using the ulnar artery rather than the radial artery as the source of free-flap donor vessels, this article assumes a certain importance.

V.R. Hentz, M.D.

Reference

1. Becker C, Gilbert A: The cubital flap. *Ann Chir Main* 7:13b–42, 1988.

A Comparison of Immediate and Staged Reconstruction of the Dorsum of the Hand

Sundine M, Scheker LR (Christine M Kleinert Inst of Hand and Micro Surgery, Louisville, Ky; Univ of Louisville, Ky)
J Hand Surg (Br) 21B:216–221, 1996   4–10

Background.—Reconstruction of combined dorsal hand defects involving the skin and extensor tendons with or without bony injury presents a clinical challenge. These injuries have traditionally been managed with multistaged procedures, with skin grafts or flaps first, followed by bony fixation, and finally tendon grafting or tendon transfer. However, immediate reconstruction after wide surgical débridement has also been performed. The success of traditional staged procedures was compared with that of immediate reconstruction.

Methods.—The records of 7 patients who underwent staged reconstruction and 7 patients who underwent immediate reconstruction were reviewed. All patients had severe injuries requiring flap coverage and tendon grafting or tendon transfer to restore extensor function. The groups were compared regarding the number of operations, range of motion (ROM) achieved, the time required to achieve the maximal ROM, and work status.

Results.—The immediate reconstruction group achieved maximal ROM significantly sooner than did the staged reconstruction group (214 vs. 630 days). Total active ROM was 55.4 degrees in the immediate reconstruction group and 45.9 degrees in the staged reconstruction group; the difference was not significant. The staged reconstruction group underwent an average of 4.9 operations compared with 2.1 operations in the immediate reconstruction group; the difference was highly significant. A return to active employment was achieved by 85.7% of the patients in the immediate reconstruction group and 42.8% of the patients in the staged reconstruction group.

Conclusions.—Compared with traditional staged reconstruction, immediate reconstruction significantly reduces the time to maximal motion and number of operations and results in a greater probability of return to active employment. In addition, immediate reconstruction is less costly and is associated with minimal morbidity. Wide early débridement, immediate microvascular reconstruction, and early mobilization are the critical factors of the procedure.

▶ This report is a retrospective review of 2 cohorts (both with the dorsal complex hand injuries): 1 group of 7 patients who had reconstructive surgery in a staged technique with delayed tendon grafting and bone grafting and 1 group in which reconstruction was done immediately with free-tissue transfer, immediate tendon grafting, and immediate bone grafting.

The concept of emergency or urgent free-tissue transfer was first brought to our attention by Godino[1] and further reiterated by Lister and Scheker.[2] All of us doing microvascular and reconstructive hand surgery have leaned toward that technique. This paper adds further evidence for all of us who deal with these injuries that this technique is, indeed, the proper way to handle them. The authors of this paper define emergency treatment as that done within 24 hours of injury. The results are impressive: one third as many operations, return to work 50% faster, and equal range of motion in the immediate group. There is little to argue with about this paper, which further supports the use of very aggressive immediate reconstruction in these complex injuries with equal or better results. It is important for hand surgeons to understand this. It is also important for third-party payers and workers' compensation representatives to understand that this aggressive, highly technical, and (initially) very expensive form of treatment is also time saving, cost-effective, and better for the patient.

I commend the authors on an excellent retrospective, comparative study.

N.B. Meland, M.D.

References

1. Godina M: Early microsurgical reconstruction of complex trauma of the extremities. *Plast Reconstr Surg* 78:285–292, 1986.
2. Lister GD, Scheker LR: Emergency free flaps to the upper extremity. *J Hand Surg [Am]* 13:22–28, 1988.

Latissimus Dorsi Musculocutaneous Flap Without Muscle
Angrigiani C, Grilli D, Siebert J (Buenos Aires, Argentina; New York)
Plast Reconstr Surg 96:1608–1614, 1995   4–11

Introduction.—When the bulk of the latissimus dorsi musculocutaneous flap presents a problem in reconstructive surgery, various technical modifications can be used to reduce the excessive value. A new flap technique in which the cutaneous portion of the latissimus dorsi musculocutaneous flap is based on just 1 cutaneous perforator—without muscle—is described.

Technique.—The design of the new flap was based on an anatomical study in 40 fresh cadaver specimens injected with colored latex. These investigations demonstrated the consistent presence of 2 or 3 cutaneous branches, or perforators, of the vertical intramuscular branch of the thoracodorsal artery. The largest of these, the proximal perforator, measures .4 –.6 mm in diameter. This vessel can supply a flap with dimensions of as great as 25 × 15 cm and its longitudinal axis can be oriented in any direction. The perforators are easily identified once the flap has been raised on the subcutaneous tissue above the dorsal thoracic fascia from medial to lateral. The proximal trunk of the thoracodorsal artery can be included to lengthen the pedicle, thereby facilitating the anastomosis or, in the case of island flaps, the arc of rotation. This permits a vascular

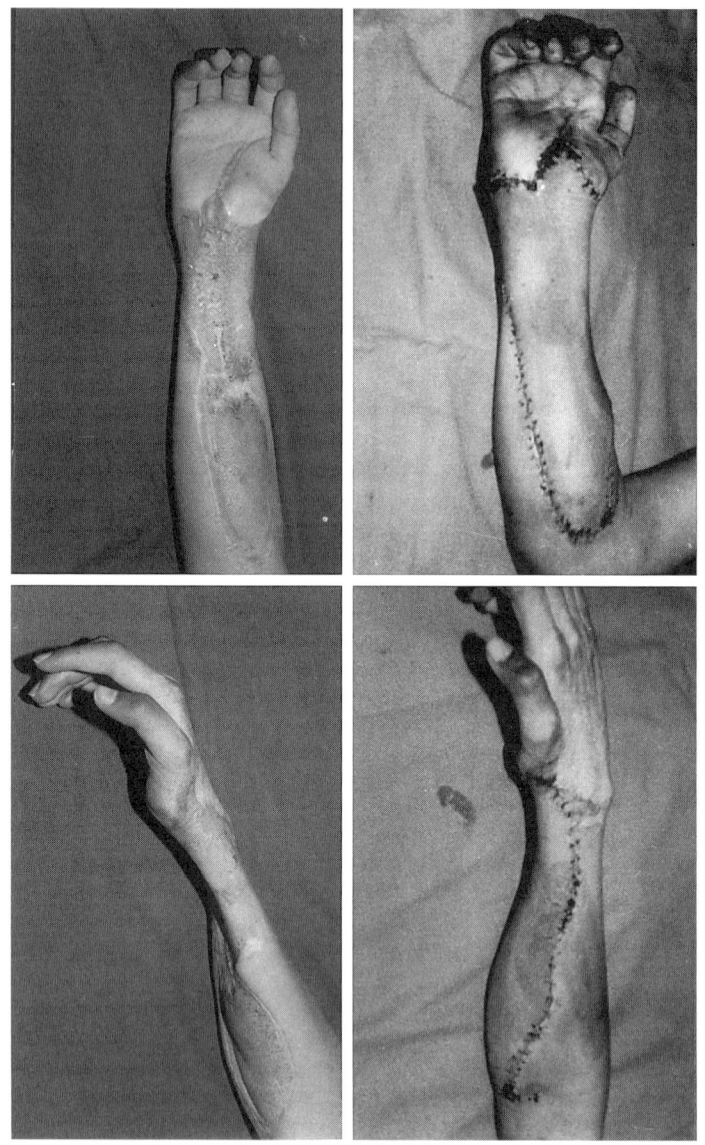

FIGURE 4.—Post-traumatic sequela on the palmar forearm. The lesion had previously been skin grafted. Flap resurfacing is necessary before tendon repair. Coverage was performed with a latissimus dorsi musculocutaneous free flap with muscle. **Top,** frontal views before and 10 days after surgery. **Bottom,** lateral views before and 10 days after surgery. (Courtesy of Angrigiani C, Grilli D, Siebert J: Latissimus dorsi musculocutaneous flap without muscle. *Plast Reconstr Surg* 96:1608–1614, 1995.)

pedicle length of 15 to 18 cm, but it does not increase the amount of transferable tissue.

Experience.—The new flap was used in 5 patients; free flaps were raised in 3 patients, and local island flaps were raised in 2 (Fig 4). The flaps averaged 20 cm in length, and all donor sites were closed, primarily without tension. No cases of ischemia, flap loss, or donor site complications occurred.

Discussion.—The skin and subcutaneous components of the traditional latissimus dorsi musculocutaneous flaps can be raised as a flap based on a single perforator of the thoracodorsal artery. The size of the skin area available for transfer with this muscle-free flap depends on the diameter of the thoracodorsal artery. Although the latissimus dorsi musculocutaneous flap remains an important flap, this and previous reports of musculocutaneous flaps without muscle suggest the need to re-evaluate the traditional concept of the musculocutaneous flap.

▶ Several papers have now suggested that the functional loss associated with complete sacrifice of the latissimus dorsi muscle is not as insubstantial as had been suggested by many previous articles. This paper describes a method of free-tissue transfer of the skin overlying the latissimus dorsi muscle based on a perforator of the thoracodorsal artery. This is a quite natural extension of our knowledge of cutaneous vasculature and parallels other similar studies that demonstrated how large skin flaps can be harvested without having to sacrifice the underlying muscle when skin is the needed tissue. The inferior epigastric and rectus abdominis flaps come to mind. Whether this flap is more safely or easily dissected than, for example, the parascapular flap, is debatable.

V.R. Hentz, M.D.

The Second Dorsal Metacarpal Artery Flap With Double Pivot Points
Karacalar A, Akin S, Özcan M (Uludag Univ, Bursa, Turkey)
Br J Plast Surg 49:97–102, 1996   4–12

Background.—Creating an island flap with a second pivot point lengthens the vascular pedicle without increasing the size of the skin incision and enables easier rotation into the recipient site. A modification of the second dorsal metacarpal artery (SDMA) flap was developed with a second pivot point around the origin of the SDMA. The results of the use of the SDMA flap with double pivot points in the hand were reported.

Technique.—A flap over the second intermetacarpal space is dissected in 2 planes: (1) at the level of the areolar tissue between the skin paddle and the paratenon of the extensor tendons to the index finger from proximal to distal and (2) at the level of the SDMA to the wrist from distal to proximal. The flap is first islanded on a pivot at the point where the recurrent cutaneous branch of the SDMA enters the skin. Once the flap is completely elevated, including the branches of the radial nerve, the main vascular pedicle, lying on the second dorsal interosseous muscle, is dissected with a cuff of muscle fascia (Fig 2).

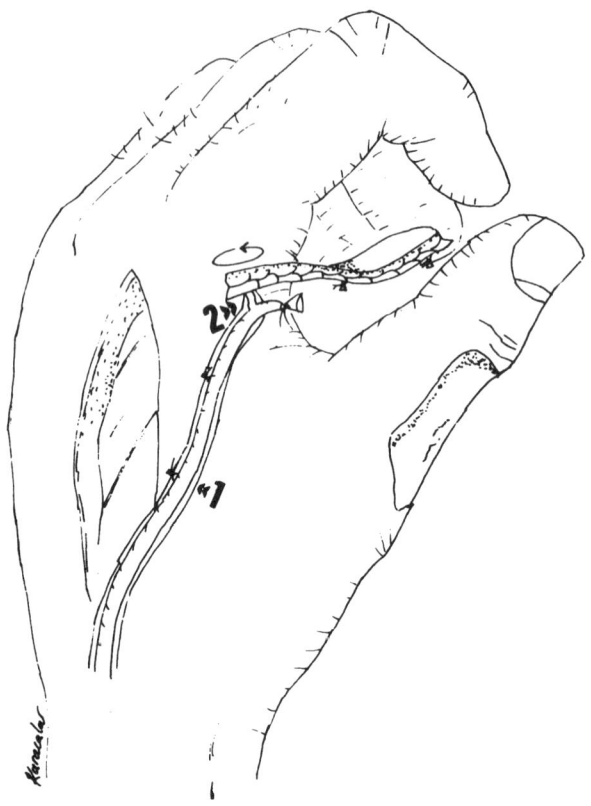

FIGURE 2.—Double pivot point flap raised on the dorsum of the hand. *1*, the second dorsal metacarpal artery and associated veins; *2*, the recurrent cutaneous branch. (Courtesy of Karacalar A, Akin S, Özcan M: The second dorsal metacarpal artery flap with double pivot points. *Br J Plast Surg* 49:97–102, 1996.)

Methods.—Thirteen patients underwent reconstruction of the thumb (10 patients), defects of the index finger (2 patients), or defects of the forearm (1 patient) with the SDMA flap with double pivot points. The patients' status was followed for 4–30 months. Sensory resurfacing in thumb reconstructions was assessed with a static 2-point discrimination test.

Results.—The flap healed well, leaving a linear, aesthetically acceptable donor scar. Static 2-point discrimination revealed good sensory response in reconstructed thumbs. No distinct dorsal hand neuromas developed.

Conclusions.—The modified SDMA flap with double pivot points has had good results in the reconstruction of sites in the hand or forearm and appears to be particularly useful in reconstruction of skin or extensor tendon defects of the thumb. Further clinical study is needed to confirm these findings and establish the flap as an alternative procedure for restoring of thumb sensibility.

▶ The second dorsal metacarpal artery flap with double pivot points is a nicely described technique for cutaneous flap coverage of primary thumb defects. The authors also state that the flap can be used in distal forearm and dorsum of hand coverage. The flap is well known to all hand surgeons because of the second dorsal metacarpal artery; however, the authors have developed a technique of lengthening this flap on the basis of the recurrent cutaneous branch of the second dorsal metacarpal artery, whereby the proximal perforators to the flap from the artery are ligated and transected and the flap is turned 180 degrees on its most distal perforator. This technique was used in 13 cases; all but 2 flaps survived. Partial skin necrosis, which eventually resulted in a healed wound, developed in the 2 flaps that did not survive. The flap is versatile and can carry the indices proprius tendon for tendon graft. The dorsal branch of the radial nerve is also available with the flap.

The paper is well illustrated, well written, and has an excellent bibliography. The technique is well described. This is certainly a nice idea for elongating antigrade flow dorsal metacarpal artery flap in thumb and digit coverage. The authors state that they did not use Doppler ultrasonography to identify the artery before surgery because the artery was present in all 13 patients; I disagree with that decision. When I use dorsal metacarpal artery flaps, I always map out the vessels with ultrasonography before making incisions because there is a small risk, perhaps 2% to 5%, that the second dorsal metacarpal artery will not be there. The most positive benefit of this flap is that it is maintained on antigrade flow and does not seem to have the propensity and problems of prolonged swelling and venous congestion that reversed flow flaps may have in this area.

N.B. Meland, M.D.

The Retrograde Radial Fascial Forearm Flap: Surgical Rationale, Technique, and Clinical Application
Braun RM, Rechnic M, Neill-Cage DJ, et al (Univ of California, San Diego)
J Hand Surg (Am) 20A:915–922, 1995   4–13

Introduction.—The use of the retrograde radial fascial forearm flap is described. This flap differs from the classical radial forearm flap in that it spares the radial artery and leaves the forearm skin intact.

Technique.—The operation is an outpatient procedure, performed with general anesthesia or brachial plexus nerve block. The surgeon applies a pneumatic tourniquet. The incision begins in the center of the palm or over the previous scar and passes proximally to the wrist flexion crease and then toward the radial border of the anterior forearm surface. When this diagonal incision reaches halfway, the incision is redirected proximally, parallel to the long axis, to within a few centimeters of the elbow flexion crease. Some fat remains on the dermal undersurface. The fat and deep fascia are developed as a long, rectangular flap based distally in the radial aspect of the distal forearm. Special attention must be paid to the lateral antebrachial cutaneous nerve and to the radial sensory nerve. The 2 parallel incisions are connected proximally to permit flap elevation. The radial artery is protected and remains below the flap. The perforating vessels in the distal forearm are necessary for flap viability. The flap is attached to the borders of the carpal canal or to soft tissue with fine, absorbable, interrupted sutures. The tourniquet can then be released and flap viability confirmed. A suction drain may be left for 24 to 48 hours. Perioperative antibiotics can be used for 24 hours. Standard skin closure is applied, and the arm is placed in a padded splint for 1 week and then examined.

Discussion.—The major theoretical complications include flap necrosis, nerve injury, infection, hematoma, and circulatory complications. In a series of 30 patients, the authors did not experience any of these complications. The postoperative scar is long and prominent. This flap is useful for revision of failed carpal tunnel operations and median nerve shielding for reconstructive surgical procedures.

Conclusions.—The retrograde radial fascial forearm flap is useful for tissue coverage of nerve, tendon, or soft tissue defects in the hand or forearm. This procedure differs from the standard radial forearm flap in that it protects the integrity of the radial artery.

▶ New anatomical analyses of upper-extremity cutaneous blood supply continue to point to a wealth of useful fascial or fasciocutaneous flaps. In fact, except for very large soft-tissue losses or perhaps composite-tissue losses, microvascular free-tissue transfer in the upper limb clearly has a diminishing role. There are very few smaller, medium-size defects located in the upper extremity that cannot be covered by one or another of these newly described flaps. The radial forearm flap either with or without skin can be used for many reconstructive circumstances without the need to sacrifice the radial artery's contribution to the circulation of the hand; this is particularly true when the radial forearm flap is used as a distally based pedicle flap.

V.R. Hentz, M.D.

Suggested Reading

Karacalar A, Özcan M: Second dorsal metacarpal artery neurovascular island flap: Clinical applications. *Eur J Plast Surg* 18:153–156, 1995.
▶ Flaps from the dorsum of the index finger based on the first dorsal metacarpal artery, such as the flag flap or the kite flap, have been advocated primarily for reconstruction of defects of the thumb. The authors point out variously configured flaps based on the second dorsal metacarpal artery (including those innervated by branches of the radial nerve) and a double flap from the dorsum of both the index and middle fingers to provide both dorsal and volar cover in thumb reconstruction. A significant drawback in using this flap for radially placed

defects is the need to divide and then to repair the extensor tendons to the index finger to allow pedicle mobilization.

V.R. Hentz, M.D.

Shibata M, Hatano Y, Iwabuchi Y: Combined dorsal forearm and lateral arm flap. *Plast Reconstr Surg* 96:1423–1429, 1995.

▶ The authors describe a unique combination *incontinuity flap* for hand reconstruction. The posterior interosseous (here termed dorsal) flap is based retrograde on the anterior-posterior communications just proximal to the ulnar head. The incontinuity lateral forearm flap is "supercharged" by anastomosing its donor posterior brachial vessel to a recipient artery. The authors demonstrate that it is unnecessary to also anastomose a vein.

V.R. Hentz, M.D.

Yao JM, Song JL, Xu JH: The second web bilobed island flap for thumb reconstruction. *Br J Plast Surg* 49:103–106, 1996.

▶ This article reports on the extension of the first dorsal metacarpal artery flap to include skin overlying the middle finger with or without the second dorsal metacarpal artery. The series documents the usefulness and reliability of this flap and shows excellent results.

C.H. Johnson, M.D.

Ghobadi F, Zangeneh M, Massoud BJ: Free fat autotransplantation for the cosmetic treatment of first web space atrophy. *Ann Plast Surg* 35:197–200, 1995.

▶ Although the transplantation of fat to restore contour is not new, it seems to be rarely applied to cosmetic disorders of the hand. The authors studied 25 patients whose first web space concavity was overcorrected by 30% with abdominal subcutaneous fat. At 5-year follow-up, the correction was well maintained.

V.R. Hentz, M.D.

Walker LG: Classification and differential diagnosis of nontraumatic fingernail deformities—Part II. *Contemp Orthop* 31:304–308, 1995.

▶ This is second in a series of 3 articles with accompanying color photographs in which the author discusses the pathophysiology and differential diagnosis of 12 of the most common nontraumatic nail deformities. An abnormal nail is a frequent cause for a visit to the hand surgeon. These 3 articles are worth keeping together in a folder in an office or clinic for easy reference.

V.R. Hentz, M.D.

Drake LA, Dinehart SM, Farmer ER, et al: Guidelines of care for nail disorders. *J Am Acad Dermatol* 34:529–533, 1996.

▶ This set of guidelines of care for nail disorders which are intended to be all-inclusive and unrestrictive, is one of a group of guidelines being written by the American Academy of Dermatology. Guidelines of care have been popular in a variety of managed care settings. Sometimes, as a result, payment is restricted for treatments not included in the guidelines. If guidelines are to be written and followed, it might be beneficial to our patients if they are prepared by physicians and specialty societies as opposed to managed care executives who may only consider cost analysis and profit.

R.K. Roenigk, M.D.

5 Tendon Trauma and Reconstruction

Early Active Mobilization for Flexor Tendons Repaired Using the Double Loop Locking Suture Technique
Groth GN, Bechtold LL, Young VL (Barnes Hosp, St Louis; Metropolitan Hand Therapy, St Paul, Minn; Washington Univ, St Louis)
J Hand Ther 8:206–211, 1995   5–1

Background.—Many of the suture techniques used during repair of flexor tendon injures do not provide sufficient strength for safe and early active mobilization. The double loop locking suture (DOLLS) technique, first described in 1990, appears to overcome this limitation, with an average in vitro strength of 4,400 g being reported. The outcomes of patients undergoing repair of the flexor digitorum profundus (FDP) tendons using the DOLLS technique were evaluated.

Patients and Findings.—Four patients with lacerations to the FDP tendon and the flexor digitorum superficialis (FDS) tendon in zone III of the left index finger (patient 1), in zone II of the right small finger (patient 2), in zone II of the long finger (patient 3), and in zone II of the small finger (patient 4) were evaluated. In all patients, the FDP tendon was repaired using the DOLLS technique, whereas the FDS tendon was repaired using a modified Kessler technique in patients 1 and 4, a figure-of-eight suture in patient 2, and an interrupted horizontal mattress suture in patient 3. At 1–4 days postoperatively, a thermoplastic dorsal blocking splint was fabricated for all 4 patients. These splints positioned the wrist in 20 degrees of flexion, the uninvolved metacarpophalangeal (MP) joints in 60 degrees of flexion, and the involved MP joints in 70 degrees of flexion, and permitted the proximal and distal interphalangeal joints full extension. In 3 patients, rubber band traction with a palmar pulley was added to keep the finger in a flexed position. Patients were advised to wear the splints at all times, with removal of the rubber band traction for flexion exercises. Early active mobilization was begun 3–7 days after surgery.

Excellent results were obtained in 2 patients, a good result in 1, and a fair result in 1 patient, according to Strickland's classification scheme. Patient 4 experienced a rupture of the FDS tendon, which had been repaired with a modified Kessler technique. The FDP tendon, however, which was repaired with the DOLLS technique, remained intact. No other complications were noted.

Conclusions.—In patients undergoing repair of flexor tendons using the DOLLS technique, early active mobilization with use of a protective splint offers effective postoperative management. Additional clinical studies are now needed to determine whether the DOLLS technique with early active mobilization provides statistically significant advantages over other surgical and postoperative treatment regimens.

▶ No conclusions can be drawn from this small sample, but the concept of some controlled active tension applied immediately at a flexor tendon repair site is gaining acceptance as we continue in our efforts to improve functional tendon gliding after repair. The authors make some good points: a stronger suture is needed for active motion protocols, passive motions should precede the active hold portion of the exercise to reduce the drag of edema and tight joint, some isolated distal interphalangeal joint motion is critical early on, and wrist position should be relaxed in the dorsal blocking splint. However, they do not measure joint angles or external load with the active hold component and only instruct the patient to hold the fingers in composite flexion "not to the extent of feeling tight." Internal tendon forces would have been imposed on the repair sites in a safer range, especially for the weaker FDS repairs, if the active hold was performed with the wrist at neutral, the digits positioned with less acute flexion angles, and external load measured with the Haldex.[1] It is unlikely that patients will consistently reproduce active forces in a safe range without specific guidelines.

The following principles need to be considered with immediate active mobilization programs:

1. The FDP and the FDS do not load share; their tensile strengths must be considered separately. The FDS repaired with a figure-of-eight or mattress suture does not have enough tensile strength to tolerate internal tendon forces generated with active motion, especially at the end arc of flexion.

2. Internal tendon forces are affected by joint angles of the wrist and digital joints, which alter the resistance of the antagonistic muscle. Tendon tensions are reduced with the wrist in neutral as opposed to a flexed position and with the digits in a position of moderate flexion (MP, 85 degrees; PIP, 75 degrees; DIP, 40 degrees).[1]

3. Active motion programs and studies of internal tendon forces are not reliable and repeatable unless the external load at the finger tip and wrist and digital joint angles are measured during testing or exercise.

4. The work of flexion, i.e., resistance to tendon gliding, will be increased by increased amounts of suture material[2]; frictional resistance produced by the digital pulleys[3]; the "compressional mechanism" of the FDP on the FDS at the chiasm[4]; the speed of exercise, the resistance of edema, hematoma, and adhesion, and joint angle position when flexion is initiated.[1]

A number of researchers have obtained excellent results with active motion programs that used conventional sutures (i.e., modified Kessler with epitenon). Increased suture material may affect the ability of the FDS and

FDP to change their shapes as they glide relative to each other at the chiasm and may make excursion through the pulleys more difficult. Increasing repair strength is important to active motion programs, but perhaps we need to look more carefully at the application of force with specific joint angles and external load as a critical part of the rehabilitation program.

R.B. Evans, O.T.R./L., C.H.T.

References

1. Evans RB, Thompson DE: The application of force to the healing tendon. *J Hand Ther* 6:266–284, 1993.
2. Aoki M, Manske PR, Pruitt DL, et al: Work of flexion after tendon repair with various suture methods. *J Hand Surg (Br)* 20B: 310–313, 1995.
3. Coert JH, Uchiyama S, Amadio PC, et al: Flexor tendon-pulley interaction after tendon repair: A biomechanical study. *J Hand Surg (Br)* 20B:5:573–577, 1995.
4. Walbeehm ET, McGrouther DA: An anatomical study of the mechanical interactions of flexor digitorum and profundus and the flexor tendon sheath in zone 2. *J Hand Surg (Br)* 20B:3:269–280, 1995.

Activity of the Extrinsic Finger Flexors During Mobilization in the Kleinert Splint
van Alphen JC, Oepkes CT, Bos KE (Univ of Amsterdam, The Netherlands; Med Centre Leeuwarden, The Netherlands)
J Hand Surg (Am) 21A:77–84, 1996   5–2

Introduction.—Primary repair and rehabilitation using early passive mobilization are the generally accepted treatments of flexor tendon injuries in zone 2 of the hand. A survey demonstrated that two thirds of hand surgeons favor the Kleinert rubber band flexion-active extension method, in which the flexor muscles relax by means of reciprocal inhibition and in which there is no profundus muscle activity. Using the original Kleinert splint and various modifications of this splint, the activity of the profundus and superficialis flexor muscles during exercise was investigated.

Methods.—Ten healthy participants had electromyographic data taken on the activity of the profundus and superficialis flexor muscles. They exercised in the original Kleinert splint and in several modifications, which varied in wrist position, position in which extension of the metacarpophalangeal joint was blocked, nature of the spring mechanism, number of fingers dynamically splinted, use of a palmar pulley, and amount of resistance.

Results.—In the majority of participants, persistent flexor muscle activity during active extension was seen. Coactivity was more often seen with the superficialis muscle than for the profundus muscle. In the slightly extended position, dynamic mobilization with the wrist did not seem to be beneficial for relaxing the flexor when compared with slight flexion under the same condition. The rate of exercises performed did not seem to influence the amount of coactivity. When extension was least resistant, the least amount of coactivity was found.

Conclusion.—During resisted extension in the Kleinert splint, the flex muscles do not relax. When active tension is least resisted, the flexor muscles are more relaxed. The amount of coactivity seems to be reduced by the use of a palmar pulley. Using the dynamic splint for early passive motion of tendon repairs may have more advantages over the Kleinert technique. The flexor muscles may not be active while the dynamic splint is being used; however, this still needs to be investigated.

▶ This study of the activity of the flexor digitorum profundus (FDP) and flexor digitorum superficialis (FDS) within the original Kleinert splint and within variations of that splint provides us with new information regarding internal tendon forces imposed on a flexor tendon repair site with postoperative rehabilitation programs. The authors have demonstrated that the theory of reciprocal inhibition (as it applies to flexor tendon passive motion protocols) proposed by Lister, et al.[1] in 1977 may be incorrect. Their study does not support the concept that the flexor muscles relax during resisted extension in the Kleinert splint. They have also demonstrated that the FDS is more active than the FDP with active extension, and that the least amount of flexor activity occurs when digital extension is least resisted.

The clinical relevance of this paper is not so much in the authors' conclusion that some active tension occurs in the flexor system with the active extension phase of "passive" motion protocols or that flexor activity is diminished by decreasing the dynamic resistance to extension, but in the demonstrated lack of activity in the FDP muscles as compared to the FDS muscles with these rehabilitation techniques.

The problem with passive protocols, especially with the original Kleinert splint, may be that the FDP probably is not subjected to enough tension or enough excursion. We should use the information gained from this study to focus more attention on the internal tension transmitted to the FDP within these postoperative protocols. The more recently described limited active motion protocols have demonstrated significant improvements in distal joint motion at the end arc of flexion as compared to passive only protocols.[2, 3] The FDP may require some active tension in the postoperative phase to maintain functional tendon gliding.

The authors comment on the rate at which exercises were performed and, on the basis of testing coactivity with 1 participant, state that the speed of exercise did not seem to be a variable. The reader should be cautioned that the speed of motion does contribute to viscous resistance and should be considered a variable with postoperative flexor tendon exercise programs. Torque increases as joint angles increase and as the speed of motion increases.[4, 5] The *work of flexion* is related to the energy required for flexion and the rate of flexion; a slower rate of flexion allows for greater relaxation of the tissues and thus lower peak forces are generated.[6] The obvious clinical implication with early motion programs is that slower motions transmit less internal tension to the repair site and are safer.

R.B. Evans, O.T.R./L., C.H.T.

References

1. Lister GD, Kleinert HE, Kutz JE, et al: Primary flexor tendon repair followed by immediate controlled mobilization. *J Hand Surg (Am)* 2:441–451, 1977.
2. Silfverskiöld KL, May EJ: Flexor tendon repair in zone II with a new suture technique and an early mobilization program combining passive and active flexion. *J Hand Surg (Am)* 19A:53–60, 1994.
3. Evans RB: Immediate active short arc motion for the repaired zone I and II flexor tendon. *J Hand Surg (Am)* submitted May 1995, under revision for resubmission.
4. Evans RB, Thompson DE: The application of force to the healing tendon. *J Hand Ther* 6:4:266–284, 1993.
5. Wainwright SA, Biggs WD, Currey JD, et al: *Mechanical Design in Organisms.* Princeton, NJ, Princeton University Press, 1976, pp. 23–29.
6. Lane JM, Black J, Bora FW. Gliding function following flexor tendon injury. *J Bone Joint Surg (Am)* 58A(7):985–990, 1976.

Biomechanical Characteristics of Suture Techniques in Extensor Zone IV

Newport ML, Pollack GR, Williams CD (Univ of Connecticut, Farmington; Texas Tech Univ, Lubbock)
J Hand Surg (Am) 20A:650–656, 1995   5–3

Objective.—Previous approaches to injuries of the extensor mechanism have sometimes yielded unacceptable clinical results, prompting the use of new or modified techniques. Poor clinical results are particularly likely to occur in the more proximal zones. The biomechanical characteristics of suture techniques commonly used in zone IV—over the proximal phalanx—were investigated.

Methods.—The study included the extensor mechanisms of 16 fresh-frozen cadaver hands. Sutured tendon specimens were prepared and mounted in an Instron Tensile Testing Machine to determine the strength of various suture techniques. The techniques were also compared regarding degree of shortening produced, metacarpophalangeal (MP) and proximal interphalangeal (PIP) joint motion after suturing, and any changes in the force required to create maximum flexion after suturing. The suture techniques studied were the modified Bunnell, modified Kessler, figure-of-eight, and mattress sutures.

Results.—None of the suture techniques produced significant tendon shortening or significant loss of flexion at the MP or PIP joints. With 8 mm of tendon shortening, flexion loss averaged only about 3 degrees at the MP joint and 12 degrees at the PIP joint. Force required to produce a 2-mm gap did not significantly differ among techniques. However, the Bunnell and Kessler techniques had greater values for failure strength than the figure-of-eight and mattress sutures (Table 3). In addition, the amount of force required to obtain maximum flexion was far less with the Bunnell and Kessler techniques.

Conclusions.—The Kleinert modification of the Bunnell technique and the modified Kessler technique appear to be the strongest suture techniques

TABLE 3.—Strength to 2-mm Gap and Failure of Tested Suture Technique

Suture	2 mm Gap	Failure
Bunnell	1202 ± 971	2255 ± 391
Kessler	1315 ± 577	2081 ± 367
Mattress	791 ± 357	1286 ± 426
Figure-of-eight	1161 ± 571	1558 ± 564

Force (g)

(Courtesy of Newport ML, Pollack GR, Williams CD: Biomechanical characteristics of suture techniques in extensor zone IV. J Hand Surg (Am) 20A:650–656, 1995.)

for repair in zone IV of the extensor mechanism. The findings of a preliminary cadaver suggest that repaired tendons can physiologically tolerate dynamic or active range of motion, under controlled conditions and in short arcs. Iatrogenic surgical factors may play little role in the suboptimal results that occur after injury to extensor zone IV; rather, adhesion formation is most likely responsible.

▶ The above abstract illustrates the shortcomings of such synopses. One of the surprising findings of this study was that shortening of the extensor tendon by as much as 8 mm produced very little loss of motion at the MP and PIP joints of a total of 15.4 degrees, on average. The force to produce this amount of flexion, however, was shown in this cadaveric study to be increased by more than 100% above that required with no shortening whatsoever.

Although the Bunnell and Kessler techniques were certainly stronger than the mattress or figure-of-eight techniques, this study indicates that over short arcs, all 4 methods will be secure.

Finally, I disagree with 1 conclusion drawn by the authors of this excellent paper: namely, that "iatrogenic surgical factors may not play a significant role in poor and fair results." Surely their findings indicate that unrestricted flexion after extensor tendon repair will result in loss of continuity in almost all repairs undertaken by the mattress or figure-of-eight techniques.

G.D. Lister, M.D.

Evaluation of Suture Caliber in Flexor Tendon Repair: Applications for Active Motion
Taras JS, Raphael JS, Marczyk SC, et al (Philadelphia)
1995 Jefferson Orthop J 24:15–19, 1995   5–4

Background.—Many studies have evaluated the mechanical effects of various techniques of flexor tendon repair. Little is known, however, about the impact of the suture caliber used for repair. The effects of suture caliber on the strength of flexor tendon repairs were studied, and a new double-grasping technique was evaluated.

Methods.—Various suture sizes were evaluated for their effects on core suture strength with the modified Kessler technique, the modified Bunnell technique, and a new double-grasping technique. In addition, the conventional running epitendinous suture technique was compared with the cross-stitch epitendinous technique. An early experience with the double-grasping and cross-stitch technique for flexor tendon repair was also evaluated.

Results.—The modified Kessler, modified Bunnell, and double-grasping techniques were equally strong when performed with suture calibers of 5-0 and 4-0. On average, for all techniques, 4-0 suture repairs were 64% stronger than 5-0, 3-0 was 43% stronger than 4-0, and 2-0 was 63% stronger than 3-0. These gains in repair strength were achieved without any increased technical difficulty. The grasping quality appeared to have a major effect on repair strength when 3-0 or 2-0 sutures were used. In this regard, the modified Kessler technique was noticeably weaker than the Bunnell and double-grasping techniques with 3-0 and 2-0 sutures. The cross-stitch technique was approximately 2.5 times stronger than the running epitendinous suture. The use of a combined double-grasping and cross-stitch technique with an active postoperative therapy protocol in 14 digits yielded an average 87% return of motion.

Conclusions.—With the modified Bunnell and double-grasping techniques of flexor tendon repair, the use of a larger suture size can increase the strength of the repair. In contrast, with the modified Kessler technique, failure may be more common when larger sutures are used. Promising results are reported with a double-grasping and cross-stitch repair followed by active mobilization. The repair strength needed for safe active digital flexion after flexor tendon repair, however, remains unknown.

▶ Bigger is not always better when tendon sutures are concerned; Kessler sutures in larger sizes tend to pull out. Of course, all these in vitro tests need to be repeated in an in vivo model before one can be certain that the larger suture/grasping technique does not have an adverse effect on blood supply, scar formation, and so forth.

P.C. Amadio, M.D.

Magnetic Resonance Imaging Scanning in the Diagnosis of Zone II Flexor Tendon Rupture

Matloub HS, Dzwierzynski WW, Erickson S, et al (Med College of Wisconsin, Milwaukee; Seattle)
J Hand Surg (Am) 21A:451–455, 1996

Background.—Magnetic resonance imaging is useful for demonstrating the fine anatomy of the hand. Although MRI has been widely used to diagnose tendon and ligament rupture in the shoulder and lower extremities, its value in the diagnosis of tendon disorders in the hand has not been fully determined.

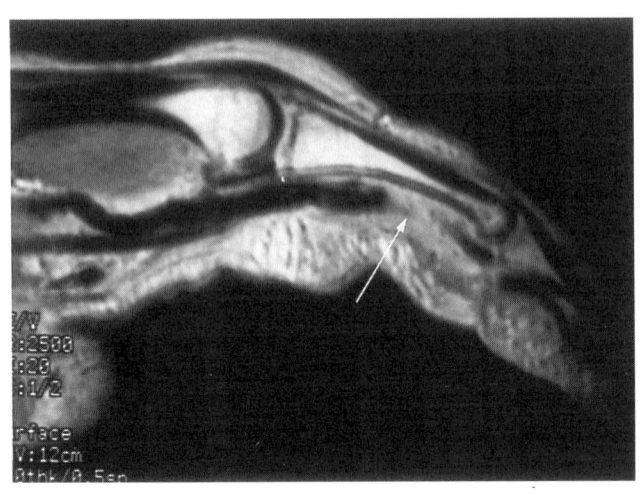

FIGURE 4.—Area of discontinuity (*arrow*) in both the flexor digitorum superficialis and flexor digitorum profundi tendons of the long finger at the level of the proximal phalanx. (Courtesy of Matloub HS, Dzwierzynski WW, Erickson S, et al: Magnetic resonance imaging scanning in the diagnosis of zone II flexor tendon rupture. *J Hand Surg (Am)* 21A:451–455, 1996.)

Methods and Findings.—Nine patients aged 16 to 37 years with suspected flexor tendon rupture were studied. All had a difficult or uncertain diagnosis. Eleven digits (16 tendons) underwent MRI. Flexor tendons were clearly seen on all MRI scans. Clinical suspicion was correlated with MRI and operative results. The diagnostic accuracy of clinical diagnosis was 60%. On MR images, ruptures were differentiated from adhesions with 100% accuracy (Fig 4).

Conclusion.—Magnetic resonance imaging, a noninvasive technique which provides good delineation of soft-tissue structures, is valuable in the early and differential diagnosis of tendon repair. It clearly demonstrates the anatomy of the flexor tendons in the hand, shows tendon rupture, and usually provides a clear differentiation from adhesions.

▶ Magnetic resonance imaging can be a valuable tool for assessing the status of a tendon or pulley. Drapé et al.[1] have shown the usefulness of MRI in assessing not only tendon rupture but also adhesions.

P.C. Amadio, M.D.

Reference

1. Drapé J-L, Silbermann-Hoffman O, Havet P, et al: Complications of flexor tendon repair in the hand: MR imaging assessment. *Radiology* 198:219–224, 1996.

Flexor Tendon Tears in the Hand: Use of MR Imaging to Diagnose Degree of Injury in a Cadaver Model
Rubin DA, Kneeland JB, Kitay GS, et al (Univ of Pennsylvania, Philadelphia)
AJR Am J Roentgenol 166:615–620, 1996
5–6

Background.—The extent of injury partly determines the choice of treatment of flexor tendon lacerations of the finger. Clinically determining the extent of injury is difficult. The value of MRI was investigated in cadavers.

Methods.—Four cadaver hands were examined. Various flexor tendon injuries were created by drawing a scalpel transversely across the volar surface. Magnetic resonance imaging of each hand was then done with the use of 2-dimensional spin-echo and 3-dimensional gradient-recalled-echo sequences. The 3-dimensional data sets were reformatted interactively along the long axis of each tendon, and the hands were dissected. Injury to each finger was classified, measured, and compared with the prospective MR findings.

Findings.—Twelve high-grade flexor tendon tears and 2 partial tears of less than 50% of the tendon area were produced. Four tendons were uninjured. Eleven high-grade lesions were diagnosed on MRI, which failed to demonstrate 1 complete tear with a separation measuring 2 mm at dissection. All intact tendons were correctly identified with MRI. The extent of 5 lesions was underestimated; none was overestimated. With the reformatted images, the number of errors that would have been made interpreting the transverse images alone were reduced (Fig 2).

Conclusions.—Different degrees of flexor tendon tears were accurately distinguished with the use of MRI. Clinical studies are needed to determine the potential of this method for noninvasively diagnosing flexor tendon injury.

▶ Magnetic resonance imaging, using sagittal, axial, or 3-dimensional techniques, and ultrasonography can both be used to evaluate the superficial tendons of the hand and wrist. The choice of technique varies with clinical features of the injury and surgical preference.

Neither technique clearly demonstrates the supporting structures (pulley systems). Real-time ultrasound, however, has the potential to show secondary changes in the tendons by using motion. We prefer MRI because of the clearly displayed anatomy and superior tissue contrast compared with ultrasound images.

T.H. Berquist, M.D.

98 / Hand Surgery

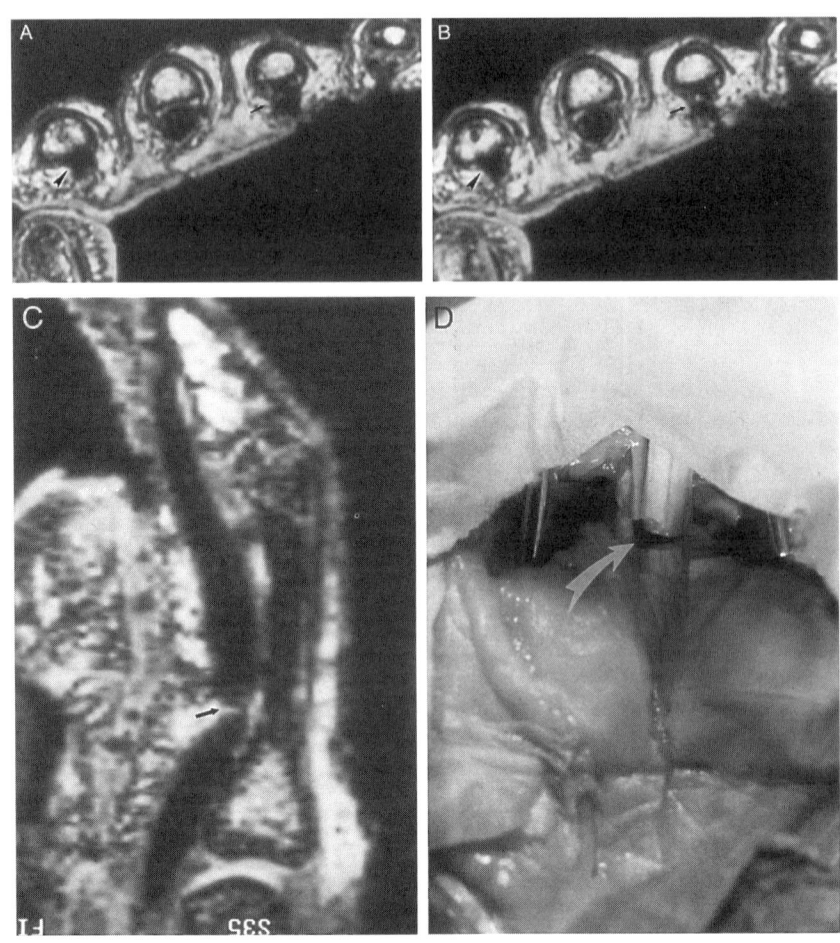

FIGURE 2.—Benefit of reformatted images. **A and B,** 2 contigious axial GRASS (gradient-recalled acquisition in steady state) images taken 1 mm apart. Note that index finger tendons have approximately 50% of their total cross-sectional area disrupted on both images (*arrowhead*), and ring finger tendons appear to have low-grade injury (*arrow*). **C and D,** reformatted image of index finger (C) demonstrates

(*Continued*)

FIGURE 2 (cont.)

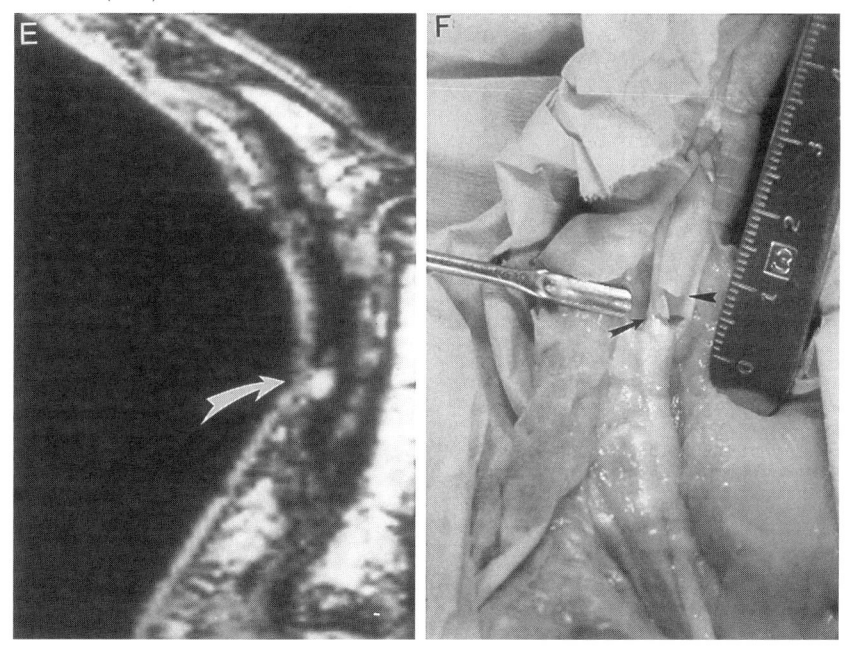

small complete tear of flexor tendons (*arrow*), which corresponds to anatomical findings (D). E, reformatted image shows that injury of ring finger (*arrow*) involves at least 50% of tendon fibers. F, photograph of ring finger at dissection shows high-grade, partial laceration: profundus tendon is completely disrupted (*arrowhead*); superficialis is partially torn (*arrow*). (Courtesy of Rubin DA, Kneeland JB, Kitay GS, et al: Flexor tendon tears in the hand: Use of MR imaging to diagnose degree of injury in a cadaver model. *AJR Am J Roentgenol* 166:615–620, 1996.)

Diagnosis of Digital Pulley Rupture by Computed Tomography
Le Viet D, Rousselin B, Roulot E, et al (Institut de la Main, Paris)
J Hand Surg (Am) 21A:245–248, 1996   5–7

Background.—Digital pulley rupture is often seen among rock climbers. Computed tomography was used to analyze digital pulley rupture after clinical and standard x-ray examination.

Patients.—Seven men who had digital pulley rupture of the nondominant hand were included. Four men were elite rock climbers. All experienced pain with a cracking sensation at injury. The patients were examined 1–3 months after injury. The initial clinical findings were pain at flexion, particularly against resistance, and abnormal palpation of the flexor tendons over the palmar surfaces of the proximal and middle phalanges. All patients underwent radiographic and CT examination. All CT scans were done in the lateral position with the proximal interphalangeal joint in flexion and the distal interphalangeal joint in extension, in a passive position and against resistance. These results were compared with those of the contralateral finger.

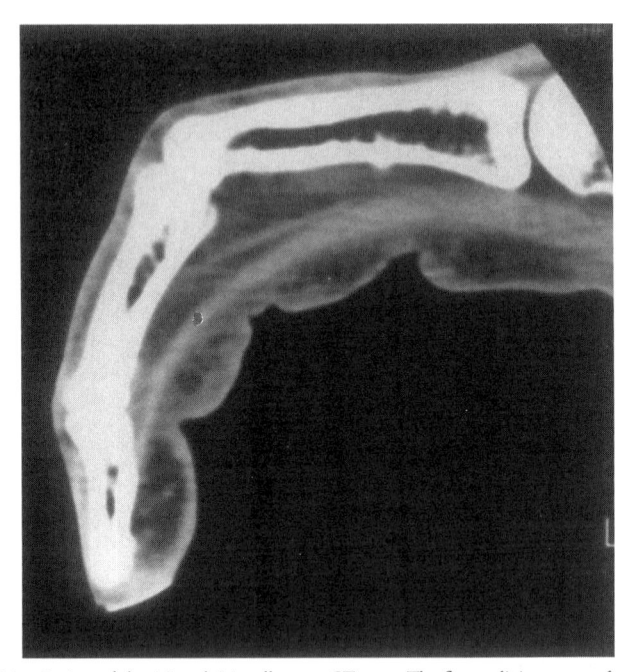

FIGURE 1.—Lesion of the A2 and A4 pulleys on CT scan. The flexor digitorum profundis tendon is bowstringing away from the proximal and middle phalanges, which suggests a rupture of the pulleys. The insertion of the flexor superficialis tendon is clearly seen at the level of the middle phalanx. (Courtesy of Le Viet D, Rousselin B, Roulot E, et al: Diagnosis of digital pulley rupture by computed tomography. *J Hand Surg (Am)* 21A:245–248, 1996).

Findings.—In 4 patients, 2 pulleys were involved at the A2 and A4 levels. In 2 other patients, only the A2 pulley was involved, and in 1 patient, only the A4 pulley was involved. Standard x-ray films did not detect abnormalities. The CT scan documented the pulley rupture in all patients. The flexor tendons did not adhere as closely to the phalanx and permitted a bowstring effect when the proximal interphalangeal joint was flexed (Fig 1). Two patients underwent surgery. The operative findings were the same as those from the preoperative CT scan. Postoperative CT scans were performed at 2 and 9 months to document repair (Fig 4).

Conclusion.—Computed tomographic scanning appears to be effective in the diagnosis of digital pulley rupture. If surgical management is indicated, CT scans can also be used postoperatively to document the success of the repair.

▶ This interesting study shows that CT can adequately image tendons and pulleys, to the extent that bowstringing and even pulley reconstruction can be clearly demonstrated. The authors note that CT has the advantage over MRI, because rapid sequence, quasidynamic imaging can be done.

P.C. Amadio, M.D.

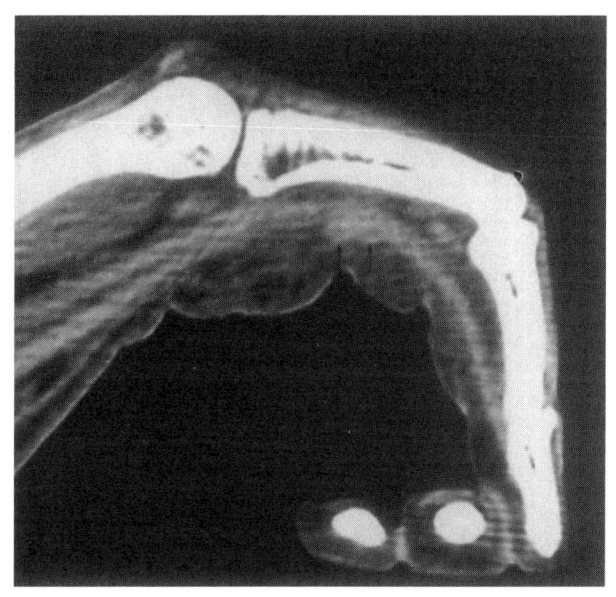

FIGURE 4.—Postoperative review at 2 months against resistance. The reconstructed pulley now keeps the tendons against the phalanges. (Courtesy of Le Viet D, Rousselin B, Roulot E, et al: Diagnosis of digital pulley rupture by computed tomography. *J Hand Surg (Am)* 21A:245–248, 1996.)

Suggested Reading

Takami H, Takahashi S, Ando M, et al: Traumatic rupture of the extensor tendons at the musculotendinous junction. *J Hand Surg* 20A:474–477, 1995.
▶ Extensor tendon rupture at the musculotendinous junction is extremely rare. The majority of "garden variety" ruptures occur at the level of the extensor retinaculum secondary to attrition or proteolytic enzymatic destruction. A musculotendinous rupture should be suspected in a gymnast with proximal forearm tenderness and digital extensor lag. An effective treatment can be anticipated by tendon transfer or side-to-side juncture. The mechanism of rupture in this location is unclear—it appears to occur after forced wrist flexion in concert with a violent extensor muscle contraction.

P.J. Stern, M.D.

Naam NH: Intratendinous rupture of the flexor digitorum profundus tendon in zones II and III. *J Hand Surg* 20A:478–483, 1995.
▶ Spontaneous intratendinous rupture of the flexor profundus (FDP) is exceedingly rare. In most cases, distal interphalangeal joint (DIPJ) flexion loss secondary to loss of FDP integrity can be attributed to a distal avulsion. If not, the treating physician must go through a mental checklist to rule out other causes, including penetrating injury (e.g., foreign body, old laceration, repeated cortisone injections), inflammatory disorders (e.g., rheumatoid arthritis), and trauma (e.g., distal radius or carpal fractures, which may cause an attritional rupture).

If exploration is being considered, the surgeon should preoperatively inform the patient of the various treatment options. In an acute setting, delayed primary tenorrhaphy may be feasible; however, a care rehabilitation program is mandatory to minimize the risk of rerupture or stiffness. One must also keep in mind that restoration of DIPJ flexion in a *chronic* setting can be complicated because a tendon graft may be necessary. Under such circumstances, DIPJ fusion or no treatment should be considered, especially in older individuals.

P.J. Stern, M.D.

Esplin VS, Tencer AF, Hanel DP, et al: Restoration of function of the thumb flexor apparatus requires repair of the oblique and one adjacent flexor tendon pulley. *J Orthop Res* 14:152–156, 1996.
▶ The title says it all.

P.C. Amadio, M.D.

Oberlin C, Atchabayan A, Salon A, et al: The by-pass extensor tendon transfer: A salvage technique for loss of substance of the extensor apparatus in long fingers. *J Hand Surg (Br)* 20B:392–397, 1995.

6 Nerve Trauma and Reconstruction

Restoration of Sensibility in the Hand After Complete Brachial Plexus Injury
Ihara K, Doi K, Sakai K, et al (Yamaguchi Univ, Japan)
J Hand Surg (Am) 21A:381–386, 1996   6–1

Introduction.—Even with ongoing advances in microsurgical reconstruction, electrophysiologic diagnosis, and other areas, complete brachial plexus palsy from traumatic avulsion of multiple cervical nerve roots continues to pose a reconstructive challenge. In the past, the emphasis has been on reconstruction of the proximal muscles, rather than sensory restoration. Previous reports have shown that it is possible to restore some useful hand function in these patients. The technique and results of surgical reconstruction of sensibility in the hand after complete brachial plexus injury were presented.

Methods.—All 15 patients had traumatic brachial plexus palsy with multiple cervical nerve root avulsions, often caused by a motorcycle accident. The patients were 13 men and 2 women (mean age, 24 years). The reconstructions were performed a mean of 4 months after the injury, and the patients' status was followed for a mean of 40 months. The basic technique of restoration of sensibility was nerve crossing to the median nerve or its lateral nerve component. Sensory reconstruction was performed along with the first or second reconstructive procedure, depending on the donor nerves used. The C5 nerve root was used as the donor nerve in the first 2 patients treated; thereafter, the supraclavicular nerve was used in 10 patients and the intercostal nerve in 3.

Results.—In 13 cases, the Tinel sign advanced gradually along the median nerve at a mean rate of 1.3 mm/day. The mean time to first recovery of sensibility was 20 months. Twelve of the 15 patients recovered limited sensibility in the distribution of the median nerve, with greatest sensitivity to pain. On Highet's S0–S4 grading system, the results were S2+ in 2 patients, S2 in 4 patients, S1 in 6 patients, and S0 in 3 patients. None of the patients had restoration of moving 2-point discrimination. Four patients had paresthesia, but there were no problems with causalgia or skin ulcers.

Conclusions.—Using the intercostal or supraclavicular nerves as donors, it is possible to restore some degree of hand sensibility in patients with complete brachial plexus injuries. Even limited recovery of hand sensibility is of value in these seriously disabled patients, whose upper extremity would otherwise be completely without feeling. Additional improvement in the restoration of hand sensibility will probably require progress in nerve regeneration and surgical technique.

▶ The emphasis in brachial plexus reconstruction has been toward restoration of motor continuity. The authors are to be congratulated on evaluating sensibility after brachial plexus reconstruction. This study reports that sensory recovery was poor (only to an S2+ level) but, in spite of this, useful in the otherwise anesthetic hand. This information should encourage us to put more emphasis toward this important, but less dramatic, component of neurologic recovery in these devastating injuries.

S.E. Mackinnon, M.D.

Use of the Phrenic Nerve for Brachial Plexus Reconstruction
Gu Yu-dong, Ma M-K (Shanghai Med Univ, China)
Clin Orthop 323:119–121, 1996   6–2

Background.—The intercostal nerves, spinal accessory nerve, and motor branches of the cervical plexus have been used for neurotization after brachial plexus injuries with nerve root avulsions. The clinical efficacy and safety of phrenic nerve neurotization for brachial plexus reconstruction were investigated.

Methods.—One hundred eighty patients underwent phrenic nerve transfer for brachial plexus injuries between 1970 and 1990. The procedure involved identifying the phrenic nerve, tracing it distally to obtain the longest possible length, and sectioning it. The surgeon coapted the proximal stump to the distal segment of the musculocutaneous nerve directly or through a nerve graft. Sixty-five patients were followed up for more than 2 years and were included in the final analysis of outcomes.

Findings.—A muscle power rating of 3 (M3) in the biceps muscle returned between 3 and 30 months, with a mean of 9.5 months. Eighty-five percent of the patients regained biceps power to M3 and improved in strength. A respiratory problem occurred postoperatively in only 1 patient and was transient. Pulmonary function tests demonstrated reduced pulmonary capacity in the first year after surgery, improving toward the end of the second year.

Conclusions.—Phrenic nerve neurotization is an acceptable option for restoring biceps function in patients with brachial plexus injury. The proportion of patients regaining biceps power to M3 and greater strength compares favorably with the outcomes of other methods. In the current series, no special motor retraining was needed.

▶ The report of recovery of M3 and greater bicep strength after transfer of the phrenic nerve to the musculocutaneous nerve in 85% of patients is truly remarkable given the small number of motor fibers in the phrenic nerve as compared to the musculocutaneous nerve. Although the author's description of operative technique seems straightforward, there must be something special these surgeons are doing to achieve these outstanding results. This manuscript is of interest to North American readers as it illustrates the unbelievable results achieved by these surgeons from Shanghai, China.

S.E. Mackinnon, M.D.

Spinal Accessory Neurotization for Restoration of Elbow Flexion in Avulsion Injuries of the Brachial Plexus
Songcharoen P, Mahaisavariya B, Chotigavanich C (Mahidol Univ, Bangkok, Thailand)
J Hand Surg (Am) 21A:387–390, 1996   6-3

Background.—Traumatic brachial plexus injuries can produce severe disability in young patients. Nerve transfer or neurotization offers the only possibility of repair, and the spinal accessory and intercostal nerves are most commonly used for this purpose. The use of spinal accessory neurotization to restore elbow flexion in patients with brachial plexus injury was evaluated.

Methods.—The experience included 216 patients with traumatic root avulsions who were treated with spinal accessory-musculocutaneous neurotization to restore elbow flexion. The patients were 208 males and 8 females, average age 26 years; 87% were injured in motorcycle accidents. One hundred fifty-eight had complete brachial plexus paralysis, and 58 had upper arm paralysis. The spinal accessory nerve was neurotized to the musculocutaneous nerve at a point just before the latter nerve entered the coracobrachialis. The connection was made using an interpositional sural nerve graft. All patients were followed for at least 2 years, with an average follow-up of 6 years.

Results.—Nearly three fourths of the patients achieved MRC III or better biceps recovery, with an average postoperative recovery time of 17 months. Waiting longer than 9 months after the injury to perform the repair increased the percentage of poor results from 26% to 63%. Patients older than 40 years were also more likely to have poor results, and none had very good results. One patient was left with postoperative weakness of the trapezius.

Conclusions.—The results of spinal accessory neurotization in restoring elbow function are at least as good as with other types of neurotization. The possibility of direct neuromuscular neurotization by rerouting the regenerating axon in the lateral antebrachial cutaneous nerve to the biceps muscle is being explored.

▶ Restoration of elbow flexion with complete brachial plexus avulsion is a challenging problem with few options for surgical intervention. The authors studied a large number of patients who underwent neurotization via nerve graft of the accessory nerve to the musculocutaneous nerve. I would choose intercostal motor nerve repair directly to the musculocutaneous nerve without the use of nerve grafts. However, the very good results presented by Songcharoen, et al., will be of interest to those doing brachial plexus reconstruction. A concern for downgrading trapezius function and compromising a subsequent shoulder fusion appears not to have been an issue in this series of patients.

S.E. Mackinnon, M.D.

Double Free-muscle Transfer to Restore Prehension Following Complete Brachial Plexus Avulsion
Doi K, Sakai K, Kuwata N, et al (Yamaguchi Univ, Ube, Japan)
J Hand Surg (Am) 20A:408–414, 1995   6–4

Introduction.—Patients with complete avulsion of the brachial plexus who undergo free-muscle and nerve transfers may have limited hand use because of failure to achieve finger extension. A second surgery allows

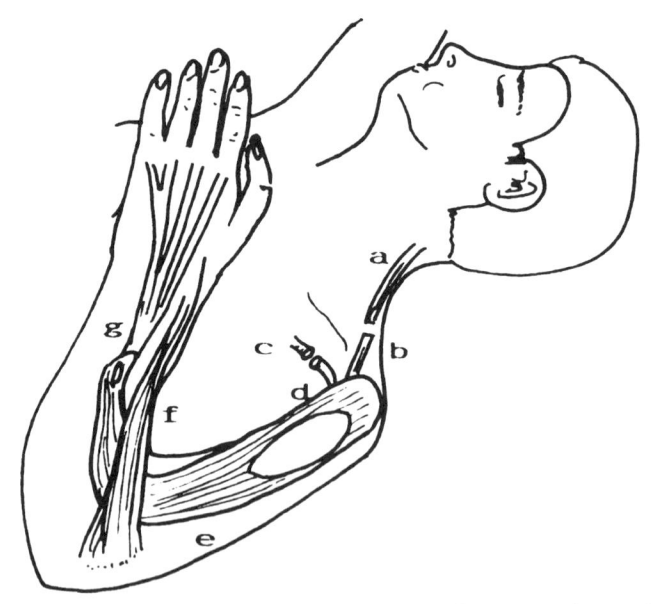

FIGURE 1.—The initial surgical procedure for reconstruction of prehension after complete brachial plexus avulsion is a free-muscle transfer to restore finger extension and elbow flexion simultaneously. Either the gracilis or the latissimus dorsi is transferred and is innervated by the spinal accessory nerve. Shown are the accessory nerve (*a*), motor branch of the muscle transplant (*b*), thoracoacromial artery and branches of the cephalic vein (*c*), nutrient artery and veins of the muscle transplant (*d*), muscle transplant (*e*), the brachioradialis and wrist extensor muscles serving as a pulley (*f*), and extensor digitorum communis tendon (*g*). (Courtesy of Doi K, Sakai K, Kuwata N, et al: Double free-muscle transfer to restore prehension following complete brachial plexus avulsion. *J Hand Surg (Am)* 20A:408–414, 1995.)

such patients to have active finger extension with a free-muscle transfer to the extensor tendons of the forearm.

Methods.—Surgical technique and outcome were assessed in 10 patients who were followed up for at least 1 year. Four patients had a combined lesion of the C5 nerve root and a preganglionic avulsion of the C6 to T1 nerve roots, 3 had complete preganglionic avulsion of the C5 to T1 nerve roots, and 3 had a postganglionic rupture injury of the C5 nerve root and a preganglionic avulsion of C6 to T1 nerve roots. The second surgery was performed 2–6 months after the first operation. In the initial surgery, the gracilis muscle was transferred in 7 patients and the latissimus dorsi muscle was transferred in 3 patients (Fig 1). The second procedure involved transfer of the gracilis muscle in 8 patients and of the ipsilateral latissimus dorsi muscle in 2 patients (Fig 2). Postoperative management consisted of immobilization of the upper limb for 4 weeks; the wrist was maintained in a neutral position and the proximal and distal interphalangeal joints were in extension. Once reinnervation of the transferred muscle was confirmed, electromyographic feedback techniques were used to train the transferred muscles to move the elbow and fingers.

Results.—With 1 exception, all musculocutaneous flaps survived without compromise. Successful revision was performed in the failed flap. In most patients, reinnervation occurred 3–8 months after surgery and was

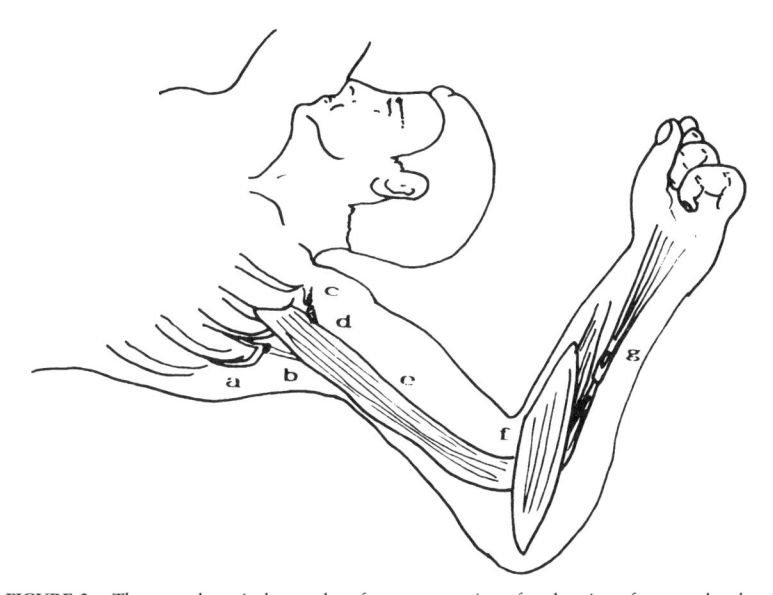

FIGURE 2.—The second surgical procedure for reconstruction of prehension after complete brachial plexus avulsion is a free-muscle transfer to restore finger flexion. Either the gracilis or the latissimus dorsi is transferred and is innervated by the fifth and sixth intercostal nerves. Shown are the fifth and sixth intercostal nerves (*a*), motor branch of the muscle transplant (*b*), thoracodorsal artery and vein (*c*), nutrient artery and veins of the muscle transplant (*d*), muscle transplant (*e*), pronator teres and wrist flexor muscles serving as a pulley (*f*), and long finger flexor tendons (*g*). (Courtesy of Doi K, Sakai K, Kuwata N, et al: Double free-muscle transfer to restore prehension following complete brachial plexus avulsion. J Hand Surg (Am) 20A:408–414, 1995.)

confirmed electromyographically. Range of voluntary elbow motion varied from 10 degrees extension to 140 degrees flexion, and the total active range of motion of the fingers ranged from 30 degrees to 110 degrees. Five patients could grasp light objects, and 4 had reasonable sensory recovery.

Conclusion.—After the additional free-muscle transfer was performed to increase hand use, 7 of 10 patients recovered elbow function and finger flexion and extension and 5 could use the hand in activities of daily living. The gracilis muscle gave better results than the latissimus dorsi muscle.

▶ The authors extended and modified previous recommendations for agressive reconstruction, primarily in young men who have complete brachial plexus avulsion injury. The authors had previously attached the free muscle used to restore elbow flexion into the radial wrist extensors but found power to be insufficient. This has been my experience in 3 attempts. The authors now attach the transfer to the finger extensors so that at least a tenodesis effect is created; they later add a second free muscle for digital prehension. There is wisdom in not asking intercostal innervation to both flex and extend the digits. The use of the spinal accessory nerve is an inprovement. The gracilis is a more predictable muscle than the latissimus dorsi. Arthrodesis of the glenohumeral joint improves the function of the transfers.

V.R. Hentz, M.D.

Early Active Mobilization After Tendon Transfers Using Mesh Reinforced Suture Techniques
Silfverskiöld KL, May EJ (Univ of Gothenburg, Sweden)
J Hand Surg (Br) 20B:291–300, 1995   6–5

Introduction.—Few reports have addressed the early postoperative management of tendon transfers, and, surprisingly, none have suggested any alternatives to immobilization for 3 weeks after surgery. Although early mobilization would be expected to decrease adhesion formation, conventional techniques of joining the tendons are too weak to withstand the strain of active movement immediately after surgery. The authors have reported the use of a mesh sleeve that joins tendon ends and thus permits early, active mobilization after direct end-to-end repairs. They have since modified their technique for use in tendon transfer and free graft reconstructions. Their experience with early active mobilization after tendon transfers is reported.

Methods.—The experience included 23 tendon transfers in the hand and forearm of 20 patients. In each case, the transfer was performed with the use of a polyester mesh sleeve to reinforce conventional suture techniques. Interlacing tendon bonds in the wrist and forearm were reinforced with 2 techniques: 1 in which a polyester mesh sleeve was fitted over and then sutured to the interlaced tendons (Fig 1A) and another in which the sleeve was applied and secured only to the tendon to be transferred (Fig 2A). The tendons were joined end to end with a mesh sleeve when the bond was

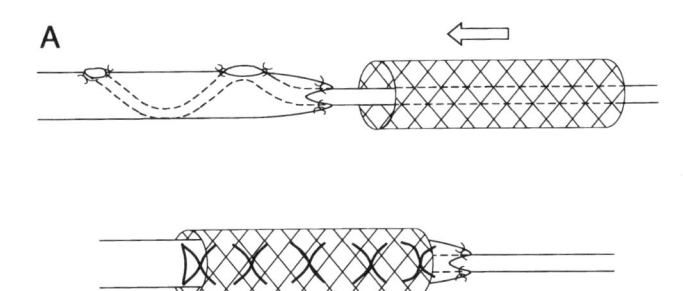

FIGURE 1A.—The "weave 1" technique for reinforcing interlacing tendon bonds. (Courtesy of Silfverskiöld KL, May EJ: Early active mobilization after tendon transfers using mesh reinforced suture techniques. *J Hand Surg (Am)* 20B:291–300, 1995.)

made in the thumb or some other more confined space. When transferred tendon was being attached to bone, the tendon end was initially reinforced with a short mesh sleeve. By the third day after surgery, all 23 transfers were mobilized with active flexion and extension.

Results.—The series included 10 transfers for extensor pollicis longus reconstruction, 4 for flexor pollicis longus reconstruction, 3 for extensor digitorum longus reconstruction, and 4 for reconstruction of wrist extension. One rupture occurred in a patient with extensor pollicis longus reconstruction, which was the result of extreme unintentional loading. One month after reconstruction, the mean final active range of motion was between 69% and 78% in the various reconstruction groups. Excluding transfers for reconstruction of wrist extension, the patients had a mean final active range of motion of 91% to 100% of the available passive range of motion. Compared with the uninjured hand, active range of motion was 75% and 100% of "normal." For wrist extension reconstructions, the mean final active range of motion was 85% of passive range of motion and at least 80% of the potentially available range of motion, given the transfers used.

Conclusions.—The combination of mesh reinforcement of suture techniques and early, active range of motion appears to offer some significant advantages for patients undergoing tendon transfers in the hand and forearm. The procedures described in this study may offer a quicker and simpler reconstruction as well as better final results. In addition to avoid-

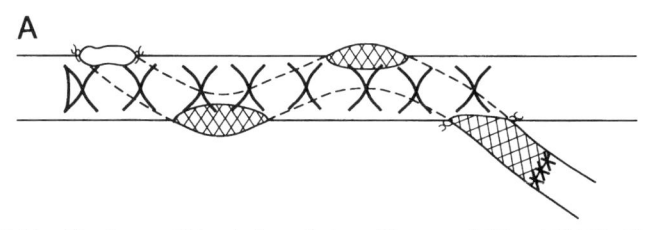

FIGURE 2A.—The "weave 2" interlacing technique. (Courtesy of Silfverskiöld KL, May EJ: Early active mobilization after tendon transfers using mesh reinforced suture techniques. *J Hand Surg (Am)* 20B:291–300, 1995.)

ing adhesions, early active motion may help to prevent muscle atrophy and joint stiffness. Perhaps most importantly, the combined technique may make it easier to perform tendon transfers with other procedures, such as synovectomy and arthroplasty in patients with rheumatoid arthritis.

▶ Operating under the assumption that early motion decreases adhesion formation around a tendon transfer junction and therefore leads to a better final range of motion, the authors presented methods of performing the tendon juncture that allow immediate active range of motion. Their proposed technique incorporates a polyester mesh sleeve into the repair site in several different fashions. One technique involves slipping the sleeve over an end-to-end repair and securing it to each tendon proximal and distal to the repair site. In another technique, they reinforce a 3-pass tendon weave with a circumferential wrap. In yet another variation, they reinforce the transferred tendon with the sleeve and then weave this covered tendon through the donor tendon. In a tendon-to-bone juncture, they recommend reinforcing the tendon with a sleeve before passing the anchoring sutures.

The authors achieved superb clinical results using 1 of the reinforcement techniques and beginning active range of motion within 3 days. Only 1 transfer ruptured, and the range of motion of the target joints was remarkably good when measured as a percentage of the available passive arc or as a percentage of the motion of the opposite uninjured side.

Wire suture markers were placed at the time of tendon repair, and elongation was radiographically monitored for 3 months. The authors report that the transfer site elongated anywhere from 1.8 mm to 6 mm, but they found no correlation between the amount of elongation and the final clinical result. Noting that they prefer to put their transfers in tightly, they claim that the elongation is beneficial to achieving the antagonistic motion. Left unanswered was the question of how much elongation is the result of the natural shifting of the repair and what amount of elongation constitutes partial failure.

In analyzing their clinical results, the authors inferred that because their rupture rate was low and the observed elongation was small, their repair must have been strong enough to allow active range of motion. Although this point cannot be refuted, the authors failed to demonstrate that their complex method which involves a large amount of foreign body and suture material, is any stronger than the currently used 4-pass weave. If their junctures are stronger, is it because of the polyester mesh or the authors' longitudinal or circumferential cross-stitch methods? A controlled laboratory study comparing traditional tendon juncture techniques and their proposed modifications should be completed before these methods are placed into widespread clinical application. Common sense and the clinical results reported here strongly suggest that early active range of motion enhances the final result after tendon transfer by decreasing adhesions, preventing joint contractures, and minimizing muscle atrophy. It will be exciting to test this hypothesis after the technical quandaries of creating an adequately sturdy tendon juncture are overcome.

T. Kiefhaber, M.D.

Outcome of Digital Nerve Injuries in Adults
Wang W-Z, Crain GM, Baylis W, et al (Christine M Kleinert Inst for Hand and Micro Surgery, Louisville, Ky)
J Hand Surg (Am) 21A:138–143, 1996   6–6

Background.—Digital nerve injury is a common civilian peripheral nerve injury. Previous research has been done on the prognostic factors correlated with good recovery, but some questions remain. The current study considered correlation with age (in adults), nerve graft vs. nerve repair in similar injuries, and degree of overlap innervation in digital nerve injury outcome.

Methods.—Sixty-seven adults with 90 complete digital nerve injuries were assessed more than 1 year after operative treatment. Both lateral aspects of the injured and contralateral uninjured digits were assessed for moving and static 2-point discrimination.

Findings.—In patients with mild crush or saw injury undergoing primary repairs, the 2-point discrimination was significantly worse than that in patients undergoing primary repair for a simple laceration. Digits undergoing primary grafting for mild crush injuries showed significantly better results than those undergoing primary repair. Two-point discrimination was better in patients younger than 40 years than in those older than 40. Two of 8 digits tested showed some overlap innervation from the uninjured side; sensation of the injured side was lost completely when the uninjured nerve of the digit was anesthetized.

Conclusions.—These findings suggest that avoiding tension at the nerve repair site in mild crush or saw injuries results in better recovery. Trimming more and grafting are apparently more effective than primary repair in minor crush-type lesions. Sensibility recovery seems better in young adults than in older adults.

▶ The authors emphasize that tension at a digital nerve repair site will significantly compromise functional recovery. This important manuscript concludes that even in mild crush injuries, primary nerve grafting has significantly better results than primary repair. This finding is in keeping with the fact that excursion of a digital nerve (1–1.3 mm) is much less than that of the nerves at the wrist (14 mm), suggesting little tolerance for the loss of even a small amount of digital nerve tissue. Allen Van Beek's report at the American Society of Reconstructive Microsurgery, in his presidential year, of very poor results after repair of digital nerve injuries in a farming population, supports the contention that in cases of other than sharp injuries, the use of a nerve graft rather than a direct nerve repair should yield better results. Implications of this study extend to the surgical management of similar injuries of all other nerves. Surgeons reluctant or untrained to perform digital nerve grafts will have to rethink their approach to these injuries.

S.E. Mackinnon, M.D.

Suggested Reading

McAllister RM, Calder JS: Paradoxical clinical consequences of peripheral nerve injury: Conduction of nerve impluses does not occur across the site of injury immediately following nerve division and repair. *Br J Plast Surg* 48:371–383, 1995.

McAllister RM, Calder JS: Paradoxical clinical consequences of peripheral nerve injury: A review of anatomical, neurophysiological and psychological mechanisms. *Br J Plast Surg* 48:384–395, 1995.

▶ Many of us have noted what appears to be an element of improved sensation occurring immediately after nerve repair. The patient reports some "feeling" in what was, before nerve repair, an anaesthetic digit or hemidigit, for example. I was taught that this resulted from conduction across the repair and that this phenomenon would disappear once wallerian degeneration of the distal segment commenced. In these 2 articles, the authors offer very convincing evidence that we must look elsewhere for an explanation of this widely observed but still mostly anecdotally reported observation.

V.R. Hentz, M.D.

Trumble TE, Kahn V, Vanderhooft E, et al: A technique to quantitate motor recovery following nerve grafting. *J Hand Surg* 20A:367–372, 1995.

▶ This technique is an excellent for beginning to compare muscle recovery after peripheral nerve injury and repair.

E. Akelman, M.D.

Omokawa S, Mizumoto S, Iwai M, et al: Innervated radial thenar flap for sensory reconstruction of fingers. *J Hand Surg* 21A:373–380, 1996.

▶ In certain select circumstances, the innervated radial thenar flap may warrant consideration for re-establishing sensibility in the severely injured finger or hand. In creating an "assist" hand, one of the elements often absent is prehension. Usually, injuries of this type are "combined" and often involve damage to the normal vascular anatomy. A preoperative arteriogram would be mandatory to be certain that the flap could be done and that it would not cause further insult to the hand. In my mind, this flap would be most useful as a pedicled flap, and would be an option to consider in addition to a neurovascular island flap.

C.H. Johnson, M.D.

7 Compression Neuropathy

A Prospective, Randomized Study With an Independent Observer Comparing Open Carpal Tunnel Release With Endoscopic Carpal Tunnel Release
Jacobsen MB, Rahme H (Central Hosp, Västerås, Sweden)
J Hand Surg (Br) 21B:202–204, 1996   7–1

Background.—Previous reports have suggested that carpal tunnel release can be safely and reliably performed by endoscopic technique. However, there have been few prospective studies to determine endoscopy's role in treating carpal tunnel syndrome (CTS). A prospective, randomized comparison of endoscopic and open surgery was performed, focusing on the outcome of return to work.

Methods.—The trial included 32 hands of 29 consecutive employed patients with idiopathic CTS. The patients were 21 women and 8 men, mean age 46 years; the diagnosis of CTS was made on the basis of clinical signs and electromyelographic changes. The patients were randomly assigned to undergo either open carpal tunnel release or endoscopic release using a 2-portal technique. The final results, including nerve conduction testing, were evaluated at 6 months. An independent, blinded observer evaluated the duration of sick leave; the study hypothesis was that endoscopic carpal tunnel release would reduce sick leave by more than 1 week.

Results.—All patients in both groups expressed satisfaction with their results. Mean sick leave was 17 days with endoscopic surgery and 19 days with open surgery, a nonsignificant difference. Neither were there any significant differences in improvement of 2-point discrimination or electrophysiologic test results. Transient numbness on the radial side of the ring finger occurred in 3 patients in the endoscopic group.

Conclusions.—Endoscopic carpal tunnel release does not reduce sick leave compared with conventional, open release in patients with CTS. The surgical results of the 2 techniques are equally good, although the endoscopic technique does carry some risk of damage to the digital nerve. The authors perform endoscopic carpal tunnel release only in carefully selected patients.

▶ Advocates of the endoscopic technique for carpal tunnel release have reported that this method offers less morbidity and a shorter return-to-work interval.[1,2] In a prospective study of patients with short open incision and active postoperative physical therapy,[3] we observed no significant morbidity and a median return-to-work interval shorter than that reported by Agee et al.[1] and comparable to that reported by Chow.[4] Jacobsen and Rahme confirmed our findings of efficacy of the open technique in their prospective randomized study of open and endoscopic cases. Recovery period aside, the more important message in the Jacobsen and Rahme paper, and ours, seems to be that the endoscopic technique is more complicated and expensive and should not be performed by surgeons inexperienced in its use. Contrarily, as stated by Jacobsen and Rahme, the conventional open technique is well proven, safe, and efficient. Decades of satisfactory outcomes with the open technique strongly suggest that endoscopic technology is better suited for procedures other than carpal tunnel release whose outcomes justify the added risks and expense associated with the endoscopic procedures.

P.A. Nathan, M.D.

References

1. Agee JM, McCarrol HR, Tortusa RD, et al: Endoscopic release of the carpal tunnel. *J Hand Surg (Am)* 17A:987–995, 1992.
2. Brown RA, Gelberman RH, Seiler JG, et al: Carpal tunnel release. *J Bone Joint Surg (Am)* 75A:1265–1275, 1993.
3. Nathan PA, Meadows KD, Keniston RC: Rehabilitation of carpal tunnel patients using a short surgical incision and an early program of physical therapy. *J Hand Surg (Am)* 18A:1044–1050, 1993.
4. Chow JC: Endoscopic release of the carpal ligament for carpal tunnel syndrome: 22-month clinical result. *Arthroscopy* 6:288–296, 1990.

A Multicenter Prospective Review of 640 Endoscopic Carpal Tunnel Releases Using the Transbursal and Extrabursal Chow Techniques
Nagle DJ, Fischer TJ, Harris GD, et al (Northwestern Univ, Chicago; Indiana Hand Ctr, Indianapolis; Philadelphia Hand Ctr, King of Prussia; et al)
Arthroscopy 12:139–143, 1996   7–2

Background.—The most common compression neuropathy of the upper extremity is that of the median nerve at the carpal tunnel. Several endoscopic carpal tunnel release techniques have been described. The surgical treatment of carpal tunnel syndrome using a modified Chow dual portal endoscopic technique was evaluated.

Methods.—Eight institutions contributed data on a total of 640 carpal tunnel releases using a dual portal endoscopic method. Seventeen percent were the original transbursal procedure described by Chow and 83% were modified extrabursal procedures.

Findings.—Patients undergoing the transbursal procedure had a complication rate of 11%, compared to 2.2% in those undergoing the extrabursal procedure. In most patients, carpal tunnel symptoms resolved by 2 weeks. By 2 months, pinch and grip strength had returned to preoperative levels. Patients receiving workers' compensation returned to work in a mean of 57 days, and those without workers' compensation returned to work in a mean of 22 days.

Conclusions.—Endoscopic carpal tunnel release can be safely and effectively performed using the dual portal extrabursal method. The perioperative and late complication rates associated with this procedure are significantly lower than those associated with the transbursal technique.

▶ The authors presented a multicenter study that clearly demonstrates that endoscopic carpal tunnel release can be done safely and effectively. Longer term reviews and longer years of experience may likely be required before 1 procedure (endoscopic) can be recommended over another. At the present time, both procedures certainly appear to be satisfactory and to be associated with a generally low incidence of complications and high incidence of success. In this particular series, the incidence of complications has not been reported to be higher with endoscopic release; in others, the incidence of complications has been higher, with potential disasters and nerve injuries. In view of this, anyone undertaking this procedure needs to have adequate training and preparation before proceeding.

R.D. Beckenbaugh, M.D.

Complete Endoscopic Carpal Canal Decompression
Okutsu I, Hamanaka I, Tanabe T, et al (Japanese Red Cross Med Ctr, Tokyo)
Am J Orthop 25:365–368, 1996   7–3

Introduction.—Endoscopic surgery for carpal tunnel syndrome differs from open surgery in that it approaches from the inside of the carpal canal to the surface and, in some procedures, releases only the transverse carpal ligament. After observing that the sectioned ends of the transverse carpal ligament were separated only 1–2 mm when this ligament alone is released, investigators sought to determine whether release of the transverse carpal ligament alone is sufficient for decompression of the carpal canal.

Methods.—An operative model, based upon 56 hands in 43 patients, was made in order to determine what constitutes complete endoscopic carpal canal decompression. The transverse carpal ligament was released first, then the transverse fibers, and, finally, the forearm fascia. Carpal canal pressure was measured using the continuous infusion technique, with the hand in a resting position and with active power grip. Preoperative and postoperative carpal canal pressure measurements could be taken within 30 minutes.

Results.—The mean preoperative carpal canal pressure was 50.1 mm Hg in the resting position. Mean pressure fell to 6.6 mm Hg immediately

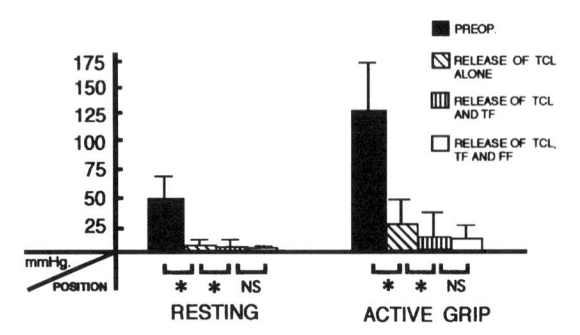

FIGURE 3. —Carpal canal pressure measurement results in 56 hands (43 patients). Complete decompression of the carpal canal was only achieved by release of both the transverse carpal ligament (TCL) and the transverse fibers (TF). Abbreviations: FF, forearm fascia; NS, not significant. *P < 0.001. (Reprinted by permission of the publisher from Okutsu I, Hamanaka I, Tanabe T, et al: Complete endoscopic carpal canal decompression. Am J Orthop 25:365–368. Copyright 1996 by Quadrant Healthcom, Inc.)

after release of the transverse carpal ligament only, to 4.8 mm Hg immediately after subsequent release of the transverse fibers, and to 4.5 mm Hg after release of the forearm fascia (Fig 3). The mean preoperative carpal canal pressure with active power grip was 125.5 mm Hg. Release of the transverse carpal ligament only, followed by release of the transverse fibers and then of the forearm fascia led to mean lowered pressures of 28.7 mm Hg, 19.8 mm Hg, and 16.3 mm Hg, respectively. For both resting position and the power active grip, the differences between preoperative data, data gathered after release of the transverse carpal ligament, and data gathered after release of the transverse fibers were statistically significant. Release of the forearm fascia produced no statistically significant change.

Conclusion.—The endoscopic procedure for carpal tunnel decompression achieves the same results as the standard open surgical procedure when it includes release of the transverse fibers as well as the transverse carpal ligament. Release of the transverse carpal ligament alone fails to provide sufficient decompression.

▶ I agree with these authors and with Cobb et al.[1] that the distal fibers of the flexor retinaculum should be released during carpal tunnel surgery. I have some concern, however, about doing this endoscopically because these fibers are superficial to, and occasionally run distal to, the superficial arch. A 2-portal approach would alllow these fibers to be released under direct vision, and I believe that such an approach would be safer for the average surgeon. It should be remembered that Okutsu first described endoscopic carpal tunnel release; his skills, acquired over more than a decade, likely exceed those of the typical surgeon doing endoscopic carpal tunnel release today.

P.C. Amadio, M.D.

Reference

1. Cobb TK, Dalley BK, Posteraro RH, et al: Anatomy of the flexor retinaculum. *J Hand Surg* 18A:91–99, 1993.

A Cadaveric Study of the Single-portal Endoscopic Carpal Tunnel Release
Van Heest A, Waters P, Simmons B, et al (Univ of Minnesota, Minneapolis; Harvard Med School, Boston; Children's Hosp, Boston; et al)
J Hand Surg (Am) 20A:363–366, 1995   7–4

Background.—Although open transection of the transverse carpal ligament (TCL) is an effective, safe approach to treating carpal tunnel syndrome, it may fail in 1 of every 5 patients. Considerable time is lost from work, and disability may be prolonged. An alternative is to release the TCL endoscopically using a single-portal technique.

Objective.—Single-portal endoscopic release was performed in 43 fresh-frozen human cadavers by surgeons who had varying experience. An average of 2 passes was needed to completely transect the TCL.

Results.—The TCL was totally released, with potentially compressing transverse fibers remaining, in 19 instances. In the remaining 24 specimens, the extent of these fibers averaged 4.4 mm. In most cases the unreleased transverse tissue was present distally, and in several cases it was clearly defined as part of the TCL. In other cases the remaining fibers represented thenar and hypothenar fascia that joined the TCL distally. The thenar fascia was partially released in nearly half the specimens. The palmar fascia was partly released in all specimens. In 1 dissection a branch of the superficial palmar arch was cut. No nerve injuries were documented, but 1 ulnar artery was transected proximally at the site of the exposing incision.

Implications.—The TCL may be released by a single-portal endoscopic approach while preserving the more superficial structures. Release is frequently incomplete, however, regardless of the surgeon's experience. The clinical significance of incomplete release, if any, is not clear.

▶ It is generally accepted that incomplete release of the TCL is an inadequate carpal tunnel release. By its very nature, endoscopic release is designed to divide less tissue than does the traditional open carpal tunnel release. Clinical studies of endoscopic release do not report a large percentage of patients with persistent symptoms,[1] and pressure studies show a decrease in carpal canal pressure after endoscopic release similar to that seen with open release.[2] After comparing clinical results with those of anatomical studies such as this, we should redefine the concept of adequate release of the TCL. The results of this study pose the question, what is the minimum release of the TCL needed to adequately decompress the median nerve? Although this study points out a discrepancy between clinical and cadaver data, it does not answer this important question.

E.R. North, M.D.

References

1. Agee J, McCarroll H, Tortosa R, et al. Endoscopic release of the carpal tunnel: A randomized prospective multicenter study. *J Hand Surg (Am)* 17:987–995, 1992.
2. Okutsu I, Ninomiya S, Hamanaka I, et al. Measurement of pressure in the carpal canal before and after endoscopic management of carpal tunnel syndrome. *J Bone Joint Surg (Am)* 71:679–683, 1989.

Prospective Comparison of Minimal Incision "Open" and Two-portal Endoscopic Carpal Tunnel Release
Hallock GG, Lutz DA (Lehigh Valley Hosp, Allentown, Pa)
Plast Reconstr Surg 96:941–947, 1995   7–5

Introduction.—Carpal tunnel release by the endoscopic approach permits a less invasive operation and allows more rapid recovery with less pain and scarring compared with conventional "open" surgery. No definitive difference in long-term relief of symptoms has been documented, but endoscopic surgery had not been compared with an open technique using a minimal incision.

TABLE 2.—Recovery of Function

Time Interval (days)	Open	Endoscopic
Between hands*		
Overall	37.9 ± 12.0 (15)†	33.2 ± 11.9 (19)
Worker's compensation	36.9 ± 12.3 (12)	35.9 ± 11.8 (15)
Nonworkers	42.0 ± 12.1 (3)	22.8 ± 3.5 (4)
Last surgery to last visit		
Overall	53.1 ± 42.4 (49)†	49.3 ± 27.2 (43)
Worker's compensation	77.2 ± 46.7 (23)	65.1 ± 21.9 (25)
Nonworkers	30.0 ± 19.5 (26)	28.8 ± 18.5 (18)
Last surgery to return work		
Overall	46.3 ± 36.9 (39)‡	39.8 ± 19.3 (25)
Worker's compensation	59.5 ± 38.2 (25)	45.9 ± 15.0 (20)
Nonworkers	22.6 ± 18.5 (14)	15.6 ± 15.5 (5)

*Only if a sequential release performed in patients with bilateral carpal tunnel syndrome.
†Values in parentheses are the number of patients in each subset.
‡Values in parentheses are the number of hands in each subset. Patients who never returned to work are not included in these data.
(Courtesy of Hallock GG, Lutz DA: Prospective comparison of minimal incision "open" and two-portal endoscopic carpal tunnel release. *Plast Reconstr Surg* 96:941–947, 1995.)

TABLE 4.—Complications

Type	Open	Endoscopic
Overall	33 (28)*	45 (32)
Worker's compensation	21 (18)	33 (23)
Nonworkers	12 (10)	12 (9)
Hypersensitive scar	19	12
Pillar pain	4	22
Incomplete symptom relief	8	5
Infection	2	2
Other	1	4

*Values in parentheses are the total number of patients with complications.
(Courtesy of Hallock GG, Lutz DA: Prospective comparison of minimal incision "open" and two-portal endoscopic carpal tunnel release. Plast Reconstr Surg 96:941–947, 1995.)

Objective.—The endoscopic and minimal open procedures were compared in a prospective series of 96 patients with medically refractory carpal tunnel syndrome. Forty-one patients with bilateral symptoms had surgery in both hands, for a total of 137 procedures: 71 of them were open procedures and 66 were closed procedures.

Methods.—The incision for open release extended from the distal margin of the transverse carpal ligament toward the distal wrist crease. Under tourniquet control, the ligament and distal deep forearm fascia were divided and an epineurolysis was done on the median nerve. The endoscopic operation used an extrabursal 2-portal technique. The deep forearm fascia was divided along with the carpal ligament. Both operations were done under local bupivacaine anesthesia, supplemented by intravenous sedation.

Results.—Two endoscopic procedures had to be converted to "open" release for technical reasons. Activities of daily living were resumed a few days earlier after endoscopic surgery, and these patients were also able to return sooner to work (Table 2). Five patients receiving workers' compensation who had closed surgery have not yet returned to work. Complications were similarly frequent in the 2 groups (Table 4). Symptoms were incompletely relieved in 11% of patients who had open surgery and 8% of those who had endoscopic surgery. In both groups the average scar was about 2 cm long.

Conclusion.—Open surgery on the carpal tunnel using a minimal incision provides results similar to those achieved endoscopically without the need for special equipment.

▶ In several studies comparing endoscopic with open carpal tunnel release, endoscopic release has been shown to result in significantly earlier return-to-work times. In this prospective study, the authors compared a dual portal endoscopic technique with a dual incision, minimally invasive "open" technique. Although many have suggested that a minimally invasive incision results in less morbidity than the traditional, more extensive, open approach, these authors have indirectly demonstrated a reduction in morbidity (compared with the more extensive, open approach) by comparing a mini-incision technique with an endoscopic technique. They have not demonstrated the inherent safety that they claim endoscopic release lacks. With endoscopy, a nerve injury rate less than 1 per 988 surgeries has been reported,[1] and the authors need more cases to show that their method is even as safe as endoscopic release. It may be, but a much larger series is needed.

E.R. North, M.D.

Reference

1. Agee J, Peimer C, Pyrek J, et al. Endoscopic carpal tunnel release: A prospective study of complications and surgical experience. *J Hand Surg* 20A:165–171, 1995.

Outcome Assessment for Carpal Tunnel Surgery: The Relative Responsiveness of Generic, Arthritis-specific, Disease-specific, and Physical Examination Measures
Amadio PC, Silverstein MD, Ilstrup DM, et al (Mayo Clinic and Mayo Found, Rochester, Minn)
J Hand Surg (Am) 21A:338–346, 1996   7–6

Purpose.—Although carpal tunnel syndrome is a common condition, its effect on health has not been fully evaluated. Many different approaches have been used to evaluate the outcomes of therapy for carpal tunnel syndrome. A standardized outcome assessment for this condition would have many important advantages, including the ability to compare the results of different studies. To standardize and generalize the measurement of outcomes of carpal tunnel syndrome, various clinical and questionnaire measures were compared.

Methods.—The study included 22 consecutive patients who were scheduled for carpal tunnel release. One day before and 3 months after their surgery, the patients completed 3 health-status assessment questionnaires for carpal tunnel syndrome: the Medical Outcomes Study 36-item short form health survey, the Arthritis Impact Measurement Scale, and the Brigham and Women's Hospital carpal tunnel questionnaire. Five physical measures commonly used to assess the results of treatment for the carpal tunnel syndrome were also evaluated: wrist range of motion, power pinch, grip strength, pressure sensibility, and dexterity. The questionnaires were compared for their responsiveness to change from before to after treatment, and their sensitivity was compared with that of the physical measures.

Results.—The postoperative assessments showed significant improvements in the pain, satisfaction, health perception, arthritis impact, and symptom scales of the Arthritis Impact Measurement Scale; in the symptom and function scales of the Brigham and Women's Hospital carpal tunnel questionnaire; and in the physical role, emotional role, and bodily pain scales of the Medical Outcomes Study short form survey. Dexterity was significantly improved on the postoperative assessment, but none of the other physical measures showed a significant change.

Conclusions.—Standardized outcome questionnaires appear to be more sensitive to the results of surgery for carpal tunnel syndrome than the widely used physical measures. A condition-specific questionnaire appears to be especially sensitive to the clinical changes produced by treatment. Future studies of the syndrome should consider using at least 1 of the instruments described; the choice may be determined by the study's specific intent.

▶ Dr. Amadio and co-workers at the Mayo Clinic have continued their interest and expertise in outcome analysis after surgical procedures in the hand and wrist. In this study of 22 patients seen and surveyed 1 day before and 3 months after carpal tunnel release, several currently utilized outcome instruments were used to gain a sense of individual relevance and application. Such objective criteria as range of motion and power pinch were also used. In this study, the condition-specific questionnaire was more sensitive to change than the more generic questionnaires; the outcome questionnaires, in general, were more sensitive to clinical change than many commonly performed physical measures of outcome.

For readers familiar with outcome analysis and the various instruments available, this report will further support the controversies surrounding generic vs. disease-specific questionnaires. This is becoming an increasingly important issue as health care providers are using information generated from these studies to make decisions regarding support for medical intervention. Thus, all investigators must make certain that the outcome tools they use accurately reflect the outcome of these specific problems. The medical neophyte might wonder whether it is more logical to have a disease-specific questionnaire than a generic questionnaire. Yes, one realizes that disease-specific questionnaires would require an inordinate amount of effort to create, and individual investigators may have their own disease-specific questionnaire, thereby limiting the ability to judge and compare results. One might suggest that the national societies involved in these surgical treatments work together to formulate, or at least agree on, standardized disease-specific questionnaires that would enhance the comparison of results.

This study had some major limitations that one must keep in mind when interpreting the results. First, the sample size was very small, and the authors do note that they did not include a concurrent comparison group. Furthermore, only 14 of the 22 patients had physical measures taken at follow-up, and a 3-month follow-up is a short time to evaluate the outcome of any intervention. One would hope that the authors will continue to investigate their patients with a considerably longer follow-up.

A second problem in such a small sample size is that the reader cannot be certain about whether the impression of outcome is influenced by the extent of the median neuropathy or the specific functional needs of the patient. A larger patient sample with more data on the specific neurologic deficits, on both physical examination and electrophysiologic study, would help readers understand the relationship between the deficits and outcome.

In summary, the authors are to be applauded for this preliminary investigational work. However, given that outcome evaluations have entered the field of hand surgery very rapidly (many of which lacked a strong foundation in the epidemiologic aspects and individual assessment tools), the readers must maintain a degree of skepticism in interpreting the data until a widespread agreement develops regarding methodology and specific instruments for evaluation.

J.B. Jupiter, M.D.

Symptoms, Functional Status, and Neuromuscular Impairment Following Carpal Tunnel Release
Katz JN, Fossel KK, Simmons BP, et al (Robert Bingham Multipurpose Arthritis and Musculoskeletal Disease Ctr, Boston; Brigham and Women's Hosp, Boston)
J Hand Surg (Am) 20A:549–555, 1995   7-7

Background.—Although carpal tunnel release is the most common hand procedure, studies of its outcome have been hampered by brief duration of follow-up and a lack of standardized measures of improvement. The rate of resolution of specific symptoms and functional limitations was measured for 2 years after carpal tunnel release in 35 patients.

Methods.—Thirty-five patients were followed prospectively from before surgery to an average of 27 months afterward. Four patients had diabetes mellitus and 4 had rheumatoid arthritis. All patients completed questionnaires and underwent measurement of grip and pinch strength and 2-point discrimination and elicitation of Tinel and Phelan signs. Although not all patients returned for each evaluation, no outcome difference was seen between those who were seen at each interval and those who missed some appointments.

Results.—Symptom scores decreased rapidly by the sixth week after surgery, then increased slightly at 2 years. Symptoms were significantly improved at 3 months and 2 years after surgery. Tingling, numbness, and nocturnal pain and numbness all improved remarkably within 3 weeks. Self-reported weakness improved most slowly and to the least degree. However, all symptoms were significantly better at 2 years. Functional scores improved more slowly but were also significantly better at 3 months and 2 years. Grip strength weakened after surgery, began to recover at 3 months, and was significantly improved at 2 years. Pinch strength improved slowly but significantly by 2 years. Two-point discrimination and the Tinel and Phelan signs improved irregularly. At 2 years, 8 patients had worse symptom scores and 3 had worse functional scores. The 4 diabetic patients followed the average pattern of improvement, but the 4 patients with rheumatoid arthritis remained more symptomatic and more functionally impaired than the group as a whole.

Conclusion.—Specific symptoms and functional impairments improve at different rates after carpal tunnel release. Pain and paresthesia improve within weeks, but functional status improves over months to years.

▶ For the worker, the term "simple carpal tunnel" has become an oxymoron. Thus, studies that provide long-term information on the outcome of patients' symptoms and function have become increasingly important. Although this study evaluated only a small number of patients, it showed the feasibility of such outcome measurements. Future studies with more patients will provide even more meaningful information.

S.E. Mackinnon, M.D.

Carpal Tunnel Syndrome in Patients Undergoing CAPD: A Collaborative Study in 143 Centers
Nomoto Y, Kawaguchi Y, Ohira S, et al (Tokai Univ, Isehara City, Japan; Jikei Univ, Tokyo; Iwamizawa City Hosp, Japan; et al)
Am J Nephrol 15:295–299, 1995   7–8

Objective.—Patients receiving hemodialysis appear to be at increased risk for carpal tunnel syndrome (CTS). Reasons for this association may include arteriovenous access, intermittent fluid overload, and localized elevations in venous pressure. Patients undergoing continuous ambulatory peritoneal dialysis (CAPD) were studied to determine their incidence of CTS.

Patients and Findings.—A 13-year review of 5,050 patients receiving CAPD from 143 Japanese dialysis centers identified only 7 patients with CTS. The incidence of CTS in patients receiving CAPD was thus 0.14%. All 7 patients were women (average age, 52 years). Carpal tunnel syndrome developed 12–108 months after the start of CAPD in 5 patients who were treated solely with CAPD. The other 2 patients had received hemodialysis for 7 to 9 years before being switched to CAPD; their CTS developed 9 years after the start of CAPD. All but 1 of the patients with CTS had no residual urine volume. Carpal bone cysts were seen in 3 of the 7 women with CTS but in none of the patients receiving CAPD who did not have CTS. Five patients underwent surgical decompression, which alleviated their symptoms dramatically. Two of 5 surgical specimens studied showed amyloid deposits, and 2 of 4 showed β_2-microglobulin.

Discussion.—Japanese patients receiving CAPD have a low incidence of CTS. The findings of this and previous studies suggest that amyloid deposits could play a major role in dialysis-related CTS. Long-term complications, including CTS and malnutrition, in patients with end-stage renal disease could result from metabolic changes occurring after the loss of residual urine.

▶ This large, multicenter study suggests that there is a much lower prevalence of carpal tunnel syndrome in patients undergoing peritoneal dialysis than in patients undergoing hemodialysis. Long-term continuous ambulatory peritoneal dialysis is used less frequently in the United States than in Japan, the source of this study. The article is valuable reading in terms of its discussions of the possible relationship between dialysis, either peritoneal or hemodialysis, and the development of carpal tunnel syndrome.

V.R. Hentz, M.D.

Outcome of Reoperation for Carpal Tunnel Syndrome
Cobb TK, Amadio PC, Leatherwood DF, et al (Mayo Clinic and Mayo Found, Rochester, Minn)
J Hand Surg (Am) 21A:347–356, 1996   7–9

Background.—Many patients continue to have symptoms after surgery for carpal tunnel syndrome. The reported prevalence of this complication ranges from 7% to 20%, the most common cause being inadequate release of the distal part of the flexor retinaculum. No large studies have addressed the results of reoperation for carpal tunnel syndrome, and the outcomes of this patient population have not been standardized. The results of reoperation for carpal tunnel syndrome in 131 patients were analyzed.

Methods.—The patients underwent a second operation for carpal tunnel syndrome between 1970 and 1990. There were 87 women and 44 men, when the second operation was performed, the median age was 52 years. Their outcomes at a mean follow-up of 11 years were evaluated by a standardized questionnaire, which asked about symptoms, functional status, and satisfaction.

Results.—Fifteen patients required a third operation, their second operation was therefore considered a failure. Although most of the remaining patients rated their procedure as at least somewhat successful, 14 said it was completely unsuccessful. Twenty-two of the 116 patients reported dissatisfaction with the results of the operation. Sixty-eight percent had residual symptoms after reoperation.

The results were significantly worse for patients who had normal results on preoperative nerve conduction tests, those who filed for compensation, and those with pain in the ulnar nerve distribution. In contrast, patients with abnormal findings on nerve conduction studies and who had not filed for compensation had the best results. Incomplete flexor retinaculum release was related to the absence of a symptom-free period after the initial release but not with the final symptoms or patient satisfaction. The type of surgical procedure performed did not affect outcome.

Conclusions.—The results of reoperation for carpal tunnel syndrome are not as good as those of primary surgery. Complete satisfaction, with no residual symptoms, will be achieved in only about one fourth of patients. In addition, poor results are obtained in about one fourth of cases. The final results are significantly better for patients with abnormal results of nerve conduction studies done before surgery.

▶ Cobb et al. have written a detailed and comprehensive analysis of the outcome after reoperation for carpal tunnel syndrome. This important article should be read by anyone involved in the surgical care of patients with carpal tunnel syndrome.

The authors' conclusions can be applied to patients being considered for primary carpal tunnel decompression. One cannot overemphasize the importance of the initial evaluation of someone suspected of having carpal tunnel syndrome. Surgeons should proceed with caution when paresthesias or pain do not follow the median nerve distribution, especially if compensation is involved. If carpal tunnel syndrome is suspected, I believe confirmatory electrodiagnostic studies are mandatory. Although carpal tunnel syndrome can exist in the presence of normal electrical studies, my anecdotal experience has been that carpal tunnel decompression done in patients with normal electrical study results has led to a significant number of dissatisfied patients. Carpal tunnel syndrome is a quality, not quantity of life problem. When elective surgery is performed, the odds for success can be maximized by proper patient selection. Paresthesias and pain not in the median nerve distribution and borderline results of electrical studies do not justify surgery. Remember that reoperation has a 25% to 40% failure rate.

P.J. Stern, M.D.

Carpal Tunnel Surgery Outcomes in Workers: Effect of Workers' Compensation Status
Higgs PE, Edwards D, Martin DS, et al (Washington Univ, St Louis, Mo)
J Hand Surg (Am) 20A:354–360, 1995   7–10

Background.—The prognosis of patients undergoing surgery for occupational carpal tunnel syndrome (CTS) may be less favorable than that for patients treated surgically for CTS in general. It is unclear whether the work itself or the enticement of financial gain is the main contributor to these less favorable outcomes. The outcomes of patients whose occupational CTS was covered by workers' compensation were compared with those of patients whose occupational CTS was not covered.

Methods.—One hundred thirteen patients with workers' compensation and 53 without workers' compensation were studied. Information was elicited regarding job status and the residual symptoms of numbness, pain, or nocturnal awakening a mean of 42 months after surgery.

Findings.—Fifty-three patients with workers' compensation and 39 without workers' compensation were working at their original jobs. Seventeen patients with workers' compensation were unemployed compared with 2 without workers' compensation; this difference was significant. Of those who changed jobs, 39 patients with workers' compensation and 2 without compensation attributed the change to CTS symptoms. Those with workers' compensation had significantly more residual symptoms than those without workers' compensation. Ninety-two of the former group and 26 of the latter group reported some residual symptoms.

Conclusions.—Although a causal relationship between workers' compensation and poor outcomes cannot be inferred from these data, they do show an association between the two. Additional, carefully designed prospective studies are needed to fully determine the reasons for the poor outcomes reported here.

▶ Although this is a case-control study, it is well done and supports other evidence showing that patients entering into the compensatory system tend to have more subjective symptoms.

M.L. Kasdan, M.D.

Long-term Results of Carpal Tunnel Release
Nancollas MP, Peimer CA, Wheeler DR, et al (State Univ of New York, Buffalo)
J Hand Surg (Br) 20B:470–474, 1995   7–11

Background.—The surgical treatment of median nerve compression in the carpal tunnel is now widely accepted and commonly performed. Although many studies have demonstrated the short-term benefits of carpal tunnel release, few reports on the long-term outcomes have been published.

Methods.—Data on 60 procedures performed in 52 patients (35 women and 17 men) were reviewed a mean of 5.5 years after surgery. Eight patients (13%) had bilateral procedures. At the time of surgery, the mean patient age was 44 years. In 42% of the patients, carpal tunnel syndrome (CTS) was job related.

Findings.—The outcomes of surgery were good or excellent in 87% of patients. The mean time to maximum improvement in symptoms was 9.8 months. Thirty percent of the patients reported strength that was only poor to fair and long-term scar discomfort. In 57% of the patients, some preoperative symptoms returned, most often pain, beginning at a mean of 2 years after surgery. Neither preoperative symptoms nor the extent of surgical dissection was associated with outcome. Twenty-six percent of the patients with job-related CTS switched from heavy to lighter work after surgery. Patients with occupational CTS improved more slowly and remained off from work longer, but the long-term subjective outcomes were the same for both groups.

Conclusions.—In this long-term assessment of the results of carpal tunnel release, morbidity from the surgical scar was significant and strength decreased. Furthermore, the delay to ultimate improvement was often long, especially in patients with job-related CTS.

▶ Although many aspects of this study can be criticized, such as relying on a patient's memory for events occurring 5 years previously, it presents an important message: The most important factors leading to long-term patient dissatisfaction are not consequences of the syndrome but rather consequences of the treatment. Efforts directed at modifying the sequelae of previous standard surgical procedures for this often time-limited condition should be applauded rather than condemned.

V.R. Hentz, M.D.

Workers' Compensation Recipients With Carpal Tunnel Syndrome: The Validity of Self-reported Health Measures
Katz JN, Punnett L, Simmons BP, et al (Brigham and Women's Hosp, Boston; Univ of Massachusetts, Lowell; Maine Health Information Ctr, Augusta)
Am J Public Health 86:52–56, 1996   7–12

Introduction.—The reluctance to use self-report measures of health-related quality of life in workers is likely based on doubts about the validity of self-report in patients receiving workers' compensation. It has been argued that these patients have incentives to amplify and seek medical care for symptoms that others manage without complaint. The reliability, validity, and responsiveness of self-report scales were compared in patients with carpal tunnel syndrome who were recipients and nonrecipients of workers' compensation.

Methods.—Both groups of patients with carpal tunnel syndrome underwent baseline physical examination and grip strength measurements, and were interviewed regarding symptoms severity, functional status, and satisfaction with outcome of surgery, if it had been performed. Patients were mailed a follow-up questionnaire 6 months after baseline.

Results.—Of 268 patients at baseline, 155 were workers' compensation recipients and 113 were nonrecipients. At 6-month follow-up, 121 recipients and 95 nonrecipients returned questionnaires. Recipients of workers' compensation were a few years younger and had somewhat worse symptom severity and functional status scores than nonrecipients. In both groups, women had worse functional status scores and lower grip strength than men. Symptom duration was significantly shorter in the recipient than in the nonrecipient group (2.2 vs. 5.6 months). Female recipients were significantly less satisfied with results of surgery and less symptomatically improved than female nonrecipients. There was no significant difference in satisfaction or symptomatic improvement among male recipients and nonrecipients. Reliability of functional status, symptom severity, and satisfaction scales for recipients and nonrecipients were nearly identical. The correlation between subjective assessment of weakness and objective measures of grip strength showed good validity and was not influenced by whether or not patients received workers' compensation. The correlations between improvements in symptom severity, functional status scores, patient satisfaction, perceived improvement in quality of life, and perceived improvement of symptoms were higher in the recipient than in the nonrecipient group.

Conclusion.—In patients with carpal tunnel syndrome, self-report measures of symptom severity, functional status, and satisfaction had comparable reliability, validity, and responsiveness in recipients and nonrecipients of workers' compensation. Self-report measures appear to be suitable for research in patients receiving workers' compensation.

Clinical Significance.—Financial incentives may influence return to work in recipients of workers' compensation. However, patients' responses to questionnaires in the research setting do not seem to be influenced by whether or not they are recipients. The inclusion of quality-of-life measures in trials of occupation-associated illness is encouraged.

▶ For those who might question the reliability of questionnaires in worker's compensation patients, here is evidence to the contrary. Differences between patients who receive compensation and those who do not may relate to different perceptions, but not to any difference in the consistency of responses.

P.C. Amadio, M.D.

Sequelae of Carpal Tunnel Surgery: Rationale for the Design of a Surgical Approach
Abdullah AF, Wolber PH, Ditto EW III (Washington County Hosp, Hagerstown, Md)
Neurosurgery 37:931–936, 1995   7–13

Introduction.—A review of various studies suggest that the sequelae of carpal tunnel surgery appear to be related to the linear vertical section of the transverse carpal ligament. It is assumed that anterior displacement of the median nerve and flexor tendons between the cut ends of the transverse carpal ligament may be responsible. In addition, the vertical incision may result in a continuous scar through the skin. On the basis of the concept of the pathogenesis of carpal tunnel syndrome, a modified approach to ligament section was designed to avoid the untoward sequelae of carpal tunnel surgery.

Procedure.—The modified approach was designed to reduce pressure in the carpal tunnel while retaining the integrity of the ligament as a barrier between the median nerve and the surface of the wrist and to preserve its function as a pulley–restraint for more efficient functioning of the flexor tendons. The crucial element of this surgical approach was a parabolic incision in the transverse carpal ligament that left a protective flap to cover the nerve and tendons within the tunnel in the area of maximum convexity of the wrist (Fig 1). By the use of narrow retractors and focused lightning, the ligament could be visualized in its entirety except sometimes for the distal 1 cm.

Results.—Compared with the sequelae observed in 770 previous patients of the same surgeon who used a vertical incision in the ligament, the

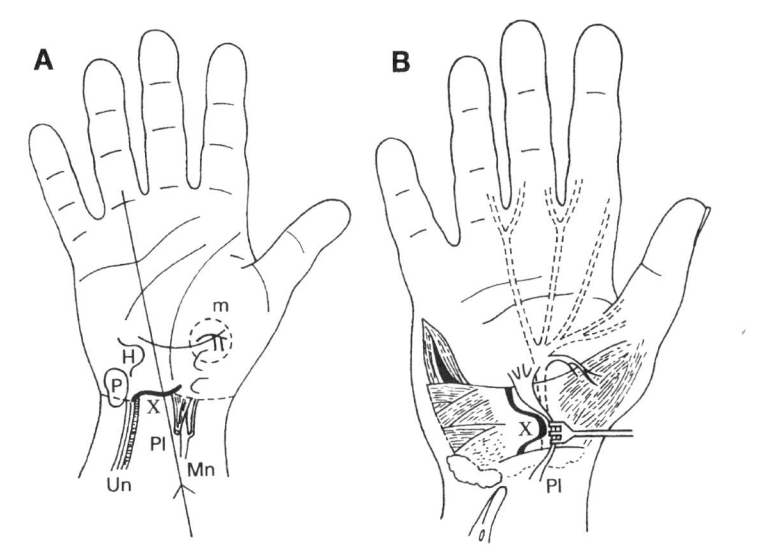

FIGURE 1.—**A,** near transverse incision at the distal wrist crease may be extended at both ends to an S incision if necessary. The direction of the *arrows* shows the line of dissection. The flaps are undetermined, and narrow right angle (Senn or Brewster) retractors are used to lift the lower flap and expose the distal area of ligament. **B,** parabolic incision in the transverse carpal ligament retains ligament flap coverage of the tunnel in area of maximum convexity of the wrist. *Abbreviations:* H, hamate; M, motor branch of median nerve; *Mn,* median nerve; *P,* pisiform; *Pl,* palmaris longus tendon ending in palmar aponeurosis; *Un,* ulnar nerve and vessels. (Courtesy of Abdullah AF, Wolber PH, Ditto EW III: Sequelae of carpal tunnel surgery: rationale for the design of a surgical approach. *Neurosurgery* 37:931–936, 1995.)

modified approach to carpal tunnel surgery significantly reduced the incidence of untoward postoperative sequelae in 100 patients. At 1 month after surgery, only 2 patients had residual numbness attributed to occasional transection of a medial branch of the palmar cutaneous nerve by the skin incision. All patients had complete relief of symptoms after 1 month, and all returned to work and normal activity.

Conclusion.—For carpal tunnel surgery, the parabolic incision accomplishes the same degree of expansion of the ligament with the same proportionate increase in the volume of the carpal tunnel as does a vertical linear incision, the former incision, however, prevents the wide gaping of the tunnel space that is associated with the latter. Although the edges are less separated in the oblique limbs, the longer incision compensates by providing a total surface area of the spread similar to that of other incisions. Furthermore, expansion of the ligament is not in 1 dimension as in the vertical incision, and the lesser spread in the oblique limbs promotes faster healing.

▶ The authors' retrospective series of 100 new cases compared with 770 historical controls has no statistical significance. No objective electrophysiologic data are presented, nor was any variable such as grip strength, pinch strength, or sensibility measured for quantitative comparison. The use of a transverse incision for open technique has long been condemned by hand surgeons but still finds popularity among neurosurgeons performing carpal tunnel release. Nevertheless, the concept of making a parabolic incision to section the transverse carpal ligament instead of a linear vertical incision merits some further study. This incision is not dissimilar to a Z-plasty lengthening of the transverse carpal ligament, but no sutures are placed to approximate the flaps. The authors have demonstrated that this can be done safely, but whether this is worth the trouble must be answered in a prospective randomized study.

R.M. Szabo, M.D., M.P.H.

Position of the Wrist Associated With the Lowest Carpal-tunnel Pressure: Implications for Splint Design
Weiss ND, Gordon L, Bloom T, et al (Univ of California, San Francisco)
J Bone Joint Surg (Am) 77-A:1695–1699, 1995   7–14

Introduction.—Treatment of carpal tunnel syndrome consists of immobilization of the wrist. Immobilization of the wrist is thought to prevent elevations of carpal tunnel pressure, thereby relieving symptoms. Many wrist splints currently available place the wrist in a position of 20 to 30 degrees of extension. However, the wrist position that results in the lowest carpal tunnel pressure is unknown. Carpal tunnel pressure was continuously measured throughout a wide range of motion of the wrist to determine the wrist position associated with the lowest carpal tunnel pressure.

Methods.—Four patients with carpal tunnel syndrome and 24 controls were studied. Patients and controls were examined by a hand surgeon for signs and symptoms of carpal tunnel syndrome, including evaluations of muscle strength, presence of thenar atrophy, and sensations to touch in the hands and fingers. Electrodiagnostic studies of the median nerve tests for the Phalen and Tinel signs were also done. Carpal tunnel pressure was measured using a pressure transducer inserted into the carpal canal through a catheter. Wrist position was measured using a 2-channel electrogoniometer. Patients and controls moved their wrist slowly in all directions through a wide range of motion. Motions and positions were repeated until the position that had the lowest carpal tunnel pressure was found. Carpal tunnel pressure and wrist position were recorded simultaneously.

Results.—For controls, carpal tunnel pressure increased as the wrist was moved away from a neutral position, resulting in a parabolic relationship. The lowest average carpal tunnel pressure was found to be 8 ± 4 mm Hg in controls, with an average position of 2 ± 9 degrees of extension and 2 ± 6 degrees of ulnar deviation. For patients with carpal tunnel syndrome, the average positions associated with the lowest pressure were similar to those observed for controls, however, the average lowest carpal tunnel pressures were significantly higher than controls, at 19 ± 2 mm Hg. As with the controls, the relationship between carpal tunnel pressure and wrist position were parabolic for patients with carpal tunnel syndrome.

No significant changes between the lowest pressure and associated positions were found during the 4-hour test period in either group.

Conclusion.—Elevations in carpal tunnel pressure at extremes of motion in patients with carpal tunnel syndrome as compared with controls have been previously reported. The results of this study indicate that carpal tunnel pressure is significantly elevated in patients with carpal tunnel syndrome even when the wrist is in positions that slightly deviate from the neutral position. Wrist splints that place the wrist in a functional position may not provide maximum benefit in the treatment of carpal tunnel syndrome. A position closer to neutral should be used for wrist immobilization.

▶ Movements of the wrist away from the neutral position and finger flexion will increase pressures within the carpal tunnel. These positions are frequently assumed during sleep and probably account for the early and common reports of nocturnal paresthesia in patients with carpal tunnel syndrome. Prefabricated wrist splints are marketed for use in a functional position of wrist extension. Physicians treating carpal tunnel syndrome must recognize that splints that position the wrist in extension will, in fact, increase pressures within the carpal tunnel and probably exacerbate the symptoms of the syndrome. Patients should be advised to straighten their wrist splints to ensure that they maintain their wrists in a neutral position. The authors are to be congratulated for bringing science to this empirical suggestion.

S.E. Mackinnon, M.D.

Restricted Motion of the Median Nerve in Carpal Tunnel Syndrome
Nakamichi K, Tachibana S (Toranomon Hosp, Minato-ku, Tokyo, Japan)
J Hand Surg (Br) 20B:460–464, 1995   7–15

Introduction.—Adhesion of the median nerve to the flexor retinaculum is often a characteristic finding in surgery for carpal tunnel syndrome (CTS). The extent to which the physiologic mobility of the nerve was decreased in CTS was studied.

Methods.—Motion of the median nerve was compared on axial ultrasonographic imaging in the midcarpal tunnel in 30 wrists of 15 women with bilateral idiopathic CTS and 30 wrists of 15 healthy women.

Results.—During passive flexion and extension of the index finger, the control wrists had transverse sliding of the nerve beneath the flexor retinaculum, a motion that was considered to be physiologic. Significantly less sliding was seen in the wrists of patients with CTS, indicating that the physiologic motion of the nerve is restricted.

Conclusion.—The decrease in nerve mobility in CTS may play a role in the pathophysiology of the syndrome. In the presence of nerve adhesions, motion of the wrist and flexor tendons might cause deformation of the nerve, stretching, or traction.

▶ The authors report decreased excursion of the median nerve at the wrist in patients with CTS compared with an age- and sex-matched control group. This simple but elegant study has implications for the pathophysiology of chronic nerve compression and postoperative management of any peripheral nerve reconstruction. The study emphasizes a nerve's need to glide through its surrounding soft-tissue bed. Recommendations for early postoperative movement after any peripheral nerve surgery are supported by these findings.

S.E. Mackinnon, M.D.

Low-dose, Short-term Oral Prednisone in the Treatment of Carpal Tunnel Syndrome
Herskovitz S, Berger AR, Lipton RB (Albert Einstein College of Medicine, Bronx, NY)
Neurology 45:1923–1925, 1995

Background.—Carpal tunnel syndrome (CTS) is a significant source of morbidity. Most patients are initially treated with conservative, nonoperative therapy. The efficacy of low-dose, short-term oral prednisone on the symptoms of CTS was examined in a randomized, double-blind, placebo-controlled study.

Methods.—Patients with mild to moderate CTS had screening that included standard medical and neurologic history, detailed neurologic examination, bilateral nerve conduction studies (NCS), and needle electromyography. Eligible participants had a 1-week therapy washout period and returned for baseline assessment, including measurement of bilateral quantitative thermal and vibratory threshold and a standard symptom questionnaire. The end point variable was the global symptom score (GSS), the mean score of 5 rated symptoms. After baseline evaluation, 6 patients were randomly assigned to receive prednisone, 20 mg daily for 1 week and 10 mg daily for the second week, and 9 patients were randomly assigned to receive matched placebo treatment for 2 weeks. Follow-up evaluations at 2, 4, and 8 weeks included neurologic examination quantitative thermal and vibratory threshold measurement, bilateral nerve conduction studies, and the standard symptom questionnaire.

Results.—Three patients were lost to follow-up and were not included in the analysis. At 2-week follow-up, significantly more improvement was detected in the treatment group by the global symptom score and self-report. Symptoms gradually began to return after discontinuation of therapy. Three patients in each group reported adverse reactions, but none discontinued therapy. Results of neurologic examination, nerve conduction studies, and measurements of quantitative thermal and vibratory measurements did not significantly change.

Conclusions.—This small controlled clinical trial demonstrated that low-dose, short-term oral prednisone therapy resulted in significant improvement in the symptoms of CTS in patients with the mild to moderate form of the syndrome. Symptoms worsened after discontinuation of therapy. Although further research is necessary to optimize this treatment, low-dose oral steroids may become an effective conservative therapy for patients with mild CTS.

▶ These results indicate that low-dose oral steroids provide effective but short-term relief of symptoms in a significant percentage of patients with mild to moderately symptomatic CTS. Many patients recoil at the suggestion of an injection into an already uncomfortable hand and wrist, and inadvertent and damaging intraneural injections still occur too frequently. However, to date, no prospective study has addressed the relative effectiveness of orally administered vs. injected steroid. The use of low-dose steroids may answer one anecdotal criticism of therapy with higher-dose steroids—the potential for the development of avascular necrosis.

V.R. Hentz, M.D.

A Comparison of Traditional Electrodiagnostic Studies, Electroneurometry, and Vibrometry in the Diagnosis of Carpal Tunnel Syndrome
Cherniack MG, Moalli D, Viscolli C (Yale Univ, New Haven, Conn; Mem Hosp, New London, Conn)
J Hand Surg (Am) 21A:122–131, 1996   7–17

Objective.—In addition to conventional nerve conduction studies for carpal tunnel syndrome (CTS), new alternative qualitative tests that use portable devices have been introduced. These tests require less training and have potentially lower costs. The results of electroneurometry, vibrometry, and conventional nerve testing, all performed on the same patients and controls, were compared.

Methods.—Nerve conduction and electroneurometer studies were performed with an electromyograph, an electroneurometer, and a vibrometer on the median and ulnar nerves of 49 patients (98 hands). Ten hospital workers (20 hands) served as the control group. The ability of each method to distinguish median nerve entrapment in CTS was tested in recognition models and analyzed statistically. Electrophysiologic thresholds for each method were established empirically.

Results.—Median nerve measurements made with the electroneurometer were more significantly associated with motor nerve conduction latencies than with sensory nerve conduction latencies. The opposite was true for vibrometry measurements. There was no association with either sensory or motor latency in the control group. Median nerve entrapment was diagnosed by conventional nerve conduction studies, with a sensitivity of 0.94 and a specificity of 0.60. Diagnosis using the vibrometer was much less sensitive but was uniformly specific. The electroneurometer provided specific (0.93–0.95) and sensitive diagnoses of median nerve entrapment. These results depended on the threshold values used. The manufacturer's recommended normal thresholds gave good correlations, but normal values selected from control populations resulted in weak correlations.

Conclusion.—Before vibrometry and electroneurometry can be used in screening for CTS, additional studies need to be conducted and techniques need to be standardized.

▶ This work contributes timely data and context to the issues of neurometry and vibrometry in screening for CTS and underscores several basic considerations. Vibrometry primarily addresses receptor injury of the fingertip and is correspondingly inadequate as a screening evaluation of intratunnel nerve function. Motor nerve assessment with neurometry omits the widely recognized sensitivity advantages of sensory fiber evaluation. Accordingly, the authors demonstrated conventional, control-based, 2-SD–threshold sensitivities of 20% at best. The insensitivities and inherent technique-dependent variabilities suggest that these methodologies do not significantly complement definitive electrodiagnostic evaluation and may compromise patient care.

P.A. Nathan, M.D.

Wrist Squareness and Median Nerve Impairment
Sposato RC, Riley MW, Ballard JL, et al (Univ of Nebraska, Lincoln)
J Occup Environ Med 37:1122–1126, 1995   7–18

Introduction.—Previous studies suggest that carpal tunnel syndrome (CTS) is more likely to occur in persons whose wrist-squareness ratio is greater than 0.7. Such a ratio is associated with median sensory latencies greater than 3.7 ms, usually a predictor of CTS. A volunteer group of 417 railroad maintenance workers was examined for the relationship between wrist squareness and the median nerve impairment typical of CTS.

Methods.—The study group consisted of 375 men and 42 women (mean age, 39.8 years). A small sliding caliper was used to measure wrist dimensions at the proximal wrist crease. Wrist squareness was defined as the ratio of wrist thickness divided by wrist width. Electrodiagnostic testing was performed on motor and sensory fibers of the median nerve. Before testing, heating pads were used to warm the hands to a temperature greater than 31°C. According to the electrophysiologic characteristics of the median nerve of the distal segment, study participants were categorized as normal or abnormal. Motor latency or sensory latency of 4.4 ms or greater was considered abnormal.

Results.—Forty of the 417 study participants (9.6%) were considered to be abnormal according to results of electrodiagnostic testing; this prevalence rate is slightly higher than the suggested CTS prevalence rate (approximately 6%) in the general population of United States workers.

Neither men nor women showed a significant linear relationship between nerve latency and squareness ratios of the wrists.

Conclusion.—This sample of workers did not exhibit an association between increasing wrist-squareness ratios and greater median motor and sensory nerve conduction latency values. The wrist-squareness ratio is therefore not clinically useful as a predictor of CTS or as a way to identify workers who have the impaired median nerve function typical of CTS.

▶ Despite providing evidence to the contrary, the authors conclude that "wrist squareness is not a useful predictor of median nerve impairment typical of CTS." In the left hands, highly significant linear correlations were seen between wrist-squareness and median nerve sensory latency ($r = .179$; $P < 0.001$) and between wrist squareness and median nerve motor latency ($r = 0.182$; $P < 0.001$).

The report lacks tables and other data that would allow the reader to verify the authors' findings and conclusions. No means or standard deviations are given for the wrist-squareness ratio (depth-width ratio). It would have been helpful to have had a 2 × 2 table (slowing versus wrist squareness) using the standard cutoff value of greater than or equal to 0.70 for the wrist-squareness ratio.

Our experience[1-3] and that of others[4-6] has been that the wrist-squareness ratio has been useful for classifying patients and hands as to median nerve slowing status. For a large group of U.S. industrial workers, patients, students, and retirees, we find a correlation coefficient of 0.222 ($R^2 = 0.049$) for the linear correlation between the wrist-squareness ratio and maximum latency difference. The relationship between wrist dimensions and maximum latency difference, which is even stronger for the sexes separately, allows us to correctly classify 66% of male hands and 68% of female hands. This finding suggests that wrist dimensions are useful predictors of the median nerve impairment typical of CTS.

P.A. Nathan, M.D.

References

1. Nathan PA, Keniston RC, Myers LD, et al: Obesity as a risk factor for slowing of sensory conduction of the median nerve in industry: A cross-sectional and longitudinal study involving 429 workers. *J Occup Med* 34:379–383, 1992.
2. Nathan PA, Keniston RC: Carpal tunnel syndrome and its relationship to general physical condition. *Hand Clinics* 9:253–261, 1993.
3. Nathan PA, Keniston RC, Lockwood RS, et al: Tobacco, caffeine, alcohol and carpal tunnel syndrome in American industry. *J Occup Environ Med* 38:290–298, 1996.
4. Radecki P: A gender specific wrist ratio and the likelihood of a median nerve abnormality at the carpal tunnel. *Am J Phys Med Rehabil* 73:157–162, 1994.
5. Johnson EW, Gatens T, Poindexter D, et al: Wrist dimensions: correlation with median sensory latencies. *Arch Phys Med Rehabil* 64:556–557, 1983.
6. Gordon C, Johnson EW, Gatens PF, et al: Wrist ratio correlation with carpal tunnel syndrome in industry. *Am J Phys Med Rehabil* 67:270–272, 1988.

Temperature Effects on Vibrotactile Sensitivity Threshold Measurements: Implications for Carpal Tunnel Screening Tests

Klinenberg E, So Y, Rempel D (Brooks Air Force Base, Tex; Univ of California, San Francisco)
J Hand Surg (Am) 21A:132–137, 1996   7–19

Background.—Multifrequency vibrometry offers promise as a technique for the screening and early detection of carpal tunnel syndrome. The vibrometer is used to measure vibrotactile sensitivity at a patient's fingertip, with sensitivities obtained at a variety of frequencies. Vibrotactile sensitivity may be influenced by many factors, however, including contact force, age, height, and skin temperature. The effect of skin temperature on vibrotactile sensitivity measurements was examined in a study of 20 adults who had no history of carpal tunnel syndrome or diabetes.

Methods.—Study participants were 11 men and 9 women (mean age, 34 years); all were actively working. Four vibratory frequencies (31.5, 125, 250, and 500 Hz) were tested on the glabrous skin on the right middle fingertip. For each frequency, 6 temperature categories were used. Initial measurements were done at room temperature. Participants then placed their fingers and hand in ice water until fingertip temperature reached 17–20°C. Vibrotactile thresholds were continuously measured until hands warmed to 32–35°C.

Results.—Lower fingertip skin temperatures were associated with decreases in vibrotactile sensitivity. In both men and women, significant subject and temperature effects were seen at all frequencies. The greatest temperature effects were observed at higher frequencies, with significant effects beginning at 29°C for 500 Hz. Temperature effects at 31.5 Hz were minimal. The effects of temperature on vibrotactile sensitivity can be substantial and may lead to false-positive results.

Conclusion.—The value of multifrequency vibrometry in the early detection of CTS depends on the measurement accuracy of each vibrotactile sensitivity threshold and the choice of cutoff points for CTS. To minimize errors, a skin temperature greater than 29°C is recommended. Fingertip temperature should be warmed so that this level is maintained during the measurement.

▶ Vibrotactile sensitivity testing appears to be gaining acceptance as a screening tool for detecting neuropathies of the upper extremity. Objective investigation of possible confounders of this form of assessment is essential if it is to be used as a screening tool for peripheral neuropathies.

The authors have appropriately raised the issue of temperature as a possible confounder of vibrotactile sensitivity testing. Their results seem to confirm that hand temperature can affect testing outcome and suggest that controlling for temperature can result in a more valid test.

The authors have pointed out many potential flaws in their investigation. Nonetheless, it seems logical to expect that temperature variations can affect this technique of sensation measurement just as temperature has been shown to affect the outcome of nerve conduction study measurements.

It is not clear from this study whether temperature variation affects the nerve as a whole or simply the receptor end organ (Meissner and Pacinian corpuscles). This raises the larger and more important question of whether the test is primarily of the sensory end organs or an assessment of the nerve itself. If vibrotactile sensation testing is primarily a measurement of sensory end organ function, it cannot be used as an independent, objective method for screening for primary nerve conditions such as carpal tunnel syndrome.

P.A. Nathan, M.D.

Electrodiagnostic Testing and Carpal Tunnel Release Outcome
Glowacki KA, Breen CJ, Sachar K, et al (Brown Univ, Providence, RI)
J Hand Surg (Am) 21A:117–122, 1996   7–20

Introduction.—Electrodiagnostic testing is often used in the diagnosis of carpal tunnel syndrome (CTS), despite the recognition that negative results do not exclude the possibility of CTS. To assess the value of electrodiagnostic testing, the eventual outcome of carpal tunnel release in patients with presumed CTS was compared with the preoperative findings of electromyographic–nerve conduction velocity (EMG–NCV) studies.

Patients and Methods.—Study participants were 167 patients (227 hands) who underwent an open carpal tunnel release. The 35 men and 132 women had an average age of 42 years. All surgeries were done by the same surgeon between 1991 and 1994. Of 93 patients who had EMG–NCV studies, 74 (99 hands) had a positive result and 22 (27 hands) had a negative result. Clinical diagnosis was based on the finding of numbness and tingling in the median nerve distribution at night or during activities of daily living and either a positive Phalen's test result or Tinel's sign at the carpal tunnel region. Four groups of outcomes were defined: complete resolution of symptoms, improvement with occasional symptoms, no change, and worse.

Results.—Nearly all patients with positive EMG–NCV results had both daytime and nocturnal symptoms and a positive Phalen's test result; 50 of 99 hands had a positive Tinel's sign. After surgery, 64 of 99 hands had complete resolution of symptoms, 28 had occasional symptoms, 5 were unchanged, and 2 were worse. Twenty-six of 27 hands in the group with negative EMG–NCV results had a positive Phalen's test result, 16 had a positive Tinel's sign, 26 had nocturnal symptoms, and 24 had symptoms with activities of daily living. Surgery was followed by complete resolution of symptoms in 16 hands, occasional symptoms in 9, and worsening symptoms in 2. Preoperative findings and outcome were similar in the group in which no EMG–NCV studies were done. Sixty-one of 101 hands had complete resolution of symptoms, 33 had occasional symptoms, 6 had no change, and 1 was worse. Symptom outcome of carpal tunnel release did not differ significantly among the 3 groups or between the workers' compensation and the non–workers' compensation subgroups.

Conclusion.—Although the reproducibility and validity of the EMG–NCV test are good, the correlation of test results with outcome from carpal tunnel release surgery has not been established. This study indicates that for patients who meet specific diagnostic criteria for carpal tunnel syndrome, EMG–NCV studies may not be necessary. The test is recommended, however, for patients with confounding symptoms or those who do not meet strict diagnostic-inclusion criteria.

▶ This article showed no correlation between preoperative electrodiagnostic test results and outcome after carpal tunnel release surgery. These outcome findings are not surprising in view of the heterogeneity of the sample and the lack of specificity of both the case definition and the electrodiagnostic measurements. In addition, several subjective factors, such as patient motivation, secondary gain, and other complex psychosocial components, are possible confounders in the relationship between use of electrodiagnosis and surgical outcome.

Historically, electrodiagnostic testing has not been considered to be a valid tool for determining functional outcome after carpal tunnel release. This article and a similar article by Shivde et al.[1] suggest that results of preoperative nerve conduction tests are not reliably associated with symptom reporting. These 2 studies share the same deficit in experimental design: lack of sensitive sensory nerve conduction measurements. Further research is needed to explore the applicability of sensitive nerve conduction measurements, such as the maximum latency difference[2,3] for predicting rigorously and systematically defined symptoms in a homogeneous sample. These methods could also be used after surgery, across increasing time intervals, to determine long-term outcome of carpal tunnel release and symptom reporting.

Outcome predictions aside, the importance of preoperative nerve conduction studies lies in their ability to confirm or rule out the diagnosis in the presence of unclear clinical findings and in determining the severity of the median nerve disease. Thus, they can aid in avoiding diagnostic and treatment decisions that are imprecise and prone to error. In the extreme, the criteria outlined in this paper are nonspecific and could define a case of carpal tunnel syndrome by the following combination: subjective tingling, a positive Tinel's sign, and an amplitude measurement of less than 20 µV. Add to this picture the possibility of secondary gain and one may come to question the generalizability of these results to the clinical setting.

The careful clinician can diagnose classical cases of carpal tunnel syndrome without electrodiagnostic confirmation, but the prudent clinician will insist on electrodiagnostic confirmation to avoid medicolegal complications. Further investigation is needed to determine whether sensitive electrodiagnostics are useful outcomes measures.

P.A. Nathan, M.D.

References

1. Shivde AJ, Dreizin I, Fisher MA: The carpal tunnel syndrome: a clinical-electrodiagnostic analysis. *Electromyogr Clin Neurophysiol* 21:143–153, 1981.
2. Kimura J: The carpal tunnel syndrome: localization of conduction abnormalities within the distal segment of the median nerve. *Brain* 102:619-635, 1979.
3. Nathan PA, Meadows KD, Doyle LS: Sensory segmental latency values of the median nerve for a population of normal individuals. *Arch Phys Med Rehabil* 69:499–501, 1988.

Carpal Tunnel Syndrome: Correlation of Magnetic Resonance Imaging, Clinical, Electrodiagnostic, and Intraoperative Findings
Britz GW, Haynor DR, Kuntz C, et al (Univ of Washington, Seattle; Seattle VA Med Ctr, Seattle)
Neurosurgery 37:1097–1103, 1995   7–21

Introduction.—Carpal tunnel syndrome is frequently diagnosed on the basis of clinical findings alone. However, the diagnosis is often confirmed using nerve conduction velocity and electromyographic studies. Findings from MRI in patients with carpal tunnel syndrome were correlated with clinical, electrophysiologic, and operative findings.

Methods.—Thirty-two patients with a clinical diagnosis of carpal tunnel syndrome in 43 wrists were studied. Five asymptomatic wrists were used as controls. All patients underwent physical examination, and severity of symptoms were graded. Sensory and motor conduction delays were evaluated and graded electrophysiologically; electromyography of the thenar eminence was also performed, and results were graded by severity. Magnetic resonance imaging was performed on all wrists in axial and coronal planes through the carpal tunnel. Operative release was performed on 27 patients, and the extent of median nerve compression was graded.

Results.—Thirty-five wrists (81%) were assessed clinically as having grade 2 carpal tunnel syndrome; 1 patient had grade 1, and 7 patients had grade 3. Abnormalities were found in 41 wrists (95%) by nerve conduction studies; denervation was found in 14 wrists (33%) by electromyographic studies. All 27 wrists in which operative release was done had evidence of median nerve compression; 19 were graded as moderate compression and 8, as severe. All 43 wrists were found to have either abnormal signal or configuration of the median nerve by MRI; median nerve signal and configuration were normal in all controls. Fifteen of 18 patients with abnormal nerve conduction had good or excellent surgical outcomes; 2 patients had poor outcomes and 1 did not complete follow-up. Good or excellent surgical outcomes were found in 5 of 9 patients who had no MRI evidence of abnormal nerve configuration; the remaining 4 had fair or poor surgical outcomes. Forty-one wrists showed increased short tau inversion recovery signal of the flexor tendon sheath. Abnormal nerve conduction was present in 39 of these wrists. Tendon sheath swelling, as evidenced by increased spacing between flexor tendons, was present in 37 of 43 wrists and was associated with abnormal nerve conduction in 35 of these wrists. Abnormal nerve conduction was also associated with bowing of the flexor retinaculum in 39 wrists.

Conclusion.—Magnetic resonance imaging findings were found to correlate well with other diagnostic findings for carpal tunnel syndrome, including clinical, electrodiagnostic, and operative findings. Abnormal nerve configuration found with MRI may help predict which patients would have the best outcomes after surgery.

▶ The authors studied a series of patients who had received clinical diagnoses of median nerve compression at the wrist. Almost all had continuous rather than intermittent symptoms, and almost all had abnormally prolonged conduction delays. By any definition, these patients had carpal tunnel syndrome. The MRI images demonstrated the mechanical deformations one would expect. That only 26% of the patients who had surgery still experienced postoperative symptoms is really quite remarkable. It is my contention that patients with median nerve compression who state that they have numb fingers (implying constantly present sensory disturbances) will, if examined or questioned closely, persist with these abnormalities for a very long time after surgery. Certainly, for most, the troubling "symptoms" may resolve rapidly. Normalcy is more unusual. It is interesting to see how clinical entities diverge in direction when prominent (some would say outspoken) hand surgeons reassess the usefulness of electrodiagnostic studies (in, for example, predicting outcome as it is typically defined today, as patient satisfaction). There seems to be little role for MRI in the evaluation of carpal tunnel syndrome.

V.R. Hentz, M.D.

Explant Culture, Immunofluorescence and Electron-microscopic Study of Flexor Retinaculum in Carpal Tunnel Syndrome
Allampallam K, Chakraborty J, Bose KK, et al (Med College of Ohio, Toledo; St Vincent Med Ctr, Toledo, Ohio)
J Environ Med 38:264–271, 1996   7–22

Objective.—Carpal tunnel syndrome (CTS) can be relieved by dividing the flexor retinaculum (FR). Although few studies have examined the role of the FR in CTS, the presence of collagen dysplasia in the FR of some CTS patients supports the theory that fibroblasts in the FR may cause tissue contraction that can create pressure on the median nerve by decreasing the volume of the CT. The explant and primary cell culture, cellular growth, immunocytochemical, fine morphologic, and biochemical properties of the FR cells from individuals with and without CTS were studied.

Methods.—Pieces of the flexor retinaculum, removed from the wrists of 4 patients with CTS (2 women) and 1 control, were cultured and examined by light, immunofluorescence, and electron microscopy. Electrophoresis and Western blot analysis were performed. Molecular weights of proteins were determined.

Results.—Bipolar, serum-dependent cells emerged in 3–7 days; control cells took much longer to become confluent. Growth rate of the CTS cells showed no lag phase, and CTS cells grew much more quickly than control cells. Both CTS and control cells demonstrated immunofluorescence reactivity to antibodies against vimentin. All stained positively for fibroblast marker but did not react in the presence of anti-α smooth-muscle actin or normal serum. Cellular outlines were irregular under electron microscopy, and long cytoplasmic extensions and pinocytotic vesicles were evident. Cytoplasm contained microfilaments with abnormal nuclei and appeared to be undergoing contraction. Well-developed rough endoplasmic reticulum, Golgi apparatus, and mitochondria were seen. Control and CTS cells reacted with antivimentin and antifibroblast markers. Molecular weights of proteins from CTS and control appeared to be the same.

Conclusion.—Cultured cells from pieces of flexor retinaculum of patients with CTS exhibit contractile properties and increased growth rate, which may explain a change in cellular reaction to injury.

▶ This study supports the hypothesis that CTS is the result of physical changes in the carpal canal. Whether the changes in the flexor retinaculum are primary or secondary (e.g., in response to synovial proliferation, and increased carpal tunnel pressure) cannot be determined by the results reported in this study. That the changes noted here are similar to those seen in response to injury also supports the hypothesis that CTS may be the result of a physiologic response to chronic tissue loading. However, the hypothesis that the flexor retinaculum may actually contract under the influence of myofibroblasts is a bit much for me; that cells contain contractile elements does not mean that they function like muscle. Similarly, that such cells are present in contracting wounds does not mean that they cause wound contraction. Gross[1] has shown that, in fact, wounds contract even when the myofibroblast-containing granulation tissue is excised daily. It is cellular migration from the wound edges, not contraction of the central granulation tissue, that closes wounds.

P.C. Amadio, M.D.

Reference

1. Gross J. Getting to mammalian wound repair. *Wound Repr Reg* 4:190–202, 1996.

Radial Tunnel Syndrome: A Retrospective Review of 30 Decompressions of the Radial Nerve
Lawrence T, Mobbs P, Fortems Y, et al (Wrightington Hosp, Wigan, England)
J Hand Surg (Br) 20B:454–459, 1995

Introduction.—The pain and sensory disturbance of radial tunnel syndrome are caused by radial nerve compression of the radial nerve by the free edge of the supinator muscle or by related structures around the elbow. The anatomy of the radial tunnel and radial nerve are well described, and surgical decompression of the radial nerve usually produces good results. However, the natural history of radial tunnel syndrome is not well understood, and the condition often goes unrecognized and neglected. Its symptoms are similar to those of tennis elbow, chronic wrist pain, and tenosynovitis, and there are no objective criteria by which to reliably distinguish between the various causes. The results of radial nerve decompression in 30 patients with radial tunnel syndrome were reviewed.

Methods.—Twenty-nine patients (16 women and 13 men, mean age, 41½ years) underwent 30 primary explorations and proximal decompressions of the radial nerve during a 15-year period. The mean delay to surgery was 3 years. The most common symptom was pain around the arcade of Frohse, commonly associated with writer's cramp. Tenderness over the radial nerve—distinct from the lateral epicondyle—was present in all cases. Distal symptoms, such as paresthesias or burning sensations, were not well localized. Most patients had manual occupations for which they required repeated pronation and supination; most had already been treated for other suspected conditions. At surgery, pronation and supination of the forearm revealed the structures compressing the radial nerve.

Results.—According to visual analogue assessments, the results were excellent in 60% of cases, good in 10%, fair in 13%, and poor in 17%. Forty-one percent of patients had no pain during all activities, 31% had pain only during their most strenuous activities, and 28% could not perform even light activity. Most patients had little improvement in paresthesia. Seven of 9 patients with poor or fair results had evidence of additional pathologic conditions. Women were more likely to be satisfied with their results than men. The results were good or excellent in 4 of 6 patients with medicolegal claims.

Conclusions.—The possibility of radial tunnel syndrome should always be considered in patients with forearm and wrist pain that has not responded to conventional therapies (Table 7). This problem may be especially likely in patients whose jobs require repetitive manual tasks. Surgery may produce fair or poor results because of an incorrect diagnosis, incom-

TABLE 7.—Possible Presentations of Radial Tunnel Syndrome

Forearm pain radiating from the elbow to the wrist
Chronic wrist pain with radial sided dysaesthesia
Dorsal, radial, and occasional thenar sited wrist pain associated with swelling
Failed tennis elbow treatment
Failed de Quervain's release
Wartenberg's neuropathy (handcuff neuritis)
Dorsal 'tenosynovitis' without crepitus or thickening
Burning pain in the forearm and hand (autonomic dysfunction)

(Courtesy of Lawrence T, Mobbs P, Fortems Y: Radial tunnel syndrome: a retrospective review of 30 decompressions of the radial nerve. *J Hand Surg (Br)* 20B:454–459, 1995.)

plete release, or irreversible nerve injury. Objective techniques are needed for accurate identification of patients with radial tunnel syndrome and localization of the compressive site.

▶ Radial tunnel syndrome is a great mimic. There is simply no easy way to explain all the symptoms attributed to this condition, which is far different from carpal tunnel or cubital tunnel syndrome. The nerve lacks cutaneously directed sensory axons that might focus the patient's attention (and therefore lead the patient to report this as a symptom); thus, we cannot rely on their presence to make the diagnosis. I have often relied on the outcome of a local anesthetic block of the radial or posterior interosseous nerve with the site of injection controlled by a nerve stimulator and hollow fine-needle electrode. A low concentration frequently results in less than profound motor block but in some patients, symptoms are completely relieved for varying periods of time.

V.R. Hentz, M.D.

Spontaneous Anterior Interosseous Nerve Palsy With Hourglass-like Fascicular Constriction Within the Main Trunk of the Median Nerve
Nagano A, Shibata K, Tokimura H, et al (Univ of Tokyo)
J Hand Surg (Am) 21A:266–270, 1996
7–24

Introduction.—Neuralgic amyotrophy, isolated neuritis, and entrapment neuropathy have been suspected as causing spontaneous anterior interosseous nerve (AIN) palsy. Results of interfascicular neurolysis in 9 patients with AIN palsy were reported.

Methods.—Of 14 patients with spontaneous AIN palsy, 5 responded to conservative treatment. The remaining 9 patients underwent surgical exploration of the AIN. The mean duration of the interval between onset of symptoms and surgery was 5 months. Eight patients experienced pain in the elbow region at a mean of 15 days before onset of palsy. The median nerve and the AIN were surgically explored from the proximal one third of the forearm to approximately 5 cm proximal to the elbow. Interfascicular neurolysis was performed under microscopic guidance when no external compression was detected.

Results.—No patients had signs of external compression. The appearance of 6 median nerves was within normal limits. Slight swelling, hardening, or adhesion to surrounding tissue at the elbow was observed in 3 median nerves. An hourglass-like fascicular constriction was observed in the fascicles of the AIN within the median nerve at 2.0–7.5 cm proximal to the elbow in 8 patients. One fascicular constriction was detected in 2 patients (Fig 1A), 2 were seen in 1 fascicle in 4 patients, 1 was found in 2 fascicles in 1 patient, and 2 were found in 2 fascicles in 1 patient. One patient with no fascicular constriction had signs and symptoms similar to those of patients with constriction. Seven of 8 patients with hourglass-like fascicular constriction were treated only with interfascicular neurolysis.

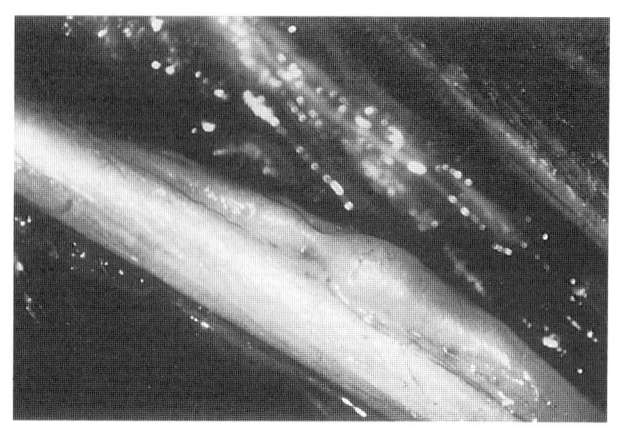

FIGURE 1A.—One hourglass-like fascicular constriction. (Courtesy of Nagano A, Shibata K, Tokimura H, et al: Spontaneous anterior interosseous nerve palsy with hourglass-like fascicular constriction within the main trunk of the median nerve. *J Hand Surg (Am)* 21A:266–270, 1996.)

The other patient underwent resection and grafting of the constricted nerve because the constriction was as severe as it would be had the fascicle been completely ruptured. Muscle strength returned at varying intervals (1.5–7.5 months) after surgery in all patients.

Conclusion.—External neurolysis alone is not sufficient for thorough exploration of the AIN in patients with spontaneous AIN palsy. Interfascicular neurolysis should be done. Nerve grafting is unnecessary in treating this lesion. Recovery in this patient cohort was considered to be good. It was not known whether the good recovery was spontaneous recovery or a result of the interfascicular neurolysis. Further investigation is needed.

▶ This fascinating report suggests that AIN palsy is not caused by either compression in the forearm or a spontaneous neuritis; rather, it is the result of a focal constrictive neuropathy of unknown cause, located 5–7 cm proximal to the elbow. I have seen a similar constriction in the radial nerve above the elbow when I was exploring a spontaneous radial neuropathy that developed some weeks after surgery. I must say that I would have some trepidation in exploring the nerve and, if finding nothing, going further proximal and even doing an intrafascicular exploration; however, I will certainly give the matter some thought when next faced with an AIN palsy that has not improved with observation.

P.C. Amadio, M.D.

Early Versus Late Range of Motion Following Cubital Tunnel Surgery
Warwick L, Seradge H (Tulsa, Okla; Hand Ctr of Oklahoma, Oklahoma City)
J Hand Ther 8:245–248, 1995
7–25

Background.—At present, the optimal time to begin rehabilitative therapy after cubital tunnel release with medial epicondylectomy remains unclear. Although various recommendations have been proposed in the literature, these lack statistical support and seem to be based on the authors' personal preferences. A prospective case study was therefore performed to determine which therapeutic strategy would provide the best outcomes for active range of motion of the elbow after decompression with medial epicondylectomy.

Patients and Methods.—Fifty-seven patients undergoing cubital tunnel release with medial epicondylectomy in a 24-month period were included in the study. Patients were randomly divided into 2 groups, with 29 patients (mean age, 45 years) placed in group 1 and 26 patients (mean age, 38 years) placed in group 2. Patients in group 1 began performing active and passive range-of-motion exercises 14 days after surgery and attended an average of 12 sessions, whereas those in group 2 began exercises 3 days postoperatively and attended an average of 12.3 sessions. Various rehabilitative modalities also were used for both groups, including hot or cold packs, ultrasound, whirlpool, and transcutaneous electric nerve stimulation. Goniometric measurements of elbow flexion and extension were done initially and at the discharge evaluation, with a loss of 5 degrees or more in elbow active extension defined as significant.

Results.—All patients had normal flexion, pronation, and supination. In both groups, immediate postoperative evaluation of active range of motion was not statistically significant. Final elbow range of motion for extension in groups 1 and 2 was, however, significant, with 52% of the patients in group 1 demonstrating flexion contractures of more than 5 degrees compared to only 4% of patients in group 2. In group 1, the mean, median, and mode for active extension were 11, 10, and 0 degrees, respectively. Corresponding figures for patients in group 2 were 1, 0, and 0 degrees. Grip strength and/or other functions of the upper extremity were not adversely affected by early initiation of exercise. Group 2 patients also returned to work at a mean of 2.2 months postoperatively, compared to a mean of 4 months among patients in group 1. No significant differences in pain ratings were noted between groups, and the use of rehabilitative modalities did not appear to affect range-of-motion outcomes in either group. Nine of 11 patients in group 2 who did not receive any modality achieved full range of motion.

Conclusions.—Early initiation of rehabilitation therapy significantly decreases the likelihood of postoperative flexion contracture of the elbow and leads to better postsurgical outcomes in patients undergoing cubital tunnel surgery with medial epicondylectomy. Range-of-motion exercises begun as early as the first postoperative day are recommended to help prevent loss of motion and reduce flexion contractures.

▶ This study demonstrates the importance of timing and very early therapuetic intervention after cubital tunnel release and medial epicondylectomy. Patients who initiated therapy by the second postoperative day were significantly improved with regard to range of motion and return to work compared with patients who initiated therapy at 14 days. The authors concluded that the institution of range-of-motion exercises immediately postoperatively is more effective in preventing flexion contractures of the elbow than is delayed treatment. I would suspect though that the statistic from this study that is the most relevant in today's managed cost environment is that the patients who delayed treatment by 2 weeks also delayed return to work by an additional 2 months.

One of the most frustrating problems within the new managed care environment is the delay in approval for therapy. It is not uncommon for third-party payers to delay approval for therapy as much as 2 or 3 weeks after physician referral, leaving the patient without the proper supervision during the early stages of wound healing. The problem of bureaucratic delay is now occasionally compounded in my practice by the adjuster's request for studies that validate the use of modalities, splinting, and frequency of treatment for the specific diagnosis. This information is not available for many treatment regimens. Therapists are now finding themselves in the uncomfortable position of having limited research and outcome data to provide statistical support for treatment modalities and timing and duration of treatment.

This study of functional results after cubital tunnel and medial epicondylectomy provides exactly the kind of statistical data that we need to support our position as we bargain with the insurance adjuster over the right to treat their claimant and our patient. I will fax this article after my next telephone call to the adjuster representing my next patient with cubital tunnel release. Come to think of it, I'll send a copy to the employer as well.

R.B. Evans, O.T.R./L., C.H.T.

Anterior Submuscular Transposition of the Ulnar Nerve for Cubital Tunnel Syndrome
Pasque CB, Rayan GM (Univ of Oklahoma, Oklahoma City)
J Hand Surg (Br) 20B:4–447–453, 1995   7–26

Background.—Cubital tunnel syndrome, caused by ulnar nerve entrapment at the elbow, is characterized by pain, paresthesia, hypoesthesia, and motor dysfunction in the nerve's distribution. Surgery is occasionally necessary if nonoperative treatment fails. The results of 1 procedure, anterior submuscular transposition of the ulnar nerve with Z-lengthening of the flexor-pronator muscle origin, were evaluated.

Methods.—A group of 48 patients (50 affected limbs) answered a detailed questionnaire and underwent extensive assessment of their postoperative status. Surgical outcome was graded as excellent, good, fair, or poor, on the basis of a combination of subjective and objective findings.

Results.—The nature and duration of preoperative symptoms and treatment, including surgery, were not significantly related to postoperative outcome. After surgery, 26 patients (27 limbs; 54%) were completely satisfied and 18 patients (19 limbs; 38%) were satisfied but had reservations. Four patients (8%) were dissatisfied, 2 of whom were still pursuing workers' compensation litigation. Before surgery, 54% of patients had a poor functional grade and 46% had a fair functional grade. After surgery,

26% had an excellent grade, 58% had a good grade, and 16% had a fair grade. Most patients experienced significant improvement in motor and sensory function. After surgery, 92% of patients had no limitations in activities of daily living. Time to return to full activity averaged 6 weeks and return to work averaged 9 weeks. Patient status with regard to workers' compensation litigation was not significantly related to postoperative grade or patient satisfaction. Seven complications occurred, including 2 subcutaneous hematomas, 2 flexor-pronator origin ruptures caused by falls, 1 case of medial antebrachial cutaneous neuralgia, 1 symptomatic scar, and 1 case of reflex sympathetic dystrophy.

Conclusion.—Anterior submuscular transposition with Z-lengthening of the flexor-pronator origin achieves satisfactory results in the surgical treatment of cubital tunnel syndrome.

▶ Problems relating to cubital tunnel syndrome are recognized with increasing frequency, yet the surgery for this condition continues to be problematic. Thus, the authors are to be congratulated on their efforts to report the results of their surgery. They report that although only 54% of their patients were completely satisfied with the results of this surgery, 90% would have the operation again, even knowing their long-term results. Studies such as these, which solicit patients' subjective feedback regarding surgical outcome, provide useful information for patients contemplating this type of surgery.

S.E. Mackinnon, M.D.

Suggested Reading

Atrosh I, Johnsson R, Ornstein E: Radial tunnel release: Unpredictable outcome in 37 consecutive cases with a 1–5 year follow-up. *Acta Orthop Scand* 66:255–257, 1995.
▶ The authors concisely reviewed their series of 37 radial tunnel syndrome decompressions. Their percentage of successful results (33⅓ %) is lower than in most published series of radial tunnel syndrome. I share their frustration that diagnostic criteria are not always reliable and that results are not always predictable. Perhaps using the transbrachioradialis muscle-splitting approach would yield improved results and fewer complications.

W. Engberger, M.D.

Seror P: The value of special motor and sensory tests for the diagnosis of benign and minor median nerve lesion at the wrist. *Am J Phys Med Rehabil* 74:124–129, 1995.
▶ The American Association of Electrodiagnostic Medicine (AAEM) Quality Assurance Committee did an extensive literature review of the value of nerve conduction studies for the evaluation of patients with carpal tunnel syndrome. Their report[1] concluded that median sensory nerve conduction studies (NCS) are more sensitive than motor NCS. The median sensory conduction from wrist to digit is less sensitive compared with palmar study across the carpal tunnel (palm–wrist), median to ulnar (wrist–digit), and median to radial (wrist–digit 1) comparative tests. This study strengthens the conclusion drawn by the AAEM.

P. Wu, M.D.

Reference

1. Jablecki CK, Andary MT, So YT, et al: Literature review of the usefulness of nerve conduction studies and electromyography for the evaluation of patients with carpal tunnel syndrome: AAEM Quality Assurance Committee. *Muscle Nerve* 16:1392–1414, 1993.

Okutsu I, et al: What is endoscopic surgery in carpal tunnel syndrome? *J Jpn Soc Surg Hand* 12:391–394, 1995.

▶ Arthroscopic surgery for carpal tunnel syndrome is drawing attention to hand surgeons. The authors developed a Universal Subcutaneous Endoscope system and first reported the results of arthroscopic surgery for carpal tunnel syndrome in 1986.[1] Since then the authors noticed that the carpal canal pressure mesured in resting hand position showed lower than normal pressure after the release of the transverse carpal ligament (TCL), and that there were several cases that did not show low carpal canal pressure in the active hand grip position. The authors confirmed that carpal canal pressure showed lower than normal pressure in any hand position after the release of both TCL and the distal holdfast fibers of the transverse carpal ligament (DHFTCL), which he named. It will be necessary to clarify whether there are any anatomical differences between the DHFTCL and the distal portion of the flexor retinaculum named by Cobb, and the deep layer of the midpalmar fascia named by Zancolli.

S. Ishii, M.D.

Reference

1. Okutsu I, Ninomiya S, Natsuyama M, et al: Subcutaneous operation and examination under universal endoscope. *Nippon Seikeigeka Gakkai Zasshi* 61:491–498, 1987.

Lehtinen I, Kirjavainen T, Hurmem, et al: Sleep-related disorders in carpal tunnel syndrome. *Acta Neurol Scand* 93:360–365, 1996.

▶ The study is somewhat flawed, and gives no relevant new information regarding diagnosis or management of carpal tunnel syndrome; nevertheless it is a fascinating introduction to the study of sleep disorders and will be of interest to any who wish to determine the effect of neuro-musculo-skeletal disorders on sleep patterns. The interesting results regarding patterns of sleeplessness even when merged with the results of the same questionnaire for patients with carpal tunnel syndrome and the results of sleep studies on an aliquot of these patients, do not tell us anything new about the syndrome. There is a great deal of information, however, about studying sleep disorders, particularly those that result from neuro-musculo-skeletal problems. Any investigator who is interested in pursuing the effect of such disorders on sleep would do well to review this paper and its references.

J.H. Dobyns, M.D.

Worseg AP, Kuzbari R, Korak K: Endoscopic carpal tunnel release using a single-portal system. *Br J Plast Surg* 49:1–10, 1996.

Kluge W, Simpson RG, Nicol AC: Late complications after open carpal tunnel decompression. *J Hand Surg (Br)* 21B:205–207, 1996.

8 Wrist

General

Triradiate Skin Incision for Dorsal Approach to the Wrist
Barbieri CH, Mazzer N (São Paulo Univ, Brazil)
J Hand Surg (Br) 21B:21–23, 1996   8–1

Introduction.—Most previous reports have described a longitudinal straight incision for procedures involving a dorsal approach to the wrist. The incision and its length may vary when used for different indications. An alternative, triradiate incision for the dorsal approach to the wrist was described.

Technique.—The incision, centered over Lister's tubercle, consists of 3 rays separated by 120 degrees. The proximal ray goes down the longitudinal axis of the radius for 3–5 cm, while one distal ray is directed toward the radial styloid process and the other toward the ulnar styloid process for 3 cm each (Fig 1). As the incision is deepened, the main longitudinal trunks of the dorsal wrist veins are identified and preserved, as are the terminal sensitive branches of the radial and ulnar flaps. A triangular operating field is created by undermining and eversion of the 3 flaps. A longitudinal incision of the extensor retinaculum between the third and fourth extensor compartments is performed. A distally based rectangular capsular flap may be used to approach the carpus.

Experience.—The triradiate incision has been used in 32 patients with various wrist problems. The incision was simple to use, and the dorsal veins and nerve branches were easily found and preserved. The triangular operating field provided good access to all structures on the dorsal aspect of the wrist, and did not have to be overextended proximally or distally to relieve tension on the wound edges. The longitudinal ray sometimes had to be extended as far as 7 cm. The incision was healed within 10 days in all patients, with no signs of vascular impairment. There were 2 instances of subcutaneous hematoma, which were managed by needle aspiration. Five patients had moderate temporary edema. The skin healed uneventfully in all patients, though 8 had some degree of hypertrophic scarring.

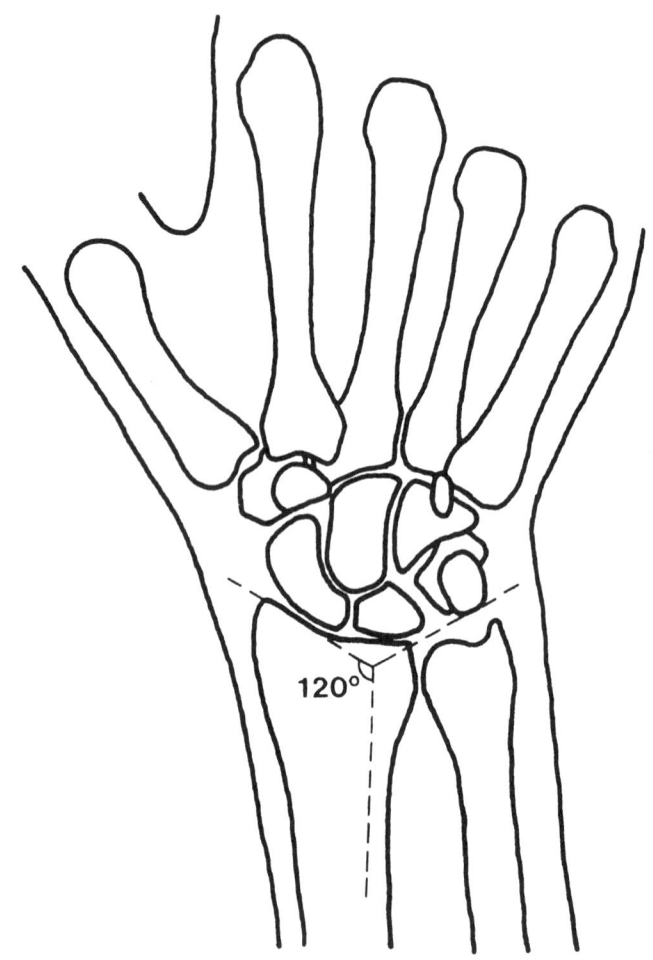

FIGURE 1.—Schematic drawing of the triradiate incision. (Courtesy of Barbieri CH, Mazzer N: Triradiate skin incision for dorsal approach to the wrist. *J Hand Surg (Br)* 21B:21–23, 1996.)

Conclusion.—A triradiate incision for operations on the dorsal aspect of the wrist yields a wide triangular surgical field with a very low complication rate. It offers several advantages over longitudinal straight incisions and their variants, and provides excellent cosmetic results in most cases.

▶ The concept of the triradiate skin incision is useful for most dorsal exposures to the wrist region. I have been using a modification of this incision which was taught to me by Peter Carter, M.D., in which the distal limbs are a continuous curvilinear incision, leaving a distally based flap. Most procedures are easily approached through the transverse limb, and one always has the option of extending the incision proximally through the longitudinal limb. Because of concern about the viability of the flaps at the corners of the incision, it is advisable to handle these with care, including placement of sutures in lieu of instruments for flap margin manipulation. The incision line can generally be drawn within the natural contour of the wrist extension creases, and it is advisable to use the landmarks of the radial and ulnar styloid processes for the lateral and medial limits of the incision, respectively. The results are cosmetically pleasing with minimal scar formation, which serves to optimize functional recovery.

R.A. Berger, M.D., Ph.D.

Does the Normal Contralateral Wrist Provide the Best Reference for X-ray Film Measurements of the Pathologic Wrist?
Schuind F, Alemzadeh S, Stallenberg B, et al (Cliniques Universitaries de Bruxelles, Belgium)
J Hand Surg (Am) 21A:24–30, 1996   8-2

Introduction.—Normal reference values can be useful in the identification of various osteoarticular deformities, provided that the variability in the general population remains within narrow limits. At the wrist, however, interindividual variability is high and patients can have mild deformities even when radiographic measurements are normal. A study of 20 volunteers with normal wrists examined the hypothesis that in unilateral diseases, the normal contralateral wrist should be used as a reference for evaluating the pathologic wrist.

Methods.—Study participants were divided into 4 groups according to age (20–39 and 40–60 years) and sex; 16 were right-handed, 2 were left-handed, and 2 were ambidextrous. All had posteroanterior and lateral radiography done in both wrists, including the metacarpals. A single observer obtained the following measurements: radial inclination and palmar tilt of the distal radius; ulnar variance; length of the third metacarpal; carpal height and carpal height ratio; carporadial and carpoulnar distances and ratios; and radiolunate, scapholunate, and capitolunate angles.

Results.—The carpal height ratio and carporadial ratio were statistically significantly higher in men than in women; women had a higher capitolunate angle. Older persons showed a significant decrease in the scapholunate angle. For the study group as a whole, the only difference between measurements made from the right and left radiographs was in the carporadial ratio, which was statistically significantly higher on the right side. Measurements made on the dominant side did not significantly differ from those on the nondominant side. Correlation varied for individual right vs. left wrist measurements. Correlation was good for length of the third metacarpal joint; carpal height; and the radiolunate, scapholunate, and capitolunate angles, almost no correlation was seen for the radial inclination angle. Correlation was poor for both the distal radius palmar tilt and ulnar variance.

Conclusion.—In unilateral wrist diseases, the normal wrist can provide reference values for carpal height and carpal angles. For radial inclination, palmar tilt, and ulnar variance, however, normal values obtained from databases may be preferable.

▶ Schuind and colleagues have attempted to validate the assumptions that many clinicians make—that the contralateral, normal wrist should be used as a reference for assessing radiographic features of a wrist that has some type of malady, whether it be traumatic, inflammatory, or developmental. Although the study sample was relatively small (20 volunteers), the correlation between right and left sides was high ($R > 0.88$). In addition, it was interesting that anthropomorphic differences were seen between the sexes—the carpal height and carpal to radius ratios were lower and the capitolunate angle was higher in women than in men. Their findings that scapholunate angle decreased in older persons is also of some interest; these findings should be correlated with the attritional changes related to age that we previously reported in a study of cadavers. Interestingly, the authors found that radial inclination, palmar tilt, and ulnar variance could just as easily be compared with normal values obtained from databases. I commend the authors on their study and would encourage them to continue to monitor these types of variables, to expand their sample size, and to entertain collaborative studies that could compare various populations worldwide.

S.F. Viegas, M.D.

Carpal Bone Anatomy Measured by Computer Analysis of Three-dimensional Reconstructions of Computed Tomography Images
Patterson RM, Elder KW, Viegas SF, et al (Univ of Texas, Galveston)
J Hand Surg (Am) 20A:923–929, 1995
8–3

Objective.—A reference database of carpal bone morphologic characteristics would be helpful in diagnosing and planning treatment for wrist injuries. Few 3-dimensional imaging studies of the wrist have been done that allow measurement of anatomical variables of the wrist. Anatomical measurements of cadaver and patient wrists were generated using an automated program to construct 3-dimensional images from computed tomographic (CT) scans of the wrists.

Methods.—Transverse CT images of 35 wrists, including 9 paired wrists, from 21 cadavers and 14 patients (12 female), aged 17 to 89 years, were processed using a software program that generated 3-dimensional reconstructions of the wrist. Volume, surface area, maximum length, surface area of bone, maximum length or antipodal axis of each bone, intercarpal distances, and 3-dimensional carpal height ratio (the latter was determined by the formula L_1/L_2, where L_1 = minimum 3-dimensional distance between the 4th metacarpal joint and the radius and L_2 = maximum 3-dimensional length of the capitate) were calculated.

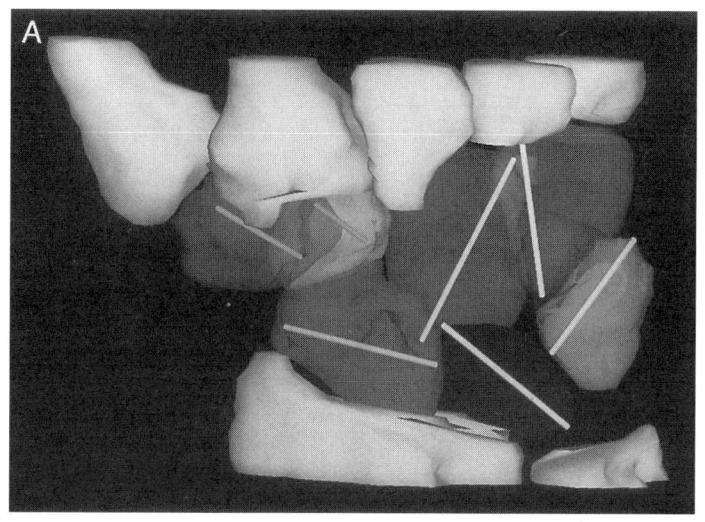

FIGURE 2.—A, Dorsal view of a 3-dimensional display of a right wrist with the maximum length axis displayed for each carpal bone. (Courtesy of Patterson PM, Elder KW, Viegas SF, et al: Carpal bone anatomy measured by computer analysis of three-dimensional reconstruction of computed tomography images. *J Hand Surg (Am)* 20A:923–929, 1995.)

Results.—No differences were seen between cadaver and patient carpal bones or between left and right wrists whether matched or not. Volume and length of carpal bones in male wrists were significantly larger than bones in female wrists. Bone size decreased as follows: capitate, hamate, lunate, pisiform, scaphoid, trapezium, trapezoid, and triquetrum (Fig 2). The mean 3-dimensional carpal height ratio was 30.4 mm. The mean ratio divided by the capitate length was 1.08.

Conclusion.—This 3-dimensional study provides information about the morphologic characteristics and spatial relationship among the carpal bones.

▶ This elegant study provides more accurate and precise quantitative information about the size, shape, and relationship of each carpal bone to the remainder of the wrist. The authors have also described a new index, the 3-dimensional carpal height index. They feel this index is more accurate and precise than the 2-dimensional indices described by Youm, et al[1] and Nattrass, et al.[2] Furthermore, as they point out, the index may allow obtaining dynamic studies in patients or normal volunteers to accurately measure wrist kinematic behavior noninvasively in vivo. Whether this technique will move beyond the research stage in our present fiscally constrained atmosphere remains to be seen. Nevertheless, this is an important study.

L.K. Ruby, M.D.

References

1. Youm Y, McMurtry RY, Flatt AE, et al: Kinematics of the wrist: I. An experimental study of radial-ulnar deviation and flexion-extension. *J Bone Joint Surg (Am)* 60:423–431, 1978.

2. Nattrass GR, King GJ, McMurtry RY, et al: An alternative method for determination of the carpal height ratio. *J Bone Joint Surg* 76A:88–94, 1994.

A Modified Approach to the Flexor Surface of the Distal Radius
Allen PE, Vickery CW, Atkins RM (Bristol Royal Infirmary, England; Univ of Bristol, England)
J Hand Surg (Br) 21B:303–304, 1996   8–4

Purpose.—In standard operative approaches to the flexor surface of the distal radius, the surgical plane developed runs close to either the radial artery or median nerve. A new approach between the flexor pollicis longus and flexor carpi radialis was evaluated to determine whether it could protect the radial artery and median nerve.

Methods.—Dissections were performed in 23 cadaver arms. In 13 specimens, the flexor carpi radialis muscle was dissected to examine its nerve supply. In the remaining specimens, an incision was made over the tendon of the flexor carpi radialis, which was retracted toward the radius to protect the radial artery. A surgical plane was then developed between the flexor carpi radialis tendon and the flexor pollicis longus, which was retracted toward the ulna to protect the median nerve. This exposed the pronator quadratus, which was incised on its radial border to expose the distal radial shaft. Further dissections were performed to define the feasible proximal limit of this approach.

Results.—The flexor carpi radialis nerve supply arose in the forearm from the median nerve 31 mm below the intercondylar line and entered the muscle 66 mm below the intercondylar line. This branch usually arose from the ulnar side of the median nerve. The point at which the flexor carpi radialis nerve supply entered the muscle was less than one third of the way between the intercondylar line and the wrist. The proximal limit of the approach was found to be 123 mm from the wrist, or about as far as the junction of the proximal and middle thirds of the radius.

Conclusions.—With this modified approach to the flexor surface of the distal radius, the median nerve and radial artery are protected by muscles or tendons, thus reducing the chances of injuring them. Because the approach is a direct one to the midline of the flexor surface, it provides much better exposure for buttress plate fixation. It can be safely extended as far proximally as the junction of the middle and proximal thirds of the radius.

▶ The authors have described an alternative approach to the anterior surface of the distal radius by dissecting in the plane between the flexor carpi radialis and flexor pollicis longus. The apparent goal of this approach is to protect the radial artery from injury, which they believe is at risk with the standard Henry approach in the interval between the flexor carpi radialis and the radial artery. Although the anatomical documentation in this manuscript is sound, I caution readers to consider several points before abandoning the Henry approach for this new surgical exposure technique. First, I believe that, with careful dissection, the radial artery is not at substantial risk of injury through the standard Henry approach, and can be adequately protected by simply observing good surgical technique. Second, I have never experienced any difficulty in adequately exposing the distal radius through the Henry approach, and find it easily extensile proximally, which may present a substantial limitation with this new technique. Finally, I believe that the palmar cutaneous branch of the median nerve is at substantial risk with this new technique because of its direct proximity to the medial border of the flexor carpi radialis tendon. If injured, this may result in substantial morbidity, which can be avoided altogether by continuing to use the approach of Henry.

R.A. Berger, M.D., Ph.D.

A Dynamic Biomechanical Study of Scapholunate Ligament Sectioning
Short WH, Werner FW, Fortino MD, et al (State Univ of New York, Syracuse)
J Hand Surg (Am) 20A:986–999, 1995   8–5

Introduction.—There is confusion as to which ligament combinations must be injured to effect specific wrist instability patterns. The outcome of sectioning the scapholunate interosseous ligament (SLIL) on the biomechanics of the scaphoid and lunate was evaluated by using 3 different technologies.

Methods.—Radiographs were taken to rule out pre-existing bony abnormalities in 6 fresh cadaver arms that were amputated at midhumerous level. A 3 SPACE tracker was used to amass translational and angular measurements for the scaphoid, lunate, and wrist positions. Thin, tactile TekScan robotic pressure sensors were used to monitor the pressure in the radiocarpal and ulnocarpal joints. A wrist joint simulator was used to dynamically move the wrist. Pilot investigations were conducted with each of these technologies for calibration and determination of accuracy of data collected. The 3 technologies were combined for continuous and simultaneous monitoring of pressure and position while the wrist was moving. Measurements were recorded before and after sectioning of the SLIL. Specimens were dissected at completion of the experiment.

TABLE 1.—Portion of Wrist Flexion Extension Motion During Which Scaphoid Flexion Statistically Significantly Increased After Sectioning of the Scapholunate Interosseous Ligament

	Type of Cyclic Wrist Motion	
Direction of Wrist Motion	± 30° Flexion/Extension	30° Extension to 50° Flexion
Moving from maximum flexion to maximum extension	Maximum flexion to 4° and 13° extension to maximum extension	Maximum flexion to 1° flexion
Moving from maximum extension to maximum flexion	14° flexion to maximum flexion	21° extension to 8° extension and 12° flexion to maximum flexion

(Courtesy of Short WH, Werner FW, Fortino MD: A dynamic biomechanical study of scapholunate ligament sectioning. J Hand Surg (Am) 20A:986–999, 1995.)

TABLE 2.—Portion of Wrist Radial—Ulnar Deviation Motion During Which Scaphoid Flexion Statistically Significantly Increased After Sectioning of the Scapholunate Interosseous Ligament

Direction of Wrist Motion	Type of Cyclic Wrist Motion: ± 10° Radial/Ulnar Deviation
Moving from maximum radial to maximum ulnar deviation	7° ulnar to maximum ulnar deviation
Moving from maximum ulnar deviation to maximum radial deviation	Maximum ulnar deviation to 4° ulnar deviation

(Courtesy of Short WH, Werner FW, Fortino MD: A dynamic biomechanical study of scapholunate ligament sectioning. J Hand Surg (Am) 20A:986–999, 1995.)

Results.—Positions of the scaphoid and lunate were determined to be dependent on wrist position and direction of movement (Tables 1 and 2). Sectioning the SLIL did affect the position of the scaphoid and lunate during wrist motion. The primary motions of the scaphoid and lunate were flexion and extension. When the SLIL was sectioned, the scaphoid supinated less, or had more pronation. After SLIL sectioning, no changes in scaphoid radial–ulnar deviation or lunate radial–ulnar or pronation–supination could be determined.

Before the SLIL was sectioned, the magnitude and distribution of pressure across the wrist joint changed depending on wrist position and whether the wrist was going into flexion or extension. The pressure in the radiocarpal and ulnocarpal joints was redistributed after SLIL sectioning. There was a tendency for pressure to shift from the radioscaphoid fossa to the radiolunate fossa. Pressure was concentrated in the radioscaphoid fossa, and relatively less pressure was seen in the radiolunate and ulnocarpal fossae when the intact specimen was placed in radial deviation (Fig

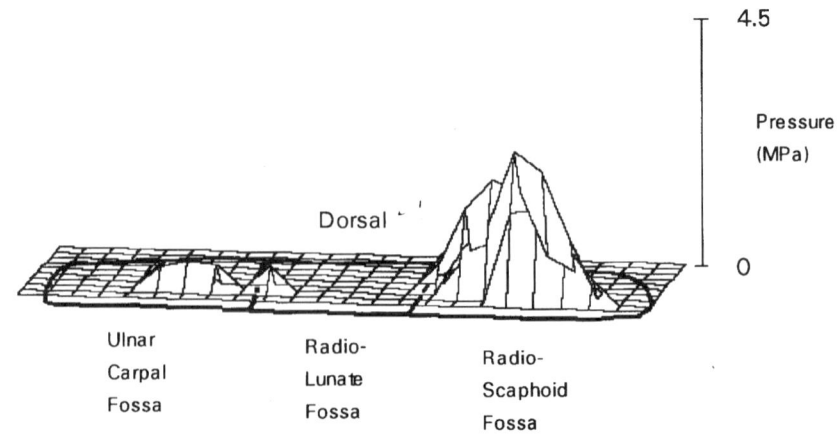

FIGURE 14.—Wire diagram plot of the pressure distribution in the radiocarpal and ulnocarpal joints of an illustrative intact forearm, with the wrist in 9 degrees of radial deviation, just before the wrist reached maximum radial deviation. (Courtesy of Short WH, Werner FW, Fortino MD: A dynamic biomechanical study of scapholunate ligament sectioning. J Hand Surg (Am) 20A:986–999, 1995.)

14). Radioscaphoid pressure decreased and radiolunate pressure increased when the wrist was moved into ulnar deviation. Computed tomography done after ligament sectioning showed normal relationships among the carpal bones.

Conclusion.—This was the first investigation to simultaneously observe carpal bone position and radiocarpal and ulnocarpal joint pressures during wrist motion. Findings indicate that carpal bone position depends on wrist position and direction of motion. These results support the hypothesis that carpal kinematics are altered significantly with complete tear of the SLIL. The extent of this change can probably produce pain and instability in the affected wrist.

▶ This study uses 3 different technologies to attract the scaphoid and lunate during wrist motion after sectioning the SLIL. One of these technologies is a space age device that enables fighter pilots to aim guns and missiles that operate with an electromagnetic field source. This study demonstrates that the SLIL is an important ligament and stabilizer of the scapholunate joint. After the ligament was sectioned, simultaneous radiocarpal and ulnocarpal joint pressures were concurrently measured during wrist motion. The analysis of the data supports the conclusion that pressure distribution in the radiocarpal and ulnocarpal joints is altered after sectioning of the complete SLIL. This is an important article that helps illuminate the kinesiology of the scaphoid and lunate after ligamentous failure.

P. Dell, M.D.

Wrist Kinematics During Pitching: A Preliminary Report
Pappas AM, Morgan WJ, Schulz LA, et al (Univ of Massachussets, Worcester; New Haven Orthopedic Group, Hamden, Conn)
Am J Sports Med 23:312–315, 1995   8–6

Background.—Wrist kinematics during the pitching cycle have not been described in the literature. Characterization has been difficult because of the joint's small size, high angular velocity, and distance traveled during the pitching motion. These technologic problems were overcome by adapting a recently developed computerized motion analysis system to significantly increase data capture rate.

Methods.—The computerized hand and wrist motion analysis system can capture data at a rate as high as 1,000 Hz. Five right-handed professional pitchers performed 75 pitches for analysis of wrist flexion and extension. For each pitch, a graph was constructed of wrist position vs. time. None of the pitchers reported changes in ball handling resulting from wearing the spandex glove (with digit tips free) used in the motion analysis system. The goniometer is attached to a processing module in a waist pouch, which is connected to the computer interface with a 10-foot cord.

Results.—A reproducible analysis of motion was produced for most pitches, and 4 phases of wrist motion were identified: (1) the cocking phase, which is the motion of the wrist as it moves into maximum exten-

TABLE 1.—Phases of the Pitch

	Cocking	Acceleration	Deceleration	Recovery
Range of motion (deg)	32.4 (±7.8)	94.2 (±1.8)	43.4 (±3.3)	91.0 (±10.2)
Time (msec)	218.9 (±40.1)	105.2 (±10.8)	863.3 (±40.3)	582.7 (±91.6)
Angular velocity (deg/sec)	148.5 (±25.8)	1084.9 (±121.5)	50.2 (±2.9)	165.3 (±15.2)

(Courtesy of Pappas AM, Morgan WJ, Schulz LA, et al: Wrist kinematics during pitching: A preliminary report. *Am J Sports Med* 23:312–315, 1995.)

sion; (2) the acceleration phase of ball propulsion; (3) the deceleration phase after the ball is released, during which the wrist progresses through flexion and wrist velocity consistently decreases; and (4) the recovery phase as the wrist returns toward neutral. For each phase of the pitch, average values for wrist range of motion, length of phase, and angular velocity were calculated (Table 1).

Discussion.—The phases that the wrist repeats in a reproducible fashion during the pitching cycle have not been previously described. Attempts at assessing wrist kinematics with high-speed cinematography led researchers to believe that the wrist did not flex past a neutral position. The ability to quantify this wrist motion and to correlate it with shoulder and total body motion may be useful both in development of pitching technique and in evaluation of injury.

▶ This is the first study to quantify wrist motion during pitching. This advance is the result of computer technology interfaced with a sensing glove that oviates the need for more cumbersome external devices such as an electrogoniometer. The technique has promise and can be applied to other situations. By measuring and further quantifying wrist function in a dynamic way, we can improve our understanding of wrist physiology, pathology, and perhaps treatment.

L.K. Ruby, M.D.

Carpus

The Gross and Histologic Anatomy of the Scapholunate Interosseous Ligament
Berger RA (Mayo Clinic/Mayo Found, Rochester, Minn)
J Hand Surg [Am] 21A:170–178, 1996
8–7

Background.—Although it is believed that the scapholunate interosseous ligament is a strong ligament that connects the carpal scaphoid and lunate bones, there are no detailed reports of normal or variant anatomy. No information is available on the histology of age-related degenerative changes that can occur in the most proximal region of the ligament. Direct repair of the scapholunate interosseous ligament is recommended for scapholunate dissociation, but this is based on the assumption that the ligament tissues will heal and are strong enough to hold sutures securely during healing. No detailed gross anatomical or histologic descriptions of

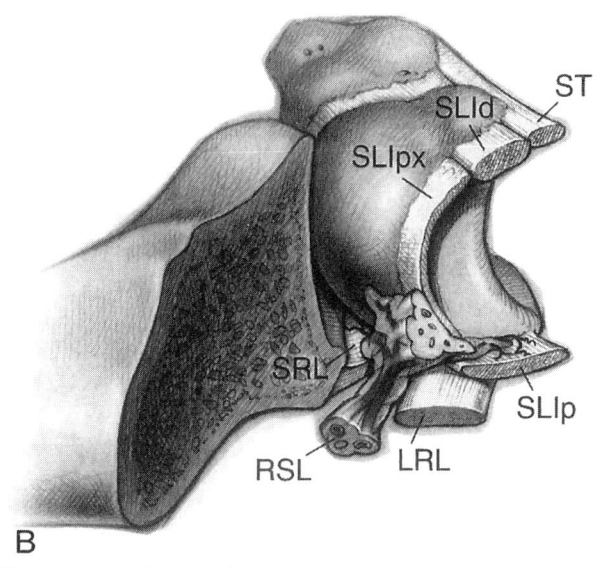

FIGURE 3B.—Interpretive drawing of the relationship between the radius and the scapholunate interosseous (*SLI*) from a radial and slightly proximal perspective. The radius is depicted with the radial styloid region excised. This interpretation is based on the findings of the gross anatomy study and is intended as an orientation device. With the scaphoid removed, the subdivisions of the scapholunate interosseous ligament can be appreciated, as can its relationship to surrounding capsular ligaments. The lunate remains, serving as an attachment for the palmar capsular ligaments, including the long radiolunate (*LRL*) and short radiolunate (*SRL*) ligaments. The scapholunate interosseous ligament is divisible into 3 regions: dorsal (*SLId*), proximal (*SLIpx*), and palmar (*SLIp*). The radioscapholunate ligament (*RSL*) is a neurovascular pedicle that separates the palmar and proximal regions of the scapholunate interosseous ligament. Palmar (*p*) and dorsal (*d*) scaphotriquetral ligament fibers form distal extensions of the scapholunate ligament. (Courtesy of Berger RA: The gross histologic anatomy of the scapholunate interosseous ligament. *J Hand Surg [AM]* 21A:170–178, 1996.)

this ligament have been done to support these assumptions. The gross and histologic anatomy and any regional anatomic differences of the scapholunate interosseous ligament were described.

Methods.—In 21 fresh and 16 fixed adult cadaver wrists, the scapholunate interosseous ligament was studied by gross dissection and serial histologic sections in transverse, sagittal, and coronal planes.

Results.—The scapholunate interosseous ligament can be divided into 3 regions: dorsal, proximal, and palmar (Fig 3B). The dorsal region is thick and consists of short, transverse collagen fibers. The proximal region is chiefly composed of fibrocartilage and a few superficial longitudinal collagen fibers. The proximal region may extend distally into the scapholunate joint space, resembling a knee meniscus. The proximal and palmar regions are separated by the radioscapholunate ligament, which can extend distally to cover the dorsal surface of the palmar region of the scapholunate interosseous ligament. The palmar region is thin and consists of oblique collagen fascicles that are dorsal to and separate from the long radiolunate ligament.

Discussion.—The scapholunate interosseous ligament is a complex structure that connects the dorsal, proximal, and palmar edges of the scaphoid and lunate bones. The proximal region is composed of fibrocartilage and has few superficial longitudinal collagen fibers. Further analysis of the morphology of this ligament is needed to assess the subregions for mechanoreceptors.

▶ This excellent work, initially presented in 1992, clearly shows that the central, intraarticular portion of the scapholunate complex is not ligament but rather fibrocartilage. It has little mechanical strength. Other than serving as a barrier of questionable importance between the radiocarpal and midcarpal joints, this fibrocartilaginous segment has no role to play in scapholunate interaction and apparently no role in determining scapholunate stability. Unfortunately, it is this structure that is visualized arthrographically and arthroscopically. The mechanically important structures are in the capsule, especially dorsally. It is no wonder, then, that tears in the scapholunate seen arthrographically or arthroscopically do not always correlate with symptoms or signs of instability. Tear of this fibrocartilaginous membrane would seem a probably necessary but definitely not sufficient condition for scapholunate instability. Caveat emptor!

P.C. Amadio, M.D.

Influence of Joint Laxity on Scaphoid Kinematics
Garcia-Elias M, Ribe M, Rodriguez J, et al (Hosp General de Catalunya, Barcelona, Spain;)
J Hand Surg (Br) 20B:379–382, 1995   8–8

Background.—Radioulnar deviation may produce various types of normal carpal bone behavior. Compared with normal wrists, excessively lax joints are more likely to develop symptoms if they become overloaded or injured. This could result from either biological or mechanical factors. The link between joint laxity and the kinematic behavior of the scaphoid during radioulnar deviation was evaluated.

Methods.—Sixty normal volunteers underwent assessment of hand and wrist laxity by 4 clinical tests, the results of which were summed to give a global laxity score. Scaphoid motion was assessed using posteroanterior radiographs of the dominant wrist obtained with the wrist in full radial deviation and in full ulnar deviation. These films were used to calculate indexes of scaphoid flexion, inclination, and kinematics.

Results.—Women had greater global wrist laxity scores than men. The direction of scaphoid motion and the amount of wrist laxity were significantly and linearly related. In wrists with greater laxity, the scaphoid rotation produced by lateral deviation occurred mainly along the sagittal plane of flexion and extension—there was little accompanying lateral deviation. For participants with less laxity, rotation occurred mainly along

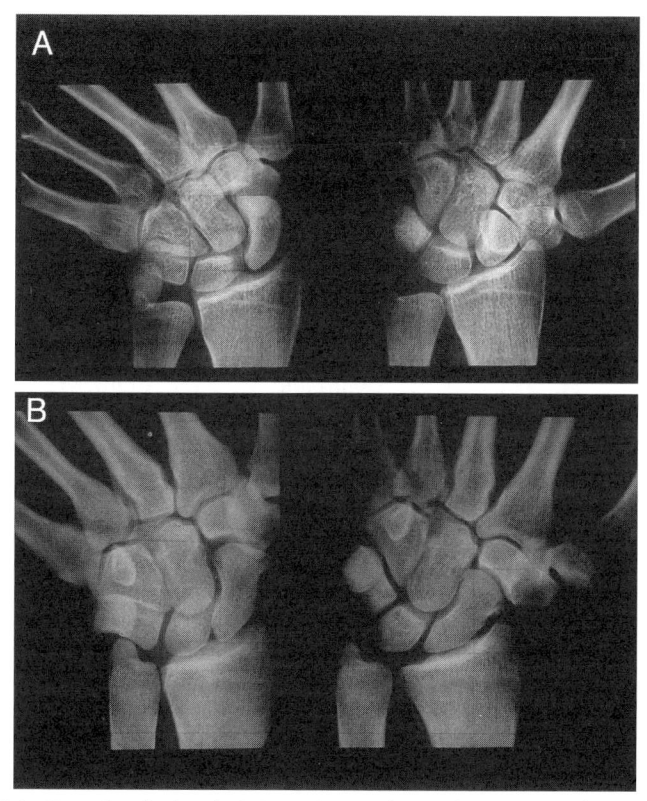

FIGURE 4.—Dynamic radioulnar deviation projections showing the 2 extremes of scaphoid behavior. A, the scaphoid tends to flex rather than deviate in a 34-year-old man with a wrist laxity score of 69 points (scaphoid flexion index, 33%; scaphoid inclination index, 20%). B, the scaphoid tends to deviate rather than flex in a 38-year-old man with a wrist laxity score of 33 points (scaphoid flexion index, 2%; scaphoid inclination index, 35%) (Courtesy of Garcia-Elias M, Ribe M, Rodriguez J, et al: Influence of joint laxity on scaphoid kinematics. *J Hand Surg (Br)* 20B:379–382, 1995.)

the frontal plane of radioulnar deviation. In these cases, flexion extension was minimal (Fig 4).

Conclusions.—Carpal kinematic characteristics appear to be directly related to wrist laxity. Participants with more lax wrists demonstrate scaphoid rotation in the sagittal plane with minimal lateral deviation. The findings may help to explain why patients with lax wrists are more likely to experience capsuloligamentous injuries than patients with tighter wrists, in whom scaphoid rotation follows the opposite pattern. Increased out-of-plane scaphoid rotation could be an important factor in vulnerability to overload or injury.

▶ This very brief report (barely 3 pages) challenges the common concept of carpal kinematics. The lax wrist typically has a scaphoid that flexes and extends on radial–ulnar–radial deviation (the common concept) whereas more inately stable joints demonstrate little flexion or extension and more radial–ulnar shift of the scaphoid. In the lax wrist, scaphoid movement satisfies the columnar theory of carpal kinematics; in the more stable wrist, it satisfies the tenets of the row theory. What is the implication of these findings on provocative tests such as the scaphoid "shift" test of Watson or the scaphoid "thrust" test of Belsky?

V.R. Hentz, M.D.

Positive Ulnocarpal Stress Test
Nakamura R, et al (Nagoya Univ, Japan)
J Jpn Soc Surg Hand 12:18–20, 1995
8–9

Methods.—Thirty-five patients who had persistent ulnar wrist pain after conservative treatment and who had positive ulnocarpal stress test results underwent radiographic examination, bone scan, MRI, radiocarpal arthrography, and arthroscopy.

Results.—Radiographs revealed lunate ulcer or cyst in 7 patients (20%), and accumulation of isotope in ulnar wrist was confirmed in 16 of 17 patients (94%) by bone scanning. Magnetic resonance imaging showed low signal on a T1-weighted image of the lunate ulnar in 4 of 27 patients (15%). Arthroscopy revealed triangular fibrocartilage (TFC) perforation or wear in 21 of 35 patients (60%), lunate fibrillation or ulcer in 14 patients (43%), lunotriquetral ligament (LTL) tear or wear in 11 patients (37%), synovitis in 2 patients, chondromalacia of ulnar head in 3 patients, joint mouse in 1 patient, and joint fibrosis in 1 patient. Established diagnoses were TFC injury in 5 patients, LTL injury in 5 patients, TFC and LTL injury in 2 patients, ulnocarpal abutment syndrome in 19 patients, arthritis in 2 patients, joint mouse in 1 patient, and posttraumatic joint fibrosis in 1 patient.

Conclusion.—The ulnocarpal stress test is sensitive to arthroscopic pathologic conditions, including TFC injury, LTL injury, and ulnocarpal abutment syndrome.

▶ Diagnosis and treatment of ulnar wrist pain are major topics in the field of hand surgery. Although the ulnocarpal stress test (Palmer's procedure) is widely used in hand clinics, sensitivity of this test has not been evaluated.

The authors analyzed the pathologic findings in 35 patients who had persistent ulnar wrist pain after conservative treatment and had positive ulnocarpal stress test results. Arthroscopic examination revealed some pathologic changes in 34 of 35 patients (97%). Pathologic findings observed arthroscopically included the following: TFC tear and wear, 60% of patients; lunate chondromalacia, 43%; and LT ligament tear and wear, 37%.

The ulnocarpal stress test may be as sensitive as arthroscopy, but it will be necessary to estimate how many patients with negative ulnocarpal stress test results have arthroscopic pathologic conditions in order to evaluate the reliability of this manual test.

S. Ishii, M.D.

Dynamic Scapholunate Instability: Results of Operative Treatment With Dorsal Capsulodesis

Wintman BI, Gelberman RH, Katz JN (Massachusetts Gen Hosp, Boston; Washington Univ, St Louis; Brigham and Women's Hosp, Boston; et al)
J Hand Surg (Am) 20A:971–979, 1995
8–10

Purpose.—The nonoperative treatment of symptomatic dynamic scapholunate instability is not always successful. Dorsal capsulodesis to stabilize the scaphoid in patients with chronic static scapholunate instability was first described in 1987. The technique was subsequently used to treat acute static and chronic dynamic types of scapholunate instability. In this study, dorsal capsulodesis was used to treat acute dynamic scapholunate instability.

Patients.—During a 5-year period, dorsal radioscaphoid capsulodesis was performed in 6 men (7 wrists) and 13 women (13 wrists) whose age ranged from 15–55 years. The interval from initial injury or symptom onset to operation ranged from 3–61 months. All patients had undergone mandatory nonoperative therapy for at least 12 weeks. The diagnosis of acute dynamic scapholunate instability was confirmed with the scaphoid shift test. Seventeen patients (18 operated wrists) were reexamined and surveyed with a self-administered follow-up questionnaire at a mean of 34 months after operation.

Results.—Subjective symptoms of scapholunate instability such as wrist clicking or clunking and wrist pain, were significantly alleviated after dorsal radioscaphoid capsulodesis (Table 1). Most patients were satisfied with the results; of the 17 evaluated patients (18 wrists), 15 stated that they would undergo the operation again, 1 would not, and 1 was unsure. Objective assessment revealed that wrist motion in extension, ulnar deviation, or radial deviation did not change significantly but that wrist stability was significantly improved, as confirmed by the scaphoid shift test and an average loss of 12 degrees of flexion (Table 2). Postoperative wrist function was improved to the extent that 15 of the 17 patients could

TABLE 1.—Symptom Severity Data

	Preoperative	Postoperative	*P* Value
Pain frequency*	8.8 ± 1.3	3.7 ± 3.1	< .000001
Pain duration*	7.3 ± 3.2	3.8 ± 3.4	< .01
Pain severity*	5.4 ± 1.8	2.4 ± 1.9	< .0001
Night pain	9 of 18 patients	1 of 18 patients	< .01
Grip weakness	5.5 ± 3.2	2.7 ± 2.4	< .01
Decreased wrist motion	4.9 ± 3.2	4.6 ± 2.6	> .05
Clunking frequency*	6.5 ± 4.1	1.0 ± 1.8	< .0001
Clunking severity	5.6 ± 3.2	1.1 ± 1.7	< .0001

Note: All categories scored on a 0–10 scale; higher numbers indicate increased symptom severity. Associated labels not shown.
* Original data transposed to a 0–10 scale to facilitate comparison.
(Courtesy of Wintman BI, Gelberman RH, Katz JN: Dynamic scapholunate instability: Results of operative treatment with dorsal capsulodesis. *J Hand Surg (Am)* 20A:971–979, 1995.)

TABLE 2.—Physical Examination Data

	Preoperative	Postoperative	P Value
Extension	60° ± 17°	68° ± 12°	> .05
Flexion	63° ± 18°	51° ± 15°	< .05
Radial deviation	17° ± 8°	19° ± 5°	> .05
Ulnar deviation	33° ± 13°	39° ± 13°	> .05
Grip strength (% of normal)	73% ± 32%	87% ± 18%	> .05
Key pinch (% of normal)	80% ± 32%	97% ± 12%	> .05
Scaphoid shift test	20 of 20 positive	1 of 18 positive	< .0001

(Courtesy of Wintman BI, Gelberman RH, Katz JN: Dynamic scapholunate instability: Results of operative treatment with dorsal capsulodesis. *J Hand Surg (Am)* 20A:971–979, 1995.)

resume their previous occupations, although 7 did so with some restrictions. The average interval from operation to return to work was 12 weeks. None of the patients were receiving or were about to receive workers' compensation.

Conclusions.—Dorsal radioscaphoid capsulodesis of the wrist substantially improves the quality of life for most patients with dynamic scapholunate instability that has not responded to a trial period of conservative management.

▶ The exact anatomical disruption that results in dynamic scapholunate instability remains unclear. Some measure of injury to the scapholunate interosseous ligament, radioscapholunate ligament, dorsal radial carpal ligament, and radioscaphocapitate ligament are necessary to destabilize the scaphoid. Dorsal radioscaphoid capsulodesis provides a check to prevent excessive flexion of the scaphoid. This paper reports excellent results in a series of 20 patients who were followed up for a mean of 34 months. Diagnosis was made in several ways, but the authors recommend a good clinical examination as the keystone of diagnostic procedures. This is an important paper, even though the duration of follow-up is somewhat short. Alternate types of stabilization of the scaphoid, which includes intercarpal arthodesis, remain unsatisfactory in terms of patient acceptance and limitations. Proximal row carpectomy is a good way to relieve pain but, of course, does not retain normal anatomy.

P. Dell, M.D.

Autografts From the Foot for Reconstruction of the Scapholunate Interosseous Ligament
Svoboda SJ, Eglseder WA Jr, Belkoff SM (Univ of Maryland, Baltimore)
J Hand Surg (Am) 20A:980–985, 1995   8–11

Purpose.—Disruption of the scapholunate interosseous ligament (SLIL) is a commonly encountered injury. Current SLIL repair techniques include direct ligament repair, with or without dorsal capsulodesis or plication of the joint capsule, tendon grafting, and limited carpal arthrodesis. How-

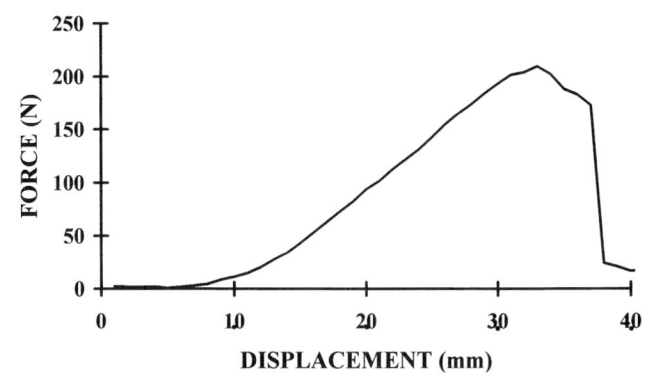

FIGURE 2.—Typical graph of force vs. displacement obtained from one scapholunate interosseous ligament complex. (Courtesy of Svoboda SJ, Eglseder WA Jr, Belkoff SM: Autografts from the foot for reconstruction of the scapholunate interosseous ligament. *J Hand Surg (Am)* 20A:980–985, 1995.)

ever, none of these techniques provide a painless wrist with good stability. The use of ligament autografts to repair the disrupted dorsal portion of the SLIL has been proposed. This study compared the mechanical properties of the SLIL and those of 3 potential autograft ligament complexes from the foot.

Methods.—Six pairs of matched cadaveric hands and feet were obtained from male cadavers, aged 51–68 years. The SLILs were harvested as bone–ligament–bone complexes. The 3 ligament complexes harvested from cadaver feet were the dorsal metatarsal ligament of the fourth and fifth metatarsals, a dorsal tarsometatarsal (TMT) ligament, and the dorsal calcaneocuboid ligament. Each ligament complex was mounted on an Instron materials-testing machine and deformed until ligament failure or bony avulsion occurred. Ligament stiffness and ligament failure load were determined from force-vs.-displacement curves (Fig 2).

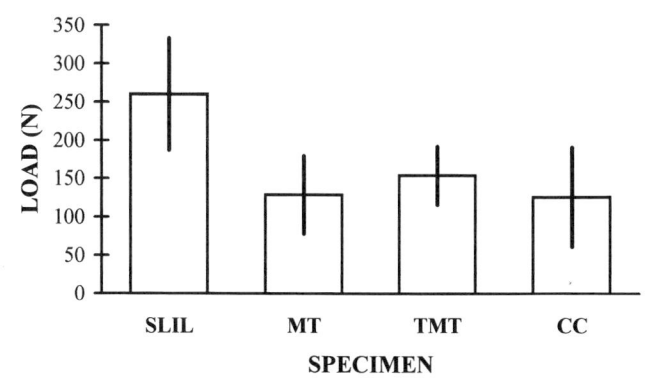

FIGURE 3.—Mean failure loads ± SD for the scapholunate interosseous ligament (*SLIL*) and each of the candidate autografts ($n = 12$). *Abbreviations: MT*, metatarsal; *TMT*, tarsometatarsal; *CC*, calcaneocuboid. (Courtesy of Svoboda SJ, Eglseder WA Jr, Belkoff SM: Autografts from the foot for reconstruction of the scapholunate interosseous ligament. *J Hand Surg (Am)* 20A:980–985, 1995.)

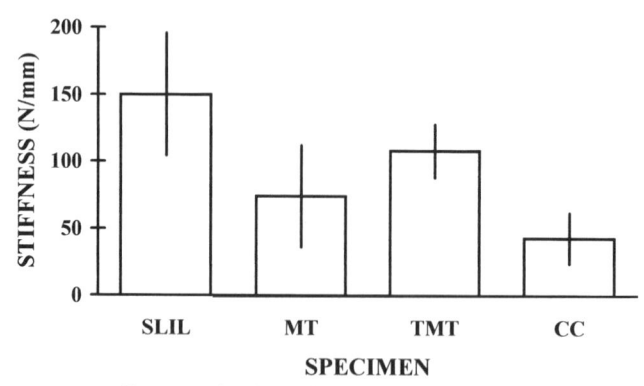

FIGURE 4.—Mean stiffness ± SD for the scapholunate interosseous ligament (*SLIL*) and each of the candidate autografts ($n = 12$). *Abbreviations: MT*, metatarsal; *TMT*, tarsometatarsal; *CC*, calcaneocuboid. (Courtesy of Svoboda SJ, Eglseder WA Jr, Belkoff SM: Autografts from the foot for reconstruction of the scapholunate interosseous ligament. *J Hand Surg (Am)* 20A:980–985, 1995.)

Results.—All specimens failed in the ligamentous substance and none by bony avulsion. The mean failure loads for all 3 candidate autografts were significantly lower than for the SLIL (Fig 3). The mean stiffness value for TMT ligaments did not differ significantly from that for the SLIL, but mean stiffness values for the metatarsal and calcaneocuboid ligaments were significantly lower than that for the SLIL (Fig 4).

Conclusions.—Of the 3 potential autograft ligament complexes tested, the TMT ligament is biomechanically the most similar to the intact SLIL. However, other issues, such as the effects of TMT ligament removal on normal foot function, need to be investigated before TMT ligament autograft can be used to repair a ruptured SLIL in the clinical setting.

▶ This article raises the possibility of clinical application of bone ligament bone preparations obtained from the foot. This is a preliminary study whose technique has not been applied clinically. The technique is designed to determine the mechanical properties of the scapholunate ligamentous complex and 3 potential autografts from the foot. Although none of the selected autografts had a mean failure load similar to that of the scapholunate ligament, the TMT ligament was approximately 60% of the scapholunate ligament. The scapholunate ligament was approximately 30% stiffer than the TMT ligament. It is unknown whether the autograft would achieve the strength and stiffness necessary for normal wrist function, but the concept is extremely important and awaits clinical application.

P. Dell, M.D.

A New Operation for Scapholunate Dissociation: Proposal of a New Surgical Technique for Carpal Instability With Scapholunate Dissociation [11 cases] [in French]

Brunelli GA, Brunelli GR (Clinique Orthopédique de l'Université de Brescia, Italia)
Ann Chir Main 14:207–213, 1995 8–12

Introduction.—The need for repair of a ruptured scapho–trapezium–trapezoid ligament in patients with scapholunate dissociative carpal instability has only recently been recognized. This ligament is a short fibrous complex located at the distal part of the scaphoid at the base of the second metacarpal and is attached to the trapezium and trapezoid. A new surgical procedure for the correction of carpal instability with scapholunate dissociation is described.

Technique.—Access is obtained by dorsal and volar incisions. To restore normal function to the scaphoid, all scar tissue formed in the space between the scaphoid, the trapezium, and the trapezoid that was created by the subluxation is resected. The fibrous sheath of the flexor carpi radialis is cut at the level of the radial–triquetral ligament to allow removal of the scar formed in the space between the scaphoid and the lunate. A tunnel is drilled in the distal pole of the scaphoid, and a slip of flexor carpi radialis is passed through it (Fig 2). The slip is pulled so that the scaphoid is reduced to its

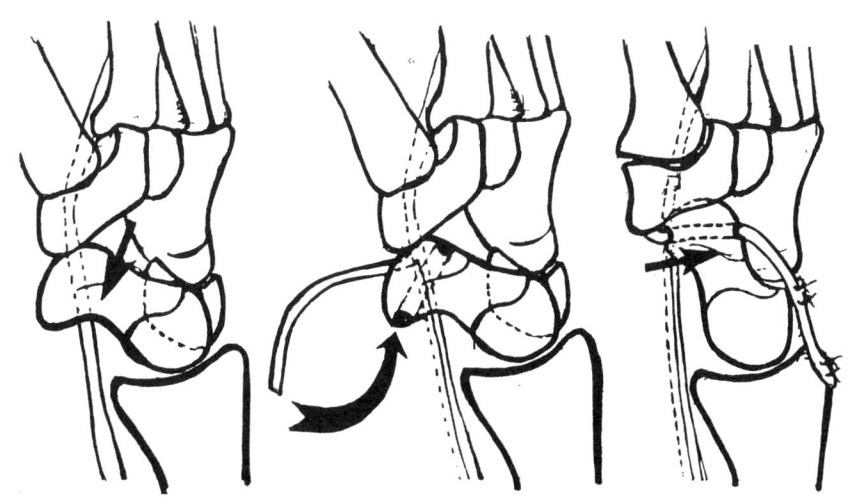

FIGURE 2.—Sketch of the operation. **Left,** the scaphoid is flexed. **Middle,** a slip of flexor carpi radialis is prepared, as is a tunnel in the distal pole of the scaphoid. **Right,** the slip has been passed through the tunnel, pulled distally, reducing the scaphoid to its position and sutured to the dorsal and ulnar edge of the radius. (Courtesy of Brunelli GA, Brunelli GR: A new operation for scapholunate dissociation: proposal of a new surgical technique for carpal instability with scapholunate dissociation (11 cases). *Ann Chir Main* 14:207–213, 1995.)

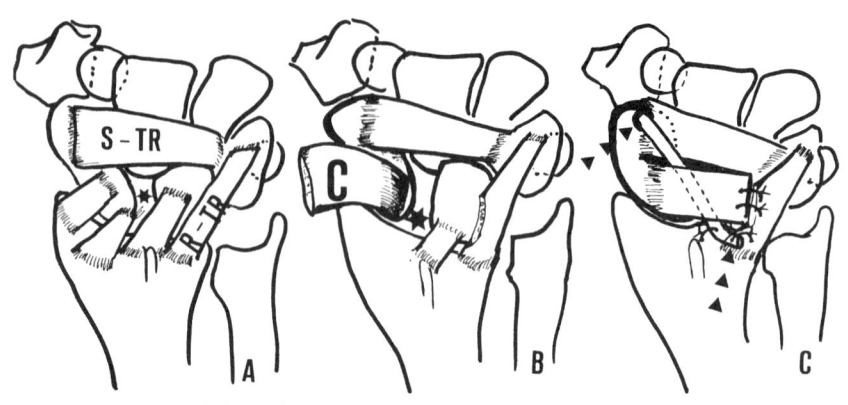

FIGURE 3.—A, scapholunate dissociative carpal instability *asterisk*. B, the capsule (*c*) is cut at the level of the radial–triquetral ligament, which allows removal of the scar formed in the space between scaphoid and lunare. C, The slip of flexor carpi radialis protruding from the tunnel made in the distal pole of the scaphoid is pulled to reduce the scaphoid to its position and is sutured to the dorsal ulnar edge of the radius. The capsule is sutured back to the radial–triquetral (*R-TR*) ligament. *Abbreviation*: *S-TR*, scapho-triquetral ligament. (Courtesy of Brunelli GA, Brunelli GR: A new operation for scapholunate dissociation: proposal of a new surgical technique for carpal instability with scapholunate dissociation (11 cases). *Ann Chir Main* 14:207–213, 1995.)

correct position. The slip is then sutured to the dorsal ulnar edge of the radius with 1 or 2 Kirschner wires, which are removed after 25 days (Fig 3).

Patients.—The operation has been performed in 11 patients. Duration of follow-up ranges from 6 months to 2 years. At the follow-up examination, none of the scaphoid reductions had been lost. Wrist mobility in flexion was limited to an average of 25 degrees. Grip strength was reduced by an average of 35% compared with the contralateral hand but was improved by 50% when compared with preoperative grip strength. All 11 patients were very satisfied with the results and have gone back to work. Only 1 patient has occasional wrist pain, which can be controlled with oral medications.

Conclusions.—Early follow-up data suggest that this new operation for correcting carpal instability with scapholunate dissociation gives satisfactory results. If the long-term results confirm the early findings, this technique may well replace more complicated tendinoplasties and limited wrist fusions.

▶ The Brunellis (father and son) have described an interesting approach to the stabilization of acute and chronic rotatory subluxation of the scaphoid. Use of both volar and dorsal exposure of the scaphoid's multiple articulations allows the scaphoid to be sufficiently freed from scar, which is especially important in chronic dissociation. The wrist is immobilized for only 25 days; rehabilitation is then begun. This is a considerably briefer period than that currently recommended for the dorsal capsulodesis procedure. Only 11 cases were followed, some for only 6 months. Wrist flexion is significantly limited, averaging only 25 degrees.

V.R. Hentz, M.D.

Triquetrohamate Arthrodesis for Midcarpal Instability
Rao SB, Culver JE (Cleveland Clinic Found, Ohio)
J Hand Surg (Am) 20A:583–589, 1995   8–13

Introduction.—In midcarpal instability, pain on the ulnar side of the wrist and a weak grip are accompanied by abnormal midcarpal joint motion. From the lateral perspective, the proximal row of carpal bones lags behind and remains flexed as the wrist is moved from radial to ulnar deviation and then suddenly snaps into extension, producing a painful "clunk." Surgery may be warranted when conservative measures fail to relieve the symptoms.

Patients.—The results of triquetrohamate arthrodesis were examined in 10 patients with midcarpal instability who had surgery (1 of them in both wrists) from 1981 to 1988. Ulnar wrist pain, weak grip, and decreased motion were consistent findings and interfered with daily activities. There was tenderness dorsally over the triquetrohamate joint, and midcarpal joint motion was excessive on anteroposterior stress testing. Range of motion was reduced in all patients. Cineradiography confirmed asynchronous motion of the carpal bones.

Management.—All patients had tried conservative measures, and 2 had undergone soft-tissue stabilization procedures with no relief of symptoms. The joint was exposed by a dorsal approach. Exploration revealed localized synovitis and, in some cases, superficial erosion of the opposed cartilage surfaces of the triquetrum and hamate. The joint cartilage and subchondral bone were totally removed, and cancellous bone from the distal radius was packed into the defect. Kirschner wires or staples were used for internal fixation.

Results.—After an average follow-up interval of 26 months, 2 wrists had excellent results; 4, good results; 3, fair results; and 2, poor results. Pain was relieved in 7 of the 10 patients. Range of motion decreased after surgery, especially in flexion, but grip strength improved steadily. Bony union was achieved in an average of 9½ weeks, but 2 nonunions occurred. No patient exhibited degenerative changes.

Conclusion.—Triquetrohamate arthrodesis reliably stabilizes the midcarpal joint, but not all patients have a good clinical outcome.

▶ The authors described 11 wrists with midcarpal instability treated by stabilization with intercarpal arthrodesis, (specifically, triquetrohamate). Only slightly more than 50% of their results were good to excellent, despite successful union in all but 2 cases and a relatively short duration of follow-up (average, 26 months). These results are not dissimilar from those reported for other limited carpal arthrodeses. Why do some patients with successful arthrodeses continue to have pain? Possibilities include incorrect diagnosis, multiple problems, scarring from surgery, and psychological factors. In addition, the surgeon may have failed to diagnose and treat all of the painful wrist conditions. For instance, if radiocarpal chondromalacia, ulnar impingement, or nonassociated volar carpal ligament injuries accompany the midcarpal instability, will these conditions become more painful or symptomatic after midcarpal stabilization? Perhaps prearthrodesis wrist arthroscopy could provide an answer.

E.R. North, M.D.

Arthroscopic Management of Partial Scapholunate and Lunotriquetral Injuries of the Wrist
Ruch DS, Poehling GG (Wake Forest Univ, Winston-Salem, NC)
J Hand Surg [Am] 21A:412–417, 1996   8–14

Background.—Arthroscopy has enabled the accurate characterization and effective treatment of a variety of soft-tissue lesions. Although much is known about the mechanism of injury, kinematics, and treatment of complete injuries to the intrinsic ligaments of the wrist, very little is known about incomplete injuries to these structures. The outcomes of patients undergoing arthroscopic débridement of isolated partial scapholunate or lunotriquetral ligament injuries with no evidence of instability were documented.

Patients and Findings.—Fourteen patients treated for mechanical wrist pain of more than 6 months' duration were included. Ages ranged from 17 to 59 years. At a minimum of 2 years after treatment, the patients were interviewed and underwent physical and radiographic assessment. Eleven patients had complete relief of symptoms and were able to return to work within 7 weeks of operation. The remaining 3 patients reported occasional, mild wrist pain. Two returned to work a mean of 6.5 weeks after surgery, and the third returned after 1 year. No patient had a significant loss of grip or pinch strength. No abnormalities were found on radiographic films and dynamic examinations under fluoroscopy. Thirteen patients were highly satisfied with the results of treatment, but 2 still occasionally had mild wrist pain.

Conclusion.—Incomplete ligamentous wrist injuries are a possible cause of painful crepitance. Arthroscopic débridement can improve outcomes. In the current series, 13 of 14 patients had excellent pain relief and an early return of wrist function.

▶ This article evaluates a discrete subgroup of patients with persistent mechanical wrist pain of longer than 6 months' duration secondary to partial tears of the scapholunate or lunotriquetral ligament. The finding that mechanical débridement by arthroscopy provides good short- and intermediate-term palliation is significant and is supported by other clinical reports. These data also suggest that partial tears of intercarpal ligaments do not necessarily progress to complete tears in 2 years. These data *cannot* be extrapolated to the unstable wrist.

L.A. Koman, M.D.

Carpal Instability and Scaphoid Pseudoarthrosis
Martin MA, Hernández C, Hurtado P, et al (Hosp Universitario, Valladolid, Spain)
Rev Esp Cir Mano 50:25–32, 1995
8–15

Introduction.—The natural course of nontreated scaphoid pseudarthrosis has been a matter of concern for many authors in recent years. The relationship between the pseudarthrosis of the scaphoid with carpal malalignment and degenerative arthritis was studied.

Patients.—Thirty-six wrists in 36 patients with a pseudarthrosis of the scaphoid were reviewed. In 27 cases, the fracture was in the middle third; in 8 cases, in the proximal pole; and in 1 case, at the tubercle. The time of evolution of the pseudarthrosis ranged from 1 to 16 years, with an average of 5.7 years. The following carpal misalignments were observed: a dorsiflexed intercalated segment instability (DISI) deformity superior to 10 degrees in 80.5% of the patients, a carpal collapse superior to 0.48 (Youn Y et al: *J Bone Joint Surg,* 1978) in 36.1% of the wrists, and ulnar translation of the carpus superior to 5 mm in 27.7% of the wrists.

Conclusion.—A carpal collapse with DISI deformity is the most common misalignment observed. In a few cases, it was present in the early stages, regardless of the scaphoid displacement, and was probably secondary to an associated ligamentous injury. The DISI deformity has a tendency to increase, being present in 95.5% of the cases who had a pseudarthrosis for more than 3 years. Degenerative arthritis had a direct relationship to the passing of time, being present in 97% of the cases of pseudarthrosis after 5 years, and in all cases of more than 10 years' duration. Degenerative arthritis presented at an earlier stage in older patients, especially in those who had performed heavy labor, as well as in those with a greater displacement of the bone fragments. There was no direct relationship between degenerative arthritis and the degree of DISI deformity, nor between ulnar translocation of the carpus and the degree of DISI deformity or degenerative arthritis.

▶ The authors have done a very detailed study of 36 cases of scaphoid pseudoarthrosis, confirming the opinion of most authors that the natural course of this pathologic condition is a progressive carpal collapse and degenerative arthritis. Based on these findings, all scaphoid pseudoarthrosis should be treated as early as possible, even if patients are asymptomatic.

A. Lluch, M.D., Ph.D.

Internal Fixation of Acute Stable Scaphoid Fractures in the Athlete
Rettig AC, Kollias SC (Methodist Sports Medicine Ctr, Indianapolis, Ind)
Am J Sports Med 24:182–186, 1996   8–16

Introduction.—Scaphoid fractures are commonly treated with casts and usually require 9–12 weeks for healing. Although playing casts may be appropriate for athletes desiring to return to play, open reduction and internal fixation can offer an early return to sports requiring maximal manual dexterity. The 12 athletes reported here were treated with Herbert screw fixation for acute mid-third scaphoid fractures.

Methods.—Patients ranged in age from 17–31 years; 8 participated in basketball, 2 in baseball, and 2 in archery. All were treated within 4 weeks of the injury. The fractures were nondisplaced in 10 cases and minimally displaced in 2. Most surgical procedures were performed through a volar Russe-type approach. Patients wore a short arm-thumb spica splint for 7–10 days, followed by a resting splint and a program of stretching and strengthening at home. Return to sports was approved when the patient could participate without pain or use of a supportive device. During the healing period, the patients were regularly examined for grip strength, range of motion, and point tenderness.

Results.—With an average follow-up of 2.9 years, 11 of the 12 athletes had radiographic union of the fracture. Average time to union was 9.8 weeks. Range of motion of the wrist was symmetrical in 9 of 12 patients, and 10 had grip strength equal to or greater than the injured side. Archers returned to their sport at an average of 3.5 weeks after surgery; basketball players required 6 weeks and baseball players 5.8 weeks. Except for the patient with nonunion—a basketball player with insulin-dependent diabetes—patients were pleased with the surgical results.

Conclusion.—For athletes who desire an early return to sports and accept the risks of surgery, internal fixation of an acute mid-third scaphoid fracture is a viable alternative to cast treatment. The procedure was safe and the outcome excellent in this small series of patients, but longer follow-up is advisable before internal fixation is widely recommended in such cases.

▶ Although these authors rightly state that cast treatment remains the treatment of choice for undisplaced scaphoid fractures, one wonders how many readers will accept the idea that the authors truly believe what they say, given their use of surgical management for this group of mostly high school and college age athletes. I am, myself, somewhat concerned about the cost-benefit ratio in such cases. Getting a player back in 6–10 weeks (the results here in all but 4 cases) vs. 9–12 weeks (what they quote for nonoperative management) seems a small benefit, perhaps in most cases, not worth the cost in terms of dollars and the risk of complications of surgical treatment.

I have no quibble with the authors' approach, when applied to the professional athlete. My concern is for the vast number of recreational and amateur participants who may be convinced, to their potential detriment, to have the "treatment of the stars" by an overenthusiastic surgeon supported by literature such as this. Our sports medicine colleagues have been down this road already with the anterior cruciate; our spine colleagues may be treading it with internal fixation for low back pain. Should hand surgeons follow?

P.C. Amadio, M.D.

Radio-lunate Arthrodesis for Distal Radial Intraarticular Malunion
Saffar P (Institut Français de Chirurgie de la Main, Paris)
J Hand Surg [Br] 21B:14–20, 1996   8–17

Background.—Radiolunate arthrodesis has been used in rheumatic patients with ulnar shift of the carpus but is used only rarely in patients with traumatic wrist injuries. Patients with distal radial intra-articular malunion treated with the radiolunate limited arthrodesis were reviewed.

Technique.—By using a dorsal approach, articular cartilage remnants are excised from the proximal lunate and the lunate fossa. Normal carpal height and scaphoid alignment are created with manual distraction. A corticocancellous graft from the iliac crest or the proximal end of the ulna is placed in a trough in the distal part of the radius and the dorsal part of the lunate to maintain the restored carpal height. Internal fixation can be performed with 2 or 3 screws, a plate, or staples. The joint is immobilized until union is achieved. Daily rehabilitation is used to establish full range of motion.

Methods.—The records of 11 patients with painful intra-articular distal radial malunions who underwent radiolunate arthrodeses between 1983 and 1991 were reviewed. Examination of preoperative radiographs, revealed a mean articular step-off of the distal radius of 4.4 mm and irregular contour of the lunate fossa in all patients. The scapholunate interval was normal in 3 patients and was greater than 2 mm in 2 patients, greater than 3 mm in 3 patients, and 5 mm in 1 patient. Eight of 9 patients had volar intercalated segment instability (VISI). The distal radioulnar joint was destroyed in 3 patients, irregular in 1 patient, and incongruent in 5 patients.

Results.—Pain was reduced in all patients. The average range of motion was 33 degrees flexion, 39 degrees extension, 17 degrees radial deviation, and 29 degrees ulnar deviation. Strength improved from 45% to 57% of the opposite side. At the final follow-up examination, 5 patients had VISI; in 4 patients, the lunate was in neutral position. Dynamic radiographs showed perilunate motion of the carpus (Fig 5, C and D). Union was achieved in 10 of the 11 patients within 45–90 days. Nonunion in the remaining patient was treated with plate fixation and graft. Eight patients returned to their previous work, and 2 returned to lighter work.

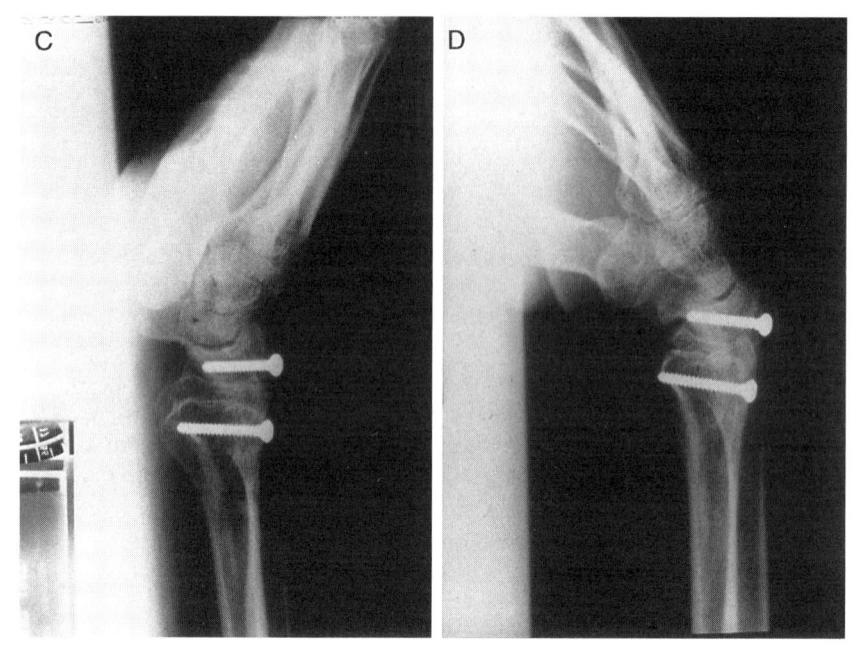

FIGURE 5, C and D.—Dynamic radiographs after radiolunate arthrodesis. (Courtesy of Saffar P: Radiolunate arthrodesis for distal radial intraarticular malunion. *J Hand Surg* 21B:14–20, 1996.)

Conclusions.—Radiolunate arthrodesis is appropriate for treating distal radial intra-articular malunion of the radial lunate facet with or without dorsal subluxation of carpus to restore carpal height, realign the scaphoid, relieve pain, restore strength and motion, and prevent further osteoarthritis. Because abnormalities of the distal radioulnar joint may necessitate associated procedures, preoperative analysis should also include planning for these additional treatments.

▶ When intra-articular malunion results in radiocarpal arthritis, limited radiolunate or radioscapholunate arthrodesis is a good alternative to complete wrist fusion or wrist arthroplasty. The former limits motion more than a limited fusion, and the latter is almost always doomed to failure for this indication.[1]

P.C. Amadio, M.D.

Reference

1. Amadio PC, Botte MJ: Treatment of malunion of the distal radius. *Hand Clin* 3:541–560, 1987.

Can a Day 4 Bone Scan Accurately Determine the Presence or Absence of Scaphoid Fracture?
Murphy DG, Eisenhauer MA, Powe J, et al (Univ of Western Ontario, Canada)
Ann Emerg Med 26:434–438, 1995   8–18

Objective.—Scaphoid fracture can be very difficult to diagnose in patients with acute wrist trauma. Many patients in whom scaphoid fracture is suspected will have the wrist immobilized for 10–14 days, at which time the fracture may be apparent on radiography. As many as 85% of such patients will eventually prove to have no fracture. Although bone scanning can confirm the presence or absence of scaphoid fracture after 10–14 days, few studies have looked at its use in the period just after injury. The ability of a bone scan performed 4 days after injury to predict the presence or absence of suspected scaphoid fracture was evaluated.

Methods.—The prospective study included 99 patients, aged 16 years or older, who were seen in the emergency department with "clinical scaphoid fracture." The criteria for this diagnosis were the presence of "snuffbox tenderness" in a patient whose mechanism of injury was consistent with scaphoid trauma but whose initial radiographs were normal. All patients underwent immobilization in a thumb spica cast. Four days after injury, patients had bone scanning of both wrists. Clinical examination and radiographs were repeated on the 14th day. The results of the bone scans were compared in blinded fashion with the final diagnosis.

Results.—Thirteen patients had scaphoid fractures, and all were correctly identified by the bone scan obtained on day 4. However, the early bone scans gave false-positive results in another 7 patients. The day 4 bone scans had a sensitivity of 100%, specificity of 92%, positive predictive value of 65%, negative predictive value of 100%, and accuracy of 93%. These scans also identified many other types of fractures, including fractures of the triquetra, distal radius, capitate, hamate, trapezoid, trapezium, and metacarpals, some of which had not previously been suspected.

Conclusions.—In patients with acute wrist trauma, bone scans obtained on the 4th day after injury can accurately rule out the diagnosis of scaphoid fracture. However, because false positive scans are common, day 4 bone scanning cannot reliably confirm this diagnosis. Early bone scans may also identify other, previously unsuspected fractures of the wrist, which are surprisingly frequent in this patient population.

▶ The literature suggests that perhaps 15% of patients with acute scaphoid fractures have initial false negative findings on initial radiography. This is the impetus for treating patients who have clinical signs but indeterminant radiographic findings of a scaphoid fracture by immobilization for 10 to 14 days and re-examination. The literature also suggests that as many as 85% of these patients do not have a fracture of the scaphoid and thus may have been needlessly immobilized. Unfortunately, although this study demonstrated that a negative early bone scan accurately ruled out a fracture of the scaphoid, the utility of a positive scan was less clear (positive predictive value of 65%). An interesting observation was the incidence of other initially undetected fractures of the carpus recognized by bone scan in this sample. It is unclear whether the examination is cost-effective in terms of limiting the number of unnecessarily immobilized wrists that prevent the patient from returning to work.

V.R. Hentz, M.D.

Non-union of the Scaphoid: Revascularization of the Proximal Pole With Implantation of a Vascular Bundle and Bone-grafting
Fernandez DL, Eggli S (Lindenhof Hosp, Bern, Switzerland)
J Bone Joint Surg (Am) 77-A:883-893, 1995   8-19

Introduction.—Because conventional autogenous nonvascularized bone-grafting procedures have poor results in patients with nonunions of the scaphoid with avascular necrosis of the proximal fragment, other procedures have been proposed, including the implantation of a vascular pedicle or vascularized bone graft. The experience with surgical treatment of 11 nonunited scaphoid fractures with an avascular proximal segment by combining implantation of a vascular pedicle and a corticocancellous strut of autogenous bone graft is described.

Patients.—Avascular necrosis was confirmed in 11 ununited scaphoid fractures by both radiographic criteria (increased bone density, loss of normal trabecular appearance, collapsed subchondral bone, cystic changes, and deformed osseous segment) and clinical criteria (sclerotic bone with no bleeding after débridement). Nonunion of the scaphoid had been present for an average of 14 months. Six patients had undergone a previous unsuccessful surgical procedure.

Surgical Procedure.—The wrist capsule is opened along the long axis of the scaphoid; the radial nerve and the radial arterial nutrient branches are protected. The sclerotic surfaces of the nonunion site are débrided. A cavity is drilled in the central portion of the avascular proximal fragment, as is a trapezoidal trough on the dorsoradial aspect of the distal fragment. A corticocancellous peg graft matching the prepared defect of the scaphoid is cut from the iliac crest. The scaphoid fragments are separated. The graft is first inserted into the central cavity of the proximal fragment, then reduced into the trough of the distal fragment, with 1 or 2 Kirschner wires used for stabilization (Fig 2). A vascular pedicle consisting of the second intermetacarpal artery and its venae comitantes with a thin layer of perivascular areolar tissue is dissected, elevated, passed through a 2.7-mm hole drilled in the proximal pole of the scaphoid just ulnar to the bone graft, and tied with a suture over the palmar antebrachial fascia. The wrist is immobilized for 8 weeks after surgery; the Kirschner wires are then removed.

Results.—Of the 11 nonunions, 10 healed an average of 10 weeks after the Kirschner wires were removed; 1 patient had a persistent nonunion.

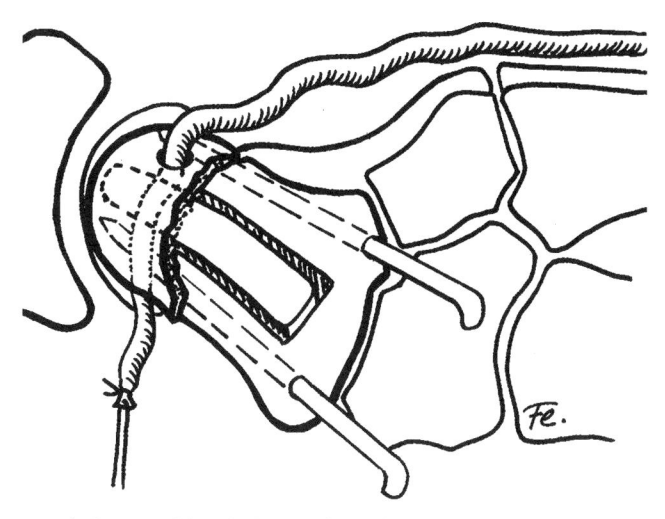

FIGURE 2.—The location of the inlay bone graft and the vascular pedicle as well as the ideal position of the Kirschner wires for fixation of the nonunion. (Courtesy of Fernandez DL, Eggli S: Non-union of the scaphoid: Revascularization of the proximal pole with implantation of a vascular bundle and bone-grafting. *J Bone Joint Surg (Am)* 77-A:883–893, 1995.)

One patient had radiographic union but persistent pain. According to the Mayo Clinic wrist scoring system, the overall functional result was excellent in 3 patients, good in 3, fair in 3, and poor in 2. Subsequent arthrodesis of the radioscapholunate joints in 1 patient, total arthrodesis of the wrist in 1, and styloidectomy in 1 produced satisfactory results.

Conclusions.—This technique, which combines inlay bone grafting, internal fixation, and implantation of a vascular bundle, is a promising alternative to vascularized bone-grafting procedures in patients with nonunion of the scaphoid with an avascular proximal fragment but no evidence of periscaphoid degenerative changes.

▶ This paper addresses a difficult but not uncommon clinical situation—patients with scaphoid nonunions and avascular necrosis of the proximal pole. In addition, more than half of the patients in this series had undergone previous unsuccessful surgery. Their technique is clearly described and illustrated. A combination of inlay corticocancellous iliac bone graft stabilized with Kirschner wires and a vascular pedicle into the avascular proximal pole was used. The dual factors of stability and vascularity are appropriately emphasized.

The union rate of at least 90% in this difficult group of patients rivals the results in other series of uncomplicated nonunions. This is an important paper. Certainly, most surgeons have had success treating avascular non-unions with conventional techniques, but the union rate does not approach the results in this series.

W. Engberger, M.D.

Nonunion of the Carpal Scaphoid: Results of Internal Fixation With Anatomical Staples (43 Cases) [in French]
Savornin C, Esling F (Hôpital Begin, Paris)
La Main 1:29–37, 1996
8–20

Purpose.—The surgical treatment of pseudarthrosis of the carpal scaphoid always involves the use of a bone graft and an osteosynthesis method. There is agreement on the need for using bone grafts, but not on what constitutes the ideal fixation method, as none of the available techniques are ideal. The initial results obtained with a new anatomical staple for stabilizing the scaphoid are presented.

Methods.—The shape of the staple reflects the morphology of the scaphoid. The shape and precise angulation of the design were derived from cadaver studies. The staple comes in 7 sizes and is made of titanium. Before the staple can be placed, any dorsal intercalary segment instability (DISI) must be corrected. This is done by inserting a radio-lunate pin and repositioning the semilunate bone. Restoration of the normal scaphoid anatomy with an iliac bone graft before insertion of the staple is essential if callus formation is to be avoided (Fig 2).

Patients.—Between 1987 and 1994, 52 men and 1 woman, aged 14–57, with pseudarthrosis of the carpal scaphoid were operated on by this technique, and 43 of them were evaluable after a mean follow-up of 24 months. All except 1 of the re-evaluated pseudarthroses had consolidated after an interval of 3–12 months. One pseudarthrosis consolidated after reoperation with the same technique. The height of the scaphoid had returned to normal in 32% of the patients, was increased by at least 10% in 50% of the patients, and was decreased by at least 10% in 18% of the cases. The overall results were good or very good in 83.7% of the cases.

Conclusions.—The newly designed anatomical staple enables proper fixation for the pseudarthroses of the scaphoid, whatever their localization, except for the type I Schernberg pseudarthroses.

▶ Staple fixation of scaphoid fractures is becoming common in Europe. This paper reviews the technique and results in a large series. The staples are of

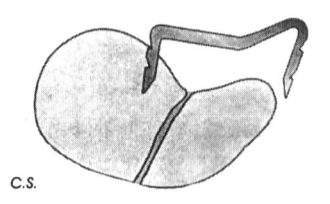

Unacceptable position of the staple and scaphoid before reduction of "D.I.S.I."

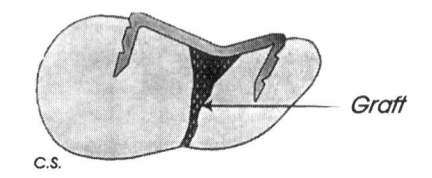

Acceptable position of the staple and scaphoid after reduction of "D.I.S.I."

FIGURE 2.—A, placement of the staple impossible before reduction of the dorsal intercalary segment instability (DISI) and the scaphoid. B, placement of the staple possible after reduction of the DISI and the scaphoid. *Abbreviation:* C.S., carpal scaphoid. (Courtesy of Savornin C, Esling F: Pseudarthrose du scaphoïde carpien: Résultat de la stabilisation par agrafe anatomique. *La Main* 1:29–37, 1996.)

a special design that is not available (to my knowledge) in the United States, but one suspects they will eventually appear on this side of the Atlantic. I believe they would be worth a try.

P.C. Amadio, M.D.

Vascular Bundle Implantation Into Bone for Aseptic Necrosis of the Lunate
Guo J-h (East-South Hosp, Fu Jian, People's Republic of China)
Ann Plast Surg 36:133–138, 1996   8–21

Objective.—The operative technique and clinical results of vascular bundle implantation into bone were presented for 11 cases of aseptic necrosis of the lunate bone. Also described were the anatomical studies that preceded introduction of the procedure at the study institution in April 1986.

Technique.—The procedure is performed with the patient under axillary nerve block anesthesia and a pneumatic tourniquet. An S-shaped incision is made on the dorsum of the wrist joint and the dorsal carpal ligament incised longitudinally. The tendon of the extensor digitorum communis muscles is retracted ulnarly and the tendon of the extensor pollicis longus retracted radially.

A single vascular bundle consisting of the ramus lateralis or the ramus medialis of the ramus carpeus dorsalis of the interosseal anterior artery and vein, together with a few perivascular connective tissues, is isolated, ligated, and severed at its distal end. Sufficient length is allowed for insertion into the lunate bone. The 2 ligated ends are then tied to straight needles and ligated to the skin, with a button padded to immobilize the vascular bundle. Patients wear a plaster cast, applied from the metacarpophalangeal joint to the forearm, for 4 weeks.

Results.—The 11 patients ranged in age from 19 to 24 years and had jobs requiring moderate-to-heavy labor. Symptoms of wrist pain were reported as an average of 12.8 months duration before the operation. With an average of 36 months of follow-up, outcome of vascular bundle implantation was judged excellent in 9 cases and good in 2. Those with excellent results were free of wrist pain, regained at least 75% of normal grip strength, had normal flexion-extension of the wrist, and were able to return to work. Roentgenograms showed no sclerosis of the lunate bone and normal architecture and bone density of the lunate. Patients with good results continued to have slight pain with wrist activity and mildly diminished motion, but had regained 70% to 75% of normal grip strength; roentgenogram findings were normal.

Conclusion.—Transplantation of a vascular bundle containing an artery and its accompanying vein achieved good results in patients with aseptic necrosis of the lunate bone. Necrotized lunate bones were seen to have healed on roentgenograms, and most patients were free of symptoms.

▶ I agree that vascular bundle implantation is a useful therapy for Kienböck's disease, particularly for stages II and IIIA, in the ulna-neutral wrist. This paper supports that thesis, but, unfortunately the quality of the x-ray film reproductions makes it impossible to confirm the author's interpretation of the quality of the bone stock at final follow-up.

P.C. Amadio, M.D.

Ulnar Lengthening and Radial Recession Procedures for Kienböck's Disease: Long-term Clinical and Radiographic Follow-up
Trail IA, Linscheid RL, Quenzer DE, et al (Mayo Clinic, Rochester, Minn)
J Hand Surg [Br] 21B:169–176, 1996   8–22

Objective.—Long-term clinical and radiologic outcome was reported for 20 patients who underwent ulnar lengthening or radial recession for treatment of Kienböck's disease. These joint levelling procedures were found to yield good subjective clinical results at earlier follow-up.

Methods.—Sixteen patients had undergone ulnar lengthening procedures and 4 were treated with radial recession. The average age at diagnosis was 26.9 years and the average follow-up was 11 years. Preoperative tomograms were available for 14 patients; all 20 patients had new trispiral tomograms of the wrist in anteroposterior and lateral projections. Follow-up x-ray evaluation included analysis of ulnar variance, radiologic

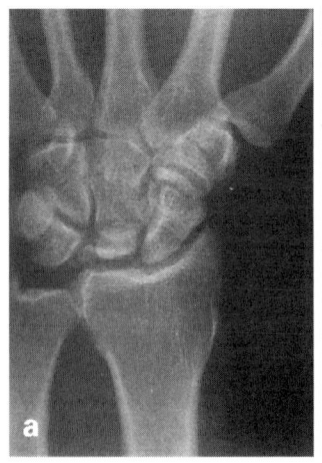

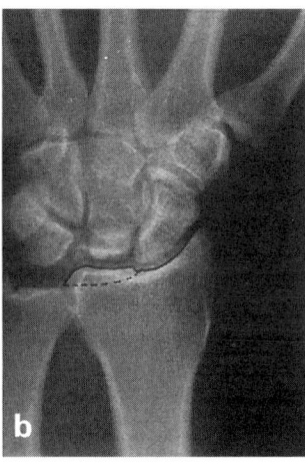

(*Continued*)

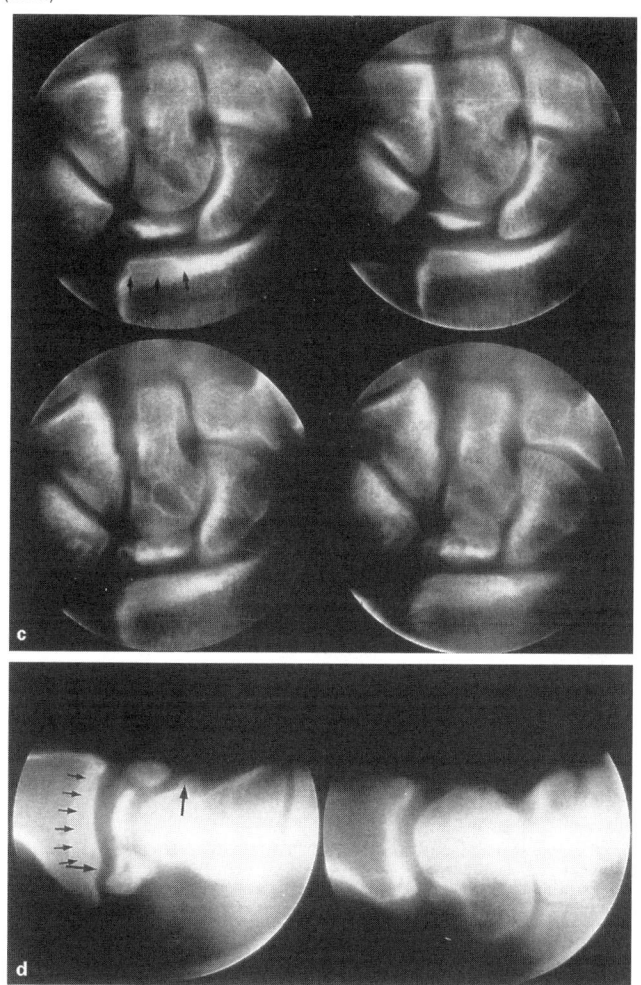

FIGURE 5.—Fourteen-year follow-up ulnar lengthening. **a** and **b**, enchondral remodeling of lunate fossa outlined. **c** and **d**, trispiral tomograms. **c**, anteroposterior shows lunate fossa projection at several levels. **d**, lateral views. Enchondral growth beneath lunate fossa (**left**) designated by *proximal arrows*. Note fragmentation and lunate collapse. There is some scaphoid fossal growth palmarly. (Courtesy of Trail IA, Linscheid RL, Quenzer DE, et al: Ulnar lengthening and radial recession procedures for Kienböck's disease: Long-term clinical and radiographic follow-up. *J Hand Surg (Br)* 21B: 169–176, 1996.)

staging, and determination of radioscaphoid and radiolunate angles and carpal height.

Results.—Ulnar lengthening averaged 4 mm and radial recession averaged 2 mm. There were 14 additional procedures, including 11 simple plate removals. Earlier follow-up (average, 28.5 months) had shown 19 of 20 patients to be subjectively improved. Eleven years after the procedures, 15 were able to work full-time, without restrictions, at their original jobs. All reported less pain in the operated wrist than before surgery, 17 believed that the operated wrist was stronger, and 16 believed that range of motion was improved. Clinical examination confirmed significant increases in the arc of wrist extension and flexion and in grip strength. Thirteen patients had new bone formation at the lunate fossa of the radius (Fig 5), a finding not present in any cases preoperatively, and 12 showed osteoarthritic changes. Four of 9 patients with lunate bone fragmentation before surgery were seen to have partial resolution at long-term follow-up. Ulnar variance averaged +0.6 mm at follow-up, compared with +1.9 mm postoperatively. Carpal height did not change significantly.

Conclusion.—All 20 patients who underwent a joint levelling procedure for Kienböck's disease reported subjective improvement at an average of 11 years postoperatively. There appeared to be no deterioration in results, compared with earlier follow-up. Radiologic examination, however, indicated continuing fragmentation, cysts, and nonunion of the lunate fractures.

▶ Little has been written on the long-term follow-up of treated Kienböck's disease, and nothing with this degree of tomographic detail. Joint levelling may help symptoms, but there is little evidence that the lunate can restore itself after this treatment. Thus, although joint levelling is currently the benchmark procedure for most hand surgeons, there is clearly room for improvement.

P.C. Amadio, M.D.

Scaphocapitate Arthrodesis for the Treatment of Kienböck's Disease
Sennwald GR, Ufenast H (Chirurgie St Leonhard, Gallen, Switzerland)
J Hand Surg (Am) 20A:506–510, 1995   8–23

Introduction.—The surgical treatment of Kienböck's disease is often scaphotrapezium–trapezoid arthrodesis (STT). The results of scaphocapitate arthrodesis as an alternative treatment for patients with advanced Kienböck's disease were assessed in a retrospective study.

Methods.—Ten patients with grade III and 1 patient with grade II Kienböck's disease were treated surgically by scaphocapitate arthrodesis. The lunate was not removed and the scaphocapitate joint was subjected to arthodesis at a radioscaphoid angle of 50 degrees. Preoperative and follow-up radiographic evaluations were performed and rehabilitation was initiated 6–10 weeks after surgery.

Results.—Grip strength and mobility in patients receiving scaphocapitate arthrodesis were reduced by 28% and 52% respectively when compared with the side not affected by Kienbock's disease. Pain resolved in all but 1 patient: this patient had previously undergone ulnar lengthening and had demonstrated a positive variance and impingement. Before scaphocapitate arthrodesis, the ulnar on the affected side of these patients was shorter by 2 mm. The radiolunate and radioscaphoid angles of the patients were reduced slightly by scaphocapitate arthrodesis; the mean postsurgical radioscaphoid angle was 51 degrees.

Discussion.—These patients had preoperative variance of the ulnar similar to that seen in other studies. The mean postoperative grip strength of 83% (compared with the unaffected side) is similar to grip strength after a STT, but the residual flexion–extension after scaphocapitate arthrodesis was diminished when compared with patients who had STT. This finding was attributed to the differences in wrist kinetics after each procedure. Because pain is significantly alleviated after scaphocapitate arthrodesis, this procedure is recommended for patients with advanced Kienböck's disease.

▶ One patient in this study had stage II Kienböck's disease. I would have excluded this patient from the study, which would have left 10 patients. The duration of follow-up is adequate but relatively short. The scaphocapitate fusion rate was high, and the authors did not specify what "on load only" meant in patients who had pain "on load." These results are similar to those reported for proximal row carpectomy, scaphotrapezial trapezoid (SST) arthrodesis, and radial shortening. However, the authors' comment regarding the development of radioscaphoid arthritis is premature. In fact, their 1 illustration does show radioscaphoid sclerosis and cyst formation. Because no good studies on the natural history of Kienböck's disease have been done, the best controls are comparisons with other operative series for the treatment of late-stage Kienböck's disease. However, most of the limited intercarpal arthrodeses that have been reported have had variable success rates in terms of union and pain relief when performed for intercarpal instability. In addition, all of these procedures significantly alter normal wrist kinematics and loading patterns; and longer follow-up is necessary to determine whether this procedure deteriorates with time.

L.K. Ruby, M.D.

Proximal Row Carpectomy With Partial Capitate Resection
Salomon GD, Eaton RG (St Luke's–Roosevelt Hosp, New York)
J Hand Surg [Am] 21A:2–8, 1996   8–24

Background.—Advanced radioscaphoid degenerative arthritis is often treated with proximal row carpectomy (PRC). However, the finding of radiolunate, especially lunocapitate, degenerative changes is considered a contraindication to PRC. The PRC technique has been modified by including resection of a portion of the projecting proximal dome of the capitate to create a broader stable radiocarpal pseudarthrosis (Fig 4). The results of this modified technique were reviewed.

Technique.—A dorsal transverse incision is used to expose the operative area. After excision of the superficial extensor retinaculum, the finger and wrist extensors are retracted. A capsular inci-

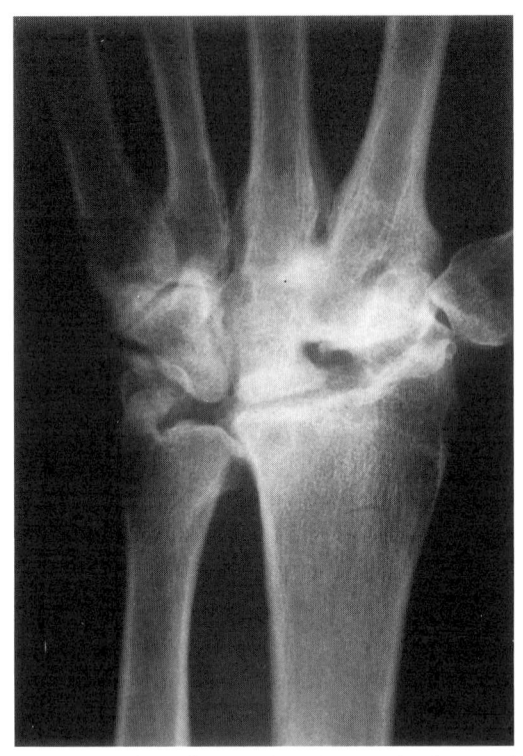

FIGURE 4.—Posteroanterior radiographic view obtained 91 months after a proximal row carpectomy with capitate leveling. The proximal capitate is now wide and flat and essentially congruous with its radius interface. (Courtesy of Salomon GD, Eaton RG: Proximal row carpectomy with partial capitate resection. *J Hand Surg (Am)* 21A:2–8, 1996.)

sion is made transversely along the dorsal lip of the radius to create a distally based dorsal capsular flap. Excision includes the proximal two-thirds of the scaphoid, all of the lunate and triquetrum, the impinging portion of the distal scaphoid, and the projecting proximal capitate in line with the proximal articular surface of the hamate. The capsular flap is then sutured across the base of the newly created distal carpal row to the volar capsule. The radiocarpal joint is temporarily stabilized with Kirschner wires and a short arm cast, which are removed in 3 weeks. A removable splint is worn for 7–10 days during progressive rehabilitation.

Methods.—Of 17 patients who underwent modified PRC, 12 were examined after an average follow-up of 55 months, and 10 had chronic scapholunate advanced collapse deformity. Seven of these 10 patients had lunocapitate arthritis, and 3 had radiolunate degenerative changes.

Results.—Pain relief was excellent in 7 patients, good in 4, and fair in 1. Nonsignificant improvement was seen in active extension and total active range of motion, and significant improvement was seen in active flexion and grip strength. The patients returned to work or full activity in an average of 14 weeks, and grip strength and range of motion progressively increased for as long as 1 year.

Conclusions.—A modified PRC with partial resection of the capitate can result in satisfactory motion improvement and pain relief even in patients with radiographic evidence of lunocapitate or radiolunate joint degenerative changes.

▶ It is unfortunate that almost one-third of this small series of 17 patients did not complete follow-up, for this potentially diminishes the validity of the authors' conclusions regarding this procedure. Fortunately, within the remaining 12 patients is a core of 10 who deserve our attention; those with periscaphoid osteoarthritis secondary to either chronic scapholunate dissociation or to nonunions of the scaphoid and those with associated midcarpal (lunocapitate) collapse. To treat this condition, the authors propose a modification of the classic PRC that involves partial resection of the head of the capitate and the interposition of a dorsally based capsular flap between radius and carpus. Compared with other procedures, (particularly those involving partial arthrodesis), this operation is attractive for several reasons: (1) a shorter period of postoperative rehabilitation; (2) a potential for greater residual range of motion; (3) a faster return to work and normal activities; (4) a simpler operation, and (5) fewer potential complications. The appeal of the procedure is enhanced by the encouraging results shown in this study, both in relieving pain and in maintaining or improving range of motion.

The procedure has some drawbacks. Although postoperative motion was excellent, 5 of the 10 patients had either the same or less motion after surgery. In addition pain was relieved, but 4 of the 10 had either frequent pain (1 patient) or pain with exertion (3 patients). Furthermore, the long-term survival of a pain-free function was questionable, judging by the appearance of the wrists in the radiographs published (see Fig 4). More significant, however, was the use of this procedure in 7 typical scapholunate advanced collapse deformities with serviceable radiolunate joints. In my experience it does not make sense to sacrifice a normal radiolunate joint, and substitute it for an abnormal one. Therefore, although this operation is worth adding to our surgical armamentarium, its indication may best be limited to wrists for which a PRC is considered and in which the articular surfaces of both the radius and the head of the capitate are abnormal.

J. Taleisnik, M.D.

Motion-preserving Procedures in the Treatment of Scapholunate Advanced Collapse Wrist: Proximal Row Carpectomy Versus Four-corner Arthrodesis

Wyrick JD, Stern PJ, Kiefhaber TR (Univ of Cincinnati, Ohio)
J Hand Surg (Am) 20A:965–970, 1995   8–25

Background.—The scapholunate advanced collapse (SLAC) wrist is the most common pattern of degenerative arthritis at this site. Both motion-preserving and motion-sacrificing operations have been proposed. Two of the most frequently used motion-preserving procedures are proximal row carpectomy (PRC) and scaphoid excision with "4-corner" arthrodesis of the capitate, lunate, hamate, and triquetrum. Excellent results have been reported for both procedures. Four-corner arthrodesis preserves significant motion while redirecting force across the uninvolved radius-lunate joint. These 2 operations were compared in patients who had SLAC wrist and did not respond to conservative measures.

Patients.—Seventeen patients underwent 4-corner arthrodesis; their status was followed for a mean of 27 months. Ten patients underwent PRC on 11 wrists; their status was followed for a mean of 37 months. In both groups, most patients had a SLAC wrist secondary to scapholunate dissociation.

Results.—Five patients had severe pain after 4-corner arthrodesis. Only 2 wrists in the PRC group were mildly painful. The total arc of motion was 64% of the normal side after PRC and 47% after arthrodesis. Grip strength averaged 94% and 74% of normal, respectively. Evaluation using the criteria suggested by Minami et al. (*J Hand Surg* 13A:660–667, 1988) showed that all 11 wrists in the PRC group, but only 12 of 17 in the arthrodesis group, had a successful outcome.

One patient in each group exhibited degenerative changes at follow-up but was asymptomatic. Three patients who underwent arthrodesis had nonunions, but only 1 was symptomatic. Two patients who had persistent pain after 4-corner arthrodesis were converted to total wrist arthrodesis. One patient in the PRC group had a pin-track infection, and 1 required reoperation to retrieve a pin that had migrated.

Conclusion.—Proximal row carpectomy is currently the preferred motion-preserving operation for the SLAC wrist, except when advanced capitolunate arthritis is present.

▶ The authors compare a short to intermediate follow-up of PRC with scaphoid excision and 4-corner arthrodesis in the treatment of SLAC wrist. In general, results after PRC were more predictable, preserved a greater percentage of normal motion, produced greater grip strength, and resulted in less need for later reoperation than did scaphoid excision and 4-corner arthrodesis. This finding led the authors to recommend PRC as the preferred procedure, provided that the capitate lunate joint is free of degenerative change in the SLAC wrist. Although this work begins to suggest that scaphoid excision and 4-corner intercarpal fusion may well be the true salvage procedure, with PRC a preferred primary treatment, the follow-up in both groups is quite short, and differences in morphology of the proximal capitate head (e.g., single arc of curvature vs. spade shaped) were not considered. Longer follow-up and more critical assessment of capitate morphology to compare the durability of the radiolunate vs. radiocapitate articulations in each of these procedures will be required to determine the preferred primary procedure for reconstruction of SLAC wrist.

V.D. Pellegrini, Jr., M.D.

Avulsion Fractures of the Volar Aspect of Triquetral Bone of the Wrist: A Subtle Sign of Carpal Ligament Injury

Smith DK, Murray PM (Mecklenburg Radiology Associates, Charlotte, NC; Wilford Hall Med Ctr, San Antonio, Tex)
AJR 166:609–614, 1996
8–26

Introduction.—Triquetral bone fractures have been classified as type 1, which are isolated avulsion or shear fractures that involve the dorsal cortex, and type 2, which are comminuted fractures of the triquetral body. Previous reports have suggested that there may be a third type that involves the volar aspect of the triquetral bone. Five avulsion injuries of the volar aspect of the triquetral bone, which were missed on initial plain radiographs and were associated with significant ligament injury and carpal instability, were reported.

Methods.—Five men, aged 20–28 years, were included. All were injured by falling on an outstretched hand during sports, mainly basketball. In each case, the initial 3-view radiographic series obtained in the emergency department was normal. One to 16 weeks later, an 8-view instability series was performed in all patients. Stress videofluoroscopy and arthrography were performed in 4 patients, CT was performed in 1, and MRI was performed in 4.

Findings.—In all 5 patients, the instability series recognized a fracture that involved the radial aspect of the volar surface of the triquetral bone. In addition, lunotriquetral joint instability was demonstrated by stress videofluoroscopy. Scapholunate joint instability was present in 1 patient as well. Arthrography revealed tearing of the lunotriquetral ligament in 4 of 4 wrists and an associated tear of the scapholunate ligament in 3 of 4. In all 4 wrists examined by MRI, a volar capsular ligament attached to the avulsed bone fragment was seen. Treatment consisted of prolonged splinting in 3 patients and arthroscopic debridement in 2. At a minimum follow-up of 1 year, all 5 patients had varying degrees of pain and instability.

Conclusions.—Avulsion fracture of the radial aspect of the volar triquetral bone is described as a subtle sign of significant injury to the ligaments that govern motion of the triquetral bone (Fig 6). These injuries are easily missed on initial plain radiographs; their true extent is defined only on an instability series and subsequent imaging studies. Patients who have this

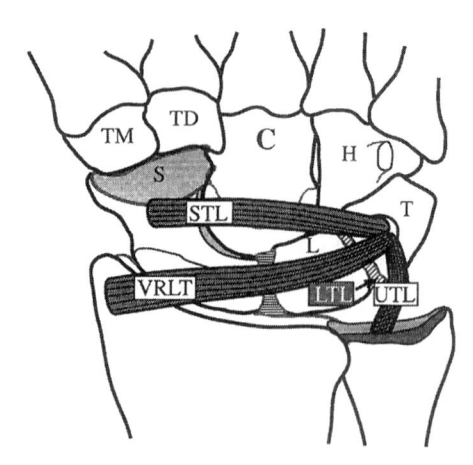

FIGURE 6.—Drawing of major volar carpal ligaments that attach to triquetral bone. *Abbreviations: STL*, volar scaphotriquetral ligament; *VRLT*, volar radiolunotriquetral ligament; *UTL*, ulnotriquetral ligament; *LTL*, lunotriquetral ligment; *TM*, trapezium; *TD*, trapezoid bone; *C*, capitate bone; *H*, hamate bone; *S*, scaphoid bone; *L*, lunate bone; *T*, triquetral bone. (Courtesy of Smith DK, Murray PM: Avulsion fractures of the volar aspect of the triquetral bone of the wrist: A subtle sign of carpal ligament injury. *AJR* 166:609–614, 1996.)

type of fracture should receive further evaluation for associated ligamentous injury and carpal instability. The optimal treatment remains to be determined.

▶ The triquetral fracture described above appears to be an excellent clue to lunotriquetral ligament tear and dissociation. Looking for this small avulsion fragment should become routine in wrist injury examinations. If found, it may present an opportunity to repair this lesion, which often otherwise causes a serious instability problem. The so-called volar scaphotriquetral ligament is not recognized by all experts in the field, but certainly the volar aspect of the lunotriquetral ligament is an important strong stabilizer of the ulnar aspect of the carpus.

R.L. Linscheid, M.D.

The Carpal Boss: A 20-year Review of Operative Management
Fusi S, Watson HK, Cuono CB (Yale Univ, New Haven, Conn; Univ of Connecticut, Hartford)
J Hand Surg (Br) 20B:405–408, 1995   8–27

Purpose.—The term "carpal boss" refers to a bony protuberance on the dorsal aspect of the hand caused by accessory ossicles in the carpal and tarsal areas. An ossicle in the area of the quadrangular trapezoid-capitate-metacarpal joint—the os styloideum—may cause repetitive stress that results in degenerative arthritis. Patients who have this problem will seek treatment because of pain during and after exertional activity of the hand.

```
Sclerotic Bone
+/- Accessory
Ossicle                              Inadequate Excision
                                     Adequate Excision

Metacarpal                                   Carpal
  Bone                                        Bone

            Normal Articular Cartilage
```

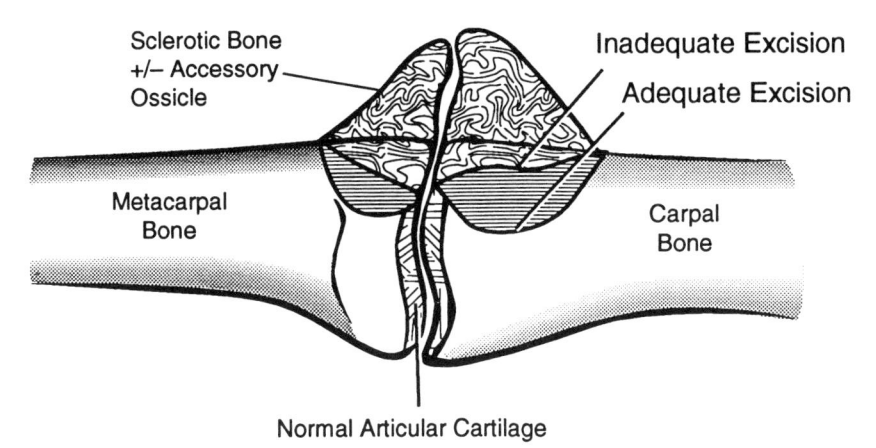

FIGURE 3.—Operative technique: Successful excision requires excavation of all the sclerotic bone and cartilage leaving a slight concavity in the cancellous bone adjacent to the normal articular surfaces. (Courtesy of Fusi S, Watson HK, Cuono CB: The carpal boss: A 20-year review of operative management. *J Hand Surg (Br)* 20B:405–408, 1995.)

The long-term results of a large series of patients who underwent surgery for symptomatic carpal bosses were described.

Patients.—Sixty-one men and 55 women (mean age, 32 years) who underwent surgery for a symptomatic carpal boss from 1969 to 1989 were included. Twenty-eight patients (24%) had a history of significant trauma, usually blunt trauma to the dorsum of the hand or wrist. Carpal boss was diagnosed by the presence of a bony protuberance of the carpometacarpal region at the base of the index and middle finger metacarpal bones; the diagnosis was confirmed by the carpal boss radiographic view. Operative treatment involved excision of the localized bony lesion and any associated degenerative arthritis. Excision continued until normal articular surface and adjacent cancellous bone was reached (Fig 3). The patients' status was followed for a mean of 42 months.

Outcomes.—There were no cases of wound infection or hematoma. At surgery, 63% of patients were found to have a bony anomaly at the region of the quadrangular joint. Ninety-four percent of patients obtained complete symptomatic relief from surgery. The remaining 7 patients had recurrent or persistent symptoms related to their carpal boss; in 5 of these patients, the symptoms recurred within 2 years after surgery. Six patients underwent reoperation, with more extensive removal of bony sclerosis and cartilaginous degeneration. The second operation produced relief of symptoms for all patients.

Discussion.—With adequate initial excision, most patients will gain complete relief of symptoms. Recurrent or persistent symptoms may result if the initial operation is inadequate; in these cases, complete excision of sclerotic bone and cartilage is necessary.

▶ A symptomatic metacarpal boss that requires surgical treatment is a relatively rare problem. From 20 years of his busy practice, the senior author gleaned these 116 cases, an average of 6 cases each year. It is interesting that none of these patients required fusion of the carpometacarpal joint to treat persistent symptoms or to manage progress degeneration of the joint. Too aggressive excision of the joint can result in destabilization of the joint, with the development of excessive motion and subsequent degeneration. As with the common dorsal wrist ganglion, the mere presence of a mass is not sufficient indication for surgery.

V.R. Hentz, M.D.

Arthrography of the Wrist: Assessment of the Integrity of the Ligaments in Young Asymptomatic Adults
Kirschenbaum D, Sieler S, Solonick D, et al (Robert Wood Johnson Univ, New Brunswick, NJ)
J Bone Joint Surg (Am) 77–A:1207–1209, 1995   8–28

Introduction.—The value of wrist arthrography is limited because the prevalence of asymptomatic ligament perforations is unknown. Degenerative perforations of wrist ligaments are common after age 49. The prevalence of perforations of wrist ligaments among asymptomatic young and middle-aged adults was analyzed.

Methods.—Arthrography of the wrist was performed in 38 men and 14 women (mean age, 28 years). All but 4 were right-hand dominant. The right wrists of 23 participants and the left wrists of 29 were randomly chosen for arthrography. Medical history and physical examination of both upper extremities were conducted. The examination included measurement of active motion with a goniometer, strength testing with a dynamometer, ballottement testing for impingement, and palpation for wrist tenderness.

Results.—Communication of the contrast material was observed in 14 of 52 wrists (27%). Multiple communications were observed in 4 wrists that had a positive arthrogram result. The most common finding in 6 of 14 wrists that had a positive arthrogram result was a perforation of the triangular fibrocartilage alone. Other perforations included scapholunate ligament alone (2 wrists), lunotriquetral ligament alone (2), triangular fibrocartilage and the scapholunate and lunotriquetral ligaments (2), triangular fibrocartilage and the scapholunate ligament (1), and triangular fibrocartilage and the lunotriquetral ligament (1). There were no significant differences in range of motion or grip strength between wrists that were examined arthrographically and the contralateral wrists. No ballottement or tenderness were noted in any wrists. There were no significant differences in range of motion, grip strength, hand dominance, or sex between participants who had wrists with perforation and those who did not. The wrists that had perforation had a slightly larger positive ulnar variance, compared with those that did not.

Conclusion.—The usefulness of arthrography of the wrist may be limited. Ligament perforation is a common finding in young asymptomatic adults. A positive arthrography result should be correlated with other clinical parameters.

▶ This excellent article should be read and digested. It is widely known that age-related attritional perforations of wrist ligaments are common. In fact, by age 50, at least 50% of wrists have perforations of the scapholunate ligament, lunotriquetral ligament, or triangular fibrocartilage complex. This article shows that more than 27% of young asymptomatic adults aged 20–35 years have "abnormal" arthrographic communications. This figure is probably low, as only radiocarpal injections were used. It is important to understand that arthrograms of the wrist represent only roentgenographic data. Any clinical decisions concerning diagnosis and treatment of wrist pain requires a synthesis of history, physical examination, and roentgenographic studies.

W. Engberger, M.D.

Evaluation of Selective Wrist Arthrography of Contralateral Asymptomatic Wrists for Symmetric Ligamentous Defects
Yin YM, Evanoff B, Gilula LA, et al (Beijing Inst of Traumatology and Orthopaedics, People's Republic of China; Washington Univ, St Louis,)
AJR 166:1067–1073, 1996
8–29

Background.—Wrist arthrography is the most sensitive imaging method for diagnosing defects of intercarpal ligaments and triangular fibrocartilage, particularly when performed in conjunction with multiple-compartment injections. Bilateral symmetric defects occur frequently and are believed to be signs of aging, whereas unilateral asymmetric defects are suspected of causing pain. The findings of wrist arthrography with complete bilateral 3-compartment injections or with separate-compartment injections were compared prospectively.

Methods.—Wrist arthrography with bilateral 3-compartment injections was performed in 62 patients with chronic wrist pain during a 5-month period. The results obtained in each wrist with 3-compartment injections were compared with those obtained with single-compartment injections. Three examiners recorded the numbers of bilateral intercarpal ligament and triangular fibrocartilage communicating defects seen.

Results.—Forty of the 62 patients had communicating defects, including 31 bilateral symmetric or asymmetric defects and 9 unilateral defects. Bilateral 3-compartment injections revealed 110 communicating defects in these 40 patients, with 59 defects in the symptomatic wrist and 51 in the asymptomatic wrist. Eighty defects were bilateral (60 symmetric and 20 asymmetric), and 30 were unilateral (19 symmetric and 11 asymmetric).

In the symptomatic wrists, radiocarpal injection alone revealed 45 of the 59 defects, midcarpal injection alone revealed 50 defects, and distal radioulnar injection revealed 13 defects. Of the 42 intercarpal ligament communicating defects, 40 were shown with midcarpal injection and 30 were shown with radiocarpal injection. Of the 17 triangular fibrocartilage communicating defects, 15 were detected with radiocarpal injection, 10 were detected with midcarpal injection, and 12 were detected with distal radioulnar joint injection.

In the asymptomatic wrists, midcarpal injection revealed 45 of the 51 communicating defects, radiocarpal injection revealed 39, and radioulnar injection revealed 11. Of the 15 triangular fibrocartilage communicating defects, 13 were detected with radiocarpal injections, 9 were detected with midcarpal injections, and 9 were detected with distal radioulnar compartment injections.

Conclusions.—The symmetry of communicating defects should be investigated with selective injection of the same compartment in the asymptomatic wrist. Midcarpal injection is recommended for investigation of intercarpal ligament abnormalities. However, radiocarpal injection is recommended for investigation of combined intercarpal and triangular fibrocartilage communicating defects. When radiocarpal injection yields inadequate information on the asymptomatic wrist, injection of multiple compartments is indicated.

▶ Magnetic resonance imaging has replaced many arthrographic techniques. However, wrist arthrography still offers many advantages over MRI, including video motion studies, stress studies, and diagnostic injections to confirm the site of symptoms.

The authors evaluated asymptomatic and symptomatic wrists using the 3-compartment injection technique. This technique is costly and time-consuming. However, it is important that their data revealed that a single midcarpal injection of the asymptomatic wrist demonstrated lunotriquetral and scapholunate defects; thus, multiple injections were not indicated in the asymptomatic side.

The use of bilateral injections and whether all 3 compartments require injection routinely are controversial. I do not support comparison arthrography except in complex cases or unusual circumstances.

T.H. Berquist, M.D.

Suggested Reading

Siegel JM, Ruby LK: Midcarpal arthrodesis. *J Hand Surg* 21A:179–182, 1996.
▶ This review adds further information to the evidence that midcarpal arthrodesis does not reliably eliminate pain. It does, however, have a high rate of union and preserves one half of the motion and grip strength as compared with the opposite side. In the properly selected and counseled patient, midcarpal arthrodesis is a reasonable first step procedure, if one recognizes that one third to one half of these patients may need to proceed to total wrist arthrodesis.

C.H. Johnson, M.D.

Chaise F, Bellemère P, Friol J-P, et al: Le collapsus carpien post-traumatique avancé: A propos de 30 cas traités par scaphoïdectomie complète et arthodèse capitolunaire (Scapholunate advanced collapse of the wrist: Results of 30 cases treated by scaphoidectomy and capitolunate arthrodesis). *La Main* 1:91–97, 1996.

▶ This series stresses 2 interesting points. First, an isolated intracarpal arthrodesis between the lunate and the capitate is sufficient and healed in all the cases without needing to be enlarged to the "4 corners." Second, results close to the fourth row carpectomy are claimed, as shown in this large series. It seems logical to propose this operation to patients who have a destroyed lunocapitate joint with good mobility. However, one may favor first row carpectomy in stiff joints with posttraumatic arthritis limited to the scaphoid area.

G. Foucher, M.D.

Weiss A-P, Akelman E, Lambiase R: Comparison of the findings of triple-injection cinearthrography of the wrist with those of arthroscopy. *J Bone Joint Surg Am* 78A:348–356, 1996.
▶ As with many other comparison studies of diagnostic tools for the wrist with pain, there are far too many variables. Also data is presented that does not entirely support conclusions. This is the type of article that should be read in full and not in abstract form.

J. Taleisnik, M.D.

Watson HK, Monacelli DM, Milford RS: Treatment of Kienböck's disease with scaphotrapezio–trapezoid arthrodesis. *J Hand Surg (AM)* 21A:9–15, 1996.

Pelto-Vasenius K, Hirvensalo E, Böstman O, et al: Fixation of scaphoid delayed union and non-union with absorbable polyglycolide pin or Herbert screw. *Arch Orthop Trauma Surg* 114:347–351, 1995.

Foster RJ: Stabilization of ulnar carpometacarpal dislocations or fracture dislocations. *Clin Orthop* 327:94–97, 1996.

Hanel DP: Primary fusion of fracture dislocations of central carpometacarpal joints. *Clin Orthop* 327:85–93, 1996.

Distal Radius

Results of Combined Internal and External Fixation for the Treatment of Severe AO-C3 Fracture of the Distal Radius
Bass RL, Blair WF, Hubbard PP (Univ of Iowa Hosps and Clinics, Iowa City)
J Hand Surg (Am) 20A:373–381, 1995   8–30

Background.—Although combined internal and external fixation for distal radius fractures has been reported previously, the indications, methods, and outcomes have not been documented. A specific surgical strategy in a homogenous population with AO-C3 fractures of the distal radius was presented.

Technique.—After the dorsal rim of the radius and articular surfaces of the fragments are visualized, an anterior approach is taken through the flexor carpi radialis sheath. The surgeon mobilizes all fragments for reduction but does not release the anterior radiocarpal ligaments. An Orthofix small-body fixator is then applied to the index metacarpal and distal radius. Open techniques are used to expose the bones. The surgeon then applies longitudinal traction along the forearm and locks the fixator in place. Fluoroscopy of the wrist in posteroanterior, lateral, and oblique projections is done to confirm optimal position of the hand relative to the forearm. The cortical shell and articular surface of the radius are realigned under direct vision through both incisions, and the fragments are reduced and fixed in an anterior to dorsal and proximal to distal sequence. This sequence enables the surgeon to restore the length of the comminuted metaphyseal-diaphyseal segment and then align the articular fragments anatomically. Fixation is done with smooth pins. Neutralization plates or interfragmentary screws may be needed for certain fracture patterns.

Patients and Outcomes.—Thirteen fractures were repaired in 12 patients; the patients' status was followed for a mean 27 months. Average wrist motion was 60 degrees of flexion and 45 degrees of extension. Mean grip strength in the injured extremities was 83% of the uninjured side. Outcomes were excellent or good in 10 wrists.

Conclusions.—At long-term follow-up assessment, clinical results in these patients were very good. Although complete restoration of palmar tilt was difficult, even with this extensive surgical approach, there was no significant loss of position from the immediate postoperative radiographic evaluation over the long term.

▶ This article identifies a surgical procedure that can be effective in severely comminuted fractures. The average total tourniquet time of 3 hours 45 minutes attests to the difficulty of this procedure. The use of volar and dorsal approaches is significant. A volar buttress plate is often beneficial, as mentioned but not shown. Although an external fixator is a helpful adjunct in the treatment of these fractures, it may not always be needed.

J. Rayhack, M.D.

In-the-socket Osteosynthesis for Unstable Extremity Fractures of the Distal Radius: Preliminary Technique and Results [in French]
Nonnenmacher J (CRAM AM de Strasbourg, France)
La Main 1:23–27, 1996
8–31

Background.—The comminuted distal radial fractures are divided into 3 types: unstable anterior, unstable posterior, and complex fractures involving both anterior and posterior instability. In France, unstable anterior

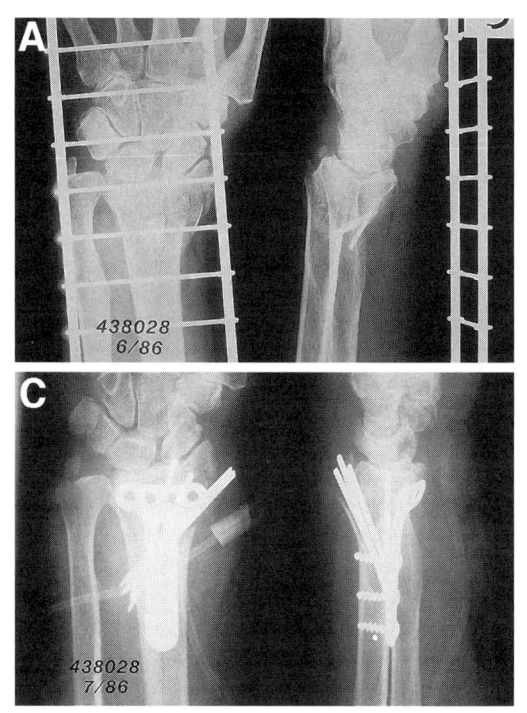

FIGURE 1.—Posterior-type crosswise articular fracture. **A**, initial status. **C**, osteosynthesis "in the socket." (Courtesy of Nonnenmacher J: L'ostéosynthèse 'en vasque' dans les fractures instables de l'extrémité distale du radius; Technique et résultats préliminaires. *La Main* 1:23–27, 1996.)

fractures are often treated with anterior plate osteosynthesis, unstable posterior fractures with Kapandji pin fixation, and complex fractures with external fixation. The preliminary results of an internal fixation method as an alternative for treating complex comminuted distal radial fractures were reported.

> *Technique.*—The procedure is performed in 3 steps. As a first step, a preformed, T-shaped plate is inserted via the anterior route. If possible, screws are placed in the distal fragment to preserve the height of the radius. At this time, the screws that fix the plate to the proximal fragment are not completely tightened. For the second step, 3 pins, each 2 mm in diameter, are inserted through short incisions on the opposite side of the anterior plate. Finally, the screws in the anterior plate are tightened, the 3 pins are cut under the skin, and the incisions are closed with drainage (Fig 1). A palmar splint is used while the incisions are healing. Mobilization

and hand therapy are started immediately after the operation. The pins are removed after 6 weeks, and the plate is removed a year later.

Patients.—This new operation was performed in 19 women and 6 men, aged 33–86 years, with anteriorly and posteriorly displaced distal radius fractures. The clinical results were very good in 8 patients (32%), good in 14 (56%), and unsatisfactory in 3 (12%). The radiologic results were very good in 7 patients (28%), good in 11 (44%), and unsatisfactory in 7 (28%).

Discussion.—The advantages of this procedure are that internal fixation avoids hypercorrection resulting from epiphyseal displacement in the palmar direction and restores the proper articular surface. Further studies are needed to determine whether the use of external fixation in comminuted distal radial fractures can be limited to the most severe cases.

▶ Management of the most severely comminuted distal radius fractures is problematic. Specifically, there is a gray zone between fractures that can be managed by internal fixation alone and those that require a combination of internal and external fixation. I have had good success with the latter construct, and go to it readily. For those who prefer to keep their fixation on the inside, this dorsal/palmar technique provides another option.

P.C. Amadio, M.D.

Fracture of the Distal Radius: A Prospective Comparison Between Trans-styloid and Kapandji Fixations
Lenoble E, Dumontier C, Goutallier D, et al (Henri Mondor Hosp, Creteil, France; Saint Antoine Hosp, Paris)
J Bone Joint Surg (Br) 77B:562–567, 1995   8–32

Introduction.—In patients aged older than 50 years, one sixth of all fractures involve the distal radius. These fractures are commonly treated by percutaneous Kirschner (K)-wire fixation, but there have been few prospective evaluations of the results achieved with different durations of immobilization. Two common methods for the treatment of posteriorly displaced distal radial fractures, trans-styloid and Kapandji K-wire fixation, were compared.

Methods.—Ninety-six patients who had extra-articular or intra-articular fractures of the distal radius with a dorsally displaced posteromedial fragment were included. Patients who had comminuted fractures that were not amenable to K-wire fixation and those who had more than 2 intra-articular fractures were excluded. Posteroanterior, lateral, and axial traction radiographs were obtained before reduction to ascertain the feasibility of reduction and the extent of the fractures. The methods of Castaing and Frykman and the AO system were used to classify the fractures. By the latter classification, there were 29 A2, 13 A3, 28 C1, and 26 C2 fractures.

Forty-two patients (mean age, 57 years), underwent trans-styloid K-wire fixation followed by 45 days' immobilization in a short-arm cast. The other 54 patients (mean age, 58 years), underwent Kapandji fixation with immediate mobilization. In this group, the K-wires were removed after 45 days with the use of local or regional anesthesia. Two 1.8-mm K-wires were used for both types of fixation.

Results.—The K-wires were removed an average of 44 days after trans-styloid fixation and 47 days after Kapandji fixation. Patients who had Kapandji fixation were more likely to have pain and reflex-sympathetic dystrophy. They also had better range of motion, although this difference was no longer significant by the 6-week evaluation. The patients in the Kapandji fixation group had better radiographic reduction, although they had some loss of reduction and increased radial shortening in the first 3 months after surgery. By the 2-year evaluation, the 2 groups had comparable clinical results.

Conclusions.—Trans-styloid fixation followed by a period of immobilization and Kapandji fixation with immediate mobilization give similar final results in patients who have fractures of the distal radius. The better early range of motion with Kapandji fixation is obtained at the cost of increased pain. With Kapandji fixation, the intrafocal location of the K-wires appears unable to resist the forces associated with early mobilization or to avoid secondary displacement. Trans-styloid fixation appears to offer better control of radial shortening.

▶ This article does a good job of comparing 2 types of percutaneous pinning techniques of the distal radius. A more meaningful evaluation, however, of pinning techniques for the distal radius fracture would compare the efficacy of surgeries performed solely on unstable or potentially unstable fractures. Because of philosophical differences, French surgeons frequently pin fractures that are routinely treated with reduction and casting by American surgeons, who are under increasing financial pressure to avoid surgical procedures, especially those associated with 2 procedures, like the Kapandji technique.

J. Rayhack, M.D.

Internal Fixation of the Distal Radius: A Comparative, Experimental Study
Rader CP, Räuber C, Rehm KE, et al (Univ of Cologne, Germany)
Arch Orthop Trauma Surg 114:340–343, 1995   8–33

Background.—Distal radial fractures that might dislocate are generally treated surgically. A wide range of internal fixation devices have been tried, but none has proved to be a superior method. Only plate fixation has provided stable motility. A number of widely used internal fixation procedures were compared.

Study Plan.—Sixty cadaver radii from individuals who did not have extensive osteoporosis were evaluated. An extra-articular extension fracture was simulated by a diagonal dorsal wedge osteotomy of at least 45 degrees. The "injuries" were treated with a T-plate; 3 Kirschner (K)-wires, 1.8 or 2.5 mm in diameter; 3 polylactide rods, 2 or 2.7 mm in diameter; or 3 polyglycolide rods, 2 mm in diameter. The forces needed to compress the internal fixation by 2, 4, and 6 mm were recorded.

Results.—Plate fixation ensured the most stability. Under 4 mm of compression, the thicker K-wires provided 10% more stability than did the thinner wires. Fixation with 2.7-mm polylactid rods resulted in slightly more stability than 1.8-mm K-wires under 4 mm of compression. Short polylactide pins and polyglycolide pins were much less stable than were plate fixation. Several polyglycolide rods fractured under stress; none of the other materials underwent this change.

Clinical Application.—Studies have begun to evaluate the use of 2.7-mm polylactide pins in patients who have dislocated distal radial fractures. The first 5 patients gave no evidence of foreign-body reaction, and none had secondary dislocation.

▶ This article compares different cadaveric fixation techniques with metal pins vs. bioabsorbable pins and rods that have a modified screw design. Most surgeons have abandoned bioabsorbable pins because of their poor fixation and tendency to cause seromas. We anticipate human studies from the authors.

A.L. Ladd, M.D.

A Comparison of Early and Late Reconstruction of Malunited Fractures of the Distal End of the Radius
Jupiter JB, Ring D (Massachusetts Gen Hosp, Boston)
J Bone Joint Surg (Am) 78A:739–748, 1996   8–34

Background.—The decision to reconstruct a malunited fracture of the distal end of the radius is based primarily on impaired wrist function, pain, or cosmetic deformity assessed long after the injury. Many patients function adequately after delayed intervention, despite residual deformity. However, a delay in intervention may also result in soft-tissue maladaptation and dysfunction of the radioulnar joint. Reconstructing malunion at an earlier stage may facilitate definition and correction of malalignment through the original site of the fracture, may enable avoidance of maladaptive soft-tissue contracture and the development of distal radioulnar joint dysfunction, and may reduce the period of disability.

Methods.—The outcomes of 10 patients with a malaligned fracture of the distal end of the radius treated with early reconstruction were compared retrospectively with the outcomes of 10 patients undergoing late reconstruction for functional limitation after complete healing of a fracture of the distal end of the radius in a malreduced position. Early reconstruction, performed at a mean of 8 weeks after injury, consisted of an osteotomy through the site of the fracture, autogenous cancellous iliac crest bone-grafting, and internal fixation. Late reconstruction, done at a mean of 40 weeks after injury, consisted of an osteotomy, corticocancellous bone-grafting, and internal fixation. The status of the early and late treatment groups were followed for an average of 48 and 34 months, respectively.

Findings.—After early reconstruction, average wrist flexion was 45 degrees; wrist extension, 52 degrees; forearm pronation, 79 degrees; and forearm supination, 77 degrees. The corresponding values for the late treatment group were 42, 45, 77, and 68 degrees. Grip strengths after early and late reconstructions were 42 and 25 kg, respectively. Mild pain in the radiocarpal joint was reported by 1 patient in each group. Outcomes were excellent in 7 patients and good in 3 patients after early reconstruction. After late reconstructions, outcomes were excellent in 1 patient, good in 7, and fair in 2. One patient undergoing early reconstruction had a complication: rupture of the extensor pollicis longus tendon 12 weeks after treatment. Two patients in the late treatment group had complications: persistent pain at the donor site of the iliac crest bone graft in 1 and a delayed union requiring a second procedure in the other.

Conclusion.—Early and late reconstructions of malunited fractures of the distal end of the radius appear to produce comparable outcomes. Early reconstruction is technically easier and decreases the length of disability in patients with radiographic signs predicting persistent functional limitation.

▶ One might have hoped that earlier treatment of impending nonunion might have improved outcome. Instead, this comparative study suggests that the only advantage to early surgery may be the time saved. So, if one can be *certain* that osteotomy will be needed, surgery should be considered as soon as that certainty is determined. The cases of severe malalignment in young adults come clearly to mind, as do those with intra-articular malalignment. Lesser degrees of malalignment in older patients present a different scenario: In many instances, the final anatomical result can be predicted but not the final *functional* result. In such circumstances, one can at least wait, safe in the knowledge that if surgery is needed later, the results will be comparable to those of an earlier intervention.

P.C. Amadio, M.D.

Anatomical and Functional Results Five Years After Remanipulated Colles' Fractures

Hove LM, Fjeldsgaard K, Skjeie R, et al (Haukeland Univ, Bergen, Norway; Bergen Legevakt, Norway)
Scand J Plast Reconstr Hand Surg 29:349–355, 1995

Patient Population —In a prospective series of 530 patients treated in various ways for Colles' fracture, secondary displacement developed in 28 patients after the fracture was immobilized in plaster. These patients represented 8% of all those whose fractures were reduced. The fractures were remanipulated and splinted in a new case for 4 more weeks. Remanipulation was generally performed when there was more than 10 degrees of dorsal angulation or 5 mm of radial shortening. The status of 26 patients was followed for 5 years after injury.

Outcome.—Radial length was significantly less after remanipulation. Dorsal angulation was significantly less after initial reduction, after remanipulation, and at follow-up compared with the initial angulation. Radial angulation averaged 22 degrees at follow-up. Seven patients had moderate osteoarthritic changes. Mean grip strength was 94%, and mean range of motion was 88% of that on the uninjured side. The functional results were graded as excellent in 13 patients, good in 7, fair in 5, and poor in 1. Total pronation and supination at follow-up correlated with initial radial length and dorsal angulation. Total movement in all directions correlated with initial radial length.

Conclusions.—Selected patients who have moderately displaced Colles' fractures are effectively treated by remanipulation and fixation in plaster. The extent of initial dislocation predicts the final range of motion, but there is little correlation between the anatomical outcome and the final functional results.

▶ The authors have chosen to describe the distal radius fractures in this study by the eponym "Colles' fractures," thus confusing the reader's attempts to analyze this article. As a result, many patient populations with different fracture characteristics are included. The "loss" of reduction is relatively loosely defined and thus applies to only 8% of the original fractures. Other studies report up to 30%. Importantly, however, the study shows that remanipulation has its merits in improving dorsal angulation but, predictably, has no significant effect.

A.L. Ladd, M.D.

Redisplaced Unstable Fractures of the Distal Radius: A Prospective Randomised Comparison of Four Methods of Treatment
McQueen MM, Hajducka C, Court-Brown CM (Royal Infirmary of Edinburgh, Scotland)
J Bone Joint Surg Br 78B:404–409, 1996 8–36

Objective.—Unstable fractures of the distal radius that have redisplaced can be difficult to manage. Closed remanipulation and casting are still used at many centers, but results can be poor. Other proposed treatments include external fixators of the wrist with articulation, bone grafting, and corticocancellous wedge grafting. Four methods of treatment for redisplaced unstable fractures of the distal radius were compared in a randomized trial.

Methods.—The study included 120 consecutive patients with unstable fractures of the distal radius. In all cases, the reduced position of the fracture could not be held in a forearm cast. The patients were 107 women and 13 men (average age, 63 years); 60% of the fractures were intraarticular. The patients were randomly assigned to 1 of 4 treatment groups: group 1, closed rereduction with forearm casting; group 2, open reduction and bone grafting; group 3, closed rereduction and external fixation; and group 4, closed rereduction and external fixation with mobilization of the wrist at 3 weeks. Radiographic and functional outcomes were evaluated at 6 weeks, at 3 and 6 months, and at 1 year after injury.

Results.—Because the results of external fixation were similar with or without wrist mobilization, the two groups were merged for further analysis. Dorsal angulation was best corrected with open reduction and bone grafting; mean volar tilt at 1 year was 3 degrees, significantly better than in the other 3 groups. Although 10 of 30 patients in group 2 regained normal volar tilt, 7 were either overcorrected or later collapsed into further volar tilt. Correction of the dorsal angle was better with external fixation than with remanipulation but worse than with open reduction and bone grafting. The dorsal angulation results were the worst in group 1, but there were no significant differences in radial shortening. Forty-two percent of patients showed some carpal malalignment after union, and 24% of wrists with normal carpal alignment showed malunion.

Grip strength and the ability to perform activities of daily living improved over time, with no significant differences between groups. Ranges of motion improved rapidly for the first 3 months, followed by slower recovery for as long as 1 year. Carpal malalignment was significantly associated with diminished recovery of grip strength and range of motion. The overall complication rate was 64%. The malunion rate was 45% and the pin track infection rate was 5%.

Conclusions.—The functional results of redisplaced unstable fractures of the distal radius are similar, whether treatment consists of closed rereduction and casting, open reduction and bone grafting, or closed external fixation. Open reduction and bone grafting appears to improve angulation of the distal radius on radiographic studies. Carpal malalignment has a negative effect on the final functional outcome.

▶ McQueen, Hajducka, and Court-Brown have once again extended their substantial experience to address contemporary issues related to fractures at the end of the radius. In this prospective study, the authors investigated 120 patients with fractures of the end of the radius that were defined as unstable because they redisplaced after a closed manipulative reduction and plaster support. The types of treatment included remanipulation in plaster, open reduction and bone grafting, and closed external fixation (with and without mobilization of the wrist at 3 weeks). The authors carefully followed the patients for as long as 12 months after injury with functional and radiographic criteria. Their results suggest that functional results at 1 year did not statistically differ among the 3 groups; however, the main influence on the final outcome was radiographic evidence of carpal malalignment.

Readers should keep several issues in mind when evaluating this clinical study. First, on a positive note, a prospective randomized study is always worth its weight in gold. The numbers drop off a bit because follow-up is inadequate and, in certain situations, there are questions as to whether enough patients have been studied to truly give an understanding of outcome. For example, although the authors suggest that open reduction offers a chance at anatomical restoration, 10 of 30 patients in this group had either a loss of position or over correction. Thus, fewer patients with anatomical reposition could be evaluated from this basis. When these variables then become present in smaller numbers, the authors might well have done a multivariate analysis to begin to look at some of the issues, even stratified to each group. By the same token, one must applaud their use of the concept of a prospective randomized study.

A second, positive note is that the authors examined both radiographic and functional criteria. It is often unappreciated that the end of the radius is indeed the seat of the wrist and that function, rather than radiographs, should be the hallmark of outcome. With this in mind, the authors' results, which support the fact that alteration in the support of the carpus may well be the most important factor in determining a successful or untoward outcome, represents another nail in the coffin for those who have a nihilistic attitude towards these injuries, suggesting that anatomy is not really important. Although the authors did not evaluate the function of the distal radioulnar joint, which is also very important in managing and assessing outcome of these fractures, this, too, represents an articular aspect to these injuries.

The authors point out that they have followed patients for 12 months, and it is possible that a longer follow-up might change the basis of their observations—in due course, one might see a greater effect of carpal malalignment compared with anatomical restoration. This certainly has been our experience; 18 months to almost 2 years is needed, particularly when articular displacement has occurred before outcome is recognized. Having said that, an important caveat for the reader to consider when addressing these issues with their patients is the reality that it will take quite a long time for outcome to be reached. The data generated in this study go a long way toward supporting this observation, and are perhaps also relevant when evaluating previous publications in terms of length of follow-up.

This study has some limitations that the reader should keep in mind when assessing these data. First, the authors used an *AO* classification to identify fractures: it is quite evident that 60% were intra-articular fractures. Many have come to realize that intra-articular fractures may represent compression of the articular surface by the carpus, with or without associated intercarpal ligament problems. In effect, these may represent injuries entirely different from the extra-articular fractures that occur with a bending or tension mode of failure. The inability to stratify these carefully is a problem for the discriminating reader or for the reader dealing with a particular patient. It has been well recognized that plaster alone, or external fixation using ligamentotaxis, will not effectively support disimpacted articular fragments, and late settling of the articular realignment is commonplace. Thus, persons dealing with these fractures should consider the extra-articular fractures to be entirely different from the impaction-compression type injuries to the end of the radius.

Second, suggesting that anatomical restoration with surgical treatment and bone grafting may not be any more effective than alternative, less-invasive treatments, belies the fact that the execution of this procedure may have been the problem rather than the treatment option. The authors note that 30% or more of their patients had had a problem with either overcorrection, which considerably increased the volar tilt, or late settling. It is not surprising that instability occurred with placement of a large corticocancellous graft and support with a single pin. Many have recognized that, once surgical treatment is in effect, the internal pin fixation must be neutralized, preferably with an external fixator or with a plate. The authors cite a study by Leung et al.,[1] who used surgical treatment with cancellous bone graft and an external fixator, with excellent control over their reconstruction. Because the authors combined the results of all the patients in this group in their reporting of radiographic and functional outcome (giving mean values), it is hard to know the exact relationship between those who had a restored anatomy and those who did not.

Finally, readers should consider the enormous incidence of identified complications. Certainly, one could not believe that these fractures are benign injuries given such a high rate of complications. The authors note that 64% of their patients had a complication of either the fracture or of the operation. The relatively high number of dystrophic or neurologic symptoms supports a careful investigation of whether there is median nerve compression; this might be addressed with early intervention.

In summary, readers should keep the results of the authors' prospective study in mind when addressing these displaced fractures. These fractures are difficult to maintain with any other method but internal fixation. Whether this is done by closed manipulation and percutaneous pins or open reduction and careful internal fixation depends on the fracture, patient cohort, and physician's experience. When a redisplacement is allowed to remain, altered function is very likely, regardless of the age of the patient. As our patients continue to be more active in their later decades, we are once again faced with the need to maintain a sufficient anatomy to permit functional capacity of the hand and wrist.

J.B. Jupiter, M.D.

Reference

1. Leung KS, Shen WY, Tsang HK, et al: An effective treatment comminuted fractures of the distal radius. *J Hand Surg (Am)* 15:11–17, 1990.

Intracarpal Soft-tissue Lesions Associated With an Intra-articular Fracture of the Distal End of the Radius
Geissler WB, Freeland AE, Savoie FH, et al (Univ of Mississippi, Jackson; River Oaks Hosp, Jackson, Miss; Orthopaedic Research of Virginia, Richmond)
J Bone Joint Surg Am 78A:357–365, 1996

Background.—The pattern of injury, presence of associated soft-tissue trauma, and specific method of treatment may influence the outcomes of fracture of the distal end of the radius. The association of skeletal and articular anatomical restoration after a fracture with eventual outcomes has been well documented. However, the prevalence of associated injury of the supporting soft-tissue structures in the wrist has not been studied thoroughly. The occurrence and severity of soft-tissue lesions in the wrist in association with displaced intra-articular fractures of the distal end of the radius were reported.

Methods and Findings.—Sixty patients with a displaced intra-articular fracture of the distal end of the radius underwent manipulative reduction and internal fixation under fluoroscopic and arthroscopic guidance. Seven fractures were Association for the Study of Internal Fixation (AO/ASIF) type B1, 2 were B2, 3 were B3, 13 were C1, 12 were C2 and 23 were C3. Sixty-eight percent of the patients had soft-tissue injuries of the wrist. Twenty-six of these 41 patients had tears of the triangular fibrocartilage complex; 19, of the scapholunate interosseous ligament; and 9, of the lunotriquetral interosseous ligament. Two soft-tissue injuries were documented in 13 patients. Intracarpal soft-tissue injuries occurred most often with fractures of the lunate facet of the distal articular surface or radius.

Conclusion.—In this series, many patients with a displaced intra-articular fracture of the distal end of the radius had tears of the carpal interosseous ligaments and triangular fibrocartilage complex. The presence of partial or complete ligament tears that are not detectable on standard radiography may explain why some patients continue to have symptoms even after the fracture is healed anatomically. Clinicians should always consider the possibility of a soft-tissue injury associated with a fracture of the distal end of the radius.

▶ This excellent study draws our attention to the intra-articular soft-tissue injuries associated with distal radius fractures. The study not only classifies the severity of the intra-articular distal radial fracture according to the AO system but also offers a classification system to assess the severity of the soft-tissue ligament injury. This classification is inexact, particularly in defining stage I and stage II lesions, and is particularly limited to the intrinsic scapholunate and lunotriquetral ligaments compared with the volar extrinsic ligaments. The paper provides an excellent description of the arthroscopic technique in approaching distal radial fractures. No treatment results are presented.

The findings of this study document the high prevalence of ligament and triangular fibrocartilage injury that is associated with intra-articular distal radial fractures. Such injuries were present in 68% of these fractured wrists. Triangular fibrocartilage injury was the most common (43%), with peripheral tears predominating. Interestingly, two thirds of the ulnar styloid fractures had dissociated triangular fibrocartilage tear, proving that an avulsion fracture of the ulnar styloid is likely to be associated with a triangular fibrocartilage injury. This finding may also be one reason the ulnar styloid fracture in itself is considered to carry a worse prognosis than that of distal radial fractures without associated ulnar styloid fracture.

Damage to the intrinsic scapholunate or lunotriquetral ligaments was present in 60% of fractured wrists. Such ligament injuries were commonly associated with more complex intra-articular fractures. The radial styloid fracture had a 50% incidence of a concomitant scapholunate lesion. Thirteen radiographs were not helpful in identifying such injuries; only 37% had scapholunate gaps greater than 4 mm or scapholunate angles greater than 70 degrees. None of the lunotriquetral injuries showed a VISI collapse deformity. Several immediate questions arise. Are these radiographically silent intrinsic lesions significant? Will they heal with the treatment required for the distal radial fracture? Should they be treated separately either with an arthroscopic reduction and pinning or an open repair at the time of the initial surgery? Do they bode a poor clinical result or worse prognosis? The answers to such questions require an outcome study. It is hoped that the office will follow this series and sometime in the future be able to correlate the result with the amount of ligament damage reserved.

Some caveats. The average age of the patient with fracture in the study was young (median age, 32 years). In other words, this series contained many patients with normal bone subjected to a significant forceful injury to the wrist. These patients differ from the "Colles' type" distal radial fractures seen in older persons, in which the bone is softer, the fracture pattern is often less frequently nonarticular, and the injury forces are less. The degree of associated intra-articular soft-tissue injury in this older group is probably less extensive. It should also be emphasized that the extra-articular soft-tissue injury in this young fracture group is greater with a higher incidence of traumatic carpal tunnel syndrome, tendon injury, and finger stiffness.

In summary, this study highlights the usefulness of wrist arthroscopy in evaluating intra-articular distal radial fractures as identified in the high frequency of triangular fibrocartilage and ligamentous injury associated with such fractures. It does not answer the critical question, as to the prognostic significance of the soft-tissue lesions for treatment and for functional results.

A.L. Osterman, M.D.

Distal Radial Fractures "Loco Typico": Arthroscopic Diagnosis and Minimally Invasive Treatment of Additional Lesions [in French]
Seibert FJ, Fellinger M, Grechenig W, et al (Universitätsklinik für Unfallchirurgie, Graz)
Arthroskopie 8:273–280, 1995 8–38

Background.—Fractures of the distal radius are associated with a high percentage of cases with soft-tissue lesions and intra-articular pathology. When closed reduction is performed, the intra-articular pathology remains unrecognized, as one may concentrate only on the bony alignment, hoping that with a correct reduction of the bony elements, the soft-tissue lesions may heal by themselves.

Methods.—The radiocarpal joints of 18 patients (aged 18–82 years) were examined arthroscopically after reduction of the radius fracture. Arthroscopy of the wrist was performed 1 to 17 days after the initial trauma or accident.

Results.—Twenty combined lesions were found. Five were chondral fractures of the proximal pole of the scaphoid, 10 were ruptures of the scapholunate ligaments, and 5 were lesions of the fibrocartilage complex. Arthroscopic control of the reduction of a distal radius fracture by routine procedure is recommended, particularly in patients younger than 40 years.

▶ The experience of the authors can be confirmed. In an urban population where life expectancy is quite high and the mechanisms for preventing accidents are highly developed (as in the case of urban agglomerations in central Europe), trauma, in general, and the fractures of the distal radius become more and more rare. In addition, most patients have high expectations concerning the quality of the therapy and are not willing to accept residual problems. Therefore, I would recommend arthroscopic control as a routine procedure after reduction of the radius. However, at this time, the criteria for patient selection still must be established by centers specializing in arthroscopy, as the prognosis of the distal radial fracture must still be improved.

Priv. Dr. Med. C.L. Jantea

X-ray Film Measurements for Healed Distal Radius Fractures
Kreder HJ, Hanel DP, Mckee M, et al (Harborview Med Ctr, Seattle; St Michael's Hosp, Toronto; Massachusetts Gen Hosp, Boston; et al)
J Hand Surg (Am) 21A:31–39, 1996

Introduction.—Assessment of treatment success and functional outcome for distal radius fractures requires a standardized method of measuring deformity. Guidelines were therefore developed for measuring 8 anatomical parameters at the distal radius. These guidelines were evaluated for interobserver and intraobserver consistency and tolerance limits computed for the accuracy of each measurement.

Methods.—After a pilot study designed to judge the clarity of directions and the number of x-ray films that could be studied without undue fatigue, 16 different raters at 3 centers followed detailed instructions and diagrams for measurements of 6 healed distal radius fractures. Anteroposterior and lateral x-ray films were provided and raters asked to measure 8 parameters: step deformity, gap deformity, radial angle, radial length, radial shift, ulnar variance, palmar tilt, and dorsal shift. The same raters provided repeat measurements 2 to 4 weeks later. Rater agreement was quantified according to the intraclass correlation coefficient (ICC).

Results.—Inter-rater consistency was high for ulnar variance, palmar tilt, and radial shift (overall ICC = 0.82, 0.74, and 0.67, respectively). There was moderate agreement for radial length and dorsal shift (overall ICC = 0.44 and 0.42, respectively). Measurements of radial angle, gap, and step deformity showed only fair agreement (overall ICC = 0.38, 0.35, and 0.27, respectively), even among more experienced raters. Intraobserver consistency ranged from 0.85 for ulnar variance to 0.22 for step deformity. For most parameters, the rater's degree of experience had no effect on intraobserver consistency. All raters, however, had difficulty measuring radial angle, gap, and step in a consistent manner. It was determined that 2 randomly chosen clinicians measuring step and gap deformity on a random x-ray film would differ by more than 3 mm at least 10% of the time; repeat step or gap measurements by the same observer would differ by more than 2 mm at least 10% of the time.

Conclusion.—There are many possible sources of measurement variability and error in x-ray films of healed distal radius fractures. Among these sources are limb positioning, accuracy of the measurement equipment, differences between observers, and inconsistency of a given observer. Even experienced clinicians using standardized guidelines do not produce identical findings. For conclusions of research to be valid, all measurements should be performed by a single well-motivated observer, blinded to patient outcome, who follows a specific and detailed algorithm.

▶ This excellent article suggests that we are better at measuring angles than we are at measuring gaps or stepoffs. The angle issue has been well studied in other contexts, particularly for carpal instability and spinal deformity. It seems that—even with clear, understandable, well-defined rules—

interobserver eyeballs will vary by 5–10 degrees, and goniometer placement may add another 5 or 10 degrees on top of that, giving an average of about 10–15 degrees difference between repeated or interobserver measurements. Gaps and steps are more problematic because they are rarely uniform in 3 dimensions. A gap or step may vary from 0 to 5 mm as one goes from 1 side of the fracture to the other. Should we be concerned with the maximum, the minimum, or the average? Which is easiest to measure? Even with large interobserver variation, with gaps it is likely that *all* are equally right and equally wrong.

All that being said, this paper makes it clear that we should spend more time coming to agreement on what we mean by gap and step and how best to measure them. I believe that, ultimately, a standard tomographic cut will have to be used for these measurements.

P.C. Amadio, M.D.

Relative Articular Inclination of the Distal Radioulnar Joint: A Radiographic Study
Sagerman SD, Zogby RG, Palmer AK, et al (Hand Surgery Assoc, Arlington Heights, Ill; State Univ of New York, Syracuse)
J Hand Surg (Am) 20A:597–601, 1995   8–40

Introduction.—Because symptomatic ulnar impingement developed in a patient who underwent ulnar shortening for symptomatic ulnar abutment syndrome, 100 randomly selected normal wrist radiographs were examined to determine the relative articular inclination of the distal radioulnar joint. This parameter might affect the results of ulnar shortening.

Methods.—The standardized wrist films were measured for ulnar variance and the inclination of the sigmoid notch of the distal radius and the ulnar seat of the ulnar head (Fig 2). Two angles based on the longitudinal shaft of the ulna were constructed. Sigmoid inclination and ulnar seat inclination were determined by regression analysis, and each inclination was compared with ulnar variance and patient age.

Results.—The patients were aged 16–76 years (mean, 39.4 years). Ulnar variance ranged from −3.8 to 3.8 (mean, 0.05); sigmoid notch inclination, from −24.3 to 26.8 (mean, 7.7); and ulnar seat inclination, from −13.8 to 40.5 (mean, 21.0). In all but 1 wrist, the ulnar seat showed a positive inclination. The sigmoid notch was inclined distally toward the ulna (positive angle) in 81 wrists. In all but 2 patients, the inclination angles were different. There was moderate correlation for both the sigmoid notch angle and the ulnar seat angle and ulnar variance. These angles appeared to decrease as ulnar variance became more positive. Neither inclination angle correlated with patient age.

Discussion.—The opposing articular surfaces of the distal radioulnar joint did not prove to be parallel. Although the relationship between the inclination of the articular surfaces may be consistent, there is considerable variability in the magnitude and direction of the angles. A change in the

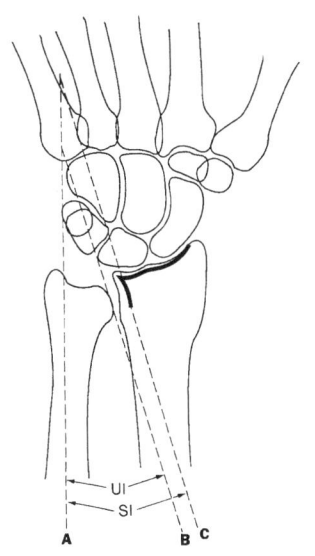

FIGURE 2.—Coronal plane diagram of the forearm shows the lines used to construct the various angle measurements. The ulnar seat inclination (*UI*) is the angle drawn between the longitudinal shaft of the ulna (A) and the tangent to the ulnar seat (B). The sigmoid notch inclination (*SI*) is the angle drawn between the longitudinal shaft of the ulna and the tangent to the sigmoid notch of the radius (C). (Courtesy of Sagerman SD, Zogby RG, Palmer AK, et al: Relative articular inclination of the distal radioulnar joint: A radiographic study. *J Hand Surg (Am)* 20A:597–601, 1995.)

relative length of the radius or ulna is therefore likely to alter the alignment and mechanics of the distal radioulnar joint. Problems may develop after ulnar shortening in patients who have large differences in the inclination of their joint surfaces.

▶ The authors extend previous work that examined the relationship between the 2 articular surfaces that compose the distal radioulnar joint. They comment that shortening the ulna, as a treatment for ulnar impaction, may create problems at this joint, proving once again that "there is no free lunch." This disturbance may be responsible for the patient who loses significant supination after osteotomy and shortening. They suggest caution in choosing ulnar shortening when the 2 measured angles vary greatly and when the normal inclination is reversed. Perhaps such patients are better candidates for a distal excision, as advocated by Feldon.[1, 2]

V.R. Hentz, M.D.

References

1. Feldon P, Terrono AL, Belsky MR: Wafer distal ulna resection for triangular fibrocartilage tears and/or ulna impaction syndrome. *J Hand Surg (Am)* 17:731–737, 1992.
2. Feldon P, Terrono AL, Belsky MR: The "wafer" procedure: Partial distal ulnar resection. *Clin Orthop* 275:124–129, 1992.

The Effect of Dorsally Angulated Distal Radius Fractures on Distal Radioulnar Joint Congruency and Forearm Rotation

Kihara H, Palmer AK, Werner FW, et al (State Univ of New York, Syracuse)
J Hand Surg (Am) 21A:40–47, 1996

Background.—Malunion of a distal radius fracture can cause significant pain and disability. These malunions may appear on radiographs as altered dorsal tilt, radial inclination, or ulnar variance. The effects of dorsal tilt on function and on the distal radioulnar joint (DRUJ) biomechanics were investigated in a cadaver study.

Methods.—Six amputated cadaveric upper extremities were stripped of skin, subcutaneous tissue, and muscle. The forearms were suspended in a biomechanical testing device that allowed force application with cables. Motion of the distal radius relative to the distal ulna was measured with electromagnetic motion-measuring devices in neutral rotation, in maximum pronation, and in maximum supination with and without the application of a 3-pound force to the dorsal aspect of Lister's tubercle or the palmar aspect of the radius. Malunion was simulated by making dorsal wedge osteotomies of the distal radius and positioning the radius at 10-degree increments of dorsal angulation. The measurements were repeated in all rotation positions at each angulation.

Results.—The alignment of the DRUJ visibly worsened with increasing dorsal angulation. The amount of pronation was decreased significantly with a 30-degree change in angulation, as did the amount of supination. Supination was also decreased after the triangular fibrocartilage complex (TFCC) or the TFCC and the interosseous membrane (IOM) were sectioned. Diastasis of the DRUJ after extension of the distal radius fragment increased with increasing dorsal angulation. In some arms, the diastasis was reduced after the TFCC was sectioned. Sectioning of both the TFCC and IOM resulted in significantly increased radial diastasis. Only sectioning of the IOM significantly increased palmar displacement in all rotation positions.

Conclusions.—Residual dorsal tilt in malunions of distal radius fracture can cause DRUJ incongruence, which may cause a disruption of the interosseous membrane. Corrective osteotomy may be indicated in patients who have this type of malunion.

▶ The authors are to be commended for a very nice study that analyzes the effect of dorsally angulated distal radius fractures on DRUJ congruency and forearm rotation. We have performed previous studies to analyze the effects of distal radius fracture malunion on proximal wrist joint contact areas and pressures. It is interesting that the degree of dorsal angulation at the DRUJ that resulted in significant changes in the radioulnar joint congruency coincided with the degree of deformity noted in our previous work,[1] in which significant changes in contact area and pressures occurred at the proximal wrist joint. The current study showed that 20 degrees of dorsal angulation of the distal radius from its original alignment resulted in the most dramatic changes in the congruency of the DRUJ. Our previous study showed, in fact, that 20 degrees in either palmar or dorsal position resulted in changes in the location of the contact areas and features of both contact areas and pressures in the proximal wrist joint. Their findings that dorsal angulation of the distal radius resulted in increased interosseous membrane tightness and subsequent limitation of pronation and supination of the forearm are quite logical but are important nonetheless to demonstrate and highlight. In distal radius fractures, the progressive disruption of the secondary constraints of the DRUJ after fracture and further deformity of the distal radius includes the distal portion of the interosseous membrane. The authors found that DRUJ dislocation did not occur until both the TFCC and interosseous membrane were sectioned.

This information further indicates that if DRUJ dislocation is seen clinically, it should be presumed that the TFCC and distal portion of the interosseous membrane are disrupted until proved otherwise. In a similar sense, our previous work revealed that we could not obtain displacements of the distal radius involving shortening greater than 4 mm or angulation greater than 20 degrees with the ulnar styloid and TFCC intact. This implies that if you do get this degree of shortening or angular deformity of the distal radius, you should presume that the TFCC is disrupted, even in the absence of an ulnar styloid fracture.

The authors should also be commended for emphasizing that distal radial malunion does result in DRUJ incongruency when assessing the appropriateness of DRUJ arthroplasty. The alignment and any malalignment of the distal radius that will result in distal radioulnar incongruency must be evaluated and considered in the treatment plan.

In regard to ulnar impaction that results from radial shortening, I believe that the extent to which a patient can tolerate radial shortening without the development of ulnar impaction syndrome depends, in part, on the baseline ulnar variance that the patient had before the fracture. Specifically, if a patient's normal ulnar variance is -2 mm, they would tolerate, for example, 2 mm of radial shortening much better than would a patient whose normal ulnar variance was $+2$ mm. I congratulate the authors not only for the completion of an excellent study, but also for their efforts to incorporate and integrate the information they gained into the clinical assessment and treatment of distal radius fractures.

S.F. Viegas, M.D.

Reference

1. Pogue DJ, Viegas SF, Patterson RM, et al: The effects of distal radius fracture malunion on wrist joint mechanics. *J Hand Surg* 15A:721–727, 1990.

Suggested Reading

Baratz ME, Des Jardins JD, Anderson DD, et al: Displaced intra-articular fractures of the distal radius: The effect of fracture displacement on contact stresses in a cadaver model. *J Hand Surg* 21A:183–188, 1996.

▶ An anatomical reduction of any fracture, including distal radius intra-articular fractures is generally the goal of treatment. Practically, however, the important questions are what degree of alignment is needed, and what lack of alignment would result in significantly abnormal load mechanics and subsequent degenerative changes in the wrist. Previous work, including work performed in our laboratory, has analyzed varying degrees of radial shortening, loss of radial inclination, and palmar tilt, and their results on contact areas and pressures within the wrist joint. The authors in this study have turned their attention to simulated intra-articular fractures with simulated displaced fractures of the lunate fossa. Their studies included 8 cadavers with 0–3 mm of depression of displaced lunate fossa fractures loaded with 100 newtons of force through flexor and extensor tendons. They found significant increases in contact stresses dealing with depressions of as little as 1 mm of the lunate fossa. They found that with increasing degrees of displacement of the lunate fossa, the contact area shifted toward the fracture line. Work by Wagner, Tencer, Kiser, and Trumble[1] used a similar experimental model with cadaver specimens loading 155 newtons of force through flexor and extensor tendons. They studied both simulated lunate fossa fracture displacement, and scaphoid fossa fracture displacement. They found that statistically significant changes of increased pressure in the scaphoid fossa occurred only with 3 mm of depression of the lunate fossa, and were noted only with the wrist in a neutral position. Scaphoid fossa depression, however, had more significant effects with even 1 mm of depression. These changes included an increase of load in the lunate fossa in neutral and radial deviation postures of the wrist. Contact areas increased in the lunate fossa in ulnar and radial deviation with 1 mm of scaphoid fossa depression and in all loading positions with 3 mm of scaphoid fossa depression.

Previous studies of displaced intra-articular fractures in the ankle and the resulting effect on load mechanics were generalized to other joints to suggest that 2 mm or more of displacement should be treated to obtain better fracture reduction. This work offers information in the simulated cadaver model, which suggests that an intra-articular fracture of the distal radius with a step-off of as little as 1 mm may benefit from improved fracture reduction, if possible. The work of Wagner, et al.[1] suggests that depression of the scaphoid fossa may result in more statistically significant changes in the load mechanics of the wrist at less fracture displacement than in lunate fossa fracture depressions. It continues to be important to look at clinical studies to validate the recommendations gained by and based on these kinds of biomechanical studies. These cadaver studies, however, offer a wonderful experimental model which allow us to both limit and control the variables which may contribute to poor functional outcomes of distal radius intra-articular fractures.

S.F. Viegas, M.D.

Reference

1. Wagner WF, Tencer AF, Kiser P, et al: Effects of intra-articular distal radius depression on wrist joint contact characteristics. *J Hand Surg* 21A:554–560, 1996.

Hutchinson DT, Strenz GO, Cautilli RA: Pins and plaster vs. external fixation in the treatment of unstable distal radial fractures: A randomized prospective study. *J Hand Surg* 20B:365–372, 1995.

▶ The authors have updated the use of pins and plaster, demonstrating in a prospective study that the results are comparable to those of external fixation.

Moving?

I'd like to receive my *Year Book of Hand Surgery* without interruption.
Please note the following change of address, effective:

Name: _____

New Address: _____

_____

City: _____ State: _____ Zip: _____

Old Address: _____

_____

City: _____ State: _____ Zip: _____

Reservation Card

Yes, I would like my own copy of *Year Book of Hand Surgery*. Please begin my subscription with the current edition according to the terms described below.* I understand that I will have 30 days to examine each annual edition. If satisfied, I will pay just $75.95 plus sales tax, postage and handling (price subject to change without notice).

Name: _____

Address: _____

City: _____ State: _____ Zip: _____

Method of Payment
○ Visa   ○ Mastercard   ○ AmEx   ○ Bill me   ○ Check (in US dollars, payable to Mosby, Inc.)

Card number: _____ Exp date: _____

Signature: _____

LS-0908

---

*Your Year Book Service Guarantee:

When you subscribe to the *Year Book*, we'll send you an advance notice of future volumes about two months before they publish. This automatic notice system is designed to take up as little of your time as possible. If you do not want the *Year Book*, the advance notice makes it quick and easy for you to let us know your decision, and you will always have at least 20 days to decide. If we don't hear from you, we'll send you the new volume as soon as it's available. And, of course, the *Year Book* is yours to examine free of charge for 30 days (postage, handling and applicable sales tax are added to each shipment.).

BUSINESS REPLY MAIL
FIRST CLASS MAIL   PERMIT No. 762   CHICAGO, IL

POSTAGE WILL BE PAID BY ADDRESSEE

Chris Hughes
Mosby-Year Book, Inc.
161 N. Clark Street
Suite 1900
Chicago, IL 60601-9981

NO POSTAGE
NECESSARY
IF MAILED
IN THE
UNITED STATES

BUSINESS REPLY MAIL
FIRST CLASS MAIL   PERMIT No. 762   CHICAGO, IL

POSTAGE WILL BE PAID BY ADDRESSEE

Chris Hughes
Mosby-Year Book, Inc.
161 N. Clark Street
Suite 1900
Chicago, IL 60601-9981

NO POSTAGE
NECESSARY
IF MAILED
IN THE
UNITED STATES

Mosby
Dedicated to publishing excellence

Radiographic results are slightly better than those of external fixation. Although both pins and plaster have high complication rates, both are very cost-effective.

A.L. Ladd, M.D.

Jantea C, Baltzer A, Strauss M: Arthroskopische Rekonstruktion radialseitiger Läjonen des Discus ulnocarpalis. *Arthroskopie* 8:288–293, 1995.
▶ Several studies have confirmed the importance of the fibrocartilage complex (FCC) for the force transmission through the ulno-carpal joint. The authors introduce a surgical technique for refixation of the FCC to the radial insertion. They report their experience with 12 patients who were observed in an open prospective study since 1990 (follow-up, 2–4 years). Depending on the thickness of the FCC, the suture used can be passed either through a part or the whole core of the FCC. Patients with an ulna plus situation were excluded from this type of operation, as reattachment of the FCC to the radius is not possible. A resorbable suture was used for the reconstruction of the FCC.

There were no permanent complications after the operation; however, 1 patient had to undergo additional surgery after 3 months because of persistent pain in ulnar deviation. The clinical results are encouraging, but even with good short-term results, a final conclusion cannot be made. Because the protocol presented is that of an open prospective study, we hope to see another later report 5 years after the operation.

This study remembers the trend observed in arthroscopic surgery of meniscal tears in the knee joint. After the "resection period" in the '80s, more and more surgeons began reconstructing the meniscus of the knee joint arthroscopically by quite genious suture techniques in order to prevent problems resulting from its resection.

Priv. Dr. Med. C.L. Jantea

Milliez PY, Dallaserra M, Dujardin F: Instabilité des fractures de l'extrémité inférieuredo radius: Classification analytique àvisée thérapeutique. *Int Orthop (SICOT)* 20:15–22, 1996.
▶ This paper proposes that distal radius fractures be classified based on displacement (direction and degree), articular (radiocarpal) involvement, and metaphyseal comminution. A toal of 4 levels of each are described, giving a classification with 64 possible types!

P.C. Amadio, M.D.

Marx RG, Axelrod TS: Intraarticular osteotomy of distal radial malunions. *Clin Orthop Rel Res* 32:152–157, 1996.

Hauck RM, Skahen J, Palmer AK: Classification and treatment of ulnar styloid nonunion. *J Hand Surg* 21A:418–422, 1996.

Distal Radioulnar Joint

The Pronator Quadratus Interposition Transfer: An Adjunct to Resection Arthroplasty of the Distal Radioulnar Joint

Ruby LK, Ferenz CC, Dell PC (Tufts–New England Med Ctr, Boston; Univ of Florida, Gainesville)
J Hand Surg (Am) 21A:60–65, 1996   8–42

Background.—Ulnar head resection is a time-honored procedure for treating painful traumatic and arthritic conditions of the distal radioulnar joint. However, several adverse sequelae have been associated with this operation, mostly resulting from the instability of the ulna remnant relative to surrounding structures, such as the radius and extensor tendons. A surgical technique to prevent and treat this problem was described.

Technique.—With the patient under axillary block or general anesthesia, the surgeon makes an incision over the distal ulna, starting just distal to the ulnar head and extending 5–6 cm proximally along the ulnar shaft (Fig 1, A). Protecting the dorsal sensory branch of the ulnar nerve, the surgeon approaches the distal ulna subperiosteally between the fifth and sixth extensor compartments of the wrist. The distal ulna is then resected according to surgeon preference. The current authors performed an oblique metaphyseal osteotomy, with the bevel facing the radius, smoothing all sharp edges with a rongeur. A curved osteotome can be used as a knife for

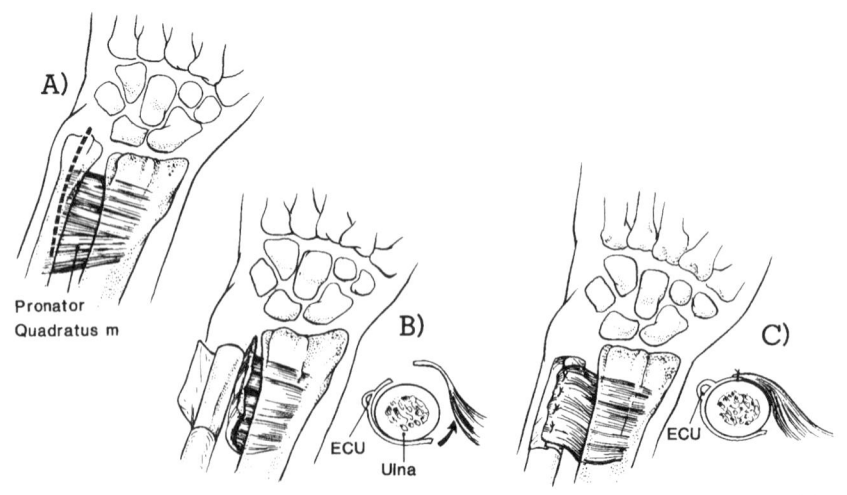

FIGURE 1.—Drawing of the pronator quadratus transfer (dorsal view). **A,** incision (*dotted line*) of skin and periosteum. **B,** periosteal flap is created and pronator is delivered through the interosseous space. **C,** pronator is sutured to the periosteal flap to stabilize the distal ulna. *Abbreviation: ECU,* extensor carpi ulnaris. (Courtesy of Ruby LK, Ferenz CC, Dell PC: The pronator quadratus interposition transfer: An adjunct to resection arthroplasty of the distal radioulnar joint. *J Hand Surg (Am)* 21A:60–65, 1996.)

detaching the deep aspect of the muscle and its fibrous origin. The pronator quadratus muscle belly is then delivered through the interosseous space and brought to the dorsum of the ulna. The surgeon elevates a cuff of periosteum and extensor carpi ulnaris tendon sheath from the bone (Fig 1, B). With the patient's forearm supinated and the distal ulna in a reduced position, the surgeon sutures the pronator quadratus origin to the extensor carpi ulnaris tendon sheath with maximal tension in a figure-eight or horizontal mattress manner (Fig 1, C). Standard closure is performed.

Patients and Outcomes.—Sixteen wrists in 15 patients underwent this procedure between 1985 and 1989. Indications included pain in the distal radioulnar joint from osteoarthritis, post-traumatic arthritis, and incongruity. Mean follow-up was 8 years. Seven patients had previously had failure of ulna head resection, and 8 had this procedure concomitantly with ulnar head resection. Only 1 failure occurred in the primary group and 2 occurred in the secondary group. No complications were directly associated with pronator transfer.

Conclusion.—Pronator quadratus interposition is a safe, relatively effective, technically straightforward technique that can be used as a salvage procedure in some patients with failed distal radioulnar resection arthroplasties. Pain can be reduced and grip strength improved in such patients. This technique may also have a role in primary ulnar head resection arthroplasty.

▶ Instability associated with resection of the distal ulna can now be effectively treated by pronator quadratus transfer as described by Ruby and co-authors. Most of the patients in the series had previously had failed distal ulna resections (Darrach procedures); in others, the procedure was done for the first time. We agree with the recommendations and operative procedure described by the authors, pointing out similar good experience by R. K. Johnson.[1] The pronator quadratus muscle, acting both as a stabilizer and soft tissue interposition, has definite advantages over other procedures to prevent radioulnar impingement. In my own experience, it is a very good adjunctive primary procedure and also a good alternative for salvage cases.

W.P. Cooney III, M.D.

Reference

1. Johnson RK: Muscle tendon transfer for stabilization of the distal radio-ulna joint. *J Hand Surg* 10A:437, 1985.

Matched Hemiresection Interposition Arthroplasty of the Distal Radioulnar Joint
Bain GI, Pugh DMW, MacDermid JC, et al (Univ of Western Ontario, London, Canada)
J Hand Surg (Am) 20A:944–950, 1995   8–43

Objective.—The subjective, objective, functional, and radiographic film results of a modified hemiresection interposition arthroplasty of the wrist were reviewed retrospectively.

Methods.—Surgery was performed on 55 wrists in 52 patients, aged 16–81 years, for pain caused by derangement of the distal radionuclear joint. Follow-up data were obtained for 49 patients.

> *Technique.*—The fifth extensor compartment is divided, the extensor digiti minimi is retracted, and the dorsal capsule and adherent infratendinous portion of the extensor retinaculum are divided 1 mm from the radial insertion. The distal ulna is then similarly resected, and the ulna-based retinaculum flap is mobilized and sutured to the 1 mm flap.

Results.—Pain improved in 35 patients, remained the same in 10, and worsened in 4. Forty-one patients were satisfied with the outcome, and women were significantly more satisfied than men. Supination and pronation improved from 54 degrees and 67 degrees to 72 degrees and 72 degrees, respectively. Patients needed 53% longer to turn smaller objects and 86% longer to turn larger objects. Complications included 1 wound infection, 1 case of reflex sympathetic dystrophy, and 1 neuroma. Four patients required reoperation for ulnar-carpal impaction. One patient experienced persistent pain. There was no correlation between pain improvement or patient satisfaction and subjective, objective, functional, and radiographic results.

Conclusion.—Pain was the primary indication for surgery. This technique does not result in increased tendon dysfunction or distal ulnar instability. Objective and functional deficits that remained after surgery were poorly correlated with patient satisfaction and pain relief. Ulnar-carpal impaction was the most common complication.

▶ This is a well-done retrospective clinical review of a modified hemiresection interposition arthroplasty procedure for a painful distal radioulnar joint. One advantage of this paper is consistency in the technique, because 1 surgeon performed all the procedures. There are adequate numbers to substantiate the data, and both the objective and subjective evaluations were well done. The retrieval was high, with only 6 of 55 patients lost to follow-up. Several observations can be drawn from this study. First, the single best correlation with patient satisfaction is pain relief. In my experience, this is a common, if not universal, theme with most wrist procedures. Second, the overall results are similar to most of the other techniques described of arthroplasty of this joint. Third, the hemiresection interposition technique has the added potential complication of styloid carpal abutment, which is avoided by a more generous resection, such as the Darrach. I agree that an attempt to interpose tissue between the resected ulna stump and the radius, and with dorsal transfer of the extensor carpi ulnaris tendon and sheath, to help prevent radioulnar impingement and improve stability is a worthwhile endeavor (although it is difficult to prove by published data). I would have preferred that the study not mix rheumatoid arthritis with post-trauma patients, but the results did not substantiate any significant difference between the 2 groups. Nonetheless, the authors describe another variation on the technique of ulna resection arthroplasty with very good (approximately 80%) successful results.

L.K. Ruby, M.D.

A Modified Darrach Procedure for Treatment of the Painful Distal Radioulnar Joint
Sotereanos DG, Leit ME (Univ Orthopaedics Inc, Pittsburgh, Pa)
Clin Orthop 325:140–147, 1996

Purpose.—The Darrach distal ulnar resection has been considered the surgical procedure of choice for patients with pain and instability of the distal radioulnar joint. More recent procedures, i.e., the Bowers hemiresection interposition arthroplasty and the Watson matched distal ulna resection, were designed to preserve the styloid attachment of the triangular fibrocartilage complex. Each of these procedures is effective, though with inherent pitfalls and complications. Results of a modified Darrach procedure for patients with painful distal radioulnar joints were assessed.

Technique.—The modified technique, which included extensor carpi ulnaris stabilization, was designed to treat ulnar abutment, radioulnar joint pain and impingement, and dorsal subluxation of the ulna in a single operation. The distal ulna was approached using a dorsal, vertical incision, through the fifth and sixth compartments of the extensor retinaculum. The ulna was shortened about 1 cm, the same amount of the proximal extent of the sigmoid notch of the radius. The extensor carpi ulnaris tendon was split from about 5 cm proximal to the resected end of the distal ulna to the base of the fifth metacarpal. A 1/8-inch bicortical drill hole was then made in the distal ulna, and the radial tendon slip was passed through it and pulled taut with the wrist in ulnar deviation. The tendon slip was sutured to itself with the ulna held volar; before closing, the surgeon ensured a smooth arc of motion without impingement.

Experience.—The modified Darrach procedure was performed in 16 wrists of 15 patients with pain of the distal radioulnar joint. The patients, average age 38 years, were followed up for 28–47 months. In 6 cases, the modified Darrach procedure was performed as revision surgery. All patients but 1 had marked reduction in pain postoperatively. Forearm pronation/supination increased by an average of 53 degrees, wrist flexion/extension by 25 degrees, and grip strength by 29 lb. Five of six workers' compensation patients were able to return to their jobs.

Conclusions.—The modified Darrach procedure described combines the advantages of several other techniques for distal radioulnar joint pain. The relatively simple operation, which combines distal ulnar resection with stabilization of the extensor carpi ulnaris and radial oblique osteotomy, is useful for primary and revision surgery. In almost all patients, the procedure provides good improvement toward pain-free motion and increased grip strength.

▶ The authors have clearly demonstrated in their patient population that supplementing the traditional Darrach resection of the distal ulna with stabilization with an extensor carpi ulnaris tenodesis was successful in achieving excellent pain relief and apparent stability. Their study included, however, only 2 patients with preoperative instability of the ulna, and as a rule, if an ulna is unstable preoperatively (after a Colles' fracture with ulnar plus deformity), the resected ulna will also be unstable postoperatively. In this patient population, the preferred choice of treatment is restoration of radial length with radial osteotomy to establish ulnar stability.

R.D. Beckenbaugh, M.D.

Dynamic Radio-Ulnar Convergence After the Darrach Procedure
McKee MD, Richards RR (St Michael's Hosp, Toronto; Univ of Toronto)
J Bone Joint Surg (Br) 78B:413–418, 1996   8–45

Introduction.—In patients with traumatic injuries of the distal radioulnar joint, excision of the distal ulna—known as the Darrach procedure—can increase range of motion and reduce pain. However, recent reports suggest that this operation provides good results only about half the time. One potential problem is an ulnar impingement syndrome caused by painful pseudarthrosis between the ulnar stump and the distal radius. The prevalence and clinical significance of ulnar impingement are unknown. Patients who had undergone the Darrach procedure were studied to determine the prevalence of dynamic radioulnar convergence and impingement and its effects on the final results.

Methods.—Twenty-three patients who had undergone a total of 25 Darrach procedures for traumatic or posttraumatic conditions of the wrist were studied. The operations had been performed a mean of 75.5 months previously, at which time the patients' mean age was 61 years. During a clinic visit, each patient completed a history and a questionnaire on patient satisfaction and activities of daily living, and had a detailed physical examination. In addition, standardized radiographs of both wrists were

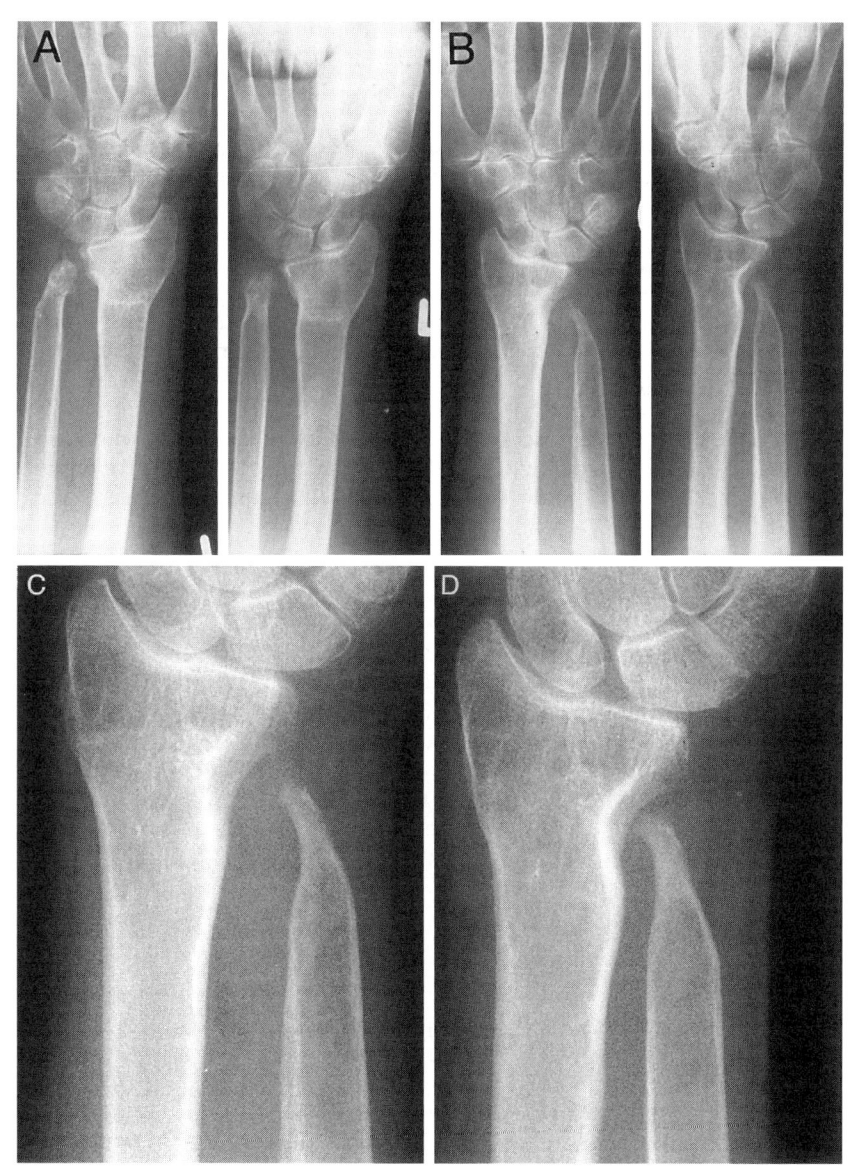

FIGURE 3. —Radiographs in the resting position (left) and during maximal grip (right) of a patient with bilateral distal radial malunion after fractures, in whom bilateral Darrach procedures were performed. On the left side (A), a conservative resection of the distal ulna was performed, and there is no evidence of dynamic radioulnar convergence. On the right (B), after a more extensive distal ulnar excision, there is dynamic radioulnar convergence with impingement, as seen by sclerosis and scalloping of the distal radius. The left wrist was rated as "good" and the right as "poor." Figures C and D show the ulnar convergence area in B in more detail. (Courtesy of McKee MD, Richards RR: Dynamic Radio-Ulnar Convergence After the Darrach Procedure. *J Bone Joint Surg (Br)* 78B:413–418, 1996.)

obtained, including "resting" views and "dynamic" views with the hand in maximal grip. On the radiographic analysis, dynamic radioulnar convergence was defined as convergence of the distal ulnar stump toward the distal radius during maximal grip.

Results.—Dynamic radioulnar convergence was noted in 14 wrists, including 5 wrists with dynamic radioulnar impingement, in which the bones were actually touching (Fig 3). However, only 2 patients were symptomatic. Dynamic radioulnar convergence had no apparent effect on grip strength, pinch strength, range of motion, or wrist score. It was more likely to be found in patients who had a greater length of distal ulna excised. Nineteen of 23 patients were satisfied with their surgical results.

Conclusions.—Many patients who have undergone the Darrach procedure show radiographic evidence of dynamic radioulnar convergence, or even impingement. However, this condition is rarely symptomatic. For older adults with pain and loss of movement related to traumatic or posttraumatic injuries of the wrist, distal ulnar resection provides reliable results. The excision should include the minimal amount of distal ulna needed to restore full rotation.

▶ This paper nicely documents the occurrence, findings, and pathomechanics of post-Darrach ulnar impingement. The range of clinical results is spread to mostly favorable outcomes. There was little mention of the painful snapping problem seen with pronosupination that has been the primary symptom in our failed ulnar head resections.[1] We agree that narrowing of the interosseous space is less with minimal resection, but found that this did not preclude impingement symptoms, especially in younger patients. The Chamay method of addressing ulnar translation was overlooked in the references. Although most outcomes are indeed satisfactory, this paper fails to address the marked difficulty in treatment of the persistently painful ulnar impingement syndrome.

R.L. Linscheid, M.D.

Reference

1. Bieber EJ, Linscheid RL, Dobyns JH: Failed distal ulna resections. *J Hand Surg (Am)* 13:193–200, 1988.

The Stabilizing Mechanism of the Distal Radioulnar Joint During Pronation and Supination
Kihara H, Short WH, Werner FW, et al (State Univ of New York, Syracuse)
J Hand Surg (Am) 20A:930–936, 1995   8–46

Introduction.—Opinions diverge regarding which structures are most important in stabilizing the distal radioulnar joint (DRUJ). Roles of the stabilizing structures of the DRUJ during pronation and supination were observed during a biomechanical cadaver investigation.

Methods.—Seven fresh-frozen upper extremities amputated at the midhumerus were examined radiographically for pre-existing pathology. Specimens were placed in a loading apparatus. A 3 SPACE motion tracker measured the amount of pronation and supination and the relative motion of the radius with respect to the ulna. Measurements were taken with the forearm in neutral pronation, supination, maximum supination, and maximum pronation. The dorsal radioulnar ligaments (DRUL) of the triangular fibrocartilage complex (TFCC), the palmar radioulnar ligaments (PRUL) of the TFCC, the distal interosseous membrane (d-IOM) including the pronator quadratus, and the entire IOM were evaluated to determine DRUJ instability on the wrist mechanics. In 1 group of 3 forearms, either the DRUL or the PRUL and the corresponding half of the articular disk of the TFCC were cut. The second cut disrupted the remaining radioulnar ligament and remaining half of the articular disk. The pronator quadratus and d-IOM were then cut to the level of the proximal pronator quadratus. Dissection was completed with sectioning of the remaining IOM. In the remaining 4 forearms, the d-IOM was sectioned, followed by the remaining IOM. Then, either the DRUL or the PRUL and the corresponding half of the articular disk were cut. The remaining radioulnar ligament and remaining half of the articular disk were then cut. The amount of subluxation was measured for each loading condition and increment of sectioning by measuring the displacement of the radius that occurred relative to the ulna. The dorsal or palmar displacement of Lister's tubercle and amount of diastasis of the radius were measured on each cross-sectional view.

Results.—Joint stability was not appreciably changed after cutting only the DRUL and PRUL. The DRUJ remained stable after sectioning 2 of any 4 structures. The DRUL was observed to be more important than the PRUL in stabilizing the DRUJ in pronation when the IOM was disrupted first. In addition, the PRUL was more important than the DRUL during supination. Only when all 4 structures were sectioned did dislocation and diastasis occur.

Conclusion.—The roles of the DRUL and PRUL in stabilizing the DRUJ when the IOM was intact could not be defined. After disruption of the IOM, the DRUL was more important than the PRUL in stabilizing the DRUJ in pronation, and the PRUL was more important than the DRUL in supination. The DRUL, PRUL, d-IOM, and entire IOM were all important in stabilizing the DRUJ in the dorsal, palmar, and lateral directions.

▶ Although this experiment has the limitations of any cadaver study, and it did not include the extensor carpi ulnaris tendon or the extensor carpi ulnaris sheath, it appears that for complete instability of the DRUJ to occur, the entire IOM, pronator quadratus, DRUL, and PRUL must be incompetent. Further, the DRUJ remains in a reduced position in neutral and supination, even if all 4 structures are compromised, if no stress is applied. This is useful clinical information when treating a complete DRUJ dislocation. However, it is still unclear which structure, the DRUL or PRUL, is more important in preventing dorsal or palmar DRUJ subluxation in full supination and pronation. Even though the study agrees with Schuind et al.,[1] it contradicts af Ekenstam et al.[2] This paper may be more important to the biomechanician than the clinician, but it is still of interest.

L.K. Ruby, M.D.

References

1. Schuind F, An KN, Berglund L, et al: The distal radioulnar elements: A biomechanical study. *J Hand Surg (Am)* 16A:1106–1114, 1991.
2. af Ekenstam F, Hagert CG: Anatomical studies on the geometry and stability of the distal radioulnar joint. *Scand J Plast Reconstr Surg* 19:17–25, 1985.

Traumatic Avulsion of the Triangular Fibrocartilage Complex at its Ulnar Insertion: Treatment by Reinsertion and Hemiepiphyseal Osteotomy at the Distal Ulna [in French]
Sennwald G, Fischer M (Chirurgie Saint-Léonard, Saint-Gall, Switzerland)
La Main 1:39–46, 1996
8–47

Introduction.—The triangular fibrocartilage complex (TFCC) has a major role in wrist function. Triangular fibrocartilage complex lesions, whether caused by trauma or overuse, have been classified by Palmer. In a type 1B Palmer lesion, avulsion of the disc from its attachment on the ulna causes wrist instability and disabling pain. The lesion is diagnosed by clinical examination, and the diagnosis is confirmed by arthrography when it shows infiltration of contrast medium at the insertion point. A new method for repairing a type 1B Palmer lesion was described.

Technique.—The procedure involves combining reinsertion of the TFCC with a hemi-epiphyseal osteotomy at the distal end of the ulna. The purpose of the osteotomy is to free the TFCC for easy access and expose a well-vascularized osseous surface for its reinsertion. A zig-zag incision centered over the head of the ulna is used. This type of an incision leaves a strip of retinaculum extensorum intact, thus avoiding the risk of iatrogenic injury to the disc during repair.

Patients.—The procedure was used in 8 men and 1 woman, aged 17–58 years, who had sustained type B1 Palmer lesions. All patients were manual laborers who had been unable to work, even though the dominant hand was involved in only 3 of the 9 patients. The cause of injury in all cases was a fall with the hand in hyperextension. The mean interval between the first occurrence of symptoms and the first consultation was 43 months.

Results.—After a mean follow-up period of 33 months, all patients had been able to resume some manual work, either part-time at the same job or a new job that was less demanding on the wrist. The pain was significantly diminished, and the average score on the Culp index achieved was 79 points. One patient had secondary clinical failure resulting from incorrect surgical technique. The patient refused reoperation.

▶ I believe this technique may be useful in cases where peripheral TFCC detachment occurs in the presence of a long ulna. Another option would be a Feldon wafer excision or formal ulnar shortening. Of course, if the ulna is not long, arthroscopic repair is possible and probably even preferable.

P.C. Amadio, M.D.

Clinical Results of Treatment of Triangular Fibrocartilage Complex Tears by Arthroscopic Debridement
Minami A, Ishikawa J-I, Suenaga N, et al (Hokkaido Univ, Sapporo, Japan)
J Hand Surg (Am) 21A:406–411, 1996   8–48

Background.—Whether arthroscopic débridement is effective in the treatment of triangular fibrocartilage complex (TFCC) tears was determined.

Patients and Outcomes.—The records of 16 patients, aged 20–53 years, who had TFCC tears were reviewed retrospectively. Eleven patients had posttraumatic tears, and 5 had degenerative tears. Mean follow-up was 35 months. Pain, range of motion, grip strength, return to work, patient acceptance, and complications were assessed before and after surgery. Clinical outcome was poor in patients who had positive ulnar variance and lunotriquetral interosseous ligament tears. A good outcome was associated with grip strength. Results were excellent in all patients who had posttraumatic TFCC tears and poor in patients who had degenerative TFCC tears.

Conclusions.—Patients who had posttraumatic tears of the TFCC had excellent results after arthroscopic débridement. Postoperative results were fair or poor, however, in patients who had degenerative TFCC tears, ulnar abutment syndrome with positive ulnar variance, lunate chondromalacia, or lunotriquetral interosseous ligament rupture.

▶ This article supports arthroscopic débridement for symptomatic TFCC pain, with excellent results in 13 of 16 patients. In this retrospective analysis, 11 patients who had posttraumatic injuries were compared with 5 who had degenerative tears; however, the conclusions are not supported by the data presented. The sample size is too small; the entry criteria, including the definitions of posttraumatic and degenerative, are not well delineated; and the statistical analysis is inconclusive. These important data demonstrate the need to analyze management protocols prospectively. The authors' approach to the management of TFCC pain is based on their extensive clinical experience and is consistent with generally accepted principles.

L.A. Koman, M.D.

Ulnar Shortening Using the AO Small Distractor
Wehbé MA, Cautilli DA (Pennsylvania Hand Ctr, Bryn Mawr; Jefferson Med College, Philadelphia)
J Hand Surg (Am) 20A:959–964, 1995

Purpose.—Various modifications of the ulnar shortening osteotomy, which was first used in 1941 to decompress the ulnocarpal articulation in patients who had the ulnar impaction syndrome, have been described. A new ulnar shortening procedure for the treatment of ulnar impaction syndrome, using the AO small distractor for temporary intraoperative external fixation and a 2.7-mm dynamic compression plate (DCP) for internal fixation, was described.

Technique.—After the incision is made, a 6- or 7-hole 2.7-mm AO DCP is held over the exposed ulna to determine the best osteotomy site. An AO small distractor is placed across the proposed osteotomy site. Threaded Kirschner wires are inserted in its inner 2 holes and outer 2 holes to control rotation (Fig 1, A). The

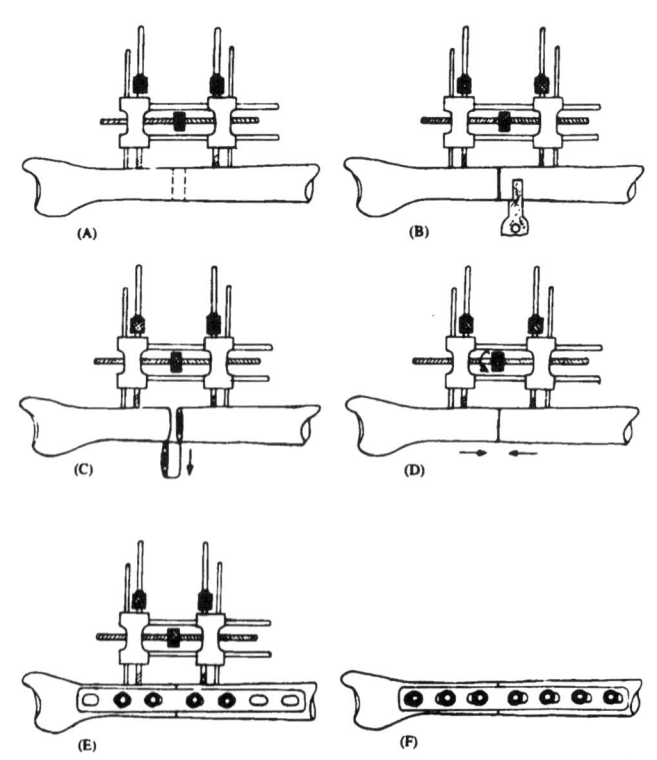

FIGURE 1.—The ulnar shortening technique. (Courtesy of Wehbé MA, Cautilli DA: Ulnar shortening using the AO small distractor. *J Hand Surg (AM)* 20A:959–964, 1995.)

fixator is pushed down, and 2 transverse osteotomies are performed (Fig 1, B). An oblique osteotomy may also be used for this technique (Fig 1, C, D). A 2.7-mm DCP is centered across the osteotomy site and fastened with 4 eccentrically placed screws, 2 on each side of the osteotomy site (Fig 1, E). The distractor and half-pins are removed, and the screws are tightened (Fig 1, F).

Patients.—Twenty-four patients, aged 18–67 years, who had ulnar impaction syndrome underwent ulnar shortening osteotomy. The preoperative ulnar variance ranged from −2 mm to +8 mm. Follow-up ranged from 8 to 74 months (average, 32 months).

Outcome.—Twenty-three patients reported complete relief of ulnar wrist pain, and 1 patient had significant but not complete relief of wrist pain. The latter patient subsequently underwent successful radioulnar joint resection. Clinical union occurred at an average of 9 weeks, and radiographic union occurred at an average of 8.8 weeks. Three patients had delayed clinical union, but all healed uneventfully with complete relief of pain. All DCPs were removed an average of 16 months after surgery. The average ulnar shortening was 3 mm, and the average postoperative variance was −2.3 mm.

Conclusions.—A new ulnar shortening technique involving a transverse osteotomy, temporary intraoperative external fixation with the AO small distractor, and internal fixation with a 2.7-mm DCP is a technically simple and effective method for treating ulnar impaction syndrome.

▶ That no nonunions occurred in this group of 24 patients who underwent ulnar shortening osteotomy certainly demonstrates that complex and expensive instruments are not necessary for success. However, although not essential, the saw guide developed by Rayhack does allow more reliably parallel saw cuts to be made.

V.R. Hentz, M.D.

Suggested Reading

Minami A, Suzuki K, Suenaga N, et al: The Sauvé-Kapandji procedure for osteoarthritis of the distal radioulnar joint. *J Hand Surg* 20A:602–608, 1995.
▶ The concept of inserting cortical bone between the distal radio-ulnar joint resected from the ulna in order to "maintain the normal radial ulnar diameter of the wrist" is intriguing. However, it is doubtful that many surgeons would rely solely on this bone without additional cancellous bone graft in order to effect union. While all 15 patients in this small series had improvement in their pain severity, this procedure should not be regarded as uniformly successful or as a panacea to the arthritic distal radio-ulnar joint.

J. Rayhack, M.D.

Adams BD, Samani JE, Holley KA: Triangular fibrocartilage injury: A laboratory model. *J Hand Surg* 21A:189–193, 1996.

▶ The mechanism for traumatic disruption of the triangular fibrocartilage is unknown. Axial loading combined with rotational torque is reported by patients but is unconfirmed by laboratory studies. In this report, Adams et al. provide the first evidence that tensile loads (lateral–medial displacement) results in avulsion of the triangular fibrocartilage from the base of the ulnar styloid. The mechanism of the more common radial-sided tears is speculated from increased strain deformations (28% radial vs. 18% ulnar) and combined loads of rotation and compression. It is not caused by distraction alone or by rotational strains of excess pronation or supination. The authors have developed an excellent experimental model demonstrating that tension changes loads within the articular disk itself. For true instability, the dorsal or palmar radioulnar joint ligaments must be disrupted. For subthreshold instability, however, central or peripheral edge tears may have occurred and may consequently produce symptoms of ulnar wrist pain.

This paper is an excellent laboratory study that confirms that rotational stress combined with compression can produce clinically symptomatic triangular fibrocartilage tears.

W.P. Cooney III, M.D.

Fellinger M, Grechenig W, Seibert FJ, et al: Arthroskopische Refixationstechniken de Discus triangularis beim frischen Handgelenktrauma (Tequniques of arthroscopic repair of the triangular fibrocartilage complex in wrist injuries). *Arthroskopie* 8:294–298, 1995.

▶ In acute injuries of the wrist, one may quite often find a tear of the fibrocartilage complex (FCC) while arthroscopy of the wrist is performed. These authors describe an arthroscopic technique for reconstruction of the FCC when a peripheral tear is observed.

In situations in which a fracture of the styloid process of the ulna is observed, the authors demonstrate a transosseous fixation technique for reattaching the FCC to its ulnar base. This technique is widely accepted in centers where wrist arthroscopy is a routine procedure.

When a discontinuity of the FCC from its insertion at the radius is observed, a transosseous reinsertion technique using one 2.5-mm drill hole through the radius is performed. The T-Fix device (Acufex Comp) is used to reattach the FCC to the radius.

The authors report their early results with 2 patients without any complication during or after the procedure. The authors insist on strict patient selection with either an ulna zero, or preferably an ulna minus, situation. Although the results are encouraging, further observation of the patients is necessary, as the T-Fix device is not resorbable and it lies within the ulnocarpal joint with a direct contact to the carpal bones.

Priv. Dr. Med. C.L. Jantea

▶ Another option, which avoids the implantation of a device, is suture repair of radial detachments of the triangular fibrocartilage, a procedure refined by Dr. Jantea over the last 6 years, with encouraging results. As noted elsewhere in this YEAR Book, TFC reattachment in the case of ulna plus is not feasible unless some sort of ulnar shortening is first accomplished.

P.C. Amadio, M.D.

Sénéchaud C, Savioz D, Della Santa D: Stabilisation de l'articulation radio-cubitale infériure par plastie ligamentaire selon la technique de Hui et Lindscheid: A propos de dix cas (Stabilization of the distal radioulnar joint by Hui-Linscheid ligamentoplasty: Report of 10 cases). *Ann Chir Main* 15:70–79, 1996.
▶ Little is written on distal radioulnar joint stabilization. This paper reviews a medium size series of reconstructions by the Hui-Linscheid method. There were 6 good results, including 1 Essex-Lopresti lesion, out of 9 cases.

P.C. Amadio, M.D.

9 Elbow

Repair of the Distal Biceps Tendon Using Suture Anchors and an Anterior Approach
Lintner S, Fischer T (Orthopaedics Indianapolis, Ind; Indiana Hand Ctr, Indianapolis)
Clin Orthop 322:116–119, 1996
9-1

Purpose.—Complete rupture of the distal biceps tendon insertion is an uncommon injury that usually occurs in middle-aged men who injure the dominant arm. A new technique for surgical repair of this injury, which involves a single, limited volar incision and implantable bone anchors, was reported.

Technique.—The technique, performed on an outpatient basis with the use of axillary block regional anesthesia, starts with an S-shaped volar incision centered on the antecubital fossa. The biceps bursa is opened to expose the ruptured tendon stump. A tag suture is placed, and longitudinal traction is applied to relax the muscle tendon unit. The cortex tuberosity is exposed with the arm fully supinated. After the tuberosity is prepared, 2 Mitek GII suture anchors with attached number 2 Ethibond sutures are placed into it. After minimal débridement, the tendon stump is held to the tuberosity with a surgical clamp, and the sutures are placed into the tendon stump with a locking stitch. The sutures are tied with the arm in 90 degrees of flexion and full supination. A posterior plaster splint is applied to maintain the elbow in this position. Each week, the elbow is extended by 10 degrees. Active range of motion from 60 degrees to full flexion begins at 6 weeks, and full active range of motion is allowed at 8 weeks.

Patients and Outcomes.—This repair was performed in 5 patients (mean age, 39 years) who had ruptures of the distal insertion of the biceps brachii. Four patients were laborers, and 1 was an athlete. All injuries resulted from an unanticipated large load applied to the arm in flexion. The repair was performed on an acute basis in 4 patients and 6 months after the injury in 1.
At a mean clinical follow-up of 2.5 years, all repairs remained intact. All patients had symmetric range of motion with no signs of nerve injury

heterotopic bone formation, or olecranon tenderness. The patients could return to their preinjury levels of activity within 5 months, and all reported satisfaction with their results.

Conclusions.—For patients who have rupture of the distal biceps tendon, this approach provides a safe and simple method of anatomical repair. The use of implantable bone suture anchors permits a small exposure and simplifies the repair. Experience suggests that the suture anchors are strong enough to maintain the anatomical repair during the healing and rehabilitation periods.

▶ This article reviews the results in 5 patients who underwent repair of distal biceps tendon rupture. The anterior Henry approach was used, and metal suture anchors (Mitek) were applied to fix the tendon end to the bone. One contribution of this article is the description of the technique for use of suture anchors. This technique has been used by a number of surgeons, but the descriptions have been primarily anecdotal. The authors comment that a lesser exposure is required than for repair that is normally performed through an anterior approach alone. They suggest that heterotopic ossification is less likely than with the 2-incision technique of Boyd and Anderson.

Some strengths and weaknesses exist. First, these patients all had an intact lacertus fibrosis, and a repair performed under such circumstances is much easier, as the bicipital aponeurosis prevents possible retraction of the tendon. This is especially important in patients who have had a rupture for 6 months. Second, the authors held the tendon stump down against the radial tuberosity while placing the suture in the tendon. They then tied the suture with the elbow at 90 degrees of flexion. This approach appears somewhat contradictory. Although I have not used this particular technique, I envision some difficulties in obtaining a very tight fixation of tendon against bone. Other investigators have also had this concern, and the authors do not convince us not to be concerned about this potential problem. If the primary advantage of this procedure is the decreased likelihood of heterotopic ossification, it would be appropriate to compare this with the technique recommended by Morrey,[1] which is an IM splitting technique for the dorsal exposure. That particular operation can be performed through a very limited combined surgical exposure anteriorly and posteriorly with minimal soft tissue dissection. The experience of Morrey, myself, and others to date with this technique has been very gratifying. The operation can be performed fairly quickly, and heterotopic ossification has not been a significant problem. Neither have nerve complications. My approach to rehabilitation for these patients is to permit immediate, passive, full motion of the elbow, including active extension and delaying active flexion for 6 weeks and flexion against resistance for 8 weeks. This allows extremely rapid return of function. There is no concern at all that the tendon will pull out of the bone when it has been sutured with 4 strands of number 2 nonabsorbable suture directly into a hole in the radial tuberosity. I am not sure whether the same degree of security exists with the Mitek suture anchors, and this point has not yet been clarified. Finally, the discussion of nonsurgical treatment is almost irrelevant. The results of surgical treatment are so excellent, and the results of nonsurgical treatment much more mediocre, that this is one of those orthopedic entities that really should only rarely even be considered appropriately treated without surgery.

Time and further experience with the different techniques will determine the usefulness and appropriate indications for this particular exposure and the use of suture anchors. One concern that I have relates to avulsion of a suture anchor, which, because of the proximity of important neurovascular structures, could theoretically cause a serious nerve injury at the time of avulsion. As usual, the implantation of metallic implants for suture fixation requires a cautious approach and concern for accurate long-term documentation.

S.W. O'Driscoll, M.D.

Reference

1. Morrey BF: Tendon injuries about the elbow, in Morrey BF (ed): The elbow and its disorders. Philadelphia, WB Saunders, 1993, pp 490–500.

Fractures of the Radial Head Treated by Internal Fixation: Late Results in 26 Cases
Esser RD, Davis S, Taavao T (Stanford Univ, Calif; Apia Natl Hosp, Western Samoa)
J Orthop Trauma 9:318–323, 1995
9–2

Objective.—The results of surgical treatment of fractures of the radial head have been variable. Although there has been a renewed interest in open reduction and internal fixation of these fractures, most studies report outcome after short-term follow-up only. The long-term results of open reduction and internal fixation of displaced and comminuted radial head fractures, using AO miniscrews, AO miniplates, and Herbert screws, were assessed.

Methods.—Twenty-six patients, aged 14–57 years, who had Mason type II, III, or IV fractures of the radial head and had undergone open reduction and internal fixation were included. The patients' status was followed for 1–14 years. Eleven patients had type II fractures, 9 had type III, and 6 had type IV. Motion, strength, stability, and pain scores were totaled and rated as excellent for 95–100 points, good for 80–94, fair for 80–94, and poor for 59 points or less.

> *Technique.*—A postlateral incision is made parallel to the humeral shaft, and the capsule, radial head, and elbow joint are exposed. Kirschner wires are used to provide temporary fixation of the fragments with AO screws, small Herbert screws, or mini AO plates for permanent fixation. Herbert screws are preferred, because it is not necessary to countersink them. Mini AO plates are used when it is necessary to remove the humeral head. Type II coronoid fractures are fixed with the use of lag screws. The wound is closed, and the arm is placed in a posterior splint for 2 weeks.

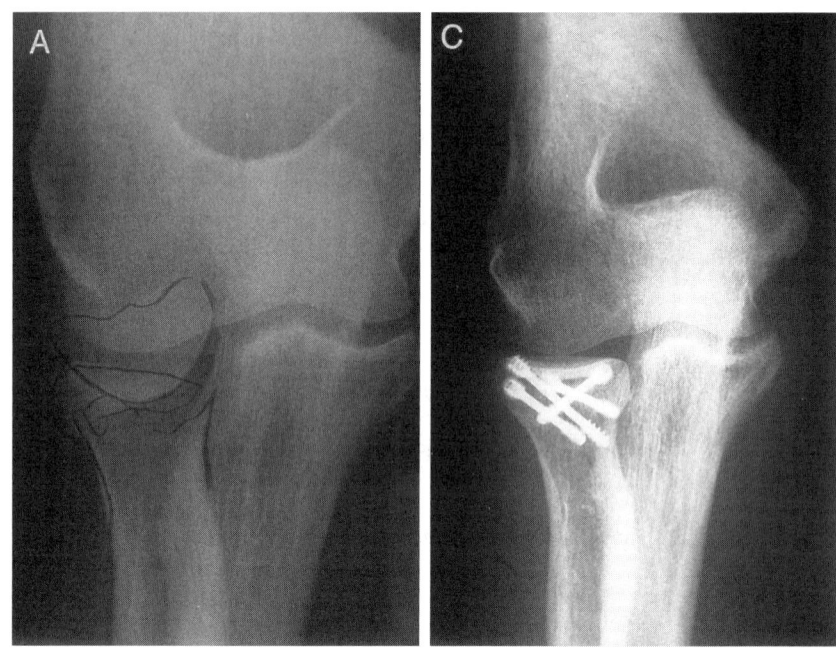

FIGURE 1.—A, anteroposterior roentgenogram shows a Mason type III severe comminuted fracture of the radial head. C, reconstruction of the head with anatomical reduction of the 5 fragments and stable fixation was achieved. Four Herbert screws were used. The patient's arm was immobilized 2 weeks in a posterior splint before physical therapy was started At 6 weeks, the patient had normal range of motion and no pain. (Courtesy of Esser RD, Davis S, Taavao T: Fractures of the radial head treated by internal fixation: Late results in 26 cases. *J Orthop Trauma* 9:318–323, 1995.)

Results.—Excellent results were achieved with Mason type II and III fractures (Fig 1), and good results were obtained with Mason type IV fractures. The results in 2 patients who had Mason type IV fractures were initially rated unsatisfactory. Delayed excision of the radial head improved in 1 patient. In the other patient, pain, but not motion, was improved.

Conclusion.—Open reduction and internal fixation of comminuted radial head fractures gave good to excellent results in most patients. The procedure improves range of motion, strength, and function and should be considered as an alternative to excision of the radial head.

▶ This long-term, retrospective study of displaced radial head fractures documents that excellent results can be expected, even if the radial head is comminuted. The Mason classification system is reviewed, and the surgical technique and results are analyzed for each type of radial head fracture. The specific instrumentation depends on the findings at arthrotomy. The authors used AO screws, mini AO plates and Herbert screws. I have found that the cannulated Herbert-Whipple screw is also quite useful. The benefits of internal fixation of these displaced fractures are numerous and should be considered before excising a fractured radial head.

W. Engberger, M.D.

Radial Head and Neck Fractures: Anatomic Guidelines for Proper Placement of Internal Fixation

Smith GR, Hotchkiss RN (Hosp for Special Surgery, New York)
J Shoulder Elbow Surg 5:113–117, 1996
9–3

Purpose.—Many studies recommend open reduction and internal fixation to preserve radiocapitellar contact in patients with displaced fractures of the radial head and neck. The internal fixation devices must be placed so that they will not protrude onto the bony surface and thus interfere with full forearm rotation. A cadaver study was performed to determine the safe limits for internal fixation devices on the surface of the radial head or neck.

Methods and "Safe Zone" Identification.—Cross-sectional dissections were performed in 6 cadaver elbows to identify a 110-degree "safe zone" of radial head surface. When viewed from a standard lateral approach, the zone was reliably confirmed relative to forearm position. The proximal radioulnar joint could not be directly visualized through the standard

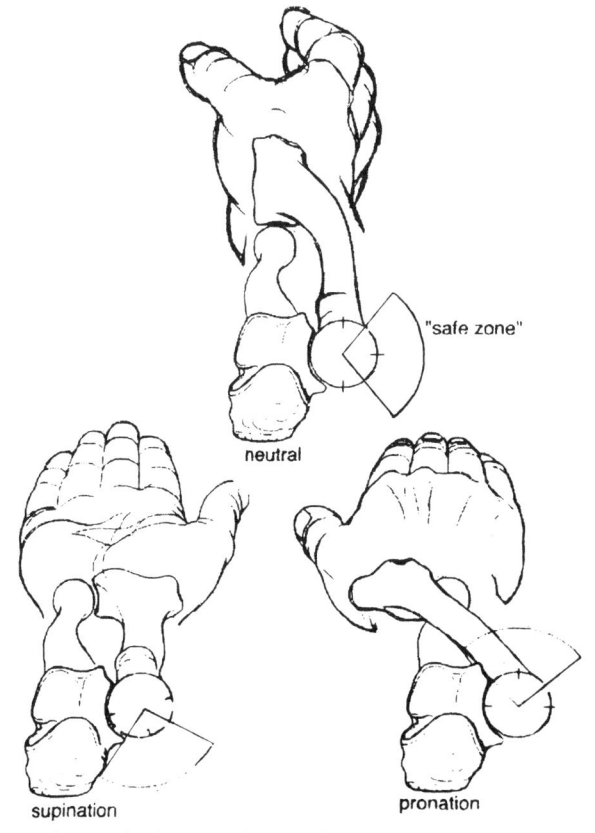

FIGURE 2.—"Safe zone" for placement of internal fixation as seen with forearm in neutral, supinated, and pronated positions. (Courtesy of Smith GR, Hotchkiss RN: Radial head and neck fractures: Anatomic guidelines for proper placement of internal fixation. *J Shoulder Elbow Surg* 5:113–117, 1996.)

lateral approach. An indirect method of identifying the zone, with the use of reference marks along the radial head and neck, was therefore devised.

Technique.—The safe zone is identified by making reference marks along the radial head and neck at a location that bisects the bone's anteroposterior distance. One mark is made with the forearm in neutral rotation, another in full supination, and a third in full pronation (Fig 2). The reference marks made with the forearm in neutral rotation and full pronation are bisected to identify the posterior limit of the safe zone. A mark made about two thirds of the distance from the mark made in neutral position to that made in full supination defines the anterior limit of the zone.

Conclusions.—This simple technique permits the surgeon to identify the safe zone for placement of internal fixation devices when operating on radial head and neck fractures. The safe zone comprises nearly one third of the circumference of the radial head.

▶ How often have we all wondered exactly what the limit is for safe placement of a screw in the radial head. When fixing radial head fractures, it is imperative to prevent placement of internal fixation such as screws and plates in the portion of the radial head that articulates with the ulna. Smith and Hotchkiss have devised a practical method for intraoperative determination of the "safe zone" for placement of such hardware. The safe zone subtends an angle of approximately 110 degrees, or about a third of the circumference of the radial head. The way to determine this is to place the forearm in neutral rotation between pronation and supination. The radial head or neck are marked laterally at the anteroposterior midpoint. The safe zone then extends 65 degrees anteriorly and 45 degrees posteriorly to this point. An easy rule of thumb for intraoperative planning is that a 90-degree angle (a quarter of the head) centered on this lateral mark plus an extra 2 to 3 mm anteriorly represents the safe zone. Understanding and adhering to these recommendations will make surgery not only safer but also easier. One caveat is that we need to recognize the possibility of penetrating the articular surface on the other side with the screws if they are too long.

S.W. O'Driscoll, M.D.

Outerbridge-Kashiwagi's Method for Arthroplasty of Osteoarthritis of the Elbow—44 Elbows Followed for 8–16 Years
Minami M, Kato S, Kashiwagi D (Hokkaido Orthopedic Mem Hosp, Japan)
J Orthop Sci 1:11–15, 1996   9–4

Objective.—The Outerbridge-Kashiwagi method (OKM) of arthroplasty for osteoarthritis of the elbow has proved very effective in restoring range of motion and reducing pain. Since 1976 OKM has been used for patients with early primary osteoarthritis of the elbow at the study institution. Long-term results in 44 elbows were evaluated.

Methods.—The analysis included 44 elbows of 44 patients followed up for more than 8 years after OKM for early-stage osteoarthritis of the elbow. There were 41 men and 3 women, average age 49 years; 39 of the patients were manual laborers. All patients had pain, with a mean limitation of 38 degrees in extension and 111 degrees in flexion. Mean follow-up was 11 years. In the OKM procedure, the olecranon and coronoid fossae were opened and all osteophytes were removed with a chisel.

Results.—At follow-up, 7 patients had no pain and 20 had only moderate pain. Pain was moderate in 9 patients and severe in 8. The patients had an average 6-degree improvement in elbow extension and an 11-degree improvement in elbow flexion. By 10 years after OKM, most patients showed radiographic evidence of progressive osteoarthritis. There were no problems with infection or ulnar nerve palsy, although 4 patients had cubital tunnel syndrome, which was treated by anterior nerve translocation.

Conclusions.—For patients with primary osteoarthritis of the elbow, OKM appears to be a simple, palliative arthroplasty technique. Pain is reduced and elbow motion improved in most patients. However, the osteoarthritic changes appear to progress in the years after surgery.

▶ This is a valuable addition to the orthopedic literature because it provides an additional emphasis on the entity and treatment of primary degenerative arthritis of the elbow. Specifically this communiqué yields worthwhile information with regard to characteristics of presentation, and equally, if not more importantly, the anticipation of long-term success of surgical intervention. It is worthwhile to note that in this sample of patients most complained of pain throughout the arc of motion (70%) and only 15% noted terminal discomfort as the major complaint. This is somewhat different from our indication for surgery in which we place particular emphasis on terminal pain and are hopeful that the arc of motion will be relatively pain-free. It should also be noted that approximately 15% did have ulnar nerve irritation at the time of presentation and an additional 10% had ulnar nerve symptoms over the next 10 years. It is also worthwhile to note that about 25% of patients had radial head involvement and over the 10-year period approximately 10% required radial head excision.

The technique of the procedure as described is somewhat different from that which we have used. Concern with regard to the use of the trephine is expressed referable to supracondylar fracture. The authors recommend removal of the osteophytes from the distal humerus with an osteotome. It would seem as though this has the possibility of creating stress risers, which may well allow potential weakening of the bone, rendering it more likely to fracture than the smooth contour provided by the trephine. We have performed approximately 50 such procedures without such fracture. By carefully defining the margins of the medial and lateral column, this complication should be minimized, yet it is worth keeping in mind. It is interesting that they do not use continuous passive motion (CPM), which we do employ, although I cannot demonstrate with scientific data that CPM treatment is of value. It is also of interest to note that these authors recommend resting the patient for 7–10 days, whereas we recommend immediate motion.

With regard to the long-term results, it is particularly curious to note that these authors demonstrate an increasing arc of motion over a 10-year period. This has certainly not been our experience. Because of the ongoing underlying degenerative changes, we have observed that the range of motion is constant for about 5 years and then begins to deteriorate.

In summary, this is a valuable contribution to our understanding. Possibly of greatest value is that this information allows us to advise our patients that approximately 50% will still be considered as satisfactory 10 years after surgery. Further, after the initial decompression procedure, progression of the disease process may involve the ulnar nerve and radial head requiring secondary intervention for both these conditions.

B.F. Morrey, M.D.

Salvage of Failed Total Elbow Arthroplasty
Ferlic DC, Clayton ML (Univ of Colorado, Denver)
J Shoulder Elbow Surg 4:290–297, 1995

9–5

Objective.—Revision of a failed total elbow arthroplasty is difficult. The salvage of 14 cases of failed total elbow arthroplasty in 12 patients was described.

Treatment and Outcome.—Three prostheses were infected. All were free of infection after the prostheses was removed and antibiotic therapy was initiated. Two elbows, however, were left unstable with poor function. Because of pain and a stiff elbow, the third patient underwent fascial arthroplasty with good results and relief of pain. Two elbows had loosening of both components and were reimplanted with Morrey-Coonrad elbows; both had good ratings. Two patients had loosening of their ulnar components; 1 underwent insertion of a Morrey-Coonrad elbow with fair results because of moderate pain, and the other was treated with a custom-made, longer, ulnar device with good results and no pain. Of the 4 elbows removed for chronic dislocation, 3 were converted to Morrey-Coonrad elbows and 1 was changed to a Triaxial elbow with a new bearing mechanism; all had good results.

Recommendations.—Revision of a failed elbow implant can be difficult. In the presence of infection, the prosthesis and all bone cement have to be removed. If failure is caused by aseptic loosening, reinsertion of new components is usually successful, although a custom prosthesis may be necessary in the presence of considerable ulnar bone erosion. Bone grafting around a prostheses or use of a humeral allograft may be considered in the presence of loosening and extensive bone destruction, although a Morrey-Coonrad prosthesis may also provide sufficient stability. Insertion of a semiconstrained prosthesis is reliable in nonconstrained elbows that fail because of dislocation.

▶ Salvage of a failed total elbow prosthesis is a special orthopedic challenge. For elbows salvaged for infection, all necrotic bone and infected tissue must be removed for success, especially if a later elbow reconstruction is being considered.[1,2] For those with aseptic loosening or instability, conversion to a semiconstrained Morrey-Coonrad elbow has been the prosthesis of choice for revision when both components are taken out. At times, bearing failure in a prosthesis design just requires replacement of the bearing, but this also gives the physician a chance to ensure that there is no malalignment that would increase the chance for failure. The elbows salvaged with removal of the prosthetic components alone may be satisfactory in terms of eradicating the infection but function poorly for motion, stability, and strength.

T. Norris, M.D.

References

1. Morrey BF, Bryan RS: Infection after total elbow arthroplasty. *J Bone Joint Surg (Am)* 65A:330–338, 1983.
2. Morrey BF, Bryan RS: Revision total elbow arthroplasty. *J Bone Joint Surg (Am)* 69A:523–532, 1987.

Short-term Complications of the Lateral Approach for Non-constrained Elbow Replacement: Follow-up of 50 Rheumatoid Elbows
Ljung P, Jonsson K, Rydholm U (Univ Hosp, Lund, Sweden)
J Bone Joint Surg (Br) 77–B:937–942, 1995

Introduction.—High complication rates have been reported with total elbow replacements in which nonconstrained and semiconstrained prostheses were used. The surgical approach used in elbow replacement is thought to be an important factor in the complication rate; the lateral approach results in fewer complications. Complications and outcomes after total elbow replacement, in which a lateral approach was used, were assessed prospectively.

Methods.—Forty-two patients underwent 50 total elbow replacements performed by a lateral approach using a capitellocondylar elbow prosthesis. Rheumatoid arthritis was present in 38 patients, and juvenile chronic arthritis was present in 4. Median follow-up was 3 years (range 2–5 years). Patients were evaluated for elbow pain, range of motion, joint stability and tenderness, swelling, and ulnar-nerve function. Radiographs obtained before and after surgery were assessed for any changes in the prosthesis.

Results.—Major complications occurred in 2 replacements. A deep hematogenous infection developed in 1 patient 12 months after surgery; the prosthesis was removed, and a resection arthroplasty was done. A second patient dislocated the prosthesis after a fall; external fixation of the lateral collateral ligament was eventually required. Early mobilization resulted in wound-healing complications in 2 elbows. Ulnar-nerve palsy occurred in 14 elbows and was permanent in 3. Lateral translocation of the ulnar component was found in 1 elbow. Reductions in visual analogue scores for pain were found at follow-up for all patients, from 7 to 0 for pain on motion and from 2 to 0 for pain at rest. Improvements in the range of flexion-extension were found in 43 elbows, with worsening in 4 and no change in 3. Before surgery, 25 elbows were considered stable or slightly unstable, and 25 were considered unstable. After elbow replacement, 49 elbows were stable or slightly unstable. Radiographs found suspected loosening of the humeral component in 1 elbow. Eight reoperations were performed; 4 for ulnar-nerve decompression, 3 for secondary wound suture, 2 for reconstruction of the lateral collateral ligament, and 1 for removal of the elbow prosthesis.

Conclusion.—Nineteen complications were reported in this series of patients with nonconstrained total elbow replacements. Most complications were minor; 14 were ulnar-nerve palsy. Outcome of elbow replacement was satisfactory for most patients in terms of pain relief, range of motion, and joint stability.

▶ The 3 noteworthy issues presented in this article include the use of an unconstrained Ewald prosthesis for rheumatoid arthritis, the lateral approach, and a complication rate approaching 40%. Neither Ewald nor Coonrad and Morrey, who used their semiconstrained elbow with the triceps-splitting approach, reported such a high complication rate.[1]

Seven of the 8 reoperations might have been avoided with the semiconstrained elbow and the posterior approach. Routine anterior transposition of the ulnar nerve should avoid the 3 permanent ulnar neuropathies. Elbow arthroplasty does not need to have this high complication rate.

T. Norris, M.D.

Reference

1. Coonrad RW, Morrey BF: Coonrad/Morrey total elbow: Surgical technique. Warsaw, Ind, Zimmer, 1989.

Fixation Strength of the Ulnar Component of Total Elbow Replacement
Zafiropoulos G, Amis AA (Derbyshire Royal Infirmary, London; Imperial College of Science, London)
J Shoulder Elbow Surg 5:97–102, 1996

Purpose.—A clinical review of 42 primary Souter-Strathclyde total elbow arthroplasties revealed 2 ulnar component fixation failures (5%) by olecranon fracture. Whether changes in the ulnar component's design or material would increase its fixation failure strength was determined.

Methods.—The normal ulnas from 15 fresh cadavers aged 55–85 years at the time of death were studied. None of the patients had had rheumatoid arthritis or had taken steroids. The articular areas of the 30 bones were replaced with 4 types of ulnar component, including a standard square component similar to that of the Souter-Strathclyde prosthesis, a long-stem component, a round-body polyethylene component, and a round-body metal-type component. All components were fixed into the bone with polymethylmethacrylate bone cement and tested to failure. Loads were applied in an anterior-posterior direction, causing bending fractures of the olecranon.

Results.—The long-stem ulnar component tended to be weaker than the standard square type, the round-body polyethylene design tended to be stronger than the standard square polyethylene type, and the round-body metal-backed component tended to be stronger than the round-body polyethylene type.

Recommendations.—The ulnar component of the elbow joint prosthesis used in total elbow arthroplasty should have a round body design with a small stem because it requires less bone excavation than a long stem. Because the difference in fixation strength between steel and polyethylene round-bodied components was not statistically significant, it is suggested to continue making the ulnar component in polyethylene because it is less costly than using a metal-backed design.

▶ This simple study provided some design considerations for improving mechanical fixation of the ulnar component of the total elbow replacement. The findings agreed well with the basic engineering principles of cantilever bending and stress concentration.

One comment made in the discussion related to the loading mode of the elbow is important and should be kept in mind when conducting such experiments of evaluating the fixation strength of implant and fracture. That is, the force across the elbow joint could be generated by the forces of either the flexor or the extensor. Stress on the olecranon and thus the failure mechanism under the action of the flexor would be significantly different from those caused by the extensor. For a complete assessment of mechanical performance of devices, both modes of loading should be considered.

K-N. An, Ph.D.

Neuroanatomy in Elbow Arthroscopy
Miller CD, Jobe CM, Wright MH (355th Med Group/SGHSB, Tucson, Ariz; Loma Linda Univ, Calif; Rush-Presbyterian St Luke's Med Ctr, Chicago)
J Shoulder Elbow Surg 4:168–174, 1995 9–8

Background.—Arthroscopic procedures of the elbow carry great potential for neurovascular injury, although most reported nerve problems have been transient and related to local anesthesia. The neuroanatomy of the elbow should be known before performing elbow arthroscopy, yet relatively few reports have addressed this topic. The neuroanatomy of the elbow during arthroscopy was studied, with an emphasis on the effects of joint insufflation and elbow position on the median, radial, and ulnar nerves. In addition, a median nerve injury that occurred from within the joint during arthroscopic synovectomy was described.

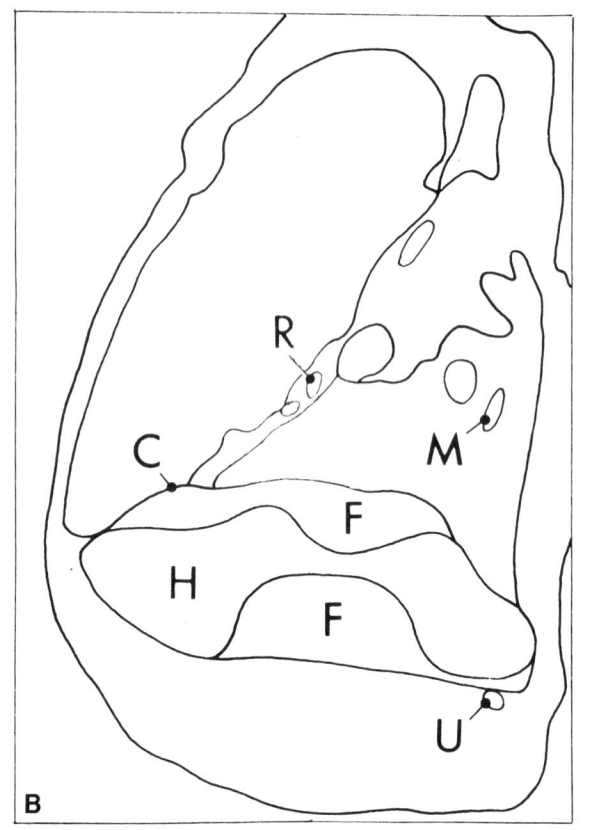

FIGURE 2.—B, explanatory diagram of a noninsufflated flexed elbow. *Abbreviations: F*, fat; *H*, bone; *R*, radial nerve; *M*, median nerve; *U*, ulnar nerve; *C*, capsule. (Courtesy of Miller CD, Jobe CM, Wright MH: Neuroanatomy in elbow arthroscopy. *J Shoulder Elbow Surg* 4:168–174, 1995.)

Methods.—Experiments were performed in 6 pairs of cadaver elbows frozen in 90 degrees of flexion and 1 pair frozen in extension. One joint in each pair was insufflated with saline solution, and each joint was sectioned at 5-mm intervals. The insufflated and control elbows in each pair were analyzed to compare differences in the capsule-to-nerve and bone-to-nerve distances for the median, radial, and ulnar nerves.

Results.—In the flexed elbows, saline insufflation increased the nerve-to-bone distance by 12 mm for the median nerve and 6 mm for the radial nerve. In contrast, insufflation had little effect on the capsule-to-nerve distance, which in some cases was as narrow as 6 mm (Figs 2 and 3). With the elbow in extension, the nerves moved closer to the bone, thereby offsetting the protective effects of insufflation.

Conclusions.—In elbow arthroscopy, elbow flexion and preinsufflation appear to be important in portal placement. In the flexed elbow, insufflation can significantly increase nerve-to-bone distances, although it has little effect on capsule-to-nerve distances. If capsular penetration or exci-

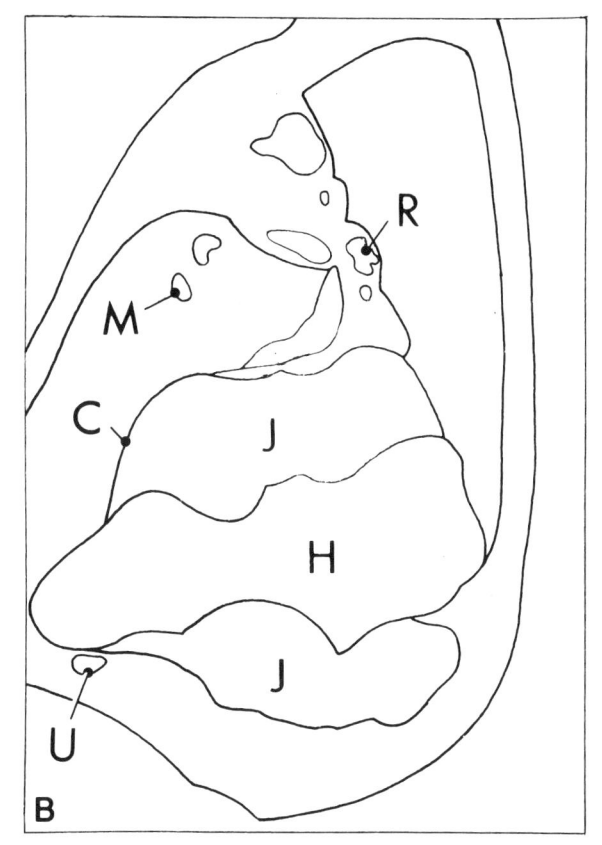

FIGURE 3.—**B**, explanatory diagram of an insufflated flexed elbow. Note that only fat exists between capsule and radial nerve and radial recurrent artery. *Abbreviations: J,* joint; *H,* bone; *R,* radial nerve; *M,* median nerve; *U,* ulnar nerve; *C,* capsule. (Courtesy of Miller CD, Jobe CM, Wright MH: Neuroanatomy in elbow arthroscopy. *J Shoulder Elbow Surg* 4:168–174, 1995.)

sion occurs during an arthroscopic procedure in the elbow, the surgeon is advised to consider converting the procedure to an open one.

▶ This excellent article addresses a very important issue: the neurovascular anatomy of the elbow and its relationship to the capsule and the underlying joint with respect to elbow arthroscopy. The senior author candidly refers to a patient of his who sustained a median nerve laceration during synovectomy for rheumatoid arthritis. This prompted the authors to study the relationship between the nerves and the capsule as well as the underlying joint. Previous studies have documented the relationship between the nerves and arthroscopic portals and instruments inserted into the elbow, but no specific relationship between the nerve and the capsule had been addressed. The authors found, as others have, that the nerves are indeed very close to the joint and can be displaced further away from the joint by distending the capsule with fluid and keeping the elbow flexed to 90 degrees. They also confirm that the radial nerve is, in fact, the closest and most likely to be injured. An important contribution is that they found that the radial nerve is within approximately 6 mm of the capsule, which puts this nerve at particular risk during capsular procedures, such as capsulectomy or synovectomy.

As with any study, there are some limitations. Their data were collected by distending the capsule at cadaver elbows and freezing them, then cutting them with a carpenter's plane at 5-mm intervals. Because these were taken perpendicular of the humerus, in reality the distance between the nerve and the capsule was at times an oblique distance rather than a perpendicular distance. Therefore, the distance between the nerve and the capsule might even be less than what they have documented. This issue emphasizes the importance of respecting the risk of nerve injuries during arthroscopic procedures, especially in any excision of soft tissues in the anterior elbow, such as capsulectomy, capsulorrhaphy (capsular release), or synovectomy. The authors also indicate that capsular contractures might decrease the ability to displace the nerves away from the elbow. In fact, we have previously documented in the arthroscopy literature that the average intercapsular volume of the elbow is reduced from an average of 23 mL for normal elbows to 6 mL for stiff elbows. Thus, it is difficult to displace the nerves away from the arthroscopic instruments and portals during arthroscopy on a stiff elbow. I am not sure that I would agree with their recommendation that arthroscopy should be aborted if capsular penetration occurs but would confirm that this is an important event to recognize and respect.

Finally, the safety and efficacy of arthroscopic capsular release remains to be determined. It is being investigated by experienced arthroscopists, but at least 1 such skilled arthroscopist has reported a permanent radial nerve injury from laceration caused by an arthroscopic capsular release. We consider arthroscopic capsular release an investigational procedure until such time as its safety has been established. It should be performed only by surgeons highly experienced in arthroscopic techniques and elbow surgery.

S.W. O'Driscoll, M.D.

Suggested Reading

Gschwend N, Simmen BR, Matejovsky Z: Late complications in elbow arthroplasty. *J Shoulder Elbow Surg* 5:86–96, 1995.
▶ The authors reviewed the major complications that occur after elbow joint replacement described in the literature in the past 10 years and contrasted this with their personal experience of almost 20 years. It seems that the major goal of this report was to highlight the authors' personal experience as superior to that reported in the literature. The value of the world's literature review is somewhat limited in that both constrained and semi-constrained devices are included and mixed. The overall complication rate of these reports is 43%, which is significantly greater than that of more recent documentation and thus does not reflect current experiences with the implants. The authors do show a distinction in their experience between a complication rate of approximately 11% in patients who have rheumatoid arthritis compared to 34% in patients who have post-traumatic arthrosis. Their reoperation rate was 8% and 31%, respectively.

Overall, although I do not consider the review of the literature to accurately reflect the current experience of most centers, the authors do appropriately highlight the major categories of problems, including ulnar neuropathy, infection, instability, and loosening. Table 5 is of some value; it contrasts the results of the collected literature with all types of designs and diagnoses with the results of their own experience in patients who have rheumatoid arthritis with those who have post-traumatic arthrosis. The authors' ultimate conclusion is that an elbow joint replacement, performed by experienced surgeons with a proven and reliable implant should be considered a successful surgical procedure with a high degree of reliability. I completely agree with this assessment.

B.F. Morrey, M.D.

Ljung P, Jonsson K, Larsson K, et al: Interposition arthroplasty of the elbow with rheumatoid arthritis. *J Shoulder Elbow Surg* 4:81–85, 1996.
▶ Relatively little is known regarding the current expectations of interposition procedures for various elbow conditions, and there has been no recent discussion regarding the use of interposition arthroplasty for rheumatoid arthritis. The experience of Ljung et al., therefore, provides a valuable benchmark not only for the procedure itself but also against which other intervention options might be considered. The sample size of 35 elbows with a median of 6 years surveillance is reasonable. The interventions took place up to 10 years ago, the first being in 1985. Thus, the technique may have changed somewhat over the past decade. Nonetheless the findings continue to be generally similar to those that have been previously reported. This includes residual problems with joint motion and stability but somewhat variable relief of pain. The complication rate of 20% is significant but is, nonetheless, considerably less than that reported in early experiences with total elbow arthroplasty. The complication rate is moderately higher than that of current experiences with prosthetic replacement for this patient population. One might also consider that approximately 50% of the patients had moderate or severe instability as a significant finding that might be considered a complication in some instances. It is of particular interest to note that almost 50% of the elbows also demonstrated progressive radiographic destruction occurring approximately twice as frequently on the humeral as on the ulnar side of the joint. As might be anticipated, one must question the viability of this procedure for rheumatoid arthritis based on the current success with joint replacement. These authors correctly identify that the results are not as predictable or as acceptable as those of total elbow replacement. They correctly recognize and recommend elbow prosthetic replacement as the treatment of choice for rheumatoid involvement of the elbow joint.

B.F. Morrey, M.D.

Partio EK, Hirvensalo E, Böstman O, et al: A prospective controlled trial of the fracture of the humeral medial epicondyle—How to treat? *Ann Chir Gyn* 85:67–71, 1996.
▶ This experience covers a relatively large sample, with treatment occurring over 6 years. It is difficult to draw too many conclusions because of the spectrum of injuries and associated injuries and the various treatment options. It appears that the most important conclusion that might be drawn was emphasized by the authors: it is possible to treat medial epicondylar fractures with absorbable implants, thus obviating the need for later removal. Instability in the presence of a resected medial epicondyle is to be expected and has been previously documented.

B.F. Morrey, M.D.

10 Neuromuscular Disorders

Tendon Transfers and Functional Electrical Stimulation for Restoration of Hand Function in Spinal Cord Injury
Keith MW, Kilgore KL, Peckham PH, et al (Case Western Reserve Univ, Cleveland, Ohio; MetroHealth Med Ctr, Cleveland, Ohio)
J Hand Surg (Am) 21A:89–99, 1996   10–1

Background.—Cervical spinal cord injury can result in the loss of hand-arm function. Electric stimulation may restore function in paralyzed muscles. Key muscles may have lower motor neuron (LMN) damage, however, which limits the effectiveness of this technique. Transfer of paralyzed but LMN-intact muscles has been proposed to provide compensatory function in the hand. A technique that uses tendon transfers, with function documented by intraoperative electric stimulation, to substitute for muscle groups with substantial LMN damage was assessed.

Methods.—Eleven patients who had traumatic cervical spinal cord injury were included. The muscle groups used for transfer were not the primary actuators of major function. The palmaris longus, the flexor carpi ulnaris, the extensor carpi ulnaris, and the brachioradialis muscle groups were typically used. The function of the transferred muscle was determined by observing the response to electric stimulation after transfer, which allowed the modeling of the amplitude, power, and line-of-force application. Each patient required several surgical procedures to provide individual augmentation of the remaining voluntary muscle function. Procedures performed included tendon transfers, side-to-side synchronization of tendons, Zancolli-lasso procedures, and arthrodesis of the thumb interphalangeal joint. The results were assessed by comparing the pre- and postoperative grades of the muscles, external transduction of muscle forces, and the joint angles obtained with electric stimulation of transferred muscles.

Results.—Forty-one procedures were performed; 38 resulted in the desired functional improvement. Tendon transfers to provide digital extension were most common and resulted in a gain of more than 1 muscle grade in 4 patients, a loss of at least 1 grade in 2, and no change in 2. Other procedures were successfully performed to provide wrist extension and finger flexion. All procedures to provide side-to-side tendon synchronization and all arthrodeses of the thumb interphalangeal joint were successful. The Zancolli-lasso procedure achieved the desired results in 2 of 3 patients.

Conclusions.—Combining tendon transfers and functional electric stimulation enhances the reconstruction of hand function in patients who have severe disabilities associated with cervical spinal cord injury and results in significant functional improvement. The use of intraoperative electric stimulation also allows the assessment of balance between the fingers during a synchronization procedure and intraoperative evaluation of the Zancolli-lasso procedure.

▶ Functional electric stimulation (FES) of certain paralyzed muscles with intact lower motor neurons can provide "another motor" for a tendon transfer in tetraplegic patients who have few muscles available. The extensor carpi ulnaris and flexor carpi ulnaris seem particularly well suited. The combination of FES with established tendon transfer techniques has simplified the application of the neuroprosthesis approach in these individuals. Improving synchronization of the fingers through cross-union of the extrinsic flexor and extensor tendons has also been useful. It is disappointing that only 2 of 8 patients obtained grade IV strength with FES and tendon transfer and that 2 patients actually lost strength after surgery. The lack of fine selective muscle control and the absence of sensory feedback certainly compromise the potential functional benefits of this technology. Concentrating on restoring wrist control and key pinch is appropriate for most patients who retain less than OCu:2 function. Although these authors continue to refine the techniques for restoration of finger control by FES, this method remains an investigational technique that requires further study at established spinal cord centers before widespread use is appropriate.

J. House, M.D.

Quantitative Comparison of Grasp and Release Abilities With and Without Functional Neuromuscular Stimulation in Adolescents With Tetraplegia

Smith BT, Mulcahey MJ, Betz RR (Shriners Hosp for Crippled Children, Philadelphia)
Paraplegia 34:16–23, 1996

10–2

Background.—A small but effective workspace can be achieved with residual arm movements in patients with midcervical level spinal cord injury (SCI). However, when active finger and thumb motion is lost, hand function must be achieved through passive grasp and release abilities or tenodesis, compensatory hand skills developed through therapy, and adaptive equipment—and manipulating objects is still often difficult or impossible. A functional neuromuscular stimulation (FNS) hand system was designed and implemented at Case Western Reserve University (CWRU).

Methods.—Five adolescents, 13–19 years old, with C5 tetraplegia were included in the study. Hand function with the FNS system was assessed and compared with tenodesis abilities using a grasp and release test especially designed for this purpose. The unilateral acquisition, movement, and release of 6 objects of varying sizes and weights were tested. In 1 session, 5 30-second trials with each object were done with and without the FNS system. The number of completions and failures were documented for each trial. The patients participated in 4–8 test sessions during 1.5–3 years. Thirty comparisons of test performance with FNS were compared with tenodesis performance and session-to-session consistency.

Findings.—In 77% of the comparisons, FNS was more effective, tenodesis was better in 17% of the comparisons, and the 2 were equal in 6%. The patients could manipulate the 3 heaviest test objects only with FNS. In 60% of the comparisons involving the 3 lighter objects, FNS was associated with significantly more trials including more completions or fewer failures. In general, performance with FNS and tenodesis was inconsistent across sessions.

Conclusions.—All patients' unilateral grasp and release abilities were significantly improved with FNS compared to tenodesis function. Variable FNS test performance from session to session appeared to be related to fluctuations in grasp strength and endurance from muscle conditioning, difficulties attaining adequate stimulated finger extension, and improvements in some patients' ability to use FNS. The variability in tenodesis test performance was mainly attributable to improved manipulation of the lightest test objects.

▶ Functional electric stimulation can be an effective method of increasing the number of muscles brought under voluntary control. The implantation of the CWRU neuroprosthesis can increase the strength of grasp and pinch as well as increase the number of hand activities that can be performed. This paper by an experienced group reviews the initial and only published clinical experience in children. The authors, in a well-designed, experimental series, evaluated the device's capabilities and studied control experiments for tenodesis movements. The utility of a new grasp and release test was evaluated for functional outcomes in tetraplegic hands. An extensive discussion of sources of variability in the data obtained from studying the tetraplegic hand during the evolution of task learning and maturation of tendon transfer surgery is a good model for future work by others. Patients show improvement beyond the training period as familiarity with new muscles allows them new strategies for task completion.

M. Keith, M.D.

Treatment of the Upper Limb in Charcot-Marie-Tooth Disease
Wood VE, Huene D, Nguyen J (Loma Linda Univ, Calif)
J Hand Surg (Br) 20B:511–518, 1995   10–3

Purpose.—Charcot-Marie-Tooth (CMT) disease, which is an inherited, degenerative peripheral neuropathy, is one of the most common neurologic diseases that require treatment. Although many reports that describe this disease and its involvement of the upper limb have appeared, few have discussed its management with tendon transfers and hand surgery. There appear to be several types of CMT disease with extremely variable clinical symptoms. The results of treatment for patients with upper extremity involvement in CMT disease were assessed.

Patients.—Thirty-seven patients who had CMT disease were evaluated by examination or questionnaire. Their average age at diagnosis was 23 years, and the average time until onset of upper limb symptoms after diagnosis was 11 years. Nine patients underwent upper limb surgery, including 3 carpal tunnel operations, 7 for opponensplasty, 10 to increase pinch, and 8 to decrease clawing. In 1 patient who had CMT subluxation and instability, first carpometacarpal arthroplasty and ligament reconstruction were performed. The results of treatment were assessed in terms of decreased nerve conduction velocity, lack of opposition, weak pinch, and clawing.

Findings.—The results were used to devise a plan for tendon transfers in CMT patients who had upper extremity involvement. Ulnar and median nerve involvement tended to progress and became severe in many patients. Radial nerve involvement, however, was uncommon. Carpal tunnel release did not appear helpful. When full-blown CMT was present, the recommended surgical treatment included fusion of the metacarpophalangeal (MP) joint of the thumb, transfer of the extensor pollicis brevis to the

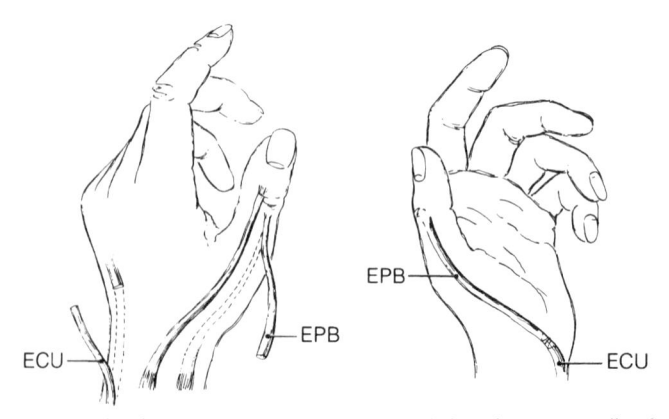

FIGURE 3.—Transfer of the extensor carpi ulnaris (*ECU*) volarly to the extensor pollicis brevis (*EPB*) gives good opposition of the thumb without the careful preparation of a pulley or special insertion. The MP joint of the thumb must be fused before the EPB is used for transfer. (Courtesy of Wood VE, Huene D, Nguyen J: Treatment of the upper limb in Charcot-Marie-Tooth disease. *J Hand Surg (Br)* 20B:511–518, 1995.)

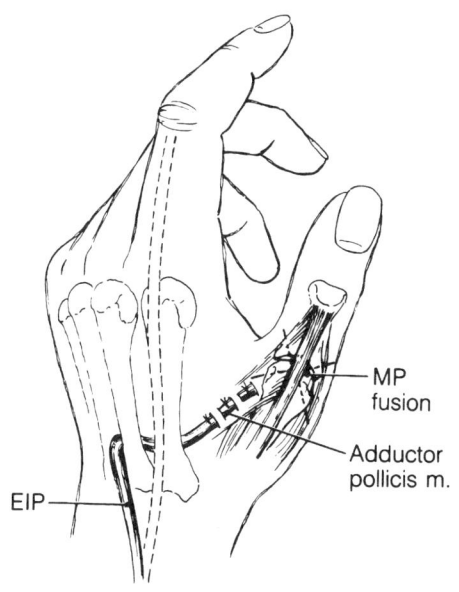

FIGURE 10.—The best procedure to restore side-to-side pinch transfer of extensor indicis around the third metacarpal into adductor pollicis. All patients who underwent this procedure were pleased with the results. *Abbreviations: EIP*, extensor indicis proprius; *MP*, metacarpophalangeal. (Courtesy of Wood VE, Huene D, Nguyen J: Treatment of the upper limb in Charcot-Marie-Tooth disease. *J Hand Surg (Br)* 20B:511–518, 1995.)

extensor carpi ulnaris for opposition (Fig 3), and transfer of the extensor indicis around the third metacarpal into the adductor pollicis for pinch (Fig 10). Transfer of a slip of abductor pollicis longus into the first dorsal interosseous by using a palmaris longus tendon graft offered an alternative procedure for pinch strength. For patients who had severe clawing, the palmaris longus could be extended with palmar fascia and used as a lasso loop procedure around the A1 pulley.

Discussion.—In properly selected patients, tendon transfers can be very helpful in the treatment of CMT disease involving the upper extremity. This surgical approach treats decreased conduction velocity, lack of opposition, weak pinch, and clawing. Many patients, however, will obtain satisfactory results with a procedure designed to increase pinch, such as fusion of the MP joint of the thumb, transfer of the extensor indicis around the third metacarpal into the adductor, and transfer of the extensor pollicis brevis into the first dorsal interosseous.

▶ This article reviews the functional results obtained from a variety of procedures used to restore a functional pinch and intrinsic balance to the hand in CMT disease. The authors provide a good discussion of the relative merits of the various tendon transfers they have used and compare the results. They emphasize that progression of the disease is likely to occur in median and ulnar innervated muscles, which will result in progressive weakness, even if the tendon transfers appear to be successful initially. The use of radial nerve innervated motors and the incorporation of stabilizing procedures, such as metacarpophalangeal fusion of the thumb and finger tenodesis to correct for clawing, are particularly useful. This article emphasizes the need to recognize the progressive nature of the disease and to use simple procedures whenever possible to help maintain function in selected patients.

J. House, M.D.

Sollerman Hand Function Test: A Standardised Method and Its Use in Tetraplegic Patients
Sollerman C, Ejeskär A (Sahlgrenska Univ Hosp, Göteborg, Sweden)
Scand J Plast Reconstr Hand Surg 29:167–176, 1995   10–4

Background.—A standardized test of overall hand function is necessary to evaluate the results of hand surgery. In 1980, a new hand function test was designed, based on the 7 most frequently used hand grips and on performance of activities of daily living. The results of this test in the evaluation of tetraplegic patients were assessed.

Technique.—The 8 most common hand grips (Fig 1) have been classified previously. A grip function test that uses the 7 most common hand grips was developed; deviations from these grips results in a lowered score on this test. The test consists of 20 subtests (Table 3), each composed of a task of daily living to be completed in 1 minute. Each is scored on a scale from 0 to 4.

Study Design.—To examine the validity of the Sollerman hand test, the test results were compared with subjective self-rating of hand function and with a disability rating scale used by Swedish insurance companies in the evaluation of 47 hands from 40 patients. Reproducibility was determined by comparing the scoring of patients by 3 clinicians who used this test. All tetraplegic patients admitted to the neurologic rehabilitation unit at Sahgrenska Hospital for reconstructive upper extremity surgery since 1985 were evaluated preoperatively by the Sollerman hand function test; these results were compared with the internationally adopted classification system.

Results.—A high correlation was observed between Sollerman test results and subjective self-rating and between test results and disability rating by insurance companies. There was a high concordance between different testers who examined the same patient with the hand function test. From 1985 to 1994, 73 arms in 59 patients were examined by the Sollerman test before surgery. There was a highly significantly positive correlation between the international classification system and the mean score on the Sollerman hand function test.

Conclusions.—The Sollerman hand function test is simple, rapid, and reproducible. It is based on activities of daily living performed with the 7 most common hand grips. This test correlates well with patient self-rating,

1. Pulp Pinch

2. Lateral Pinch

3. Tripod Pinch

4. Five-Finger Pinch

5. Diagonal Volar Grip

6. Transverse Volar Grip

7. Spherical Volar Grip

8. Extension Grip

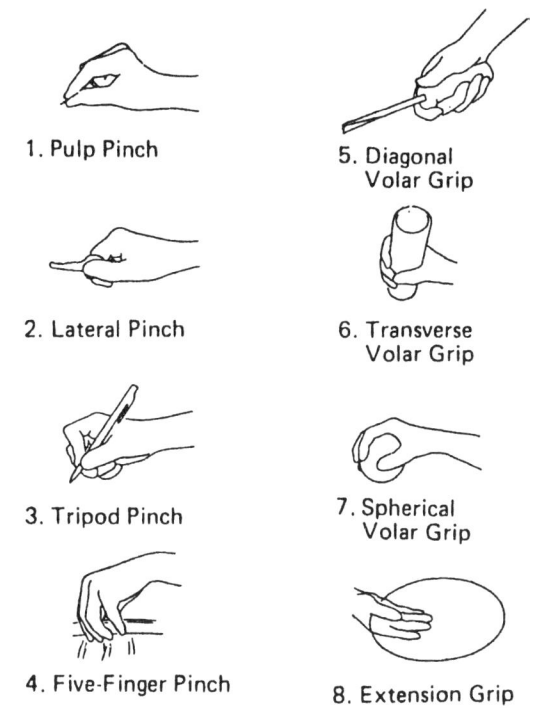

FIGURE 1.—Eight main hand grips into which a normal grip pattern can be divided: **1**, pulp pinch. The object is held between the thumb and the index or the middle finger, or both. **2**, lateral pinch. The object is held between the thumb and the radial side of the index finger. **3**, tripod pinch. The object is surrounded by the thumb, index, and middle finger. It may (but need not to have) contact with the web of the thumb. **4**, 5-finger pinch. The object is held between the thumb and the 4 fingers together. It has no contact with the palm. **5**, diagonal volar grip. The object is held with the thumb against the 4 fingers. It has contact with the palm, and its axis is diagonal to that of the hand. **6**, transverse volar grip. Same as 5, but the axis of the object is transverse to that of the hand. **7**, spherical volar grip. The object is surrounded by the thumb and the 4 fingers and has contact with the palm. **8**, extension grip. The object is held between the thumb and the 4 fingers, which are extended in the interphalangeal joints. It has no contact with the palm. (Courtesy of Sollerman C, Ejeskär A: Sollerman hand function test: A standardised method and its use in tetraplegic patients. *Scand J Plast Reconstr Surg* 29:167–176, 1995.)

TABLE 3.—The 20 Subtests That Compose the Sollerman Grip Function Test

1. Put key into Yale lock, turn 90 degrees
2. Pick coins up from flat surface, put into purses mounted on wall
3. Open/close zip
4. Pick up coins from purses
5. Lift wooden cubes over edge 5 cm in height
6. Lift iron over edge 5 cm in height
7. Turn screw with screwdriver
8. Pick up nuts
9. Unscrew lid of jars
10. Do up buttons
11. Cut Play-Doh with knife and fork
12. Put on Tubigrip stocking on the other hand
13. Write with pen
14. Fold paper, put into envelope
15. Put paper-clip on envelope
16. Lift telephone receiver, put to ear
17. Turn door-handle 30 degrees
18. Pour water from Pure-pak
19. Pour water from jug
20. Pour water from cup

(Courtesy of Sollerman C, Ejeskär A: Sollerman hand function test: A standardised method and its use in tetraplegic patients. *Scand J Plast Reconstr Surg* 29:167–176, 1995.)

the disability rating scale used by insurance companies, and the international arm classification scale in tetraplegic patients. This test appears to be the best overall hand function test available for these patients.

▶ A truly objective, reliable, and, more important, useful, measurement of hand function has been an elusive goal. Many formats have been proposed, usually directed at one diagnostic subset or another, e.g., rheumatoid arthritis. Most were designed by physiatrists or physical or occupational therapists. Sollerman is an orthopedic and hand surgeon from Göteborg, Sweden, who follows in the very large footsteps of Erik Moberg and Svante Edshage. The second author, Ejeskär, has done much to promote the Sollerman test, especially as a uniform system for assessing the functional outcome of reconstructive surgery in tetraplegic patients. The test has not been well represented in the literature because it was published as Sollerman's thesis. This article corrects this lack of availability of information and examines the application of the methodology in a series of tetraplegic patients. One criticism is that even though a test can be completed within the prescribed time, the patients scores are lowered if they use a grip that is different than that prescribed to accomplish the task.

V.R. Hentz, M.D.

Phasic Relationships of the Intrinsic and Extrinsic Thumb Musculature
Johanson ME, Skinner SR, Lamoreux LW (Shriners Hosp for Crippled Children, San Francisco)
Clin Orthop 322:120–130, 1996   10–5

Background.—Dynamic electromyography is useful in the assessment of patients who have spastic disorders and are being considered for tendon transfer or lengthening surgery. The normal phasic activity of the thumb muscles was determined during simple, reproducible activities.

Methods.—Five adults who had normal thumb musculature were included. Fine-wire electrode pairs were inserted into the extensors pollicis longus and brevis, abductus pollicis longus and brevis, flexors pollicis longus and brevis, opponens pollicis, adductor pollicis, and first dorsal interosseous. Electrogoniometers were used to record the motions of the carpometacarpal joint and interphalangeal joint of the thumb (Fig 1).

Findings.—Thumb motion during simple hand opening without resistance appeared to be accomplished mainly by extensors pollicis longus and brevis and abductor pollicis lungus. Thumb motion during hand closing seemed to be done through phasic contractions of flexors pollicis longus and brevis, adductor pollicis, and first dorsal interosseous. Pinching without force also involved phasic contraction of flexors pollicis longus, adductor pollicis, and the first dorsal interosseous muscle. In general, muscles that were silent without force became active when force was generated in pinching.

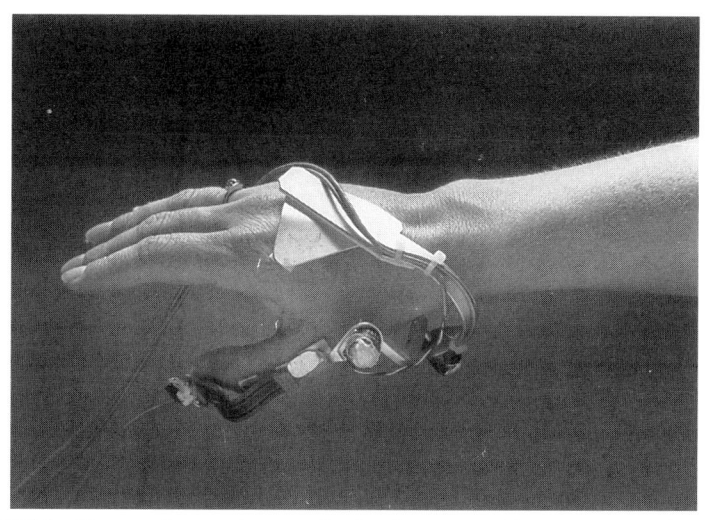

FIGURE 1.—Electrogoniometers for measuring thumb movement. The carpometacarpal joint is approximated by 2 revolute axes. Interphalangeal joint movement is measured by a strain-gauge electrogoniometer. (Courtesy of Johanson ME, Skinner SR, Lamoreux LW: Phasic relationships of the intrinsic and extrinsic thumb musculature. *Clin Orthop* 322:120–130, 1996.)

Conclusions.—These findings support the notion of individual motor strategies. Individuals who have normal thumb musculature often select different muscle combinations to achieve a functional goal.

▶ Dynamic electromyography is often useful in assessing function of spastic muscles in the lower extremity, where patterns of movement are common. This study confirms that this method is less useful in the upper extremity, because there are no predictable patterns of muscle firing associated with specific activities. Instead, individuals tend to have their own idiosyncratic way of doing things. This is good for adaptability, of course, but it does not make the surgeon's job any easier!

P.C. Amadio, M.D.

11 Cumulative Trauma Disorders

Classification Systems of Soft Tissue Disorders of the Neck and Upper Limb: Do They Satisfy Methodological Guidelines?
Buchbinder R, Goel V, Bombardier C, et al (Inst for Work and Health, Toronto; Univ of Toronto; Monash Univ, Melbourne, Australia)
J Clin Epidemiol 49:141–149, 1995   11–1

Background.—Soft-tissue disorders of the neck and upper limb are a common problem that carries substantial morbidity and expense. Although many studies have investigated the diagnosis, treatment, and other aspects of these conditions, standard labels, definitions, and diagnostic criteria are lacking. Several different classification systems for soft-tissue disorders of the neck and upper limb have been proposed. These systems were critically appraised according to methodologic criteria.

Methods.—A literature search identified 4 classification systems specifically designed to classify soft-tissue disorders of the neck and upper limb, all concerned mainly with cases arising in occupational settings. Preliminary information was found on a fifth classification system, but it was excluded from the critical appraisal. The appraisal was performed by 3 raters—2 rheumatologists and a family physician—using a standardized form. The main methodologic criteria used in the appraisal were appropriateness for purpose, content validity, face validity, feasibility, construct validity, reliability, and generalizability. Interrater agreement was assessed to establish the reliability of the appraisal form.

Results.—The critical appraisal showed good interrater reliability, with an intraclass correlation coefficient of 0.82. The purposes, intended populations, and settings of the classification systems were clear, and most were easy to understand, had clear criteria for inclusion into categories, and had clear definitions of the criteria. However, none of them included all relevant criteria and distinguished between them adequately. The 1 system that included an axis of severity did not meet criteria for content or face validity. Scientific information to justify inclusion into designated categories was largely lacking, as were data regarding construct validity and reliability. The systems varied in terms of simplicity and degree of diffi-

TABLE 3.—Critical Appraisal of Classification Systems

	Waris et al.	Viikari-Juntura	Silverstein et al.	McCormack et al.	ICD-9	No. disagreements	Score per item
Purpose							
(i) Is the purpose, population, and setting clearly specified?	Yes	Yes	Yes	Yes	N/A	—	4
Content validity							
(i) Is the domain and all specific exclusions from this domain clearly specified?	No*	No*	No*	No	No	3	0
Are all relevant categories included?	No	No	No*	No	No	1	0
(ii) Is the breakdown of categories appropriate, considering the purpose?	No	No	Partially*	No	No	1	0.5
Are the categories mutually exclusive?	No	No*	Yes*	Yes	No	2	2
(iii) Was the method of development appropriate?	No	D/K	D/K	D/K	D/K	—	0
(iv) If multiaxial, are criteria of content validity satisfied for each additional axis?	N/A	N/A	N/A	No*	N/A	1	0
Face validity							
(i) Is the nomenclature used to label the categories satisfactory?	Partially*	No	No	Partially*	No	2	1
Are the terms used based upon empirical (i.e., directly observable) evidence?	Partially*	No*	No*	Partially*	No	4	1
(ii) Are the criteria for determining inclusion into each category clearly specified?	Yes	Yes	Yes	No	No	—	3
If yes, do these criteria appear reasonable?	Partially*	No*	No*	No	D/K	3	0.5
Have the criteria been demonstrated to have validity and/or reliability?	D/K	No*	D/K	D/K	D/K	1	0
(iii) Are the definitions of criteria clearly specified?	Yes	Yes*	Yes	No	No	1	3
(iv) If multiaxial, are criteria of face validity satisfied for each additional axis?	N/A	N/A	N/A	No	N/A	—	0
Feasibility							
(i) Is classification simple to understand?	Yes	Yes	Yes	No*	No	1	3
(ii) Is classification easy to perform?	No	No	Yes	No	No	—	1
(iii) Does it rely on clinical examination alone?	Yes	Yes	Yes	Yes	D/K	—	4
(iv) Are special skills, tools, and/or training required?	Yes	Yes	Yes	Yes	D/K	—	0 (no. "no"s)
(v) How long does it take to perform?	1 hr	D/K	D/K	D/K	D/K	—	0

Chapter 11–Cumulative Trauma Disorders / 257

Construct validity							
(i) Does it discriminate between entities that are thought to be different in a way appropriate for the purpose?	D/K	D/K	D/K	D/K	D/K	—	0
(ii) Does it perform satisfactorily when compared to other classification systems which classify the same domain?	D/K	D/K	D/K	D/K	D/K	—	0
Reliability							
(i) Does the classification system provide consistent results when classifying the same conditions (test-retest)?	D/K	D/K	D/K	D/K	D/K	—	0
(ii) Is the intraobserver and interobserver reliability satisfactory?	D/K	D/K	D/K	D/K	D/K	—	0
Generalizability							
(i) Has it been used in other studies and/or settings?	Yes*	No	D/K	No	Yes	1	2
Overall score (range of scores for the 3 raters)†‡‡	7.5 (5–10)	5 (5–8)	6.5 (6–9)	3 (4–5)	1 (1)		
Overall weighted score§	3.5	1.8	2.3	1.6	1		

* Indicate responses for which there was disagreement between the 3 raters.
† Scores calculated by summing number of "yes" (1 point) and "partially" (0.5 point) responses, except for the item "Are special skills, tools and/or training required?" for which a "no" response = 1 point.
‡ Potential overall score = 21, except for McCormack, et al: potential overall score = 23.
§ Potential overall score = 7, mean score out of 1 for each category.
Abbreviations: N/A, not applicable; D/K, don't know.
(Reprinted by permission of the publisher from Buchbinder R, Goel V, Bombardier C, et al: Classification systems of soft tissue disorders of the neck and upper limb: Do they satisfy methodological guidelines? *J Clin Epidemiol* 49:141–149, 1995. Copyright 1995 by Elsevier Science Inc.)

culty. Although none called for ancillary studies, most required special training skills and several steps (Table 3).

Conclusions.—Existing classification systems for soft-tissue disorders of the neck and upper limb do not appear to meet current standards for face and content validity. There are also problems with feasibility, and the data needed to assess construct validity and reliability are unavailable. The findings question the validity of previous studies using these systems to classify soft tissue disorders of the neck and upper limb into various categories. Either the existing classification systems should be improved, or new ones should be developed to meet basic measurement criteria.

▶ We applaud efforts to bring systematized methods analysis to the study of upper extremity disorders. The proposed framework is a promising step toward understanding the similarities and differences of studies of popular and nebulous diagnostic entities. The effort of Buchbinder, et al. is timely and represents a growing research emphasis. Through these efforts, peer review and accountability will be enhanced. Regarding the classification systems in this study, areas for improvement were readily identified. The failure to meet face and content validity criteria (with concerns about fuzziness of domain and validity of detection criteria) seriously limit the utility of these classification systems. Failure to meet feasibility requirements limits dissemination.

The authors identified major shortcomings of the works under analysis concerning attention to measurement attributes and underlying assumptions of causation that are reflected in diagnostic categories. Their advice to clinicians to employ diagnostic labels based on proof is well taken.

Symptom surveys yield exaggerated population statistics while electrophysiologic measurements of the underlying disease process yield very different rates. Our work regarding carpal tunnel syndrome has taught us that incidence and prevalence rates are sensitively dependent on case definition[1].

P.A. Nathan, M.D.

Reference

1. Nathan PA, Keniston RC: Carpal tunnel syndrome and its relation to general physical condition. *Hand Clinics*; 9:253-261, 1993.

Cumulative Trauma Disorders: How to Assess the Risks
Melhorn JM (Univ of Kansas, Wichita)
J Workers Comp 5:19–33, 1995   11–2

Background.—An estimated 15% to 20% of Americans are at risk for developing cumulative trauma disorders (CTDs); these disorders represent approximately 56% of all occupational injuries. Recent research has suggested that multiple human risk factors, rather than workplace factors, are significant in predicting CTDs. A monitoring assessment program (MAP) was developed to determine individual risk level. The accuracy of the MAP in predicting CTDs was evaluated by examining its reproducibility, internal consistency, validity, and sensitivity to change.

Methods.—The MAP, consisting of a questionnaire, a physical examination, and noninvasive passive testing, was administered repeatedly to 74 persons. Reproducibility was evaluated by analyzing the test–retest agreement in 31 persons; the retest was administered 1 month after the first test. To evaluate internal consistency, individual responses to the same question in multiple monitorings were analyzed in a subgroup of 31 participants. Validity was assessed by comparing the MAP risk level values with a diagnosis of cumulative trauma established by independent physicians. Sensitivity to clinical change was evaluated by comparing serial MAP values in 2 randomly assigned groups: an exercise group and a control group.

Results.—The test–retest correlation coefficient for MAP risk levels was 92.8%. The risk level distribution had a normal, bell-shaped pattern, and these risk levels were highly accurate predictors of the probability of a CTD diagnosis, indicating good reliability. The agreement between actually diagnosed CTD cases and the probability predicted by MAP was accurate with a 95% confidence level, indicating validity. The average initial MAP risk level was 4.75. After 18 months, values were 3.75 in the exercise group and 4.70 in the control group, indicating responsiveness to clinical change.

Conclusions.—The MAP is reproducible, internally consistent, valid, and sensitive to clinical change. It therefore meets all the critical criteria for a risk assessment instrument for CTD.

▶ It has been estimated that 15% to 20% of workers are at risk for developing CTDs. Cumulative trauma disorders can account for 56% of all occupational injuries. A strategy prevention of such work-related diseases and injuries is needed. Human risk factors are unique for each person and are related to age, sex, genetics, workplace, nonwork environment, and length of activity. An index of individual risk levels can be developed by using a questionnaire, a physical examination, and nonevasive passive testing.

This study is an attempt to give employers and health care providers a tool that can help the development of occupational injuries. Under the American Disabilities Act, employment cannot be denied because of an increased risk for the development of cumulative trauma disorders. With this assessment program, however, appropriate placement can be done, and indications can be provided concerning potential disorders. Ergonomic use of the extremities and appropriate training and modification can be provided.

R.L. Horner, M.D.

Computer Mouse Use and Cumulative Trauma Disorders of the Upper Extremities

Fogleman M, Brogmus G (Liberty Mutual Research Ctr for Safety and Health, Hopkinton, Mass)
Ergonomics 38:2465–2475, 1995

Background.—With the growing presence of computers at home and in the workplace, and particularly with the adoption of the graphical user interface, use of the computer mouse and other nonkeyboard input devices is increasing rapidly. Many studies have looked at the effects of keyboard use, but little is known about the possible physical effects of mouse use. Insurance company data were analyzed to determine the contribution of computer mouse use to musculoskeletal disorders of the upper extremity.

Methods.—Insurance claims data on cumulative trauma disorders of the upper extremities (CTDUEs) from 1986 through 1993 were obtained. For each year, the number and costs of claims associated with computer use and mouse use were determined.

Results.—In 1993, mouse-related claims accounted for just 0.04% of all claims and 1.05% of CTDUE claims but 6.1% of computer claims. Mouse involvement in insurance claims rose steadily throughout the period studied. Computer-related, mouse-related, and other CTDUEs were proportionately more frequent among women, probably because of exposure. Compared with other CTDUE claims, mouse-related claims were somewhat more likely to involve strains and less likely to involve carpal tunnel syndrome. The hand, upper arm, and lower arm were more likely to be involved than the wrist.

Conclusions.—Computer mouse-related CTDUEs appear to be a small but growing problem. Further research of these problems and their management may be indicated. Assuming there is a latency period between first use of a mouse and filing an insurance claim, the number of mouse-related claims may increase rapidly over the next few years.

▶ The position of a national hand society is that, "the current medical literature does not provide the information necessary to establish a causal relationship between specific work activities and the development of well-recognized disease entities."[1] In Australia, cumulative trauma disorders have been essentially legislated out of existence with a 1987 supreme court decision. Similarly, in Great Britain, essentially all upper extremity problems except carpal tunnel syndrome related to hand-held vibratory tools have been deemed to have no relationship to work. In the United States, chronic "work-related" hand and upper extremity disorders have stimulated contentious medicolegal debates. Data continue to accumulate, suggesting that the increased exposure of computer use is associated with an increase in CTDUEs. This study suggests that prolonged use of the computer and the computer mouse can produce CTDUEs. Although there are currently few claims related to computer mouse use, it seems to be a growing problem that hand surgeons should be aware of.

S.E. Mackinnon, M.D.

Reference

1. Lister GD: Ergonomic disorders (editorial). *J Hand Surgery* 20A:353, 1995.

CTD Injuries: An Outcome Study for Work Survivability
Melhorn JM (Univ of Kansas, Wichita)
J Workers Comp 5:18–30, 1996   11–4

Background.—Work-related cumulative trauma disorders (CTDs) are an important health and safety issue of concern to business, government, and the medical profession. The cause, epidemiology, treatment, and costs of CTDs have been extensively studied, but work survivability after CTD and treatment have received little attention. A retrospective study of workers' compensation injury records investigated survivability and treatment.

Methods.—Workers' compensation injury records for a major manufacturer between 1988 and 1992 were reviewed. Data on patient age, sex, genetics (dominant hand), medical conditions, workplace and nonworkplace factors, and linked elements (medical treatment, amount of permanent physical impairment, satisfaction with the supervisor, and legal counseling) were obtained. The rates of employment in the same job at 1 and 2 years after treatment were analyzed.

Results.—At 1 year, 17% of the 109 workers were no longer employed in the same job, and 15% of these employment changes were related to injury. At 2 years, an additional 8% of employees were no longer employed in the same job, but none of these changes were related to injury. Work survivability was not significantly correlated with age, sex, genetics, job titles, or nonworkplace factors. The probability of employment at 1 year was increased with continual employment (no lost workdays) and an earlier return to work. An early return-to-work program that provided modified or transitional light work improved the probability of employment at 1 year. Work survivability was greater in those with minimal permanent physical impairment than in those with extensive impairment. Retaining an attorney was associated with reduced work survivability.

Conclusions.—Work survivability can be improved in employees with CTDs by continuation of work or providing early return-to-work programs. These programs do not appear to increase the risk for recurrent CTDs.

▶ During a 4-year period, workers' compensation injury records of a major manufacturer in the Wichita area were studied. During that time, 109 of 1,342 employees had CTD injuries. Factors such as age, sex, the dominant hand, associated medical conditions, job categories, nonwork environment, and linked elements were studied.

This study is significant because it gives statistically valid evidence of many things that hand surgeons have observed in treating workers' compensation cases. The best results are obtained in patients who return to work soon after an injury (before they have retained an attorney) and have modifications made in their job. The "work survivability" did not vary significantly for different job titles, age, or sex. This information can help guide health care workers in advising employers and employees and preventing loss of time from the job and improving the ability to continue work. In injured employees who remained at work and those who returned early, recurrence of symptoms did not increase. Staying on the job with modification of activities is shown to give the best result.

The term "work survivability" is suggested for measuring treatment outcomes for work-related injuries. Despite better employer awareness, prevention programs, and increasing government regulations, the rate of upper-extremity CTDs continue to increase.

R.L. Horner, M.D.

Work-related Upper-extremity Disorders and Work Disability: Clinical and Psychosocial Presentation

Himmelstein JS, Feuerstein M, Stanek EJ III, et al (Univ of Massachusetts, Worcester; Uniformed Services Univ, Bethesda, Md; Univ of Massachusetts, Amherst)

J Occup Environ Med 37:1278–1286, 1995

Background.—Work-related symptoms and disability are increasingly caused by upper-extremity disorders. Most work-related upper-extremity disorders (WRUEDs) are acute and self-limiting. However, a small proportion result in permanent disability, accounting for most of the cost associated with these conditions. The progression from symptoms to disability has not been well documented, and how to prevent such progression is unclear.

Methods.—One hundred twenty-four consecutive patients attending a clinic specializing in WRUEDs were included in the current study. Fifty-five patients were working at the time of the study, and 59 were unable to work. These 2 groups were similar in age, gender, and reported job demands.

Findings.—The patients unable to work had less time on the job, more operations, and a greater frequency of acute antecedent trauma. "Indeterminate" musculoskeletal diagnoses were also more common among these patients. In addition, patients unable to work reported higher levels of pain, more anger toward their employer, and a greater psychological response or reactivity to pain.

Conclusions.—These findings support a multidimensional conceptualization of inability to work that includes medical, workplace, and psychological variables. Prolonged work disability in patients with WRUEDs may be allayed by more aggressive pain control, avoiding unnecessary surgery, directed efforts to improve patients' ability to manage residual pain and distress, and attention to employer-employee conflicts.

▶ The authors have compared various characteristics of patients with WRUEDs. Work-disabled patients reported higher pain levels, more anger with their employers, more surgeries, and a greater psychological response to pain. Although this is somewhat of a "chicken-vs.-the-egg" study, the results will have important implications for hand surgeons. Besides questioning the role of surgery in these disorders, it suggests that hand surgeons interested in treating WRUEDs must increase their level of awareness of the psychological impact of chronic pain on the overall well-being of their patients. The high incidence of consultation with an attorney (62%) and litigation (46%), coupled with a high incidence of "anger with their employers," suggests that issues other than surgical problems in the upper extremity will impact patient outcome. This is an important contribution and an article of which all hand surgeons treating workers with upper-extremity complaints should be aware.

S.E. Mackinnon, M.D.

Sensitivity of the Jamar Dynamometer in Detecting Submaximal Grip Effort
Ashford RF, Nagelburg S, Adkins R (Rancho Los Amigos Med Ctr, Pasadena, Calif; Rancho Los Amigos Med Ctr, Downey, Calif)
J Hand Surg [Am] 21A:402–405, 1996   11–6

Objective.—Reliability of grip testing using the Jamar Dynamometer is determined from results of 3 trials of measurements. More than 20% variability in measurement has been assumed to indicate that the patient is not exerting maximum effort, but objective studies examining submaximal efforts have not been done. The extent to which the Jamar Dynamometer can detect a submaximal effort was studied.

Methods.—Optimal and suboptimal grip strengths were each measured 3 times in each hand in 22 healthy volunteers (7 men). The results were analyzed and compared statistically.

Results.—The average optimal and suboptimal efforts were 38.4 kg and 21.7 kg, respectively. The average range for the maximum effort was 3.8 kg (11% variability), and the result for submaximal effort was 5.4 kg (26% variability). Eight maximal trials and 25 submaximal trials had results that varied by 20% or more. Twenty maximal trials and 41 submaximal trials had results varying by 10% or more. No statistically significant differences were seen between variabilities in maximal and submaximal grip strength.

Conclusion.—The Jamar Dynamometer can be fooled by consistent submaximal grip strength efforts.

▶ It is often stated that submaximal (faked) effort on grip testing can be detected by variability of effort. This apparently is not so. I have found instrumented grip meters to be better in this regard; the slope or pattern of the increase in force with maximal effort is harder to fake. Trying multiple grip positions, preferably all 5 on the Jamar, can also help; it is also difficult for the patient to easily fake the roughly bell-shaped pattern of maximal efforts at each of the 5 positions. Usually, position 2 will be highest.

P.C. Amadio, M.D.

Reference

1. Firrell JC, Crain GM: Which setting of the dynamometer provides maximal grip strenght? *J Hand Surg (Am)* 21A:397–401, 1996.

Corticosteroid Injections in Trigger Fingers: Is Intrasheath Injection Necessary?
Taras JS, Raphael JS, Culp RW (Philadelphia)
1995 Jefferson Orthop J 24:20–22, 1995   11–7

Introduction.—A frequent ailment seen in hand surgery and general orthopedic practices is stenosing tenosynovitis of the finger or thumb flexors, commonly referred to as trigger finger. Patients with trigger finger complain of triggering, locking pain on flexion and extension, snapping, and tenderness to pressure over the A1 pulley. Injecting a long-acting corticosteroid solution into the tendon sheath once or twice is the current standard treatment for trigger fingers without fixed contracture. The true delivery of intrasynovial injections in patients treated nonoperatively has not been investigated. The efficacy of intrasynovial injection delivery for trigger finger and thumb was determined.

Methods.—Sixty patients with a total of 73 trigger fingers were randomly assigned into 2 groups: one had intrasynovial injection attempted, and the other had corticosteroid delivered into the subcutaneous tissues overlying the A1 pulley of the affected finger. Injections of 1 cc of betamethasone solution, 0.5 cc of lidocaine, and 01.5 cc of iohexal x-ray contrast solution were given to both groups. The addition of a small amount of radiopaque dye into the injection fluid was used followed by lateral and posteroanterior radiographs of the hand. Patients were followed up for an average of 11 months.

Results.—Good results were graded as complete relief of symptoms, fair results were graded as minimal pain or occasional trigger, and poor as no improvement. The intrasheath group had 34 patients with 43 trigger fingers, and they had 70% good, 12% fair, and 18% poor results. The subcutaneous group had 26 patients with 30 trigger fingers, and they had 70% good, 19% fair, and 11% poor results. The attempted sheath group showed that 27.5% of patients had introduction of the steroid completely within the tendon sheath and 66% of these had good results, according to a review of postinjection radiographs; 47% had steroid in the sheath and subcutaneous tissue (75% had good results), and 26% had no evidence of delivery of medication into the sheath (71% had good results). In the subcutaneous group, all the patients had received successful injections into the subcutaneous tissues.

Conclusion.—About half of the attempted intrasynovial injections resulted in 100% delivery of the steroid into the sheath; about a quarter resulted in infiltration of some steroid into the subcutaneous tissue; and the other quarter were totally subcutaneous. Injecting subcutaneously over the first annular pulley, thereby interfering less with tendon nutrition is recommended. Simple subcutaneous injection is also less painful.

▶ This is a prospective, randomized study, but the authors did not mention if it was blinded, or if the radiographs were reviewed by a radiologist blinded to the clinical data and not involved with the injections. The result is very interesting, however, and shows that only half of the injections went into the flexor sheath. A previous study using preoperative methylene blue injection is quoted as showing 49% success; this study additionally stressed that injection from proximal to distal was twice as effective as injection in the other direction.[1] The value of this study is that it might provide clues to the actual pathogenesis of trigger finger. One can speculate why the extrasynovial steroid can be effective. Perhaps the steroid diffuses into the flexor sheath, or acts externally by softening the thickened, fibrocartilaginous A1 pulley.

These results can be contrasted with those of a similar x-ray dye study of steroid injection localization and prospective follow-up in de Quervain's tendinitis that I recently completed; all patients in whom steroid failed to enter the first dorsal compartment failed to have relief of symptoms, compared to only 20% failure after successful injection of the abductor pollicis longus and extensor pollicis brevis compartments.

J.M. Failla, M.D.

Reference

1. Kamhin M, Engel J, Heim M: The fate of injected trigger fingers. *Hand* 15:218–220, 1983.

MRI Features in de Quervain's Tenosynovitis of the Wrist
Glajchen N, Schweitzer M (Mount Sinai Hosp, New York; Thomas Jefferson Univ, Philadelphia)
Skeletal Radiol 25:63–65, 1996   11–8

Background.—De Quervain's stenosing tenosynovitis of the first dorsal extensor compartment of the wrist is generally diagnosed clinically. The classic clinical findings include pain radiating from the radial styloid process to the thumb and into the forearm, increased pain caused by passive movement of the thumb and wrist, swelling and tenderness over the first dorsal compartment, and a positive result on Finkelstein testing. The condition may be unsuspected, however, particularly by nonspecial-

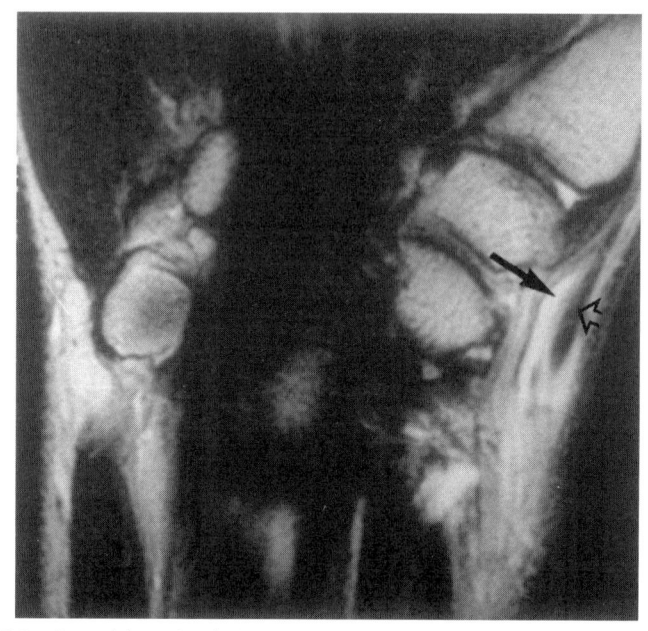

FIGURE 3.—Coronal fast spin-echo image (TR/TE 2,500/102) showing edema within the synovial sheath (*solid arrow*) or the first extensor compartment and a small amount of intratendinous high signal (*open arrow*). (Courtesy of Glajchen N, Schweitzer M: MRI features in de Quervain's tenosynovitis of the wrist. *Skeletal Radiol* 25:63–65, 1996.)

ists. The possibility of diagnosing de Quervain's tenosynovitis of the wrist with MRI was investigated.

Methods.—The MRI examinations of 5 patients seen for the evaluation of suspected de Quervain's disease were reviewed. The subsequent diagnosis was based on the clinical findings in 4 patients and the wrist arthroscopy findings in 1.

Results.—Clinical assessment confirmed the diagnosis of de Quervain's tenosynovitis in 3 patients. One patient who had the clinical features of de Quervain's disease was lost to follow-up. Diffuse synovitis was diagnosed in the patient who underwent wrist arthroscopy.

On MRI, increasing thickness of the first extensor compartment tendons was found in the 3 patients who had confirmed de Quervain's disease and in the 1 patient who had suspected de Quervain's disease. It was also found, however, in the patient who had diffuse synovitis. Peritendinous edema was found in the 3 confirmed cases and the suspected case (Figs 3 and 4). Neither surrounding subcutaneous edema nor increased signal within the tendon were reliable signs of de Quervain's disease.

Conclusions.—Magnetic resonance images that reveal thickened tendons of the first compartment of the wrist and synovial edema should suggest the diagnosis of de Quervain's tenosynovitis. The reliability of these imaging signs in this diagnosis requires further study.

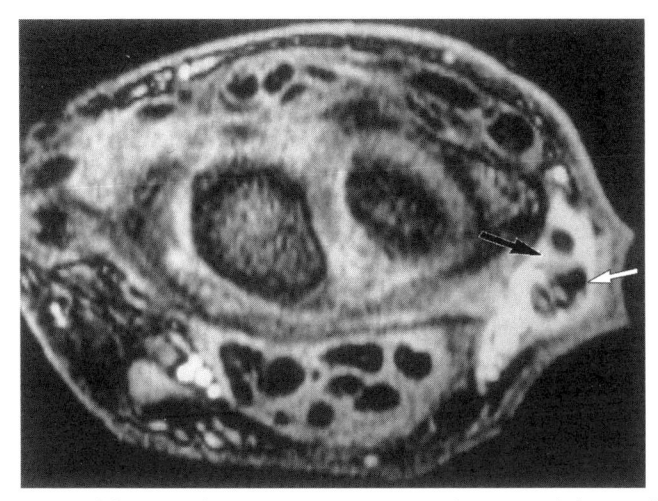

FIGURE 4.—Axial fast spin-echo image (TR/TE 3,000/102) showing marked synovial thickening (*black arrow*) with minimal subcutaneous edema (*white arrow*). (Courtesy of Glajchen N, Schweitzer M: MRI features in de Quervain's tenosynovitis of the wrist. *Skeletal Radiol* 25:63–65, 1996.)

▶ Although this study is small, it points out the utility of MRI for the detection of de Quervain's tenosynovitis. Interpreters of MRI scans need to be aware of the image features of this condition when evaluating patients who have wrist disorders.

When patients are referred for imaging because of suspected de Quervain's tenosynovitis, there are several options. Although MRI is sensitive and fairly specific, it is costly to perform. Ultrasound may be a less expressive alternative.

T.H. Berquist, M.D.

Association of Wartenberg's Syndrome and De Quervain's Disease: A Series of 26 Cases
Lanzetta M, Foucher G (SOS Main Strasbourg, France)
Plast Reconstr Surg 96:408–412, 1995   11–9

Introduction.—Entrapment of the sensory branch of the radial nerve in the forearm (Wartenberg's syndrome) has been observed in association with de Quervain's tenosynovitis. The treatment and outcome for 25 patients (26 cases) who had these conditions simultaneously were assessed.

Patients and Methods.—Twenty-one women and 4 men (mean age, 43 years) were all treated from January 1988 to July 1992. Patients referred for Wartenberg's syndrome were more likely to have the combination of conditions than were those referred for de Quervain's tenosynovitis (25 of 52 vs. 25 of 164). All patients experienced several weeks or months of pain, numbness, and tenderness or swelling. A Tinel's sign could be elicited in all patients, and a double Tinel's sign in 7. Treatment of de Quervain's disease was surgical in 15 cases, conservative in 10, and conservative and surgical in 1. Treatment of Wartenberg's syndrome was conservative in 15 cases, surgical in 10, and conservative and surgical in 1. All patients were encouraged to begin early motion after surgery.

Results.—The status of 23 patients was followed for a mean of 15 months. Of 14 patients treated conservatively for Wartenberg's syndrome, 9 (64%) had excellent or good results. Nine were managed conservatively for both conditions; 3 of these patients had excellent results, and 2 had good results. Four of 5 patients had excellent results when only de Quervain disease was treated surgically. A patient who had a poor result after conservative treatment for both conditions had an excellent outcome after surgery. Proximal neurolysis in the case of Tinel's sign in zone 1 was associated with excellent or good results, whereas fair results were consecutive to neurolysis in zone 3 in patients who had combined Tinel's signs in zones 3 and 1.

Conclusion.—The association between Wartenberg's syndrome and de Quervain's disease appears to be more common than previously recognized. Patients who have de Quervain's disease should undergo careful examination of the sensory branch of the radial nerve. Conservative treatment can be effective, but release of the first compartment is advised in cases of distal migration of Tinel's sign. It is important to rule out associated Wartenberg's syndrome before release of the first dorsal compartment.

▶ Does stenosing tenosynovitis of the first dorsal compartment lead to entrapment neuropathy of the nearby branches of the dorsal radial sensory nerve? Certainly, in long-standing cases, one can elicit a Tinel's sign by tapping over the compartment, and, frequently, the patient can detect a sensory difference between the affected and unaffected sides. Perhaps the nerve irritation then develops along the lines of a continuous minor traction injury akin to one of the purported causes of persistent median nerve symptoms in carpal tunnel syndrome. Is clinically observable irritation of the dorsal sensory branch of the radial nerve in the area of the first dorsal compartment the so-called Wartenberg's syndrome? I don't think so.

V.R. Hentz, M.D.

Low-energy Extracorporeal Shock Wave Therapy for Persistent Tennis Elbow
Rompe JD, Hopf C, Küllmer K, et al (Orthopaedic Univ Hosp, Mainz, Germany; Urologic Univ Hosp, Mainz, Germany; Inst for Med Statistics, Mainz, Germany)
Int Orthop 20:23–27, 1996   11–10

Background.—The cause and pathology of tennis elbow are still not clear. It is also unclear whether conservative treatment or surgery is best.

The efficacy of low-dose extracorporeal shock wave therapy (ECSWT) in the treatment of tennis elbow was investigated.

Methods.—Fifty patients who had had tennis elbow for at least 1 year were included in the study. All had been referred for operative treatment. By random assignment, the patients received a total of 3,000 impulses of 0.08 mJ/mm^2 (group 1) or up to 30 impulses of 0.08 mJ/mm^2 as a control (group 2). Patients were assessed after 3 and 12 weeks.

Findings.—After 3 weeks, group 1 outcomes were excellent in 8 patients, good in another 8, and acceptable in 9. After 12 weeks, outcomes in this group were excellent in 6, good in 8, acceptable in 5, and poor in 6. In group 2, outcomes were good in 5, acceptable in 8, and poor in 12 at both 3- and 12-week assessments. Four group 1 patients with poor outcomes eventually underwent a Bosworth procedure. Six months after this operation, results were good in 1 patient and acceptable in 3.

Conclusions.—Extracorporeal shock wave therapy for tennis elbow significantly reduced pain and increased grip strength. There were no adverse effects. No immobilization was needed, and working ability was not compromised. Further research on ECSWT is warranted.

▶ The treatment of chronic lateral epicondylitis is a novel use for ECSWT. In the past, ECSWT has been used for breaking up renal or gallstones. More recently it has been suggested as a treatment for bony fracture nonunion. It is theorized that the shock wave breaks up sclerotic bone ends, creating microfissures that increase blood supply to the nonunion site. I assume that the authors felt that a similar mechanism would help resolve the painful situation at the lateral epicondyle. This is essentially a form of controlled, localized trauma to the bony surface of the lateral epicondyle.

The results of this study are quite promising. They chose an especially difficult population of patients—those with unresponsive lateral epicondylitis of more than 12 months' duration—and show surprisingly good outcomes. Of course, higher numbers of patients will be needed to confirm the efficacy of this modality. However, if ECSWT does prove to benefit this condition, it raises many questions as to the treatments previously employed for lateral epicondylitis. Perhaps anti-inflammatory and stress-reducing modalities fail to get at the heart of the problem. Should we, in fact, be treating these patients with more simple, less expensive forms of localized trauma to the elbow?

K. Bengtson, M.D.

Lateral Epicondylitis: Correlation of MR Imaging, Surgical, and Histopathologic Findings
Potter HG, Hannafin JA, Morwessel RM, et al (Hosp for Special Surgery, New York)
Radiology 196:43–46, 1995

Purpose.—Lateral epicondylitis, or "tennis elbow," is usually diagnosed clinically by physical examination and treated by conservative means. Patients who do not respond to conservative management, however, may need further evaluation to identify the site of tendon injury and rule out frank rupture. The utility of MRI in the assessment of chronic refractory lateral epicondylitis was evaluated.

Patients.—Thirty-three patients who had chronic lateral epicondylitis and did not respond to conservative management underwent gradient-recalled-echo (GRE) MRI and axial and sagittal fast spin-echo sequences. The MRI scans were evaluated for changes in intratendinous signal intensity and for morphologic alteration in tendon orientation (Fig 1). Twenty patients subsequently underwent surgical débridement with or without tendon repair; 3 had elbow arthroscopy before undergoing open surgery. Surgical and histopathologic findings were compared with those from preoperative MRI.

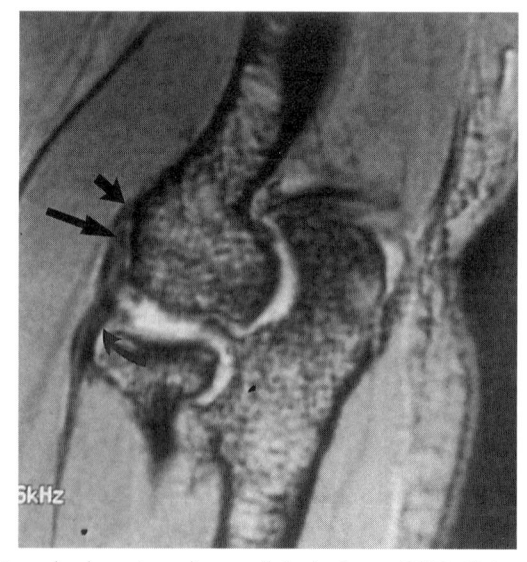

FIGURE 1.—Coronal volumetric gradient-recalled-echo image (56/20, 10-degree flip angle) of an asymptomatic woman, aged 34 years, demonstrates the normal appearance of the extensor tendons. The extensor carpi radialis brevis tendon (*long straight arrow*) lies between the extensor carpi radialis longus tendon (*short straight arrow*) and the radial collateral ligament (*curved arrow*). The tendons are oriented vertically and appear closely opposed. (Courtesy of Potter HG, Hannafin JA, Morwessel RM, et al: Lateral epicondylitis: Correlation of MR imaging, surgical, and histopathologic findings. *Radiology* 196:43–46, 1995, Radiological Society of North America.)

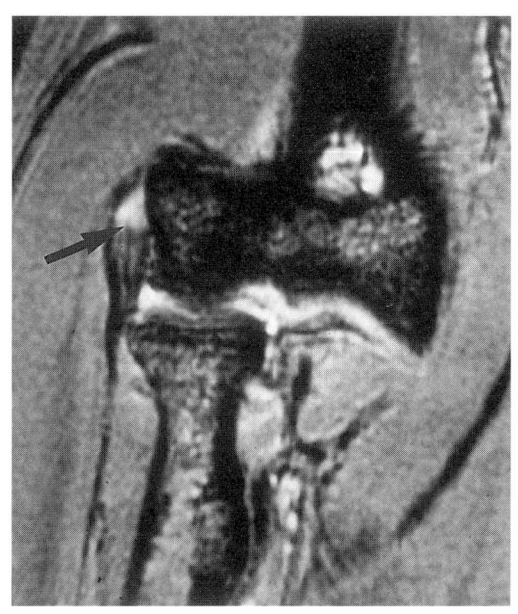

FIGURE 2.—Coronal gradient-recalled-echo image (56/18, 10-degree flip angle) of a man, aged 40 years, who had a 2-year history of elbow pain demonstrates signal hypertensity at the origin of the extensor carpi radialis brevis tendon (*arrow*), with separation between the extensor tendons and the radial collateral ligament. Severe tendon degeneration was noted at the time of surgery. (Courtesy of Potter HG, Hannafin JA, Morwessel RM, et al: Lateral epicondylitis: Correlation of MR imaging, surgical, and histopathologic findings. *Radiology* 196:43–46, 1995, Radiological Society of North America.)

Results.—Ten patients who underwent surgery had abnormal separation of the radial collateral ligament and extensor carpi radialis brevis tendon, which had been interpreted before operation as granulation tissue and inflammatory response. Tendon morphology was most easily seen on coronal GRE images (Fig 2). Frank ruptures of the extensor brevis origin and complete thickness tears were seen on the scans of 7 patients (Fig 4). All 7 cases of frank tendon rupture were confirmed at operation.

Conclusions.—Magnetic resonance imaging to investigate chronic lateral epicondylitis that does not respond to conservative management is highly recommended. The findings on MRI correlate well with surgical and histologic findings.

▶ These authors recommend MRI of the elbow in preoperative patients who have lateral epicondylitis to determine whether there are associated, intra-articular, cartilage injuries that require elbow arthroscopy as part of the surgical procedure and to evaluate the radial collateral ligament and the tendon of the extensor carpi radialis longus and brevis for tear or tendon degeneration.

G. Bergman, M.D.

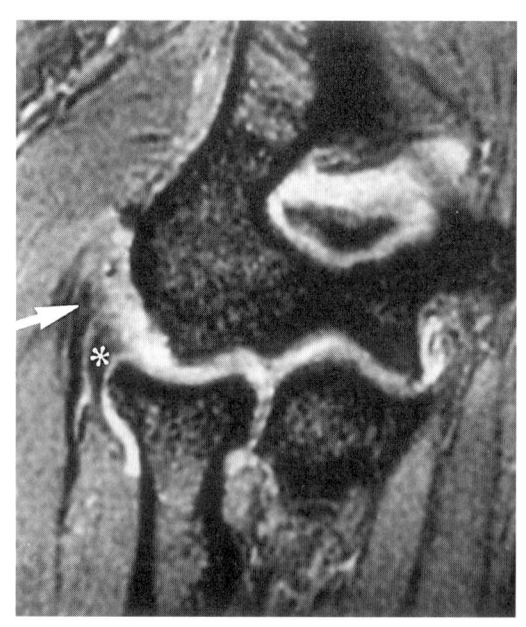

FIGURE 4.—Coronal gradient-recalled-echo image (451/20, 45-degree flip angle) of a man, aged 51 years, who had a 1-year history of lateral elbow pain and a recent increase in severity of symptoms demonstrates complete disruption of the extensor origin of the extensor carpi radialis brevis tendon (*arrow*); the retracted edge of the tendon appears focally thickened. A tear of the humeral aspect of the radial collateral ligament (*asterisk*) is also noted. Both tears were confirmed at surgery. (Courtesy of Potter HG, Hannafin JA, Morwessel RM, et al: Lateral epicondylitis: Correlation of MR imaging, surgical, and histopathologic findings. *Radiology* 196:43–46, 1995, Radiological Society of North America.)

Suggested Reading

Fransson-Hall C, Byström S, Kilbom Å: Characteristics of forearm-hand exposure in relation to symptoms among automobile assembly line workers. *Am J Industr Med* 29:15–22, 1996.
▶ The relationship of soft-tissue discomfort to the mechanical stresses of physical activity is well known to the experienced clinician. This article provides no evidence that the nonspecific symptoms reported were the result of disease or injury. There needs to be clear differentiation between the presence of symptoms and the existence of an objective injury or disease process for a study such as this to have value. As the study stands, it is no more than a survey of nonspecific symptoms which occurred in a workplace.

P.A. Nathan, M.D.

Byl N, Wilson F, Merzenich M, et al: Sensory dysfunction associated with repetitive strain injuries of tendinitis and focal hand dystonia: A comparative study. *JOSPT* 23:234–244, 1996.
▶ Anyone seriously interested in methodology for the use of peripheral sensory-motor testing to correlate with central nervous system alterations in primates, including humans, with degraded limb function would do well to review this paper and the extensive background reference material. Nevertheless, it repre-

sents a work in progress and is not ready for "prime time usage" in the day-to-day evaluation and treatment of patients.

J.H. Dobyns, M.D.

LeViet D: Tedinites et instabités du tendon cubital postérieur (extenseur carpi ulnaris, *ECU*). *La Main* 1:47–53, 1996.
▶ Subluxation and stenosing tenosynovitis of the extensor carpi ulnaris are uncommon. This nice review summarizes current thinking, and reports 16 cases.

P.C. Amadio, M.D.

Bahm J, Szabo Z, Foucher G: The anatomy of de Quervain's disease: A study of operative findings. *Int Orthop* 19:209–211, 1995.
▶ The authors could not find an anatomical predisposing factor for the development of de Quervain's disease in the 67 patients studied. They did believe that the presence of a septum in the first compartment might predispose the patient toward failure of injection, especially when the injection was made from distal to proximal. They suggest that a proximal injection might provide a better result. Study anyone?

V.R. Hentz, M.D.

12 Arthritis

Degenerative Changes of the Trapeziometacarpal Joint: Radiologic Assessment
Cooke KS, Singson RD, Glickel SZ, et al (St Luke's-Roosevelt Hosp, New York)
Skeletal Radiol 24:523–527, 1995   12–1

Background.—The trapeziometacarpal (TMC) joint is especially prone to osteoarthritis because it is subjected to a great amount of daily stress. The radiologic assessment and staging of basal joint osteoarthritis, treatments, and complications were discussed.

Radiologic Assessment.—Standard examination includes posterior-anterior oblique and lateral views of the thumb. A true lateral view, which shows superimposition of the metacarpophalangeal sesamoids, is particularly useful for identifying early degenerative changes at the dorsolateral aspect of the joint. A "stress view," which is a posterior-anterior projection of the TMC joints under lateral stress, is obtained with the plane of the thumbnails parallel to the x-ray cassette while the patient pushes the tips of the radial side of the thumb against each other. The beam is centered at the level of the TMC joint. This view displays the extent of TMC joint laxity and provides a comparison view of the other thumb. In addition, it shows an excellent posterior-anterior view of the scaphotrapezial (ST) joint.

Staging.—On the basis of radiographic findings, TMC joint osteoarthritis is divided into 4 stages. In stage 1, the articular contours are normal, although slight widening of the joint space, caused by effusion or laxity of the ligamentous support of the TMC joint, is seen (Fig 4, A). In stage 2, the joint is slightly narrowed, there is minimal subchondral sclerosis, and osteophytes or loose bodies of 2 mm or less may be present. In stage 3, the joint is very narrowed or obliterated. Findings may include osteophytes or loose bodies greater than 2 mm, subchondral cysts, sclerosis, and varying degrees of subluxation. In stage 4, the TMC joint appears as a stage 3 joint, but the ST joint is narrowed with sclerotic and cystic changes. Degenerative changes may also be apparent in other facets of the trapezium, thereby resulting in pantrapezial arthritis.

Treatment.—Initial treatment is conservative and consists of immobilization and nonsteroidal anti-inflammatory drugs, regardless of the extent of joint degeneration. For patients who do not respond, an operative

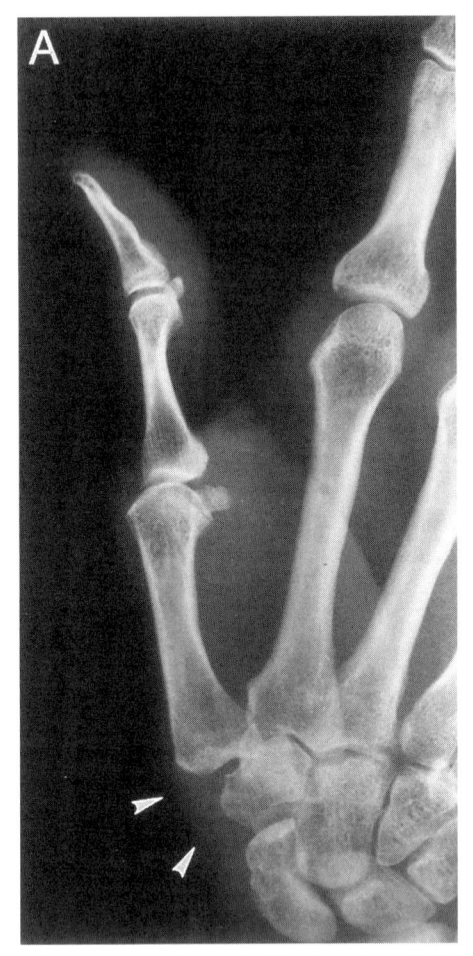

FIGURE 4.—A, stage 1: the pre-arthritic thumb. Widening of the TMC joint space is seen. The widening is apparent when compared with the rest of the carpometacarpal joint spaces. Periarticular soft-tissue swelling is distinctly evident. (Courtesy of Cooke KS, Singson RD, Glickel SZ, et al: Degenerative changes of the trapeziometacarpal joint: Radiologic assessment. *Skeletal Radiol* 24:523–527, 1995.)

procedure is selected on the basis of radiologic staging and intraoperative findings. For patients who have stage 1 osteoarthritis of the TMC joint, volar ligament reconstruction is done. For those who have stage 2, volar ligament reconstruction alone is done when articular cartilage is minimally worn or fibrillated on intraoperative inspection, and a partial trapezial resection with interposition is done along with the ligamentous reconstruction when articulating cartilages are more than minimally worn. For stage 3, arthrodesis or ligament reconstruction with partial interposition is done when the ST joint is intact, and total trapeziectomy with or without interposition is done when the ST joint shows significant degenerative changes. For stage 4, total trapeziectomy with or without interposition is done.

Surgical Complications.—All these surgical procedures can result in reduced pinch strength and range of motion. Arthrodesis often results in rigidity and poor position of the thumb. In addition, these procedures may not relieve pain. Deformation and dislocation of the prosthesis with malalignment of the thumb have been associated with interposition arthroplasties. Silicone synovitis is also of concern when silicone prostheses are used.

▶ Eaton's 4-stage classification of basal joint disease is nicely reviewed. I have often wondered whether the width of the gap that remains between base of thumb metacarpal and scaphoid after trapezial resection and interposition arthroplasty correlated with postoperative pain relief. Apparently it does not.

V.R. Hentz, M.D.

Extension Metacarpal Osteotomy in the Treatment of Trapeziometacarpal Osteoarthritis: A Biomechanical Study
Pellegrini VD Jr, Parentis M, Judkins A, et al (Pennsylvania State Univ, Hershey; Univ of Rochester, New York)
J Hand Surg (Am) 21A:16–23, 1996   12–2

Background.—The incompetence of the palmar beak ligament may initiate the progression of degenerative joint disease associated with trapeziometacarpal osteoarthritis. Metacarpal osteotomy has been used to treat advanced disease with good results. The appropriateness of this treatment, however, has not been established. The biomechanical effects of extension metacarpal osteotomy in the management of trapeziometacarpal osteoarthritis were investigated.

Methods.—The trapeziometacarpal joint contact pressures were measured with the use of ultra-low pressure-sensitive film during simulated lateral pinch in 20 cadaveric forearm specimens. In each specimen, the contact pressure pattern imprints during flexion, extension, flexion-extension, extension-flexion, static lateral pinch, and dynamic lateral pinch were analyzed before and after extension osteotomy. After testing, the trapeziometacarpal joint specimen was examined to classify the joint surfaces and capsular structures.

Technique.—Saw cuts were made 1 cm distal and parallel to the trapeziometacarpal joint, and a second was made at a 30-degree angle to the first cut to remove a bone wedge dorsally from the thumb metacarpal. The osteotomy site was closed and fixed to the metacarpal base with Kirschner wire, then rigidly fixed with screws and a mini L-plate (Fig 1).

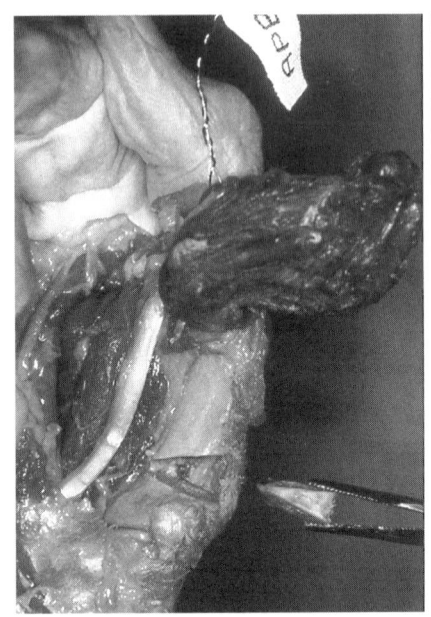

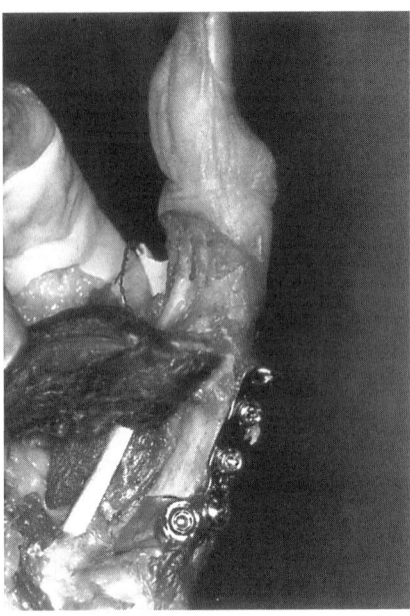

FIGURE 1.—Palmar view of the right thumb, showing the metacarpal shaft after elevation of thenar musculature for extension metacarpal osteotomy. **Left**, removal of 30 degrees, dorsally based wedge at the base of metacarpal. **Right**, closure of osteotomy and fixation with mini-plate and screws. (Courtesy of Pellegrini VD Jr, Parentis M, Judkins A, et al: Extension metacarpal osteotomy in the treatment of trapeziometacarpal osteoarthritis: A biomechanical study. *Hand Surg (Am)* 21A: 16–23, 1996.)

Results.—Examination of the joint surfaces revealed palmar compartment eburnation and degeneration of the adjacent palmar beak ligament attachment to the metacarpal in 10 specimens. Extension osteotomy resulted in redistributing the load dorsally within the trapeziometacarpal joint in all specimens that had normal joints or mild or moderate arthritis but not in those that had end-stage disease. There were no significant changes, however, in any specimens in total contact area or pressure.

Conclusions.—Performing extension metacarpal osteotomy to redistribute load away from the palmar compartment of mildly or moderately arthritic trapeziometacarpal joints has a sound biomechanical basis. This treatment may result in symptomatic improvement, but this improvement is not related to mechanical joint-surface load redistribution.

▶ This biomechanical study is an interesting extension of the senior author's study of the pathomechanics of degenerative arthritis of the trapeziometacarpal joint. The study shows some transmission of contact pressure from the palmar to the dorsal aspect of the metacarpal base in normal and moderately arthritic joints after a Wilson osteotomy. There is no change, however, in the eburnated contact areas in the more advanced disease state. Change in contact loading from the more to the lesser involved aspect of the joint may effect symptomatic relief, but an equally important feature of the procedure may be the anterior rotation of the articular surface. This provides better restraint to the radioposteriorly directed subluxation of the metacarpal base; which is thought to be the cause of the increased shear stress on the anterior facets.

R.L. Linscheid, M.D.

Results of Scaphotrapeziotrapezoid Fusion for Isolated Idiopathic Arthritis
Srinivasan VB, Matthews JP (Morriston Hosp, Swansea, Wales)
J Hand Surg (Br) 21B:378–380, 1996   12–3

Background.—Scaphotrapeziotrapezoid (STT) arthritis is characterized by tenderness over the palmar aspect of the thenar eminence and association with flexor carpi radialis tendinitis. The use of STT fusion to treat this condition was reported.

Patients.—Between 1988 and 1993, 4 men and 4 women, aged 44–70 years, who had isolated STT arthritis were assessed. The predominant symptom was pain, and the patients underwent STT fusion. The patients' status was followed 18–80 months. The operated hand was compared with the contralateral hand to assess function, pain, range of movement, grip strength, prehension, tip-to-tip pinch, and dexterity. Radiographs were used to evaluate the repair.

Results.—Four patients were free of pain after STT fusion, 3 had mild pain during specific activities, and 1 had constant pain. Hand function was good to excellent. Average grip strength was 0.8, and lateral pinch strength was 0.7 of the contralateral side. There was little difference in dexterity between the 2 sides. There was an average difference of 9 degrees of flexion-extension and 13 degrees of radio-ulnar deviation between the 2 sides. Subjective results were excellent in 5 patients; good in 2, and poor in 1. The patient with poor results had nonunion of the arthrodesis on radiographs.

Conclusion.—Scaphotrapeziotrapezoid fusion is a useful procedure in the treatment of isolated idiopathic STT arthritis. It produces good pain relief, hand function, and mobility and has a low complication rate.

▶ I agree. To me, isolated STT arthritis is the strongest indication for STT fusion, and the only one I recognize clinically.

P.C. Amadio, M.D.

Basal Joint Arthrosis: Radiographic Assessment of the Trapezial Space Before and After Ligament Reconstruction and Tendon Interposition Arthroplasty

Kadiyala RK, Gelberman RH, Kwon B (Massachusetts Gen Hosp, Boston; Washington Univ, St Louis)
J Hand Surg (Br) 21B:177–181, 1996   12–4

Objective.—Patients with basal joint arthrosis that does not improve with nonoperative treatment commonly undergo basal joint arthroplasty. At surgery, the suspensory ligaments at the base of the thumb metacarpal may be reconstructed to restore scaphometacarpal height. However, the lack of a standardized radiographic technique has made it difficult to evaluate the results of these procedures. The trapezial space ratio, a new radiographic technique for assessing the space occupied by the trapezium, was evaluated in normal participants and in patients with basal joint arthrosis.

Methods.—The trapezial space ratio was calculated by measuring the trapezial space, as defined by the distal aspect of the scaphoid and the base of the first metacarpal, and dividing it by the proximal phalangeal height. All measurements were made on routine posteroanterior radiographs of the hand and wrist. The trapezial space ratio was calculated in 100 radiographs of normal thumbs. The technique was also applied to the radiographs of 15 patients with symptomatic degenerative arthrosis of the thumb basal joint, before and an average of 2 years after ligamentous reconstruction and tendon interposition arthroplasty.

Results.—The trapezial space ratio averaged 0.476 ± 0.033 in the normal thumb radiographs, compared to 0.372 ± 0.084 in the preoperative radiographs of thumbs with basal joint arthrosis and 0.270 ± 0.078 in the postoperative radiographs. The arthritic thumbs showed a significant 22% reduction in the trapezial space ratio, compared to the normal thumbs. An additional 27% reduction was noted on comparison of the preoperative and postoperative radiographs. Thumbs operated on for basal joint arthrosis showed a 43% reduction in trapezial space ratio compared to normal thumbs.

Conclusions.—The trapezial space ratio, as defined in this study, is significantly reduced from normal in thumbs with symptomatic basal joint arthrosis. Operative treatment by ligament reconstruction and tendon interposition arthroplasty does not necessarily succeed in restoring or maintaining the thumb ray length. The study provides no information on the clinical significance of loss of height of the trapezial space.

▶ The trapezial space ratio determination is an effective method of measuring first metacarpal subsidence after one of the suspensory procedures for trapeziometacarpal degenerative joint disease. It seems unlikely that cartilage erosion alone can account for the decrease in this ratio between normal and Eaton stage III and IV joints. Change in alignment of the elements as a result of the radiodorsal subluxation of the first metacarpal, and its projection on the x-ray film may be a factor. The use of the Robert's projection may increase the sensitivity of this measurement. The lack of a significant decrease in the ratio after 18 months was somewhat surprising.

R.L. Linscheid, M.D.

Basal Joint Arthritis: Trapeziectomy With Ligament Reconstruction and Tendon Interposition Arthroplasty
Lins RE, Gelberman RH, McKeown L, et al (Massachusetts Gen Hosp, Boston; Washington Univ, St Louis; Brigham and Women's Hosp, Boston)
J Hand Surg (Am) 21A:202–209, 1996   12–5

Background.—Several earlier reports have suggested that excisional arthroplasty can effectively relieve pain associated with basal joint arthritis, as well as preserve thumb function. However, loss of thumb strength and stability can occur in patients undergoing such procedures. Reconstruction of the palmar oblique ligament using the flexor carpi radialis tendon has been proposed as a means to improve thumb function and prevent proximal metacarpal migration. A qualitative and quantitative analysis was undertaken to evaluate outcomes of patients undergoing ligament reconstruction and tendon interposition (LRTI) arthroplasty.

Patients and Methods.—Twenty-seven consecutive patients with basal arthritis of the thumb were included in the study. Ligament reconstruction and tendon interposition arthroplasty was performed on 30 thumbs. An outcomes instrument was used to assess patients' opinions about their preoperative and postoperative functional status. The presence of pain, ability to perform activities of daily living, and satisfaction with outcome were evaluated. Physical examinations also were performed at a mean of 42 months after surgery.

Results.—Twenty-four patients reported satisfaction with the relief of pain afforded by the arthroplasty. Twenty-three patients also stated that they would undergo the procedure again. Improvement in the ability to perform daily living activities was noted in 18 thumbs. Web space measurements and grip and pinch strength also were significantly improved. In preoperative radiographic studies, the trapezial space ratio averaged 0.33 in thumbs with stage III and IV degenerative arthritis. After basal joint arthroplasty, the average ratio was 0.23, representing a total decrease of 51% in the trapezial space ratio compared to normal values noted in previous studies and 33% compared to preoperative values noted in this study. At a mean of 42 months postoperatively, no significant correlation between maintenance of trapezial height and objective and subjective clinical outcomes was noted.

Conclusions.—The comparison between preoperative and postoperative trapezial space ratios indicated a significant postoperative decrease, suggesting that LRTI arthroplasty does not completely restore the trapezial space. This does not, however, appear to have a significant effect on symptom resolution or on restoration of thumb function in patients undergoing LRTI for basal joint arthritis.

▶ The authors provide detailed evaluation of both subjective and objective results, which, as previous studies have shown, indicate that first carpometacarpal arthroplasty improves the preoperative condition. Contrary to current literature supporting ligament reconstruction after trapeziectomy, the authors conclude that there is a significant loss of resected space despite ligament reconstruction, and that, regardless of the degree of trapezial space collapse, the outcomes assessment of this study show no correlation between maintenance of trapezial space and clinical outcomes.

These results in part parallel our clinical and research experience, which suggest that the results of trapeziectomy with distraction of the resected space (distraction resection arthroplasty) without ligament reconstruction is as effective as the more complex ligament reconstructive procedures. Review of our experience has shown that maintenance of the resected space is not augmented by ligament reconstruction and can more easily be accomplished by distracting the resected space via K-wire fixation for a period of 6 weeks. When compared with results in patients treated via different methods of ligament reconstruction, distraction resection arthroplasty was equivalent or superior in both objective and subjective measures.

With regard to the lack of correlation between the maintenance of the trapezial space and clinical outcome, the authors' attempt to further standardize the method of evaluating the resected space is to be commended. However, I feel that a more accurate assessment can be accomplished by obtaining radiographs of the resected space under load conditions. This would provide information as to what occurs during actual use of the thumb and allow for a more "real life" assessment as to the importance of the resected space and clinical outcome. In any event, there now appear to be increasing data that suggest that in the treatment of first carpometacarpal arthritis, more is not always better.

O.J. Moy, M.D.

First Carpometacarpal Joint Arthritis: A Comparison of Two Arthroplasty Techniques
Livesey JP, Norris SH, Page RE (Northern Gen Hosp, Sheffield, England)
J Hand Surg [Br] 21B:182–188, 1996
12–6

Introduction.—Various surgical approaches have been used to treat degenerative disease of the first carpometacarpal joint. Few investigations have compared the surgical results of 2 procedures. Reported are results of a comparison of 2-tendon arthroplasty and palmaris longus interposition arthroplasty. A method of assessment was presented.

Methods.—The 2-tendon technique was performed on 11 hands in 9 patients (group A). The palmaris longus interposition technique was performed on 8 hands in 8 patients (group B). An assessment of surgical results was designed and used for evaluation. Patients were asked to subjectively grade surgical outcome. Thumb-tip pinch and hand grip in pounds per square inch were performed using a Jamar bulb vigorometer. Dynamic function was assessed by having the patients perform fine hand movement tasks. All patients underwent radiologic assessment, including views of the trapezial space on resting and during stress to evaluate metacarpal stability.

Results.—Patients in group A reported a greater variation in subjective outcome and had less consistent pain relief compared with patients in group B. More complications occurred in group A than in group B. Group A had a higher mean power grip and mean pinch grip than group B patients. As the duration of follow-up increased, patients in group A continued to show improvement in these variables; by contrast, patients in group B did not show improvement after 1 year. Group A had better dynamic function than did group B. Radiologic assessment showed a marked tendency for calcification to increase with time in group A but not in group B. Better results were correlated with calcification within the trapezial space (this took 3 years to occur).

Conclusion.—Patients should be advised that when 2-tendon arthroplasty is done, it may take up to 3 years to achieve good subjective results. Patients in group B experienced early pain relief, fewer complications, better subjective outcome, better range of motion, less dexterity, and lower strength, than did patients in group A. Results in both groups were satisfactory. The 2-tendon technique may be more appropriate for younger, more active patients who need to regain a strong, dexterous hand. More sedate elderly patients may benefit more from the pain relief afforded by the palmaris longus technique. A multicenter trial is needed because surgery for first carpometacarpal joint is not common.

▶ This interesting paper compares a ligament reconstruction and tendon interposition (LRTI) type of procedure with simple anchovy interposition. The authors suggest that recovery after LRTI is slower but that the long-term result is better. The authors conclude with a plea for a prospective multicenter study to compare treatment options for thumb carpometacarpal surgery using standard outcome assessment. I heartily agree with that plea. There are some 2,500 subscribers to this YEAR BOOK—takers, anyone?

P.C. Amadio, M.D.

Stabilized Resection Arthroplasty by an Anterior Approach in Trapeziometacarpal Arthritis: Results and Surgical Technique
Le Viet DT, Kerboull L, Lantieri LA, et al (Hôpital Cochin, Paris)
J Hand Surg [Am] 21A:194–201, 1996   12–7

Introduction.—The benefits of surgical treatment for trapeziometacarpal joint arthritis have been shown. Many authors have described varying surgical procedures and modifications for the treatment of this condition.

Since 1986, the authors of this paper have treated trapeziometacarpal arthritis by total excision and reconstruction of the palmar ligament through the carpal tunnel and the flexor carpi radialis osteofibrous sheath. This procedure has allowed simultaneous treatment of frequently coexisting carpal tunnel syndrome with the use of only 1 excision. The technique, and its advantages and disadvantages were described.

Study Design.—From 1986 to 1992, 72 consecutive trapeziectomies were performed using the anterior approach in 57 patients (53 women and 4 men; average age, 60 years). All patients had disabling trapeziometacarpal joint osteoarthritis that was refractory to conservative treatment. All patients had coexisting pathologic conditions that involved the anterior wrist. Three patients were followed for less than 1 year and were withdrawn from the study; 59 hands in 54 patients remained for assessment. The average duration of follow-up was 44 months. Final results were evaluated by subjective and objective means. The height of the scaphometacarpal was measured after pin removal, at 6 months, and each year after that.

Surgical Technique.—The skin incision is made in the thenar crease and continues along the bulge of the flexor carpi radialis (Fig 2). A conventional carpal tunnel release is performed. The flexor carpi radialis is dislocated and the joint capsule opened. The entire trapezium is exposed and excised. The ulnar osteophyte of the trapezium and the common medial osteophyte of the first metacarpal base are also excised. The palmar ligament is reconstructed. The procedure is completed by intermetacarpal Kirschner wiring under slight traction to the first metacarpal. The thumb is immobilized in a spica cast. The splint and wire are removed after 4 weeks, and motion is initiated.

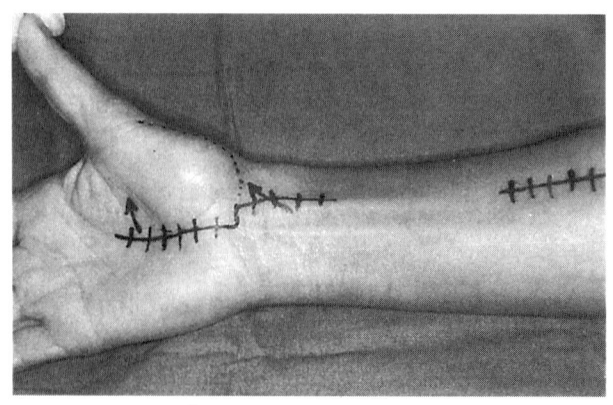

FIGURE 2.—Cutaneous incision for anterior approach. (Courtesy of Le Viet DT, Kerbouli L, Lantieri LA et al: Stabilized resection arthroplasty by an anterior approach in trapeziometacarpal arthritis: Results and surgical technique *J Hand Surg [Am]* 21A:194–201, 1996).

Results.—Pain relief was excellent in 60 hands, good in 7, and fair in 2. Thumb motion was satisfactory in 64 hands. The average strength increase was 30%. Scaphometacarpal space loss was 0.5 mm each year, so that residual space averaged 3.1 mm at 60 months. Two failures occurred in this patient group.

Conclusion.—Trapeziectomy, with an anterior approach, is the procedure of choice for disabling trapeziometacarpal joint arthritis. The treatment is effective with few complications, and permits the treatment of coexisting pathologic disorders of the wrist without additional incisions. The results remain satisfactory after 5 years of follow-up, although the scaphometacarpal space has progressively collapsed. To remedy this, the first metacarpal is no longer fixed under traction.

▶ I suppose it is good to know that one can perform trapeziectomy and carpal tunnel release through the same incision. The combination is certainly common enough. The authors suggest that in their experience, patients treated by an anterior approach have better strength than those treated by the usual lateral approach. However, a randomized trial of the 2 approaches is needed to support their opinion.

This paper continues a 30-year trend in which surgeons report their personal series of carpometacarpal arthritis surgery. Each surgeon has a little personal modification in technique or approach that he or she believes to be better than the alternatives; none has ever taken the step of comparing the results prospectively. The papers are monotonously similar: with the new XYZ procedure, pain relief was noted in 85% to 90% of patients at 2 years, pinch strength increased to 5 kg, 85% to 90% of patients were satisfied, and motion was near normal. These papers have been improved by the use of outcomes assessment (translation, we administered a questionnaire), but the fundamental flaw remains: without a prospective, randomized comparison of alternatives, we cannot say whether any of the options presented is an improvement over the others. In their discussions, most authors consider the ligament reconstruction and tendon interposition procedure the standard—why not have journals require authors of future papers about carpometacarpal surgery to compare their results to that procedure? Either that, or let everyone go their own way (and maybe save a few trees).

P.C. Amadio, M.D.

Osteotomy of the First Metacarpal for Osteoarthrosis of the Basal Joints of the Thumb
Holmberg J, Lundborg G (Lund Univ, Malmö, Sweden)
Scand J Plast Reconstr Hand Surg 30:67–70, 1996   12–8

Objective.—Although several operative techniques have been proposed for the management of osteoarthrosis of the basal joints of the thumb, there is no consensus as to the best procedure. Wedge osteotomy of the first metacarpal has been little studied, but it is a technically simple procedure that does not worsen the conditions for secondary surgery, should it be necessary. The results of wedge osteotomy of the first metacarpal in 18 patients who had osteoarthrosis of the trapeziometacarpal joint were presented.

Methods.—Sixteen women and 2 men, (mean age, 61 years) who had osteoarthrosis of the basal joints of the thumb were included. The scaphotrapezial joint were involved in 6 patients. All patients underwent a radial, 30-degree wedge osteotomy on the first metacarpal bone, approximately 1 cm from the trapeziometacarpal joint. In most patients, fixation was performed with 2 Kirschner wires and an osteosuture in the tension band position, followed by a thumb cast (Fig 1). The subjective and objective results were evaluated at a mean follow-up of 8.5 months.

Results.—Nine patients reported complete satisfaction with their surgical results, 7 were "quite satisfied," and 2 said that their condition was unchanged. None reported that their condition had gotten worse. None of the patients who were completely satisfied had scaphotrapezial joint involvement. Pain at rest was reduced in 15 patients. Grip strength on the operated side averaged 75.5%, and pulp pinch averaged 74.5% of the contralateral side. There was little change in thumb mobility.

Conclusions.—For patients who have osteoarthrosis of the basal joints of the thumb, wedge osteotomy of the first metacarpal provides a simple

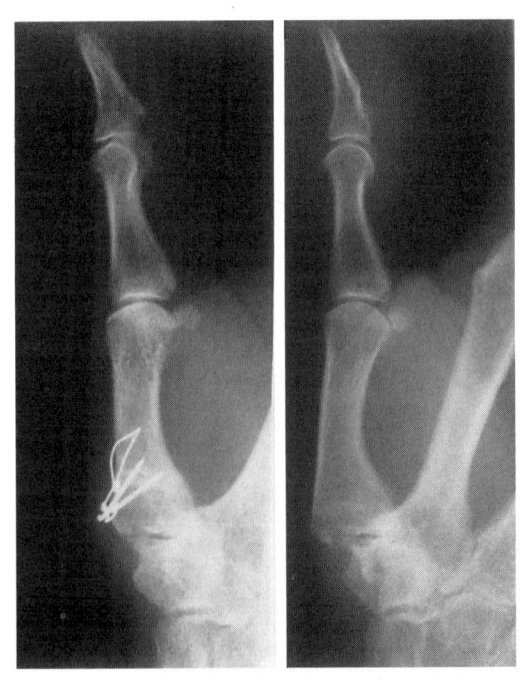

FIGURE 1.—Lateral radiograph of thumb with moderate arthrosis in the trapeziometacarpal joint before (**right**) and after (**left**) wedge osteotomy. (Courtesy of Holmberg J, Lundborg G: Osteotomy of the first metacarpal for osteoarthrosis of the basal joints of the thumb. *Scand J Plast Reconstr Hand Surg* 30:67–70, 1996.)

and safe technique for pain relief. It is especially effective in the early stages of osteoarthrosis and for patients in whom the scaphotrapezial joint is uninvolved. The pain relief obtained with this procedure may be explained by the relief of tension from the volar ligament and the shifting of stress to intact parts of the joint.

▶ This article adds another confirmational study of the efficacy of a closed wedge osteotomy of the first metacarpal for basal joint osteoarthritis which was first described by Wilson.[1] The results were largely satisfactory, even with involvement of the scaphotrapezial joint. In the discussion, the authors suggest that this procedure protects the anterior obligue ligament, whose deterioration has been well documented. It might be more logical to stress that the displacement of the articular surface in a clockwise fashion, so clearly shown in Figure 1, helps stabilize the joint from the posteroradially directed subluxing force at the joint. This displacement reduces the shear stress associated with subluxation and would appear to be more effective than trying to augment the ligament prophylactally.

R.L. Linscheid, M.D.

Reference

1. Wilson JN: Basal osteotomy of the first metacarpal in the treatment of arthritis of the carpometacarpal joint of the thumb. Br J Surg 60:854–858, 1973.

Swanson Silicone Finger Joint Implants: A Review of the Literature Regarding Long-term Complications
Foliart DE (Foliart & Associates, Moraga, Calif)
J Hand Surg (Am) 20A:445–449, 1995   12–9

Introduction.—For more than 30 years, Swanson Silastic joint implants have been used in the arthroplastic resection of finger joints. Complications associated with the Swanson Silastic finger joint implant; including particulate synovitis and lymphadenopathy, were studied.

Materials and Methods.—A literature search on the outcomes of metacarpophalangeal (MCP), proximal interphalangeal (PIP), and distal interphalangeal (DIP) Swanson silicone joint implantation was undertaken. The prevalence of 7 types of complications in 15,556 finger implants was calculated. There were 13,031 MCP implants, 2,463 PIP implants, and 62 DIP implants.

Results.—Particulate synovitis, defined by both histologic findings and by subjective findings of pain after a period of post-surgical improvement, was associated with 6 MCP and PIP implants. In addition, silicone lymphadenopathy was diagnosed in 13 patients who received MCP implants. Non-Hodgkins lymphoma was later diagnosed in 4 of these individuals. Bone resorption was found in 11 PIP implants and in 424 MCP implants. Heterotrophic bone formation and bone cysts were also reported in MCP implants. Fractures to the implants were more common in the earlier 372 Silastic implants than in the later-developed high-performance implants. Other complications associated with MCP implants included loosening of the implant and infections. Eighty-seven MCP implants were removed; the most frequent cause was fracture, and the second most common cause was infection. Proximal interphalangeal implants were removed 52 times, and DIP implants were removed 4 times. Overall, 4% of the Silastic implants were associated with bone changes, and fractures were diagnosed in 2% of them. Particulate synovitis was a complication in less than 1% of the reported cases.

Discussion.—This report may not be representative of all patients who receive Silastic implants, because not all such patients were included. In addition, because patients with advanced rheumatoid arthritis who are immunosuppressed are at greater risk of lymphoma, the finding of a relationship between silicone implants and incidence of lymphoma may be concomitant. No incidence of autoimmune disease was associated with the use of the Swanson Silastic joint implant.

▶ The author provides an exhaustive review of the literature concerning complications of flexible silicone interposition arthroplasties in the fingers. For the purpose of this report, particulate synovitis required the presence of symptoms and histologic findings on tissue sections obtained from operation; therefore, the definition of particulate synovitis is quite stringent in this review and does not include those asymptomatic patients who have previously been described with erosive bone changes noted on radiographs. Among those patients with symptoms and histologic confirmation of particulate synovitis, the prevalence was 0.046% with MCP implants and 0.16% with PIP implants, with a fourfold increase in reported prevalence of particulate synovitis with PIP joint implants. This difference may reflect the greater tendency for MCP implants to be used in the low demand rheumatoid hand, as compared with a PIP joint implant having a much greater likelihood of being used in the more active hand of a patient with erosive or inflammatory osteoarthritis. Conversely, the prevalence of bone resorption around implants was 3.25% with MCP and 0.45% with PIP implants. Fracture was noted in 2.4% of MCP and 1.6% of PIP implants. No correlation was noted between the prevalence of hematologic malignancy, such as lymphoma, and the implantation of a silicone finger prosthesis. This study was funded by Wright Medical Technology, the current owner of manufacturing rights of the silicone finger implant.

V.D. Pellegrini, Jr., M.D.

The Titanium Grommet in Flexible Implant Arthroplasty of the Radiocarpal Joint: A Long-term Review of 44 Cases
Capone RA Jr (Univ of Pittsburgh, Pa)
Plast Reconstr Surg 96:667–672, 1995

Introduction.—The use of flexible implant arthroplasty as a surgical treatment for rheumatoid arthritis (RA) of the radiocarpal joint is controversial. Failure and revision have been reported. Radiocarpal arthrodesis is often performed as treatment for RA, but postoperative motion of the joint is usually reduced. The use of protective titanium grommets in flexible implant arthroplasty was investigated.

Methods.—Forty-four flexible implant arthroplasties, with insertion of titanium grommets as a protective shield between the bone edges and the flexible hinges of the implant, were performed. The preoperative diagnoses varied, but all patients complained of significant pain. Architectural collapse was apparent, and either class III or class IV joint changes were noted on radiograph. Preoperative and postoperative grip strength and wrist extension were also assessed.

Results.—Ninety-one percent of patients reported relief of pain. By surgical design and to prolong the life of the implant, the postoperative wrist motion was restricted to 30 degrees. This restriction did not vary significantly from preoperative values and still allowed for daily activity. The grip strength of the patients who received titanium implants improved 32%. Radiographs of the joints demonstrated that alignment of the third metatarsal on the radius bone improved by 44% after surgery. No synovitis was apparent, but a sclerotic bone reaction at the interface of the bone implant increased the cortical bone width by 2.5-fold. Complications included 2 implant fractures and 2 displacements of the titanium grommets. Secondary fusion occurred in 2 instances. Eighty-seven percent of patients were very satisfied with the titanium implants.

Discussion.—The use of titanium grommets in flexible implant arthroplasty is shown to be a reasonable procedure. Complications were limited, and patient satisfaction was excellent, as pain was eliminated and everyday function was improved. Although this procedure may be refined in the future, the use of titanium grommets in flexible implant arthroplasty is a viable alternative to radial arthrodesis for patients who have RA.

▶ Although hardly a long-term follow-up of the flexible silicone implant radiocarpal arthroplasty, this work provides encouragement for use of this device in selected circumstances. Among 14 patients with a follow-up ranging from 2.7 to 7.8 years (mean, 5.1 years), there were no implant fractures and no radiographic evidence of particulate synovitis in the form of bony erosions. Even more encouraging was the observation that no adverse radiographic changes appeared in the 8 patients for whom follow-up exceeded 5 years, and clinically each wrist had maintained good function. These results are contrasted with a fracture rate of 65% among 20 implants followed for 3–9 years, as reported by Comstock et al.[1] and a fracture rate of

36% (14 of 39) in patients whose status was followed for a minimum of 3 years (average, 5.8 years), as reported by Fatti et al.[2] In this latter report, radiographic deterioration was noted in every patient, and 25% demonstrated cystic changes consistent with particulate synovitis.

Compared with previously published reports in which grommets were not used, the report by Capone may provide reason for guarded enthusiasm in a reassessment of the role of silicone interposition arthroplasty at the wrist. However, the optimism from this report is based on small numbers and awaits validation and more critical review in larger series over longer follow-up.

V.D. Pellegrini, Jr., M.D.

References

1. Comstock CP., Louis DS, Eckenrode JF: Silicone wrist implant: Long-term follow-up study. *J Hand Surg (Am)* 13A:201–205, 1988.
2. Fatti JF, Palmer AK, Greenky S, et al: Long-term results of Swanson interpositional wrist arthroplasty: Part II. *J Hand Surg (Am)* 16A:432–437, 1991.

Excision of the Distal Ulna in Rheumatoid Arthritis: Is the Price Too High?
Nanchahal J, Sykes PJ, Williams RL (Morriston Hosp, Swansea, Wales)
J Hand Surg (Br) 21B:189–196, 1996   12-11

Objective.—Resection of the distal ulna is widely performed to relieve wrist pain, and improve function and motion in patients with rheumatoid arthritis. However, some reports have suggested that removing the ulnar buttress of the wrist may actually worsen some of the deformities associated with rheumatoid arthritis. Several modifications and alternative techniques have been proposed. The results of distal ulnar resection in patients with rheumatoid arthritis were assessed radiographically and compared with the contralateral, nonoperated on wrist.

Methods.—The analysis included 40 patients with rheumatoid arthritis who underwent unilateral excision of the distal ulna. Radiographs of both wrists were obtained and compared for carpal translocation, as determined by 3 different methods: carpal height, radial deviation of the carpus, and the presence of spontaneous radiocarpal fusion or a radial shelf.

Results.—Most patients were free of pain and had improved function in the wrist that had undergone excision of the distal ulna. Reliable measurements were not possible in 1 patient with end-stage disease (Fig 2). Radiocapitate measurement proved to be the most consistent method of assessing carpal translocation. The operation was not associated with significant carpal collapse, ulnar translocation, or radial rotation of the carpus. A radial shelf or limited radiocarpal fusion developed in 61% of operated on wrists, compared to 21% of contralateral wrists (Fig 3). However, this change was not associated with any difference in carpal

Chapter 12–Arthritis / **291**

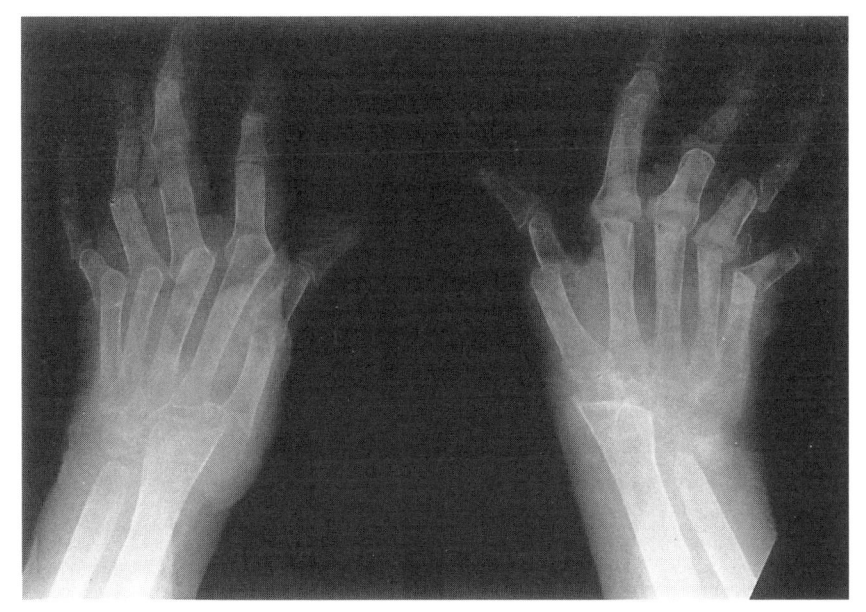

FIGURE 2.—Radiographs of a patient with end-stage (Larsen grade 5) rheumatoid disease, making measurements impracticable. (Courtesy of Nanchahal J, Sykes PJ, Williams RL: Excision of the distal ulna in rheumatoid arthritis: Is the price too high? *J Hand Surg (Br)* 21B:189–196, 1996.)

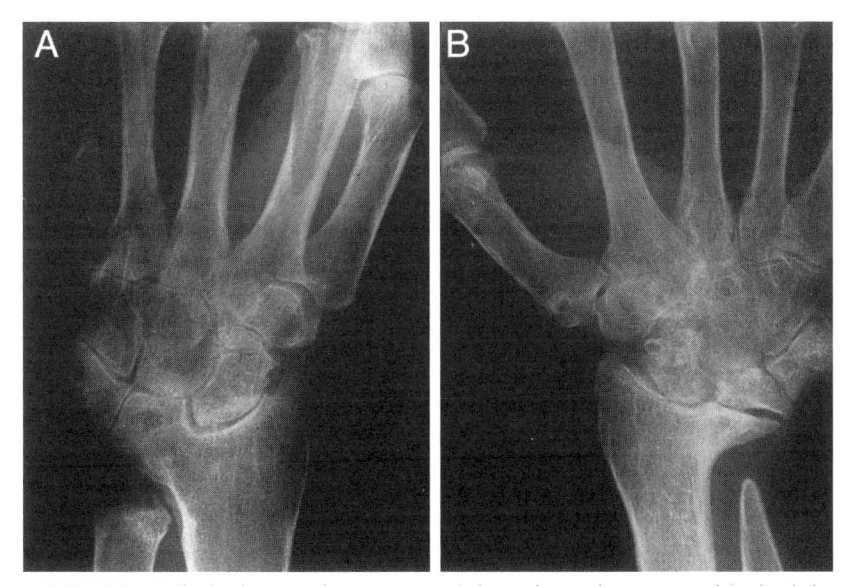

FIGURE 3.—**A**, the development of spontaneous radiolunate fusion after resection of the distal ulna. **B**, the spontaneous development of a radial shelf. (Courtesy of Nanchahal J, Sykes PJ, Williams RL: Excision of the distal ulna in rheumatoid arthritis: Is the price too high? *J. Hand Surg (Br)* 21B:189–196, 1996.)

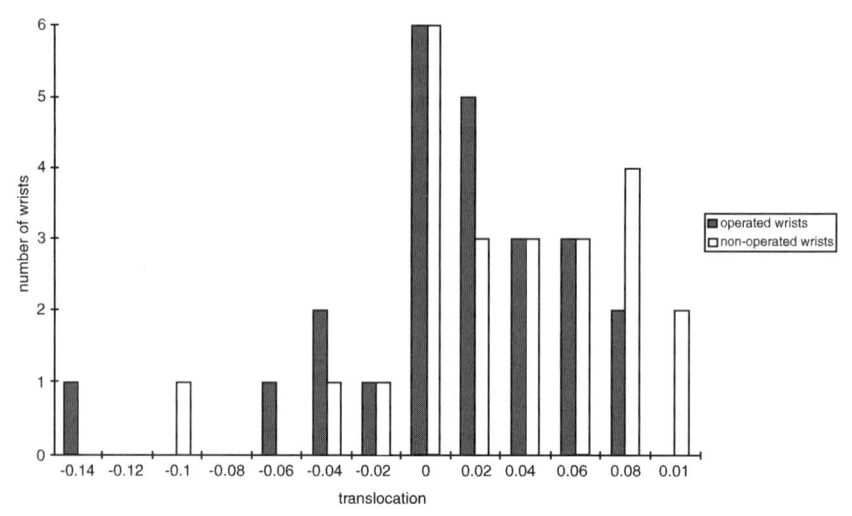

FIGURE 6.—Graphic representation of carpal tunnel translocation of patients who underwent unilateral excision. Positive values represent ulnar translocation and negative values radial translocation. There was no statistically significant difference between the operated and nonoperated wrists of each patient. (Courtesy of Nanchahal J, Sykes PJ, Williams RL: Excision of the distal ulna in rheumatoid arthritis: Is the price too high? *J Hand Surg (Br)* 21B:189–196, 1996.)

collapse or ulnar translocation between the operated on and nonoperated on wrists (Fig 6).

Conclusions.—In patients with rheumatoid arthritis, resection of the distal ulna is not associated with significant radial rotation, collapse, or ulnar translocation of the carpus. Thus the ulnar buttress is not the major structure in controlling these deformities. Although wrists in which excision of the distal ulna has been performed are more likely to develop a radial shelf or limited radiocarpal fusion, this does not reduce ulnar translocation.

▶ The authors have provided an excellent review of ulnar resection and rheumatoid arthritis. Readers should refer to the article for an excellent bibliography. Resecting the distal ulna to alleviate the caput ulnal syndrome to prevent extensor tendon ruptures is certainly valid in rheumatoid arthritis. The authors have suggested that, as there is no difference in ulnar translocation of the wrist whether the ulna is resected, the ulna itself should not be implicated as the source of the problem in ulnar translocation of the wrist, which is so often seen in combination with radial deviation and intercarpal supination in rheumatoid wrist deformity. It would be my strong recommendation in patients undergoing ulnar resection, that the radiolunate joint be stabilized to prevent ulnar translocation because the authors have shown that it occurs in both operative and nonoperative groups; this is an undesirable feature. Therefore, stabilization seems appropriate. Based on my experience with the occasional rapid deterioration of wrist position with ulnar translocation after distal ulnar resection, I now always perform a

Chamay-type radiolunate fusion in conjunction with distal ulnar resection; In so doing, one necessarily stops the progressive deformity of the wrist identified in both the operative and nonoperative groups in this study.

R.D. Beckenbaugh, M.D.

Rheumatoid Factor and HLA Antigens in Wrist Tenosynovitis and Humeral Epicondylitis

Malmivaara A, Viikari-Juntura E, Huuskonen M, et al (Finnish Inst of Occupational Health, Helsinki; Natl Public Health Inst, Helsinki; Occupational Health Care Ctr of Tampere, Finland; et al)
Scand J Rheumatol 24:154–156, 1995   12–12

Introduction.—Etiologic factors for tenosynovitis and peritendinitis of the wrist and forearm seem to be high repetition and high-force demands of work movements. Little is known about the role of host factors in these disorders, and less is known about the etiology of epicondylitis. A systemic inflammatory disorder, rheumatoid arthritis is characterized by chronic synovitis, and peritendinitis and tenosynovitis are frequently accompanying disorders. Little is known about the relationship between upper limb soft-tissue disorders and HLA antigens or rheumatoid factor. To assess whether rheumatoid factor (RF) is associated with peritendinitis or repeating tenosynovitis and whether HLA-B27 predisposes to epicondylitis, a matched case-referent study was conducted.

Methods.—Twenty workers in manually strenuous jobs with a history of at least 2 episodes of peritendinitis or tenosynovitis in the forearm or wrist, or humeral epicondylitis, were studied along with their matched referents.

Results.—In 7 of the 23 (30%) patients with tenosynovitis and in 1 (4%) of the referents, the latex agglutination test was positive for RF. In 10 of the 23 patients (43%) with tenosynovitis and 2 (9%) of the referents, IgM-RF showed up on enzyme-linked immunosorbent assay. All the patients who had positive results to the latex agglutination test also had positive results in the IgM-RF test. In 5 of the 13 workers with epicondylitis (38%) and in 1 with no such history, HLA-B27 antigen was found.

Conclusion.—An incomplete form of rheumatoid arthritis may be represented by RF-positive repeating tenosynovitis. In patients with established rheumatoid arthritis and the frequent occurrence of tenosynovitis, RF may be associated with tenosynovitis without any other clinical manifestations of rheumatoid disease.

▶ This study lends credence to the possibility of an immunologic basis for such conditions as peritendinitis in the wrist and humeral epicondylitis.

V.R. Hentz, M.D.

Quantitative Analysis of Hand Radiographs in Rheumatoid Arthritis: Time Course of Radiographic Changes, Relation to Joint Examination Measures, and Comparison of Different Scoring Methods

Pincus T, Callahan LF, Fuchs HA, et al (Vanderbilt School of Medicine, Nashville, Tenn; Ctrs for Disease Control and Prevention, Atlanta, Ga; Hosp for Special Surgery, New York; et al)
J Rheumatol 22:1983–1989, 1995

Objective.—There are several scoring methods for determining radiographic damage in rheumatoid arthritis (RA). The radiographic scoring according to the Steinbrocker, modified Sharp, and Larsen methods were compared, and articular damage to hands of patients with RA was quantitated.

Methods.—Radiographs from 210 patients were scored by each method, and joint count was determined according to the glossary of the American Rheumatoid Arthritis Association for joint tenderness, pain on motion, swelling, limited motion, and deformity.

Results.—Radiographic scores and scores for joint space narrowing, erosions, and malalignment were significantly correlated with duration of disease. Radiographic abnormalities were seen in 93% of patients who had disease duration less than 2 years. Radiographic scores were significantly correlated with joint swelling and highly significantly correlated with joint deformity and limited motion. Scores using all 3 methods were significantly correlated, particularly for limited motion and deformity and less so for joint swelling.

Conclusion.—All 3 methods provide quantitative measures of radiographic damage in the hands of patients who have RA and should be more commonly used to track progress of disease. Scoring systems should be simplified.

▶ This comparison study of the most widely used scoring systems for progression of RA in the hand and wrist shows high intercorrelation and good correlation between radiographic progression and certain clinical parameters.

G. Bergman, M.D.

Treatment of Fingernail Deformities Secondary to Ganglions of the Distal Interphalangeal Joint

Gingrass MK, Brown RE, Zook EG (Southern Illinois Univ, Springfield)
J Hand Surg (Am) 20A:502–505, 1995

Introduction.—Fingernail deformities may develop in patients who have ganglions of the distal interphalangeal (DIP) joint when cyst excision accompanies débridement of the osteocytes. Treatment of the DIP ganglions, by débridement of the osteocytes only, was investigated.

Patients and Methods.—Twenty fingernail deformities of the DIP joint were treated by removal of the osteophytes and drainage of the ganglion cyst only.

Results.—Three years after surgical treatment, there was no recurrence of ganglions in any of the digits. In most cases, resolution of the nail bed deformity resulted. In addition, joint pain was relieved in 8 of the 9 patients who had preoperative complaints of pain.

Discussion.—Intralesional injection and occlusive treatment have been reported in the treatment of DIP joint ganglions. Excision of the cyst usually leads to ganglion recurrence. It has recently become recognized that treatment of the associated osteophytes is critical. When the ganglions were not excised, residual nail deformities decreased from 36% to only 10% of patients, and the ganglions did not recur. Excision of the ganglion cyst may lead to injury of the germinal matrix, and DIP joint ganglions are best treated by débridement of the osteophytes only without excision of the ganglion cyst.

▶ This prospective review of 20 patients who had mucous cysts of the DIP joint should change the way we treat these common problems. Ganglions of the DIP joint can be successfully débrided by DIP joint osteophyte débridement alone, without excision of overlying skin and its accompanying problems.

E. Akelman, M.D.

Suggested Reading

LeViet DT, Kerboull L, Lantieri LA, et al: Stabilized resection arthroplasty by an anterior approach in trapeziometacarpal arthritis: Results and surgical technique. *J Hand Surg* 21A:194–201, 1996.
▶ This article suggests an anterior, midline, palmar approach to treat coexistent thumb carpometacarpal (CMC) arthritis and carpal tunnel syndrome (CTS). It documents nothing with respect to carpal tunnel signs, symptoms, and diagnosis. There is no mention of the clinical diagnosis or nerve conduction studies. The condition of the nerve at the time of surgery was not addressed. No postoperative results with respect to CTS outcome are presented.

In the carefully selected patient who has coexisting CTS and thumb CMC arthritis in whom conservative treatment has failed on both accounts, this approach may be useful. It would not, however, be my standard incision for treatment of basilar thumb arthritis, as it appears to have become for these authors.

C.H. Johnson, M.D.

Juutilainen T, Pätiälä: Arthrodesis in rheumatoid arthritis using absorbable screws and rods. *Scand J Rheumatol* 24:228–233, 1995.
▶ The authors described several techniques to effect fusion of the wrist and thumb using absorbable rods. All require predrilling channels for placement of the rod (an extra operative step). Results were equivalent to those obtained with more standard methods of fixation.

V.R. Hentz, M.D.

13 Tumors

Giant Cell Tumor of the Distal Radius
Sheth DS, Healey JH, Sobel M, et al (Mem Sloan-Kettering Cancer Ctr, New York)
J Hand Surg (Am) 20A:432–440, 1995   13–1

Introduction.—Giant cell tumors at the distal end of the radius present special problems because of their location, and the recurrence rate is high after treatment with curettage alone. The outcome in a large consecutive series of patients who underwent curettage and cryosurgery or en bloc excision was reviewed.

Methods.—Twenty-six of 30 patients who had undergone treatment between 1958 and 1988 were available for follow-up. There were 14 women and 12 men; their mean age was 34 years. Nine patients were referred after local recurrence of giant cell tumor of the distal radius. Tumors were classified as grade 1 in 2 patients, grade 2 in 8 patients, and grade 3 in 16 patients. Eight patients, including 5 who had previously untreated tumors and 3 who had recurrent tumors, were treated with en bloc excision of the radius. The remaining patients underwent intralesional excision with cryosurgery. All those in the en bloc excision group had reconstruction with wrist arthrodesis. Wrist arthrodesis was performed in 3 additional patients after intralesional excision because of fragmentation of the distal radius, failure of graft incorporation, and carpal collapse.

Results.—Twenty-two patients returned for physical examination, and 2 submitted follow-up x-ray films for evaluation. Follow-up information was also available from the physicians of 2 patients who had died of unrelated causes. With a median follow-up of 9 years, local occurrence was reported in 3 of 12 patients who were treated with primary curettage and cryosurgery. With repeat curettage and cryosurgery, local control was achieved in 16 of 18 primary and recurrent cases. There were no instances of local recurrence in those patients who underwent en bloc excision and arthrodesis. Complications included skin necrosis, transient nerve palsies, and fragmentation with carpal collapse in the curettage and cryosurgery group and failure of internal fixation and non-union of the graft-radius junction in the en bloc excision group. Strength and function were similar in both groups at follow-up (Table 1).

TABLE 1.—Functional Evaluation

	Pain			Return to Work	Grip strength (%)	Pinch strength (%)	Range of motion (%)	Rating*			
	None	Slight	Moderate					Excellent	Good	Fair	Poor
Currettage plus cryosurgery (11 patients)	9	2	0	10	65	68	61	1	8	1	1
Primary excision (5 patients)	5	0	0	5	64	64	N/A	0	3	2	0
Secondary excision (3 patients)	2	0	1	3	57	47	N/A	0	2	0	1
Reconstructive fusion (3 patients)	1	2	0	3	47	47	N/A	0	1	2	0

* Musculoskeletal Tumor Society rating.
Abbreviation: N/A, data not available.
(Courtesy of Sheth DS, Healey JH, Sobel M, et al: Giant cell tumor of the distal radius. *J Hand Surg (Am)* 20A:432–440, 1995.)

Conclusion.—Intralesional excision with adjunctive cryosurgery offers an effective alternative to en bloc excision of giant cell tumors of the distal radius. Although the former method of treatment can preserve the distal radius and wrist joint function, complications and recurrence remain a risk. En bloc excision is a more prudent choice for patients who have extensive cortical fragmentation and is undertaken as salvage for failed intralesional excision.

▶ We prefer to reconstruct the distal radius with a vascularized proximal fibular transfer rather than excision, bone graft, and fusion. In a small series, the average flexion-extension axis has averaged 50%.

V.R. Hentz, M.D.

Infantile Digital Fibromas
Falco NA, Upton J (Harvard Med School, Boston)
J Hand Surg (Am) 20A:1014–1020, 1995   13–2

Background.—Infantile digital fibroma is a proliferative fibrous disorder of the upper extremity that occurs in childhood. The tumor has a distinctive histology (Fig 4) and shows a predictable growth pattern. Its etiology remains unknown. The records of 8 children who were treated for multiple lesions between 1977 and 1991 were reviewed.

Patients.—Five girls and 3 boys, aged 5–68 months, were treated for 15 infantile digital fibroma lesions involving 10 separate fingers. Ten lesions involved the distal interphalangeal (DIP) joint, and 5 were proximal interphalangeal (PIP) masses. None of the lesions were attached to the extensor mechanism. All 10 DIP lesions were treated with wide excision. Eight digits were covered with hypothenar skin grafts, and the other 2 with cross-finger flaps after extensive pulp excision, collateral ligament resection, and joint exposure. The 5 PIP masses were covered with local rotation flaps or advancement flaps.

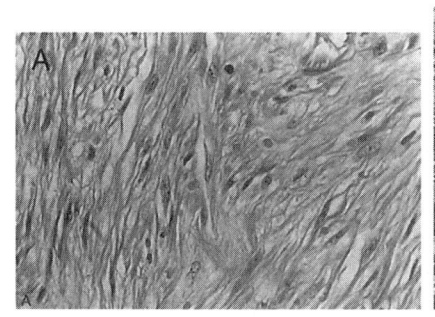

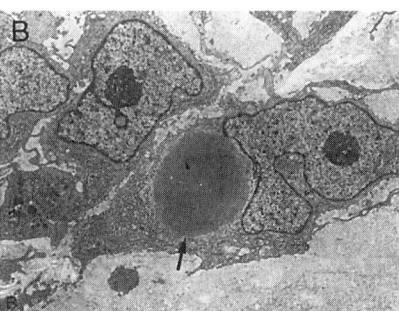

FIGURE 4.—**A**, histology reveals an irregular, wavy pattern of fibroblasts, few mitoses, and characteristic intracytoplasmic inclusion bodies. **B**, electron microscopy demonstrates an inclusion body (*arrow*) next to a nucleus. Black stain within the inclusion is artifact. (Original magnification, ×10,680.) (Courtesy of Falco NA, Upton J: Infantile digital fibromas. *J Hand Surg (Am)* 20A:1014–1020, 1995.)

TABLE 2.—Fibrous Proliferations of Infancy and Childhood

Diagnosis	Reference	Location	Recurrence
Infantile digital fibromatosis	Sakurane,[1] 1924, Reye,[3] 1965	Digits	Common
Juvenile oponeurotic fibroma/calcifying fibroma	Keasbey,[36] 1953	Palmar and plantar surfaces	Common
Infantile myofibromatosis/congenital fibromatosis	Stout,[7] 1954, Schnitka et al/,[37] 1958	Soft tissue, bone, and viscera	Rare
Infantile desmoid type fibromatosis/infantile and juvenile fibromatosis	Stout,[7] 1954	Musculature	Common
Giant cell fibroblastoma	Shmookler and Enzinger,[38] 1982	Thigh, back, inguinal region	Common
Hyaline fibromatosis	Murray,[39] 1873	Dermis and subcutis	—
Fibrous hamartoma/subdermal fibromatous tumor of infancy	Reye,[40] 1956	Axillary and inguinal regions	Rare
Fibromatosis colli	Taylor,[41] 1875	Sternocleidomastoid muscle	Rare

(Courtesy of Falco NA, Upton J: Infantile digital fibromas. *J Hand Surg (Am)* 20A:1014–1020 1995.)

Outcome.—None of the patients experienced flap or graft loss. At annual follow-up examinations for up to 14 years, none of the children showed joint distortion, and the range of motion of all involved joints has remained normal.

Discussion.—Infantile digital fibroma is one of several fibromatous disorders of childhood. Other fibrous proliferations of infancy and childhood include juvenile aponeurotic fibroma, infantile myofibromatosis, giant cell fibroblastoma, and fibrous hamartoma (Table 2). Digital fibromas should not be confused with palmar fibromatoses, which also grow rapidly and often have a histologic appearance that is consistent with fibrosarcoma. Recognition of the typical features of this tumor that distinguish it from other fibrous proliferative lesions, including malignancies with their potential for metastasis, is essential for selecting the appropriate treatment.

▶ This excellent review presents the current state of knowledge for this perplexing tumor of childhood. Although there is considered to be a high recurrent rate for this neoplasm, only 1 of 15 lesions recurred in this series.

The authors present options for reconstruction after adequate excision, and review the important characteristics that define fibromatoses. These characteristics include "(1) proliferation of well-differentiated fibroblasts; (2) an infiltrative pattern of growth; (3) the presence of a variable (but usually abundant) amount of collagen between proliferating cells; (4) a lack of cytologic features of malignancy and scanty or absent mitotic activity; and (5) aggressive clinical behavior characterized by local recurrences but without the capacity to produce distant metastases."

The fibrous proliferations encountered in this age group are nicely summarized by the authors in Table 2. In addition, the histologic characteristics are beautifully displayed in Figure 4.

Wide excision is the recommended treatment. These lesions may be technically demanding to treat and often require either skin graft or flap reconstruction.

E. Fleegler, M.D.

Angioleiomyomas of the Hand: A Report of 14 Cases
Lawson GM, Salter DM, Hooper G (Edinburgh Univ, Scotland)
J Hand Surg (Br) 20B:479–483, 1995

13–3

Introduction.—Angioleiomyoma is a rare, benign, smooth-muscle tumor. It arises from the tunica media of small veins and arteries and occurs more commonly in the lower limb. Most of these tumors are seen in patients aged 30–60 years, with a male:female ratio of about 1:2. The symptoms are classically tenderness and pain. Fourteen cases of angioleiomyomas of the hand were described.

Patients.—Between 1986 and 1994, 8 men and 6 women, aged 16–86 years, were seen with angioleiomyomas of the hand. Four lesions occurred in the dorsal aspect of the hand, and 10 occurred on the volar aspect. The mean duration was 3 years. Tenderness was present in only 6 patients. One patient had paroxysmal pain, and 10 complained of poor appearance and increasing size. All lesions were excised. On the basis of the classification of Morimoto, 5 lesions were solid, 7 were venous, 1 was cavernous, and 1 was both venous and cavernous. Five lesions had nerve fibers adjacent to or within the tumor capsule, and 3 had nerve fibers within the substance of the lesion. There was no correlation between histologic appearance and symptoms. None of the tumors recurred after excision. None of the tumors were correctly diagnosed before surgery.

Summary.—Unlike angioleiomyomas elsewhere, those that occur in the hand are less commonly painful, have an equal sex distribution, and are not predominantly of the solid type. Nerve fibers can be present within the lesion, a finding that had not previously been reported.

▶ The authors have given us another tumor to be considered in the differential diagnosis of masses of the hand and upper extremity. The lesion in question fits into more superficially located masses that may or may not cause pain and are noted to increase gradually in size, although occasionally growth can be rapid. Many of the tumors in question are painful. Therefore, when considering lesions that have these worrisome findings, it is good to have such a well-presented paper for review.

E. Fleegler, M.D.

Extradigital Glomus Tumour
Takei TR, Nalebuff EA (New England Baptist Hosp, Boston)
J Hand Surg (Br) 20B:409–412, 1995   13–4

Introduction.—Glomus tumors are relatively uncommon, solitary, small, bluish-red nodules that affect the extremities, usually the digits. Symptoms consist of a triad of pain, tenderness, and cold sensitivity. A case of an extradigital glomus tumor was described.

> *Case Report.*—Woman, 57, had chronic, severe pain and localized tenderness on the dorso-radial aspect of the distal forearm. Cold frequently exacerbated the symptoms. Under Bier-block anesthesia, surgical exploration with loop magnification identified a 4-mm glomus tumor adjacent to the superficial radial nerve. Excision of the tumor resulted in complete resolution of symptoms.

Discussion.—A review of the literature suggests that the incidence of extradigital tumors in the upper extremity may be more frequent than previously recognized. The frequency of extradigital tumors on the upper extremity varies from 11% to 65%; the forearm is the most common extradigital location. Because of its subcutaneous location in extradigital areas, the absence of objective findings often results in diagnostic delay, as evidenced by the protracted duration of symptoms. Imaging modalities may demonstrate the presence of a lesion but are not specific, which emphasizes the need for a high index of clinical suspicion. Complete excision of the tumor offers dramatic relief of pain.

▶ This thought-provoking article includes a good review of the glomus tumor. The information provided will also help in evaluating patients who complain of areas of localized pain in the upper extremity. In this reviewers opinion, when treating a mass of upper extremity when one does not have the biopsy information available to prove it is benign and not likely to spread, techniques such as the Bier-block anesthesia, which involve exsanguinating the limb and compressing the tumor, are not recommended.

E. Fleegler, M.D.

A Modified Open Palm Technique for Dupuytren's Disease: Short and Long Term Results in 54 Patients
Foucher G, Cornil C, Lenoble E, et al (SOS Main, Strasbourg, France; St Anthony's Hosp, Cheam, United Kingdom)
Int Orthop 19:285–288, 1995   13–5

Objective.—Numerous operative techniques have evolved over the years to treat Dupuytren's disease. The results of the open wound technique for the palm, fingers, or both in 54 patients who had Dupuytren's disease were reviewed retrospectively.

Methods.—Postoperative complications and risk of recurrence of Dupuytren's disease were assessed in 67 fingers of 4 women and 50 men who underwent surgery between 1984 and 1985. Twenty patients had a family history of Dupuytren's disease. Eight patients had stage 4 disease, 11 had stage 3, 25 had stage 2, and 10 had stage 1.

> *Technique.*—A transverse incision along the middle palmar crease, extended by a Bruner incision inverted at the level of the transverse incisions, was partly closed with a V-Y plasty. Transverse palmar and digital incisions were left open (Fig 1). A splint was applied for 2–3 months. Mobilization began the day after surgery.

Results.—Healing averaged 25 days, and mean time off work was 28 days. Six of 11 patients who had postoperative pain used prescription pain killers. One patient who received anticoagulants had postoperative bleed-

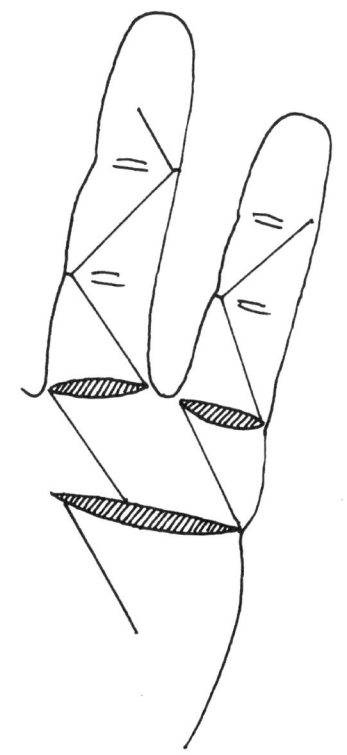

FIGURE 1.—Diagram shows the type of approach used for the ring and little fingers in which transverse and Bruner incisions are combined. The transverse incisions are left open. (Courtesy of Foucher G, Cornil C, Lenoble E, et al: A modified open palm technique for Dupuytren's disease; Short and long term results in 54 patients. *Int Orthop* 19:285–288, 1995, copyright Springer-Verlag.)

ing. There were no cases of hematoma or flap necrosis. Three patients had distal dysesthesia; 1 case was permanent. In 5 patients, reflex sympathetic dystrophy developed. There were 9 severe recurrences (disease reappearance at operative site) with extension (disease appearance distant from the operative site) and 3 without extension, 3 moderate recurrences with extension and 6 without, and 7 extensions without recurrence. Only 23% of patients required reoperation. Overall improvement of the flexion deformity was 71%. Mean time to recurrence was 3.3 years. Eighty percent of patients were satisfied, and 10% were dissatisfied. Older age, degree of proximal interphalangeal joint involvement, and disease localized to the little finger are unfavorable prognostic factors.

Conclusion.—Although this study is small, the complication rate was very low, and the operation appears to be suitable for older patients.

▶ This paper is only the second report with more than 5 years of follow-up to show the usefulness of the open palm technique. A re-emphasis on the importance of this technique is valuable. The combination of this technique with more standard incisions in the fingers is a useful additional option that I have successfully used in the past. Finally, this report is an excellent contemporary review of the current understanding of this technique and the outcome of surgical treatment of Dupuytren's disease, the complications associated with surgical treatment, and the problems of recurrence and extension.

L.C. Hurst, M.D.

Correlation of α-Smooth Muscle Actin Expression and Contraction in Dupuytren's Disease Fibroblasts
Tomasek J, Rayan GM (Univ of Oklahoma Health Sciences Ctr, Oklahoma City)
J Hand Surg (Am) 20A:450–455, 1995   13–6

Background.—Smooth muscle (α-sm) actin microfilaments can develop in specialized fibroblasts in the affected palmar fascia of Dupuytren's disease. Whether an increase in α-sm actin is associated with increased contractile forces in Dupuytren's fibroblasts was studied.

Methods.—Explant cultures of fibroblasts from the palmar fascia of 11 patients who had Dupuytren's disease and a control group of 6 who had carpal tunnel release were stained by indirect immunofluorescence to demonstrate what proportion contained α-sm actin. Fibroblasts from each patient were then cultured in stabilized lattices of type I collagen. The percentage of contraction of each fibroblast-containing lattice, after it was freed from its substratum, was measured.

Results.—Significantly more Dupuytren's fibroblasts (14%) demonstrated the presence of α-sm actin than did control fibroblasts (5%). For 6 patients who had Dupuytren's disease, more than 15% of fibroblasts were positive for the actin. Overall, there was no significant difference in the percentage of lattice contraction when Dupuytren's and control fibroblast cultures were compared. However, the lattices of the 6 Dupuytren's fibroblast cultures with greater than 15% α-sm actin expression contracted significantly more than did those of the other 5 patients or the controls.

Conclusions.—Among patients who have Dupuytren's disease, palmar fascial fibroblasts exhibit varying degrees of α-sm actin production. As the proportion of fibroblasts that produce actin increases, their ability to contract a collagen lattice increases.

▶ The authors have performed a very interesting in vitro study to quantify expression of α-sm actin in Dupuytren's (myo)fibroblasts with correlation to the amount of contractile force generated in a collagen lattice contraction assay. The authors have concluded that when more than 15% of Dupuytren's (myo)fibroblasts expressed α-sm actin, there was more significant contraction of the collagen lattice than in normal, control, palmar fibroblasts.

Drs. Tomasek and Rayan continue to add greatly to our knowledge of the molecular pathogenesis of Dupuytren's disease. There is one finding in this fine study, however, that remains unexplained. The authors found that the variation in expression of α-sm actin in Dupuytren's (myo)fibroblasts may reflect explant cultures from varying disease stages, which the authors did not predetermine. Thus, greater percentages of cells that contain α-sm actin would be expected in the proliferative and involutional, but not residual, disease stages. Future studies may determine this relationship.

The authors are to be commended on a fine study that may provide a foundation in basic science for future clinical therapy for Dupuytren's disease.

M.A. Badalamente, Ph.D.

Can Dupuytren's Contracture Be Work-related? Review of the Evidence
Liss GM, Stock SR (Ontario Ministry of Labour, Toronto; Montreal Dept of Public Health)
Am J Ind Med 29:521–532, 1996

Background.—Dupuytren's contracture (DC) affects the palmar fascia, causing thickened and contracted fibrous bands on the palmar surface of the hands and fingers. The possible involvement of acute traumatic injury or cumulative biomechanical work exposure in the cause of DC is controversial. The published literature was reviewed to investigate evidence of associations between DC and either frequent or repetitive manual work or hand vibration.

Methods.—The literature was searched by computer and manually to identify controlled studies evaluating associations between DC and manual work, vibration, or traumatic injury. The validity of the studies was assessed by 3 examiners, on the basis of 7 criteria.

TABLE 2.—Studies of Manual Work and Dupuytren's Contracture

Feature/ Study	Herzog	Early	Hueston	Mikkelsen	Bennett
Country (year)	U.K. (1951)	U.K. (1962)	Australia (1960)	Norway (1978, 1990)	U.K. (1982)
Design	Cross-sectional	Cross-sectional	Cross-sectional	Population-based survey	Cross-sectional
Study subjects	503 steel workers > 40 years old 451 miners > 40 years old	4,454 male manual workers at locomotive works (4,375 <65 years old)	530 male brewery workers	477 males, 6 females in heavy work; 2,304 males, 4,710 females in medium work; 2,285 males, 707 females in light work	216 workers at PVC bagging and packing plant
Control subjects	480 clers >40 years old	427 male office workers at same locomotive works (426 <65 years old)	550 male office workers	1,805 males, 1,104 females in non-manual work	1) 84 workers at another plant with no bagging or packing; 2) also compared with prevalence among male workers (clerical and manual) from Early (1962)
Exclusions	Not stated	Not stated	Not stated	Response rate to survey 71% for males, 82.4% for females; occupation obtained only for 13,415 of 15,950 residents examined.	No exclusions at study plant Not stated for other plant
Outcome	Presence of DC; no grading system	Presence of DC; system of staging reported	DC on examination of hands: thickening in palm either as nodule or plaque/band accepted	Examination of town inhabitants for presence of DC based on finding of nodules	DC on inspection of hands: used scheme from Early [1962]
Binding of examiners/ assessors	Not stated	Not stated	Not stated	Not stated	Not stated

Exposure	Manual vs. non-manual (clerks)	Manual vs. office workers (job title)	Presumed manual vs. office	Type of work: "heavy," "medium," "light," "non-manual"	Bagging and packing vs. 1) no bagging and packing; 2) manual and clerical workers at locomotive works (Early, 1962) Asked about tools and chemicals handled through career
Confounders measured	Age restriction; no stratification	Age	Age	Gender	Age, gender Asked about family history, past illness, injuries, alcohol
Analysis	In original: %, OR*	In original: % (relative frequency), M-H χ^2, OR*	In original: %, M-H χ^2, OR*	In original: %, M-H χ^2, OR adjusted for gender*	% and indirect standardization (morbidity ratio)
Conclusion	"Slight differences in incidence between clerks and workmen is of no significance"	Prevalence of DC no different in manual vs. office	DC prevalence no higher in brewery workers	Prevalence of DC increased with increasing heaviness of work	Prevalence of DC increased at bagging and packing plant

* By authors.
Abbreviations: DC, Dupuytren's contracture; M-H χ^2, Mantel-Haenszel chi-square; OR, odds ratio.
(Courtesy of Liss GM, Stock SR: Can Dupuytren's contracture be work-related? Review of the evidence. *Am J Ind Med* 29:521–532, Copyright 1996. Reprinted by permission of Wiley Liss, Inc., a subsidiary of John Wiley & Sons, Inc.)

TABLE 3.—Studies on Vibration and Dupuytren's Contracture

Feature/Study	Landgrot	Patri	Cocco	Thomas and Clarke	Bovenzi
Country (year) Design	Czechoslovakia (1975) Cross-sectional	France (1982) Cross-sectional	Italy (1987) Case-control	U.K. (1992) Cross-sectional	Italy (1994) Population-based cross-sectional survey
Study subjects	807 workers exposed to vibration (791 < 65 years old)	107 lumberjacks exposed to vibration	Cases: 180 cases of DC identified from 14,557 clinical files of Instituto di Medicina del Lavoro of Cagliari, 1970–1985	500 claimants considered to have VWF assessed 1988–1990 (311 aged 50–85)	570 quarry drillers and stonecarvers exposed to vibration
Control subjects	444 maintenance workers and clerical workers	115 manual workers not using vibrating devices	Controls: 180 subjects from same files without evidence of DC, matched with a case by sex, age (± 5 years), and hospitalization (± 7 days)	150 consecutive males aged 50–85 admitted to Middlesborough Hospital for elective or emergency treatment to surgical ward; none had VWF symptoms	258 stone workers (manual polishers and machine operators) not exposed to vibration
Exclusions	Not stated	Not stated	All cases of contracture included	None stated	None (all participated); random sampling of controls
Outcome	Presence of DC; grading not stated	Examination of hands (no details or grading system reported)	Cases defined by presence of definite contracture (initial stage with only nodules, isolated palmar fascia thickening or knuckle pads not considered)	Exposed: "all stages of DC from nodule to contracture". Controls: examined for presence of DC following admission	DC on examination of hands; no grading stated (on correspondence, indicated grading scheme used)
Binding of examiners/assessors	Not stated	Not stated	(Binding to case status during determination of exposure); not stated	No	Not stated (on correspondence, indicated that examiners were blinded to exposure status)

	Exposure	Vibration exposed (pneumatic tool operators, forestry, miners, stonecutters, grinders) vs. controls (maintenance workers, machine shop, clerical workers)	Vibration exposure (66 of 107 had VWF) vs. controls ("manual" workers not using vibrating devices, < 50 hours/year)	Occupational history used to establish exposure to vibration, its duration, and tools used during work activity (exposed defined as miners, hammer-drill operators, stonecutters, construction workers, saw-mill workers, sawing-machine, milling, or grinding-machine operators); photoplethysmography of fingers performed to investigate angiopathy	Vibration exposure vs. controls (102 heavy manual labor, 29 clerks and teachers, 19 semi-skilled and unskilled occupations)	Quarry drillers used rock breakers and drills; stonecarvers: some used only rotary tools (angle grinders) and others used both rotary and percussive tools (angle grinders and light stone hammers). Vibration measured in terms of hr/d, d/yr, and total years. Vibration measured on handles of representative sample of tools according to ISO 5349 under actual conditions by accelerometers to yield lifetime vibration dose
Confounders measured	Age	No age stratification; controls recruited so average age similar	Age and sex matching, alcohol	Age restriction	Age, smoking, alcohol consumption, upper limb injuries, leisure activities, other diseases
Analysis	In original: %, OR*	In original: %, OR*	OR, χ² for trend	In original: %, χ² OR*	%, OR with adjustment for age, smoking, alcohol consumption, and upper limb injuries
Conclusion	"No substantial difference in incidence of DC between various occupations"	Frequency of stage 1 DC identical among lumberjacks and manual workers; DC similar among lumberjacks with and without VWF	Statistically significant increase in risk of DC in workers occupationally exposed to vibration; a dose-response relationship between duration of employment in jobs with use of vibrating tools and risk of DC observed. Same result observed considering only miners	Prevalence of DC increased in vibration-exposed (VWF) claimants	Prevalence of DC was higher in quarry drillers (11.0%); stonecarvers using only rotary drills (6.4%); and stonecarvers using both rotary and percussive tools (12.2%) than in controls (3.5%). Prevalence and OR increased with increasing lifetime vibration dose category. However, trend statistic was not significant

* By authors.
Abbreviations: DC, Dupuytren's contracture; OR, odds ratio; VWF, vibration white finger.
(Courtesy of Liss GM, Stock SR: Can Dupuytren's contracture be work-related? Review of the evidence. *Am J Ind Med* 29:521–532, Copyright 1996. Reprinted by permission of Wiley Liss, Inc., a subsidiary of John Wiley & Sons, Inc.

TABLE 5.—Validity Assessment Results of Studies of Manual Work/Vibration and Dupuytren's Contracture

	Herzog (1951)	Hueston (1960)	Early (1962)	Mikkelsen (1978)	Bennett (1982)	Thomas and Clarke (1992)	Landgrot et al. (1975)	Patri et al. (1982)	Cocco et al. (1987)	Bovenzi et al. (1994)
Population										
Selection bias	1	1	1	2	1	2	1	1	2	2
Nonrespondent bias	1	1	1	2	2	3	1	1	2	2
Comparable groups*	2	2	2.5	1	2.5	2	2	2	2.5	3
Exposure										
Confounders	1	1	1	1	2	1	1	2	2	3
Valid exposure measures*	1	1	1	1	2	2	1	2	2	2
Outcome										
Valid outcome measures*	1	2	3	3	3	2	2	1	2	3†
Blinding of examiners	1	1	1	1	1	1	1	1	1	3†
Total (out of 21)	8	9	10.5	11	13.5	13	9	10	13.5	18

* Criteria considered most likely to compromise validity (if score of 1).
† Based on correspondence with author.
(Courtesy of Liss GM, Stock SR: Can Dupuytren's contracture be work-related? Review of the evidence. Am J Ind Med 29:521–532, Copyright 1996. Reprinted by permission of Wiley Liss, Inc., a subsidiary of John Wiley & Sons, Inc.)

TABLE 4.—Results of Studies of Manual Work/Vibration and Dupuytren's Contracture

Study	Comparison for DC	Odds Ratio	95% CI
Studies of manual exposure			
Bennett (1982)*	Bagging plant vs:		
	Non-bagging plant	5.5	0.8–36.7
	Office and manual locomotive workers	1.98	1.1–3.2
Early (1962)	Manual vs. clerical	(observed, 16; expected, 8.08)	
Mikkelsen (1978, 1990)	Males	0.98	0.6–1.7
	Heavy vs. non-manual	3.1	2.2–4.3
	Medium vs. non-manual	2.3	1.8–2.9
	Light vs. non-manual	1.9	1.5–2.4
	Females		
	Heavy vs. non-manual	21.9	0.9–230
	Medium vs. non-manual	5.4	2.8–10.9
	Light vs. non-manual	3.2	1.4–7.3
	M-H OR adjusted for gender		
	Heavy vs. non-manual	3.1	2.2–4.4
	Medium vs. non-manual	2.7	2.1–3.3
	Light vs. non-manual	2.0	1.6–2.5
Hueston (1960)	Brewery vs. office	0.9	0.6–1.4
Herzog (1951)	Steelworkers vs. clerical	1.2	0.6–2.3
	Miners vs. clerical	1.3	0.6–2.5
Studies of vibration			
Bovenzi et al. (1994)*	Quarry drillers vs. controls	2.6	1.1–6.2
	Stonecarvers vs. controls:		
	Users of rotary tools only	1.9	0.7–4.6
	Users of rotary and percussive tools	3.2	1.4–7.2
Thomas and Clarke (1992)*	Vibration-exposed (VWF) vs. hospital admissions	2.1	1.1–3.9
Cocco et al. (1987)*	Vibration exposure (DC cases vs. controls)		
	< 10 yr exposure	2.3	1.5–4.4
	11–20 yr exposure	1.7	0.9–3.4
	> 21 yr exposure	2.4	1.3–4.2
Petri et al. (1982)	Lumberjacks vs. controls (machine shop)	3.0†	1.3–6.7
Landgrot et al. (1975)	Vibration-exposed vs. controls	0.9	0.5–1.8
		1.2	0.8–2.0

* Studies meeting validity criteria.
† Chi-square for trend $P < 0.05$.
Abbreviations: DC, Dupuytren's contracture; CI, confidence interval; M-H OR, Mantel-Haenszel odds ratio; VWF, vibration white finger.
(Courtesy of Liss GM, Stock SR: Can Dupuytren's contracture be work-related? Review of the evidence. Am J Ind Med 29:521–532, Copyright 1996. Reprinted by permission of Wiley Liss, Inc, a subsidiary of John Wiley & Sons, Inc.)

Results.—Ten controlled studies were identified (Tables 2 and 3). Four of the studies satisfied the validity criteria, including 1 examining the association between DC and frequency of repetitive manual work and 3 examining the association between DC and vibration (Table 5). The study of manual work found a 5.5-fold increase in the risk for DC among bagging and packing plant workers compared with control workers. The 3 studies of DC and vibration reported an increased history of exposure to vibration at work among patients with DC compared with controls, with evidence of a dose–response relationship. The strength of the association was moderate to strong in all of the studies (Table 4).

Conclusions.—Dupuytren's contracture is associated with frequent or repetitive manual work and with hand vibration. The dose–response relationship between DC and the duration of vibration exposure suggests a causal relationship, but there is less evidence for a causal relationship between DC and manual work. More high-quality research is needed to explore the association of DC with manual work or with traumatic injury.

▶ Little, if anything, in medicine is incontrovertible, and most medical conclusions are as much a matter of opinion as of fact. With such a background plus the economics at stake, it is unlikely that this paper or any other will quiet the controversy over the factor of use-related causation of Dupuytren's contracture. It is also no surprise that the methods and conclusions of few articles on the subject can be validated. I am somewhat surprised that *any* articles survived the meticulous validation process used by the authors. It is also interesting that more articles about vibratory trauma were validated than were articles about other types of manual work. The results of the search for work-related effects on the cause of Dupuytren's contracture, although interesting, take second place to the details of search and validation of articles in the medical literature. For that alone, this is an article to be treasured.

J.H. Dobyns, M.D.

Suggested Reading

Mih AD: Desmoid tumor of the ulna in a patient with neurofibromatosis. *J Hand Surgery* 20A:1007–1010, 1995.
▶ This clear review is recommended when studying lytic bone lesions. Although rare, these tumors should be considered in the differential diagnosis of masses that cause expansion of bone with cortical thinning. Desmoid tumors can behave in a locally aggressive fashion with recurrence rates of up to 20%. The author recommends a wide or marginal resection that completely removes viable tumors cells. The paper points out that the differential diagnosis of tumors producing this appearance on x-ray film included, "nonossifying fibroma, giant-cell tumor, chondromyxoid fibroma, fibrous dysplasia, fibrosarcoma, osteolytic sarcoma, and metastatic carcinoma."

E. Fleegler, M.D.

Tubiana R: Assessment of deformity in Dupuytren's disease (in French) *La Main* 1:3–11, 1996.

▶ This classification system, described by Tubiana in 1961[1] and further refined in 1986,[2] has gained popularity in France and other European countries because of the simplicity and rapidity of its use (at least in its simplified form). It also gives a very accurate image of the contracture of each finger in a minimal space.

The main interest of this paper is the staging of thumb lesions, which had not been defined precisely before. Thumb lesions are divided into web space contractures and thumb metacarpophalangeal and interphalangeal contractures with 4 stages each. Therefore, with 2 numbers only one gets a rather accurate image of the thumb lesions.

Having personally used this staging method for over 10 years, I can only advise hand surgeons to get acquainted with it and to use it on a regular basis in their files. It saves a considerable amount of time and space, and gives a rather accurate picture of the contracture and its evolution.

C. LeClercq M.D.

References

1. Tubiana R, Michon J: Evaluation chiffrée précise de la déformation dans las maladie de Dupuytren. *Mem Acad Chir* 87:886–888, 1961.
2. Tubiana R: Evaluation des déformations dans le maladie de Dupuytren. *Ann Chir Main* 5:5–11, 1986.

Pennig D, Gausepohl T, Lukosch R: Externe Fixation zur Unterstützung der Weichteilrekonstruktion in der Handchirurgie. *Handchir Mikrochir Plast Chir* 27:264–268, 1995.

▶ The authors advocate the use of small external fixators to correct soft-tissue contractures and demonstrate effective application of gradual force in a patient with contractures of the first web space and proximal interphalangeal (PIP) joint contractures. The publication of Messina's[1] technique for preoperatively correcting the PIP contractures associated with Dupuytren's disease has stimulated interest in these techniques.

V.R. Hentz M.D.

Reference

1. Messina A, Messina J: *Ann Hand Surg* 10:247–250, 1991.

Belusa L, Selzer A-M, Partecke B-D: Die Beschreibung der *Dupuytren*-Erkrankung durch den Baselar Arzt und Anatomen Felix *Plater* im Jahre 1614. *Handchir Mikrochir Plast Chir* 27:272–275, 1995.

▶ This article contends that Felix Plater, an anatomist working in Basal realized more than 150 years before Cline, Sir Astley Cooper, or Baron Dupuytren himself, that abnormalities of the palmar aponeurosis were responsible for the disease that now carries the name "Dupuytren's" This confirms my long held belief that if you think you have discovered something new, it is probably because you can't or haven't read the German language literature.

V.R. Hentz, M.D.

Salon A, Guero S, Glicenstein J: Lipofibromatous hamartoma of the median nerve: Review of ten operated cases with a mean follow-up of eight years (in French). *Ann Chir Main* 14(6):284–295, 1995.

Usui M, Murakami T, Naito T, et al: Some problems in wrist reconstruction after tumor resection with vascularized fibular-head graft. *J Reconstr Microsurg* 12:81–88, 1996.

Weinzweig N, Culver JE, Fleegler EJ: Severe contractures of the proximal interphalangeal joint in Dupuytren's disease: Combined fasciectomy with capsuloligamentous release versus fasciectomy alone. *Plast Reconstr Surg* 97:560–566, 1996.

Van Geertryden J, Lorea P, Goldschmidt D, et al: Glomus tumours of the hand: A retrospective study of 51 cases. *J Hand Surg (Br)* 21B:257–260, 1996.

14 Congenital Problems

Characteristics of Patients With Hypoplastic Thumbs
James MA, McCarroll HR Jr, Manske PR (Univ of California, San Francisco; Washington Univ, St Louis; Shriners Hosp, St. Louis)
J Hand Surg [Am] 21A:104–113, 1996   14–1

Objective.—Thumb hypoplasia is a complex congenital disorder that is sometimes associated with other congenital anomalies and syndromes. Reported estimates of the incidence of these syndromes vary considerably. It is important to classify thumb hypoplasia according to the modified Blauth classification; some types are amenable to reconstruction whereas others are not. A large series of patients with hypoplastic thumbs was reviewed to assess the associated pathologic findings and to determine the incidence of the various types according to the modified Blauth classification.

Findings.—The review included 160 hypoplastic thumbs of 98 patients evaluated between 1923 and 1993. The patients were 62 males and 36 females; in 62 patients, both thumbs were affected. Of 139 thumbs that were classifiable according to the modified Blauth classification, 19% were types 1 and 2, 23% were type 3, and 58% were types 4 and 5.

Fifty-nine percent of patients had radial dysplasia and 86% had associated anomalies. Forty-four percent of the patients had an associated syndrome, the most common of which were the vertebral, anal, tracheoesophageal, renal, and radial limb anomaly association and the Holt-Oram syndrome. The vertebral, anal, tracheoesophageal, renal, and radial limb anomaly association was most frequent in patients with spine, genitourinary, or gastrointestinal anomalies, whereas the Holt-Oram syndrome was more likely to be seen in patients with cardiac anomalies. Other syndromes were likely to be present in patients with lower-extremity anomalies. A total of 107 operations—including 24 thumb reconstructions and 35 pollicizations—were performed in 63 upper extremities.

Conclusions.—Associated anomalies and syndromes are very common in patients with hypoplastic thumbs. All patients with hypoplastic thumbs should be carefully evaluated for these associated conditions and for bilaterality. The modified Blauth classification aids in treatment planning.

▶ The authors show 3 significant findings in their review of 160 hypoplastic thumbs over 70 years. First, the Blauth classification can be applied with benefit to almost all cases of thumb hypoplasia—only the 1 case of thrombocytopenia-absent radius syndrome showed features in the thumb that could not be categorized. The classification leads logically to the choice of treatment, but surprisingly few patients in this study received surgical correction—only 34% of the type 2 and type 3 thumbs were reconstructed, and 40% of the type 4 and type 5 thumbs underwent ablation and pollicization. Second, 86% of the cases showed other anomalies that affected all systems except the neurologic. The infant presenting with thumb hypoplasia must undergo a full physical examination and classification; in the final major observation of this paper, 43% of the children in this study were shown to have syndromes recognizable by the pediatric geneticist.

G.D. Lister, M.D.

Traitement Chirurgical des Duplications du Pouce: A Propos de 106 Dossiers (Surgical Treatment of Thumb Duplications; Based on a Series of 106 Cases)
Guero S, Haddad R, Glicenstein J (Hôpital Necker-Enfants Malades, Paris)
Ann Chir Main 14:272–283, 1995   14-2

Background.—Thumb duplication is a common congenital malformation belonging to the polydactylies. Its surgical management remains difficult, and aesthetic or functional sequelae are common. The radiology-based Wassel classification divides the thumb duplications into 7 categories. For this study, thumb duplications were divided into 2 groups: proximal duplications comprising Wassel IV, V, and VI, and distal duplications comprising Wassel I, II, and III.

Surgical Technique.—The Bilhaut-Cloquet operation is no longer performed at this institution because of numerous reported complications. Instead, the technique described by Kelikian is used, even for symmetrical distal thumb duplications. The currently used operation starts with complete resection of the hypoplastic thumb. The pulp skin is preserved and used to rebuild the paronychium and pulp of the remaining thumb. The radial part of the pulp is deliberately overcorrected but the hypertrophic appearance of the thumb normalizes as the child grows. Supplementary joint facets are resected. The capsuloligamentous apparatus is repaired with a capsuloperiosteal flap obtained from the excised thumb. The tendons are balanced and the thenar muscles reinserted.

Patients.—During the past 15 years, 95 children have undergone reconstructions of 106 thumb duplications; 11 children underwent bilateral procedures. Fifteen percent of the children sought consultation for surgical revision after undergoing unsatisfactory primary operations elsewhere. There were 55 girls and 51 boys (mean age at operation, 13 months). Presently, however, children are operated on at ages 8–10 months. Intestinal malformations were present in 30% of the patients. A family history of thumb duplications was found in 2% of the patients.

Outcome.—Nine of the 88 patients treated by primary intention had to be reoperated: 3 for instability, 5 for residual clinodactyly, and 1 for aesthetic pulp revision. Whereas the parents have been very satisfied with the outcome, the surgeons remain more critical. The overall aesthetic appearance of the reconstructed thumbs, however, has been considerably improved by the use of pulp flaps.

▶ This excellent and well-illustrated article summarizes a contemporary experience with thumb duplication. I agree with the recommendations: early surgery, avoid Bilhaut-Cloquet reconstructions, careful reconstruction of ligaments and nail fold, and tendon balancing.

P.C. Amadio, M.D.

Transposition of the Third Metatarsus for the Reconstruction of Blauth Type III Hypoplastic Thumb
Kanaya F, et al (Univ of the Ryukyus, Japan)
J Jpn Soc Surg Hand 12:776–780, 1996   14–3

Methods.—The third metatarsus, including the metatarsal head, was used for the reconstruction of the first metacarpus, including the carpometacarpal (CM) joint of Blauth type III hypoplastic thumb in 3 patients. Release of adduction contracture of the thumb, multiple tendon transfers, and free vascularized lateral arm flap for soft-tissue coverage were also done.

Results.—In patient 1 (5 years old at surgery; follow-up, 6 years), the physis of the transferred metatarsus remained open and the metacarpus grew 19 mm. In patient 2 (surgery at age 1.3 years, follow-up, 7 years), the physis closed at 6 years after 14 mm of growth. In patient 3 (surgery at age 5.7 years, follow-up, 2 years), the physis closed at 2 years after 2 mm of growth. In all patients, the proximal and distal phalanges of the hypoplastic thumb grew as much as the contralateral thumb after reconstruction of the first metacarpus. The average range of motion of the reconstructed CM joint was 32 degrees in the vertical plane and 23 degrees in the horizontal plane. These procedures could produce a functional thumb, although 2 or 3 staged surgeries were required.

▶ According to Blauth's classification, type III is a congenital hypoplasia of the thumb in which the proximal portion of the first metacarpal is deficient. Treatment for this type of condition is still disputable. Many hand surgeons prefer pollicization because the pollicized digit usually gains better function than the reconstructed hypoplastic thumb. This paper reports 3 cases of type III hypoplastic thumb treated by transplantation of the third metatarsus associated with multiple tendon transfers and free vascularized lateral arm flap. Although the authors do not mention whether the periosteum was transplanted with the metatarsus, the transplanted metatarsus could grow 11 mm, on average, after transplantation. And the reconstructed CM joints of the thumbs were stable and mobile. Photographs also show fair appearance and good function of the reconstructed thumb. This procedure seems encouraging, although technological difficulties and the requirement of stepped surgeries may be drawbacks.

Y. Ueba, M.D.

Thumb Duplication at the Metacarpophalangeal Joint: Management and a New Classification
Hung L, Cheng JC, Bundoc R, et al (Chinese Univ of Hong Kong; Prince of Wales Hosp, Shatin, Hong Kong)
Clin Orthop 323:31–41, 1996   14–4

Introduction.—The Wassel type IV deformity, in which there is duplication of the thumb at the level of the metacarpophalangeal joint, accounts for about half of cases of thumb polydactyly. The authors have been studying the surgical treatment of this condition, and their experience suggests that Wassel type IV deformities can be subdivided into 4 types. A new classification of thumb duplication at the metacarpophalangeal joint was reported, along with the results of surgical treatment in 21 patients.

Classification.—A radiographic review of 45 hands with Wassel type IV deformities led to the recognition of 4 subtypes: type IVA, hypoplastic, (12%); type IVB, ulnar deviated, (64%); type IVC, divergent, (15%); and type IVD, convergent or complex (9%). These presentations were found to have important implications for surgical treatment. The type IVD deformity was the most complicated, often associated with complex bone and soft tissue anomalies and residual deformities.

Surgical Results.—The investigators developed a surgical approach to the management of thumb duplication at the metacarpophalangeal joint. The protocol emphasized early operation by the age of 1 year, single-stage osteotomy, meticulous repair of the collateral ligaments, and reattachment of the abductor pollicis brevis tendon. This approach was followed in the management of 21 patients with an average follow-up of 5 years. One type IVA, 16 type IVB, 1 type IVC, and 3 type IVD deformities were seen. The results were satisfactory from both a cosmetic and functional viewpoint—on a 20-point scoring system, the average score was 18. The metacarpophalangeal joint was stable in all patients but 1, 15 had good range of motion, and 17 were satisfied with their results. Two cases of scar hypertrophy were seen.

Conclusions.—The new classification of thumb duplication at the metacarpophalangeal joint should aid in planning surgical treatment. Patients with a type IVB or IVD deformity with an ulnarly deviated interphalangeal joint should probably have early surgery, performed at age 6 months. Alternatively, the degree of deformity requiring surgical correction may be reduced by aggressive preoperative stretching and splinting.

▶ This group of patients is smaller than that reported from the same department in 1984 and is significantly smaller than the 237 patients described by Tada et al.[1] in presenting their system for scoring the results of surgical correction of radial polydactyly. Furthermore, the authors retrieved fewer than 50% of the Wassel type IV cases treated in their clinic. When subdivided into the classification system the authors describe, these 21 cases yielded only 1 each of types A and C and only 3 of type D, the most complex. Why, then, should the interested surgeon trouble to read this paper? The 4 categories suggested are new, comprehensive, and valid, if indeed any further classification can be tolerated. The description of the surgical procedure is detailed and proper, leading, as the authors demonstrate, to a pleasing outcome. I question the wisdom of the recommendation to implant any sizable neurovascular bundle from the discard into the retained thumb and add that it is wise to seek out anomalous lumbrical muscle bellies in all thumb duplications, especially those with a narrow first web space.

G.D. Lister, M.D.

Reference

1. Tada K, Yonenobu K, Tsuyuguchi Y, et al. Duplication of the thumb. *J Bone Joint Surg (Am)* 65A:584–598, 1983.

Long-term Results of Surgical Treatment of Thumb Polydactyly
Ogino T, Ishii S, Takahata S, et al (Sapporo Med Univ, Japan; Obihiro Kousei Hosp, Japan; Kushiro Rousei Hosp, Japan)
J Hand Surg [Am] 21A:478–486, 1996   14–5

Background.—Thumb polydactyly is a common congenital condition, and many reports of its treatment have been published. However, few objective attempts have been made to assess the results of surgical treatment. The results of treatment of thumb polydactyly in 113 hands were analyzed.

Methods.—One hundred thirteen thumbs were operated on during a 15-year period. The hypoplastic digit was removed in 109 cases; in 107 of these cases, this was a radial thumb. Four hands underwent a modified Bilhaut procedure. Other techniques included first web plasty in 26 hands, Z-plasty in 17 hands, and a rotation flap from the removed thumb in 6 hands. Almost all operations were performed by 1 surgeon. The average age at surgery was 12 months. The deformity was classified as Wassel type 1 in 3 hands, type 2 in 28, type 3 in 5, type 4 in 48, type 5 in 12, and type 6 in 9. In addition, there were 3 floating-type and 5 radially deviated-type deformities. The results were evaluated objectively and subjectively at an average follow-up of 49 months.

Results.—A modified Tada evaluation showed good results in 97 hands, fair results in 12 hands, and poor results in 4 hands. The patients or parents of the patients were satisfied with the results in 100 cases and dissatisfied in 13. The results were more likely to be unsatisfactory in hands with Wassel type 3, 5, or 6 deformity and in hands with triphalangeal-type thumb polydactyly. The dissatisfaction rate was higher when the ulnar rather than the radial digit was resected. The results were better in the second half of the 15-year period than in the first half.

Conclusions.—Surgery for thumb polydactyly provides good long-term results in most cases. The results are affected by the type of deformity, the type of surgical procedure, and the skill of the surgeon. To achieve consistently good results, the surgeon must be trained in the surgical treatment of congenital hand deformities.

▶ This paper summarizes the results of surgery in a large group of patients with thumb polydactyly. The factors that influenced the potential for a good result were the type of thumb polydactyly, the presence of a triphalangeal component, and, most importantly, the experience and skill of the surgeon.

M. Ezaki, M.D.

Traumatic Ulnar Physeal Arrest After Distal Forearm Fractures in Children
Ray TD, Tessler RH, Dell PC (Volusia Hand Surgery, Daytona Beach, Fla; Univ of Florida, Gainesville)
J Pediatr Orthop 16:195–200, 1996   14–6

Introduction.—Traumatic ulnar physeal arrest resulting from radius fractures appears to be rare; only 23 cases have been reported in the literature. Five additional cases were described.

Patients.—The medical records of patients seen between 1981 and 1991 were reviewed to identify 5 patients who had ulnar physeal arrest associated with distal radius fractures. The records and radiographs were examined to determine the type of fracture, the type of ulnar physeal arrest, and the primary and surgical treatment. In the 5 patients, the initial fractures were distal radius fracture that required closed reduction, displaced metaphyseal-diaphyseal fracture of the distal radius and a displaced Salter-Harris III fracture of the ulna, radial fracture and a Salter-Harris III or IV ulnar fracture just lateral to the ulnar styloid (Fig 3), greenstick fracture of the radius with dislocation of the distal ulna and fracture of the ulnar styloid, and fracture of the distal radial metaphysis. Ulnar physeal arrest was diagnosed from immediately after the initial injury healed to 7 years later. The radiographs showed ulnar shortening in all patients and angular deformity. Wrist motion and strength varied. Treatment included a lateral closing-wedge radial osteotomy with or without distal radioulnar joint arthrodesis with segmental ulnar resection and a Suave-Kapandji procedure.

Discussion.—Ulnar physeal arrest can occur symmetrically or asymmetrically and is typically associated with Salter-Harris injuries. Patients who

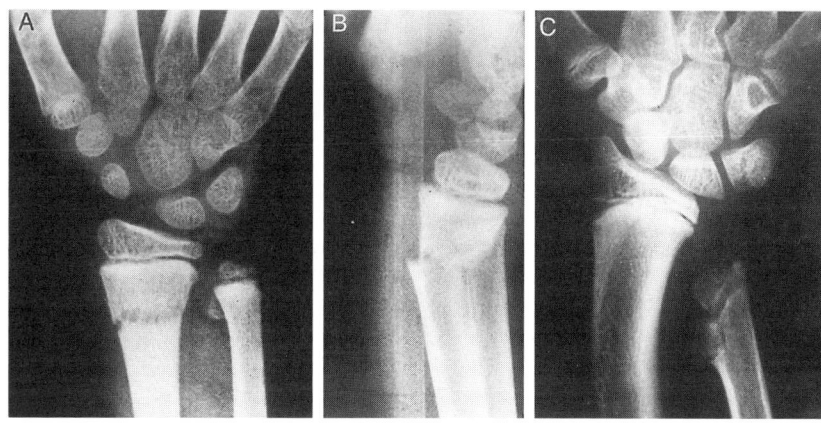

FIGURE 3.—A–C, type II distal ulnar growth arrest: predominantly lateral ulnar shortening (case 3). A, B, what appears to be a Salter-Harris IV injury of the distal ulnar physis. (Courtesy of Ray TD, Tessler RH, Dell PC: Traumatic ulnar physeal arrest after distal forearm fractures in children. *J Pediatr Orthop* 16:195–200, 1996.)

have these injuries should be carefully monitored during and after healing to detect traumatic ulnar physeal arrest early. Early treatment with radial epiphysiodesis may prevent deformity and poor wrist function.

▶ I agree that a traumatic physeal arrest of the distal ulna after a forearm fracture is rare. As the authors point out, however, this problem can occur even with undisplaced fractures. The distal ulnar physis, because of its size, is more prone to physeal arrest than is the distal radius. The 5 new cases here emphasize the need for careful follow-up, because early treatment may prevent the substantial deformities that can result. In the young child, physeal bar excisions should be strongly considered. Epiphysiodesis of the distal radius is reasonable in older children. Lengthening of the ulna is beneficial when a large discrepancy exists.

W.J. Shaughnessy, M.D.

Open Fractures of the Arm in Children
Haasbeek JF, Cole WG (Hosp for Sick Children, Toronto)
J Bone Joint Surg (Br) 77B:576–581, 1995   14-7

Background.—Open fractures of the arm in children are so uncommon that not enough cases have been reported to draw conclusions about the characteristics and treatment of such fractures. The patterns of injury and results were reviewed in a large group of children seen during a 10-year period.

Methods.—The medical records of 61 children (mean age, 9 years), treated from 1980 to 1990 at The Hospital for Sick Children in Toronto for open fractures of the scapula, clavicle, humerus, radius, or ulna were reviewed. Thirty-six injuries were caused by falls; 16, by playground accidents; and 9, by motor vehicle accidents or other causes. The late assessment was 3 years or longer after the injury. None of the patients had open injuries of the scapula, clavicle, or proximal humerus. Seventy-two percent of open fractures were Gustilo type I, 15% were type II, and 13% were type III.

Results.—Among the 15 children who had open diaphyseal, supracondylar, or T-shaped fractures of the humerus, 2 had arterial injuries and 7 had nerve injuries. All nerve injuries recovered spontaneously. Records of 13 of these 15 children included long-term assessments; 11 had excellent or good results, and 2 had fair results. Of the 46 children who had open forearm fractures, arterial injuries occurred in 1, nerve injuries occurred in 5, and a compartment syndrome occurred in 5. Only 1 child required repair of ruptured radial and ulnar arteries and median and ulnar nerves. The other children's nerve injuries healed spontaneously. Volkmann's ischemic contractures were prevented by early compartment release in 5 children. Overall, 22% of children had delayed union, nonunion, malunion, or refracture, especially those who had complicated type II or III fractures of the shafts of the radius and ulna. Probably because of thorough debridement within 12 hours of injury (and antibiotic prophylaxis), none of the children had osteomyelitis.

Conclusions.—Although short-term results were better for children who had open fractures of the humerus than for those who had open fractures of the forearm, the long-term results were excellent or good in more than 85% of children in both groups. In children who had open fractures of the mid-forearm, compartment syndrome is not sufficiently frequent to warrant routine compartment release in all cases. Injured nerves do not need to be explored if they are not in the wound and not associated with arterial injuries.

▶ Nerve injuries occurred in almost half the humeral fractures that resolved spontaneously in this study. The incidence of nerve injury was much less in forearm fractures—11%.

A.L. Ladd, M.D.

Percutaneous Kirschner-wire Pinning for Severely Displaced Distal Radial Fractures in Children: A Report of 157 Cases
Choi KY, Chan WS, Lam TP, et al (Chinese Univ of Hong Kong, Shatin, New Territories)
J Bone Joint Surg (Br) 77B:797–801, 1995
14–8

Background.—Closed reduction and application of a plaster cast are the typical treatments for distal radial fracture, a common occurrence in children. Poor results, however, particularly limited forearm rotation, have been reported in 15% to 29% of these patients. The most important predictor of poor outcome is translation of the fracture, especially if the fracture is displaced by more than half the diameter of the radius. The efficacy and safety of treatment with percutaneous Kirschner (K)-wires were evaluated for these high-risk radial fractures in children.

Methods.—Of 549 children treated with acute fractures of the distal radius, 157 had translation greater than half the diameter of the radius. Complete medical records and radiographs were available for review for 140 patients. The patients underwent closed reduction and percutaneous K-wire insertion from either the radial styloid or Lister's tubercle through the fracture site to the opposite cortex of the radius or up the medulla for at least 4 cm past the fracture site. An extra wire was inserted when additional security was needed. The patients' status was followed 13–54 months after surgery. Failure was defined as irreducibility, loss of reduction exceeding 10½ during K-wire stabilization, greater than 15½ limitation of movement in any pain, or persistent pain or deformity.

Results.—The failure rate was 14.3% in the 140 patients. Of the 20 patients who had recorded failures, 11 required open reduction and 9 had a loss of reduction exceeding 10½ in 1 plane. None of the patients had osteomyelitis, vascular complications, or premature physeal closure.

Conclusions.—The placement of percutaneous K-wires significantly reduced the failure rate in children who had high-risk distal radial fractures and did not induce premature physeal closure. This approach is therefore recommended for patients who have fracture translation that exceeds half the diameter of the radius. Open reduction is recommended when satisfactory alignment and bony apposition cannot be achieved.

▶ Like distal radial fractures in adults, these fractures in children are frequently undertreated. The authors treat the high-risk fracture (translation more than 50% of the diameter) with percutaneous pinning, which significantly reduces the failure rate.

A.L. Ladd, M.D.

Dupuytren's Disease in Children
Urban M, Feldberg L, Janssen A, et al (St Andrew's Hosp, Essex, England; Sint-Niklaas, Belgium)
J Hand Surg (Br) 21B:112–116, 1996   14–9

Background.—Dupuytren's disease is generally considered a disease of adults, although cases of this disease have been reported in teenagers. Nine cases of Dupuytren's disease that occurred in children younger than 13 years were reported.

> *Case 1.*—Boy, 9 years, had a 6-month history of flexion contracture of the right little finger. He had no history of acute trauma, but his family history included significant Dupuytren's disease. A routine fasciectomy was performed. Extension of the PIP joint deteriorated postoperatively during splinting. The boy was not cooperative, but the increasing flexion contraction may have resulted from

early disease recurrence and not splinting failure. A dermofasciectomy should have been done as the primary surgery. Histologic assessment confirmed Dupuytren's disease.

Case 2.—Boy, 10 years, had 2 asymptomatic nodules noted in the palm of the left hand. He had no history of acute trauma or family history of Dupuytren's disease. The nodules were excised, and histologic examination indicated Dupuytren's disease.

Seven other preadolescents have also had confirmed Dupuytren's disease of the hand, although no clinical information was available to the current authors. Other unproved cases have also been cited.

Conclusions.—Flexion contracture of the fingers in children may be caused by camptodactyly or, less commonly, congenital ulnar drift. Dupuytren's disease, though rare, is another cause. Dermofasciectomy may be indicated in children with histologically confirmed Dupuytren's disease and progressive finger contracture.

▶ The authors report on 9 cases of histologically proved Dupuytren's disease by combining 2 cases of their own and 7 previously reported. Dupuytren's disease in children is extremely rare, and more common causes of flexion deformity should be considered including camptodactyly, scleroderma, and congenital ulnar drift or mild arthrogryposis. Children seen with the disease may have a more aggressive form, and the authors' suggestion of dermatofasciectomy is probably justified. They also believe that the disease, rather than the child's ability to cooperate with therapy, leads to the majority of recurrences but that waiting until the child will cooperate (if possible) may be beneficial.

J.A. Katarincic, M.D.

Progressive Lengthening in the Post-traumatic Epiphysiodesis of the Distal End of the Radius
Gonzalez J, Caso J, Fontaneda JM, et al (Hosp Nuestra Señora de Aránzazu, San Sebastian, Spain)
Rev Ortop Traum 40:158–160, 1995   14–10

Introduction.—Relative shortening of the radius in relation to the ulna is a not uncommon complication after epiphyseal injuries before bone growth is completed. The classic treatment has been shortening or epiphysiodesis of the distal ulna, but in recent years, progressive radial lengthening has had many advocates.

Patients.—Two male patients, 12 and 16 years of age, underwent distal metaphyseal radial osteotomy and progressive radial lengthening with an external fixator. The preoperative radial-ulnar length discrepancies were 14 mm and 20 mm, respectively.

Results.—The length discrepancy was corrected in both cases after a period of lengthening of 102 and 98 days, respectively. In the first case (the

12-year-old), a new radial lengthening had to be done because the ulna continued to overgrow the radius by 10 mm.

▶ Progressive bone lengthening using an external fixator is a technique that has been used frequenty in recent years for treating short bones from tumor, congenital, and traumatic causes. It is a simple and noninvasive technique that provides a considerable amount of bone lengthening. Its main inconvenience is that a long period of time, under very close supervision, is needed for bone healing. Both cases presented pin tract infections which required antibiotic treatment. The authors have followed the advice of other authors, who recommend delaying the lengthening for about 10 days after the osteotomy. This will allow for periosteal and soft-tissue healing before the bone fragments are lengthened, and the gap will supposedly be filled with a periosteal sleeve that will enhance bone growth. Another advantage is that this technique will allow for more than 1 lengthening in young patients, as was the case with the 12-year-old child—unless one chooses to do a simultaneous epiphysiodesis of the distal ulna.

A. Lluch, M.D., Ph.D.

Suggested Reading

Slakey JB, Hennrikus WL: Acquired thumb flexion contracture in children: Congenital trigger thumb. *J Bone Joint Surg (Br)* 78B:481–483, 1996.
▶ I cannot gainsay the authors' contention that no *physician* has confirmed either triggering or fixed flexion of the thumb tip in a newborn without other abnormalities to account for the finding. Furthermore, I agree with their contention that the probable initiating event is a deforming interaction between the digit flexor and the pulley mechanism. Nevertheless, I have seen too many parent–child and sibling–sibling combinations of this condition to totally dismiss the possibility of some inherited propensity. Regardless, it is highly unlikely that the long accepted name of "congenital trigger digit" will be replaced by the authors' favored term or by my own, which is "flexor tendon entrapment of childhood."

J.H. Dobyns, M.D.

Ekerot L: Syndactyly correction without skin-grafting. *J Hand Surg (Br)* 21B:330–337, 1996.
▶ The design of the dorsal commissure flap is intriguing, although I personally prefer a broader central flap. In any event, for those who are still undecided, this flap design begs to be tried before one selects among the other, more standard commissure patterns. However, such a trial should not be handicapped by the author's insistence that the dorsal commissure flap avoids the use of a skin graft. If there is a fundamental principle in managing the skin envelope of syndactyly, it is that there is insufficient skin and that no amount of clever utilization of the elastic properties of dorsal skin will alter that fact. In short, for supple syndactyly webs there are many methods of redesign that create a good looking web and a minimum of tightness without a skin graft. This is never true, however, in the extended and tight syndactyly (which is common) unless there is an underlying skeletal structure to be discarded; such was the case in several of the author's patients.

The article is well illustrated, but I do not agree (from the illustrations only) that all the webs are satisfactory. Furthermore the appearance of the webs during various stretch configurations and, in particular, the feel of the webs, scars, and lines of tightness from web into palm and digits are more predictive of eventual contractures than in the static photographs usually employed. For these reasons plus the relatively short time of follow-up, I recommend that surgeons who employ this technique remain open minded about possible skin graft needs and that they employ skin grafts generously rather than *ever* closing tightly.

J.H. Dobyns, M.D.

Taniguchi K: A practical classification system for multiple cartilaginous exostosis in children. *J Pediatr Orthop* 15:585–591, 1995.
▶ Dr. Taniguchi proposes a classification system for multiple osteochondromatosis based on severity of involvement of the distal forearm. The association of other skeletal deformities and the potential for malignant transformation were identified in 41 children. Therefore this classification scheme provides information regarding severity and prognosis.

A.L. Ladd, M.D.

Ogino T, et al: Long-term results after pollicization for hypoplastic thumb: Follow-up for more than 10 years (in Japanese). *J Jpn Soc Surg Hand* 12:765–767, 1996.
▶ This paper reports the long-term follow-up results of pollicization for severe congenital hypoplasia of the thumb. Only 5 cases are reported, but all of these patients underwent operations done according to the Buck–Gramcko method and were followed up for more than 10 years. All patients used the pollicized thumb. The average pinch power of the pollicized thumb was about half that of the opposite side. Two of the 5 patients used the pollicized hand as the dominant hand. Reflecting on their vast past experience, the authors concluded that a finger with good motion before pollicization would yield better postoperative function than one with poor preoperative mobility. The authors recommend pollicization just after the age of 1 year to get good functional results.

Y. Ueba, M.D.

Nanchahal J, Tonkin MA: Preoperative distraction lengthening for radial longitudinal deficiency. *J Hand Surg (Br)* 21B:103–107, 1996.
▶ The authors have shown the benefits of preoperative distraction lengthening for congenital radial longitudinal deficiencies. Soft-tissue distraction techniques preclude the need for skeletal shortening of the ulna, thereby preserving length of the upper extremity. I concur with the authors' enthusiasm for this technique. It has become our procedure of choice for dealing with soft-tissue contracture and radial deviation of the wrist before centralization. In older children who have radial bowing of the ulna, the procedure can be combined with ulnar osteotomy and distraction to attain increased ulnar length and correction of the bowing deformity. Distraction at a rate of 1 mm/day is well tolerated but occasionally results in contractures of the finger flexors. The importance of daily stretching and therapy cannot be over emphasized.

W.J. Shaughnessy, M.D.

15 Rehabilitation, Occupation, and Sports

The Economic Cost and Social and Psychological Impact of Musculo-skeletal Conditions
Yelin E, for the National Arthritis Data Work Group (Univ of California, San Francisco)
Arthritis Rheum 38:1351–1362, 1995   15–1

Objective.—A literature review, coupled with estimates of data pertaining to health care utilization and acute and chronic disability associated with musculoskeletal conditions from the 1990–1992 National Health Interview study, was performed to evaluate the economic, social, and psychological effects of musculoskeletal conditions in the United States.

Findings.—In 1992, the cost of musculoskeletal conditions was $149.4 billion. Forty-eight percent of these costs were related to direct medical costs. Institutional care, including inpatient hospital admissions and nursing home care, was responsible for more than 50% of the direct costs. Physician inpatient and outpatient costs accounted for slightly more than one tenth of the total, suggesting that overall hospital costs could be decreased if increases in services provided by physicians and other health care professionals resulted in fewer admissions. The magnitude of costs of prepayment and administration (primarily costs of administering insurance payments) absorbed nearly as much of the total direct cost of medical care for patients with musculoskeletal disease as outpatient physician visits, underscoring the need to carefully assess such costs as part of the health care reform effort. The remainder of costs related to musculoskeletal conditions were related to indirect costs resulting from loss of wages.

The relative economic impact of musculoskeletal and associated conditions evidently is on the rise. In 1963, 1972, and 1980, the total cost of musculoskeletal conditions was equal to 0.7%, 0.7%, and 0.8% of the Gross National Product, respectively, whereas in 1992, this had increased to 2.5%.

It also was noted that individuals with musculoskeletal conditions make 315 million physician visits on an annual basis, have more then 8 million hospital admissions, and experience approximately 1.4 billion days of limited activity. Nearly 42% of individuals with musculoskeletal conditions, corresponding to more than 17 million overall, report activity restriction. Many studies also have found increased levels of psychological distress among patients with musculoskeletal conditions compared to the general population. Associations between increased health services utilization and increased levels of psychological status also have been noted.

Conclusions.—Musculoskeletal conditions are associated with considerable economic and social costs, and also account for a substantial amount of health care use and disability. Psychological status also is adversely affected. More awareness about the problems of psychological distress and social dislocation associated with musculoskeletal conditions is needed.

▶ The statistics presented in this paper regarding the economic and psychosocial impact of musculoskeletal and related conditions in America have been compiled by the National Arthritis Data Work Group and update previous studies.[1, 2]

This is a long and detailed report, which documents a substantial increase in the economic and social costs of these conditions. The relative economic impact of musculoskeletal and associated conditions has grown from 0.7% in 1963, 0.7% in 1972, and 0.8% in 1980 to 2.5% of the Gross National Product in 1992. One of the most interesting statistics is in the category of the cost of prepayment and administration (mostly the cost of administering insurance payments). This category absorbs almost as much of the total direct cost of medical care for patients with musculoskeletal disease as do outpatient physician visits.

R.B. Evans, O.T.R./L., C.H.T.

References

1. Felts W, Yelin E: The economic impact of the rheumatic diseases in the United States. *J Rheumatol* 16:867–884, 1989.
2. Yelin EH, Felts WR: A summary of the impact of musculoskeletal conditions in the United States. *Arthritis Rheum* 33:750–755, 1990.

Self-reported Physical Exposure and Musculoskeletal Symptoms of the Forearm-Hand Among Automobile Assembly-line Workers
Fransson-Hall C, Byström S, Kilbom Å (Swedish Inst of Occupational Health, Solna, Sweden)
J Occup Environ Med 37:1136–1144, 1995   15–2

Objective.—Several studies have suggested that objective and subjective signs of musculoskeletal disorders in the forearm-hand may be increased among populations exposed to highly repetitive jobs, such as garment workers and assembly-line packers. The prevalence of physical exposures and symptoms of the forearm-hand in automobile assembly-line workers (ALWs) was determined.

Methods.—Seven hundred individuals who worked for at least the past 3 months and performed assembly work were randomly selected. Of these, 393 men and 128 women (80% of sample) completed a questionnaire that focused on individual and employment-related factors, physical workload and psychosocial factors, and musculoskeletal symptoms and sick leave concerning the forearm-hand. A control group of randomly chosen men and women from the general population was also evaluated.

Results.—Both men and women in the ALW group reported significantly more symptoms from the forearm-hand within the last 7 days than did those in the control group. The prevalence ratio for male ALWs vs. controls was 2.2 and for female ALWs 2.5. Further, ALWs reported significantly higher exposures to repetitive movements, precision movements, and manual handling (less than or equal to 15 kg) than did controls. The wrist was the most commonly affected part of the forearm-hand in male ALWs, whereas the women considered the dorsal aspect to be most affected. Symptoms suggestive of rheumatoid arthritis were reported by 20% of female ALWs and by 5% of male ALWs. Male ALWs who reported more musculoskeletal symptoms were more likely to have "type A" personality and to not exercise. The prevalence of sick leave during the past 6 months attributed to symptoms of the forearm-hand was 11% for male ALWs and 27% for female ALWs, with a median number of days on leave of 8 in men and 11 in women. Compared with male ALWs, female ALWs reported more symptoms, more repetitive movements, less use of hand tools, and higher exposure to wrist extension and flexion. Obese women and those shorter than 160 cm reported more symptoms than did their counterparts.

Conclusions.—Automobile assembly-line workers appear to be a high-risk group for work-related symptoms from the forearm-hand, and women appear to be at greater risk than men. Because most studies address physical load classification in terms of coarse criteria, such as job title, exposure to physical load should be conscientiously analyzed, as women may perform different tasks than men.

▶ This paper presents several interesting and useful points regarding physical exposure and upper extremity somatic complaints in ALWs. It is particularly interesting to find that women might be exposed to more risk factors for cumulative trauma disorder, even though their job titles are the same as the men's. However, the control group in this study is older than the study group. This difference would certainly affect the comparison results.

P. Wu, M.D.

Treatment Outcome in Instrumentalists: A Long-term Follow-up Study
Lederman RJ (Cleveland Clinic Found, Ohio)
Med Probl Perform Art 10:115–120, 1995

Background.—The medical problems of musicians have only recently begun to receive attention in the literature. Few studies have reported treatment results, and even fewer have addressed long-term outcomes.

Patients and Methods.—One hundred patients, aged 11–64 years, who had been seen 5–7 years earlier at a Medical Center for Performing Artists were interviewed about their current status. Fifty-nine patients were string instrumentalists, 27 were keyboard players, and 14 were wind instrumentalists. At the time of the initial assessment, 49 patients were professional performers, 40 were students, 7 were primarily teachers, and 4 were amateurs. Symptoms had persisted from 2 days to 16 years.

Findings.—At follow-up, 54 patients were playing professionally, 14 were mainly teaching, 6 were still students, 4 continued to play as amateurs, and 22 had quit playing. Thirty-five patients were playing more than 20 hours a week; 32, 6–20 hours a week; and 33, 5 hours or less. Thirty of those who were still playing had no symptoms, 34 were better, 13 were the same, and 1 was worse. New symptoms had developed in 10 patients. Primary diagnoses were musculoskeletal in 66 patients. Eighteen patients had nerve compression syndromes, 6 had focal dystonia, and 10 had other disorders. Sixteen of 34 patients who had muscle-tendon overuse were free of symptoms, 15 were better, and 3 had new symptoms. At follow-up, the presence of symptoms was unassociated with the number of hours played. More than 80% of patients were engaged in physical and/or occupational therapy. For one third of patients, technique changes were recommended. A minority needed medication, surgery, and psychotherapy. Patients who had a shorter duration of symptoms at the initial assessment tended to be free of symptoms at follow-up, but long-term outcomes were unpredictable.

Conclusions.—Many instrumentalists who have playing-related symptoms benefit from a comprehensive assessment and carefully selected multifacted treatment program. Although relapses can occur and new symptoms develop, the long-term outcome is usually favorable, especially in patients who have regional limb or axial pain syndromes.

▶ This report from a well-known center emphasizes the role of technique in both the development and the treatment of musculoskeletal symptoms in musicians.

P.C. Amadio, M.D.

A Case-Control Study of Performance-related Hand Problems in Music Students
Manchester RA, Park S (Univ of Rochester, NY)
Med Probl Perform Art 11:20–23, 1996

Introduction.—Performance-related cumulative trauma disorders (CTDs) in musicians have been related to gender, instrument, and increased practice times. It is unclear, however, why one musician experiences an overuse problem and another does not. A case-control study tested the hypothesis that 1 or more modifiable variables might account for some of the risk for the development of a performance-related upper-extremity CTD.

Methods.—The patients were university-level music students who sought treatment for performance-related hand problems. Controls, who were matched with patients for gender, instrument, and academic year, had not reported such problems. Both cases and controls completed a questionnaire regarding performance-related hand problems, practice and performance patterns, potential preventive factors, physical characteristics, and nonperformance employment.

Results.—Over 3 academic years, completed questionnaires yielded 48 matched pairs of student musicians. Thirty-three pairs were female and 15 were male; the average age of the study group was slightly more than 20 years. Seventeen pairs played string instruments; 13, keyboard instruments; 10, woodwinds; and 8, brass. Muscle overuse syndrome was the diagnosis in 75% of cases; most of the remaining 25% had upper-extremity tendinitis. Survey responses revealed only 3 items on which cases and controls differed in a statistically significant manner. Patients played and performed more than controls during their freshman year (mean, 5.5 vs. 4.7 hours per day); patients took more practice breaks per hour during the senior year; and patients were more likely than controls to have taken Alexander or Feldenkrais lessons (67% vs. 27%). Hypermobility, previously cited as an important factor in the development of performance-related CTDs, did not differ between cases and controls.

Conclusion.—This retrospective study identified a single possible modifiable risk factor for performance-related hand injury. As freshmen, music students who reported injuries spent more hours per day practicing their instrument than matched music students who did not experience these problems. A multicenter research project may shed additional light on the subject of performance-related hand problems in instrumental music students.

▶ Relatively few studies have looked at the etiology or pathophysiology of CTDs, which is unfortunate considering the scope of this problem. The musician population is a fairly straightforward group to study because they are usually unencumbered by worker's compensation claims and secondary gain issues. On the other hand, it is usually difficult to assemble a large number of such subjects to assess, as is illustrated in the relatively small numbers in this particular study (48 matched pairs).

This study provides additional evidence for linking the risk of the development of a CTD to the number and force of repetitive movements that a musician performs. Similar conclusions have been reached in previous studies with industrial workers.[1] Although the concept seems intuitively obvious, it has been refuted by many other authors.[2] This particular article will not resolve the ongoing debate, but it is a good addition to our knowledge base regarding this controversial subject.

K. Bengtson, M.D.

References

1. Silverstein BA, Fine LJ: Cumulative trauma disorders of the upper extremity: A preventive strategy is needed. *J Occup Med* 33:642–644, 1991.
2. Hadler NM: Cumulative trauma disorders: An iatrogenic concept. *J Occup Med* 32:38, 1990.

Grip Lock Injuries to the Forearm in Male Gymnasts
Samuelson M, Reider B, Weiss D (Univ of Chicago)
Am J Sports Med 24:15–18, 1996   15–5

Background.—The 6 competitive events in male gymnastics require complex, high level skills. As high-bar routines become more demanding, many gymnasts seek ways to increase their grip strength. Leather hand grips fitted with a small dowel (Fig 1) are designed to increase the gymnast's hold on the bar but are associated with certain types of injuries, including grip lock. Surveys sent to coaches of college and high school

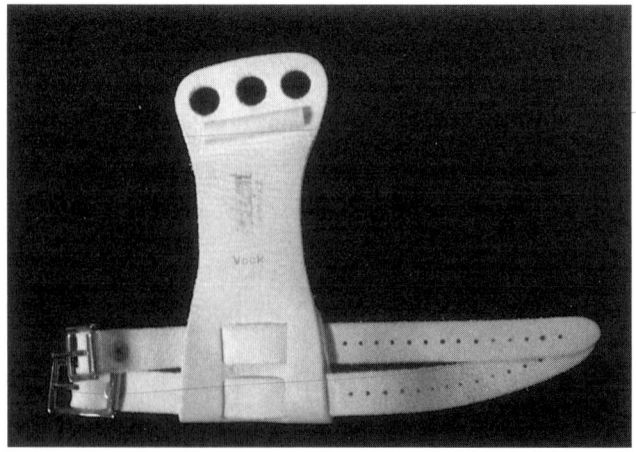

FIGURE 1.—High-bar dowel grip used in men's gymnastics. (Courtesy of Samuelson M, Reider B, Weiss D: Grip lock injuries to the forearm in male gymnasts. *Am J Sports Med* 24:15–18, 1996.)

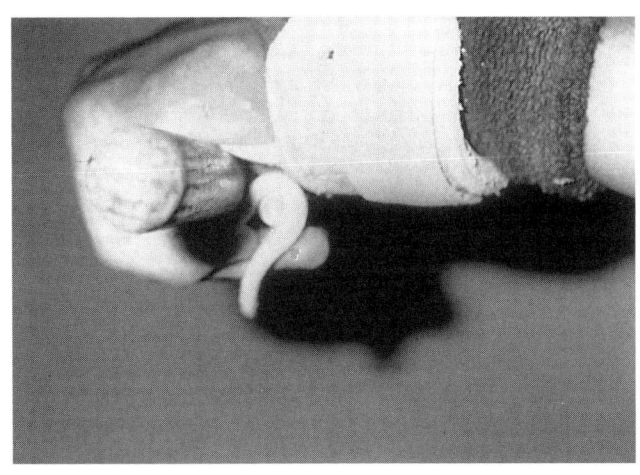

FIGURE 2.—A dowel caught between palm and bar, creating grip lock. (Courtesy of Samuelson M, Reider B, Weiss D: Grip lock injuries to the forearm in male gymnasts. *Am J Sports Med* 24:15–18, 1996.)

teams identified gymnasts who had sustained grip lock injuries. These gymnasts were questioned on the nature and outcome of grip lock injury.

Methods.—This acute injury occurs when the dowel becomes caught between the palm and the high bar. The hand locks to the bar (Fig 2) while the gymnast continues to rotate, and this movement often results in a sprain or fracture of the wrist or forearm. Data gathered included the type of injury, type of grips worn, treatment, complications, and long-term outcome.

Results.—Questionnaires were received from 38 of 61 Illinois high school coaches and from 32 of 48 college coaches. Thirty-eight grip lock injuries were reported among male gymnasts from 25 teams. Twenty-three of 25 gymnasts who could be located returned the surveys. The average age at the time of injury was 18 years. In 16 of 23 respondents, a nondominant upper extremity was injured; the most common injury site was 3–4 inches above the wrist. There were 20 fractures (8 requiring surgery) and 3 sprains. At the time of grip lock injury, 15 gymnasts were using a cubital (hyperpronated) grip and 19 were using dowel grips; 14 attributed the injury to worn or stretched grips. All respondents eventually returned to gymnastics and most reached maximum recovery within 1 year; however residual pain was reported by 14, 8 had limited wrist motion, and 7 had functional limitations.

Conclusion.—Based upon data from this survey, the incidence of grip lock injury is estimated to be 0.2% per year. Grip lock appears to occur most often during performance of cubital grip skills and is associated with serious injury. The use of dowel grips should be reserved for advanced-level gymnasts, and grips should be checked regularly for proper fit and signs of wear.

▶ Hand and wrist injuries are common in gymnasts. According to DeFiori et al.,[1] 73% of gymnasts complain of wrist pain at some point. These complaints relate not only to falls, but also to chronic traction and compression on growing wrists, and to failures of specific equipment such as the dowel grips reported here. A knowledgeable hand surgeon who deals with athletes should be familiar with the special equipment needed in the various sports and how it is used (both properly and improperly) to best manage current injuries and prevent future ones.

P.C. Amadio, M.D.

Reference

1. DeFiori JP, Puffer JC, Mandelbaum BR, et al: Factors associated with wrist pain in the young gymnast. Am J Sports Med 24:9–14, 1996.

Tonic Vibration Reflex and Muscle Afferent Block in Writer's Cramp
Kaji R, Rothwell JC, Katayama M, et al (Kyoto Univ, Japan; Takeda Gen Hosp, Kyoto, Japan; Natl Hosp for Nervous Diseases, London)
Ann Neurol 38:155–162, 1995
15–6

Introduction.—Patients who have writer's cramp, a form of focal dystonia, generally alleviate their discomfort by assuming a comfortable arm posture or applying pressure on their "hot spots." Because attenuation of pain can be attained by these methods, this type of dystonia may be influenced by cutaneous and proprioceptive sensory inputs. High-frequency vibration was used to identify the muscles involved in this focal dystonia. In addition, whether lidocaine and ethanol injections could improve the discomfort experienced by patients with writer's cramp was determined.

Methods and Materials.—Fifteen right-handed patients who had focal dystonia of the right hand were included. Tonic vibration reflexes (TVRs) were recorded in 15 controls as well as in those affected with writer's cramps. While the patients were writing, surface electromyograms were used to determine the muscle into which lidocaine was to be injected. Thirteen patients also received 99.5% ethanol in their injection.

Results.—The mean latency of TVR in 6 of the normal patients was 12.5 seconds; TVR could not be evoked in 9 controls. In 11 patients, TVR elicited dystonic movements; their mean onset latency was 2.7 seconds. Lidocaine eliminated dystonic movements in 6 patients and decreased movements in 5 of them. A slight prolongation of latency was observed when lidocaine was administered to the normal controls. Flexor carpi radialis T reflexes also diminished on injection of lidocaine. M response amplitudes were also slightly reduced. For 11 patients, handwriting scores improved after injection of lidocaine. Duration of drug action for patients who received lidocaine averaged only 6–7 hours; for those who also received ethanol, however, clinical improvement lasted an average of 12 days.

Discussion.—The dystonic movements of patients who have writer's cramps can be mimicked by a TVR and then blocked by local injection of lidocaine into the affected muscle. In patients who have writer's cramp, an increase in sensitivity of tonic muscle to vibration is observed. This abnormality may be related to an abnormal gamma drive or fusimotor mechanism. Lidocaine and ethanol injections improve the dystonia of patients with writer's cramp without sacrificing decreased muscle function.

▶ Effective, long-term treatment of writer's cramp can be challenging. As with other dystonias, the mechanism responsible for the abnormal postures and movements in this condition is not well understood. The results of this study support abnormal gamma drive as the mechanism responsible for writer's cramp. The authors also report intermediate term (5–21 days) suppression of dystonic activity after IM injection of 10% ethanol. This technique may be clinically useful for evaluating patients before longer term neurolysis or chemodenervation.

C. Burgar, M.D.

Benefits and Use of Digital Prostheses
Pereira BP, Kour A-K, Leow E-L, et al (Natl Univ, Singapore, Republic of Singapore)
J Hand Surg [Am] 21A:222–228, 1996   15–7

Background.—In patients with digital amputations, the loss of form and cosmetic appearance may be so psychologically damaging that active hand function is inhibited. Fitting a socially acceptable, custom-made prosthesis can augment microsurgical reconstruction. One clinical experience with such prostheses was reported.

Methods and Findings.—One hundred thirty-six digital prostheses were fitted in 90 patients (Fig 3). Thirty patients were followed for at least 2 years. Seventy-three percent reported using their prostheses daily, and 23% reported using them intermittently. Twenty-three percent of the patients using their prostheses occasionally had technical problems, such as loose fit and perspiration (see Fig 3).

Conclusion.—High-quality digital prostheses can restore near-normal appearance and form, improve body image, and contribute to better physical outcomes in patients with digital amputations. Careful patient selection, with special attention to patient expectations, is crucial.

▶ Custom digital prostheses of hand-colored silicone rubber, coated finally with a superficial translucent layer (which improves appearance and facilitates cleaning) were pioneered by Jean Pillet. They are now available from other sources, as noted here, but the concepts are similar. The authors imply, but do not clearly state, that the 30 patients represent all of their patients, with a minimum 2-year follow-up. If so, the acceptance rate be-

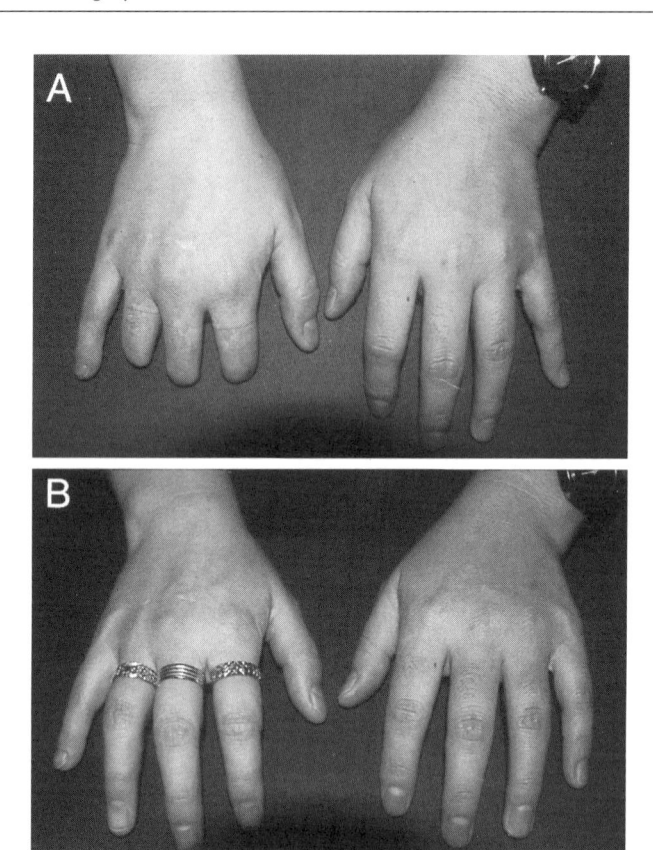

FIGURE 3.—A patient with multiple-digit amputations of the index, middle, and ring fingers at the proximal interphalangeal joint (**A**) before fitting and (**B**) after fitting. (Courtesy of Pereira BP, Kour A-K, Leow E-L, et al: Benefits and use of digital prostheses. *J Hand Surg [Am]* 21A:222–228, 1996.)

speaks excellent patient selection but, perhaps, also an effect of a cultural bias in the relative importance of having 10 digits, whether or not they move or have sensibility. Most of the amputees in my practice are farmers from the United States Midwest; few are interested in these "passive" prostheses.

As shown in the figure, the seam where the prosthesis joins the finger must be covered by a ring; for this reason, in my own practice again, women are more accepting of these prostheses, as ring wearing, especially on multiple fingers, is not as socially acceptable for men in the United States. Finally, as these authors note, with such prostheses, aesthetics is all. Fabrication of these prostheses is an art form; some prosthetists will be better at it than others. I always advise patients to see samples of the work of the prosthetist they are considering on other patients of similar skin tone before making a final decision.

P.C. Amadio, M.D.

Reliability and Validity of the Wheelchair User's Shoulder Pain Index (WUSPI)
Curtis KA, Roach KE, Applegate EB, et al (California State Univ, Fresno; Univ of Miami, Coral Gables, Fla)
Paraplegia 33:595–601, 1995   15–8

Introduction.—Shoulder pain that interferes with functional activity is a frequent problem in long-term wheelchair users. The reliability and validity of the Wheelchair User's Shoulder Pain Index (WUSPI), a 15-item self-report index developed for clinical and research use to assess pain during transfers, self-care, wheelchair mobility, and general activities, were examined.

Methods.—To establish reliability, the WUSPI was administered twice in the same day to 16 wheelchair users, aged 21–59 years, who had used a wheelchair an average of 15 years. Scores were compared with intraclass correlation. To establish concurrent validity, the index was administered to 64 long-term wheelchair users, and scores were compared with shoulder range-of-motion measurements.

Results.—Intraclass correlation for reliability was 0.99. There was a significant relationship of total index score to loss of shoulder range of motion, as shown by statistically significant negative correlations of total index scores to measurements of shoulder abduction, flexion, and extension.

Discussion.—The WUSPI shows high levels of reliability and internal consistency, as well as concurrent validity, with loss of range of motion in the shoulder. It may be useful in establishing baseline shoulder dysfunction and for longitudinal studies of musculoskeletal complications in wheelchair users.

▶ The authors use a numeric index scale to assess shoulder pain in wheelchair ambulators in an active population. The index measures shoulder pain during various activities. Obtaining the index had been previously reported by the authors, but it would have been useful to re-introduce it to understand this study better. A statistical negative correlation was shown between restrictive range of motion and shoulder pain. Its utility will likely be borne out in further studies of this very common problem that affects wheelchair ambulators.

A.L. Ladd, M.D.

Prosthetic Usage in Major Upper Extremity Amputations
Wright TW, Hagen AD, Wood MB (Mayo Clinic and Mayo Found, Rochester, Minn)
J Hand Surg (Am) 20A:619–622, 1995   15–9

Background.—Most patients who have major upper extremity amputations are candidates for a prosthesis, but most studies show rejection

TABLE 1.—Patient Data by Level of Amputation

Level of Amputation* (m)	M	F	Mean Age (years)	Follow-up Interval (years)	Reason for Amputation (no. of pts.)				No. Patients Employed After Amputation	No. Patients Phantom Pain at Follow-up Examination	No. Patients Who Stopped Using Prosthesis
					Trauma	Malignancy	PVD	Unknown			
Wrist Disarticulation (14)	12	2	55.0	17.4	14	0	0	0	14	6†	6
Below elbow (42)	37	5	55.4	19.0	32	3	4	3	33	24	3†
Above elbow (51)	43	9	48.5	16.4	36	8	1	7	36	38	29
Shoulder Disarticulation and forequarter (21)	15	6	53.0	16.7	10	8	1	2	14	18	12

* Unknown in 6 patients.
† Significant: P < 0.01.
Abbreviation: PVD, peripheral vascular disease.
(Courtesy of Wright TW, Hagen AD, Wood MB: Prosthetic usage in major upper extremity amputations. J Hand Surg (Am) 20A:619–622, 1995.)

rates close to 60%. Usage rates have increased with the arrival of the myoelectric prosthesis. The patterns of use with contemporary upper limb prostheses were evaluated retrospectively in a large group of patients seen in a referral practice.

Methods.—A chart review of patients seen from 1975 to 1987 identified 330 who had upper extremity amputations. Of these patients, 113 men and 22 women both responded to a mailed questionnaire and met the inclusion criteria. In 47%, the dominant extremity was amputated. The average age at amputation was 36 years, and the average follow-up was 12 years. Levels of amputation were as follows: 11% wrist disarticulation, 33% below elbow, 40% above elbow, and 15% shoulder disarticulation or forequarter (Table 1).

Results.—Of 113 patients (84%) who were fitted with a prosthesis, 99 (88%) obtained their prosthesis within the first year after amputation. The first prosthesis was usually body powered (82%) rather than myoelectric powered. Of the patients fitted with a prosthesis, 38% stopped using it. The most common reasons for not using the prosthesis included limited usefulness (65%), the heavy weight of the prosthesis (48%), and stump socket discomfort (30%). Prosthesis usage rates differed by level of amputation: wrist disarticulation (54%), below elbow (94%), above elbow (43%), and shoulder disarticulation and forequarter (40%). The high acceptance rates among patients who had below elbow amputation included all 5 patients who had a myoelectric prosthesis and 27 of 29 who had a conventional prosthesis. The low acceptance rate of 54% in the patients who had wrist disarticulation seemed to occur because the stump is quite functional at this level. The 4 bilateral amputees used their prosthesis. None of the 3 patients in the brachial plexus palsy group used their prosthesis. Seventy-eight percent of patients were employed before and 75% were employed after amputation.

Conclusions.—A contemporary body-powered or myoelectric prosthesis was used by nearly two thirds of the upper extremity amputees. Most below elbow amputees used a prosthesis, but less than half the above elbow amputees used one. Wrist disarticulation amputees often preferred to use the stump rather than a prosthesis. Patients who had both an above elbow amputation and a stiff shoulder or an associated brachial plexus injury were unlikely to use a prosthesis.

▶ This article provides helpful information for clinicians in assessing patients who have upper limb amputations for prescription of prostheses.

M. Leblanc, Ph.D.

Prognosis of Occupational Hand Dermatitis in Metalworkers
Shah M, Lewis FM, Gawkrodger DJ (Royal Hallamshire Hosp, Sheffield, England)
Contact Dermatitis 34:27–30, 1996
15–10

Introduction.—Metalworkers engaged in the cutting and grinding of metal components frequently have hand dermatitis. This dermatitis has been linked to the use of water-based soluble oils, which contain a wide variety of ingredients. The prognosis and responsible allergens for occupational hand dermatitis in metalworkers were studied.

Methods.—Patch testing was performed in 64 metalworkers (mean age, 46 years) who had hand dermatitis. One to 5 years later, follow-up information was gathered by a mail survey.

Results.—Thirty-seven patients had at least 1 positive reaction on patch testing (Table 1). Twenty-nine patients reacted to biocides, 20 to metals, and 19 to other oil ingredients. The survey response rate was 80%. Most patients continued to have symptoms, whether their dermatitis was of the occupational allergic, occupational irritant, or endogenous only type. In addition, the symptoms continued regardless of whether they continued to work with oils and metals. Symptoms were common even in patients who were unemployed or had changed jobs.

Conclusions.—Metalworkers who have hand dermatitis have positive results of skin tests for a wide range of metals and oil constituents. This condition has a poor prognosis; most patients remain symptomatic regardless of whether they continue to work with metals. Worker education and/or better occupational hygiene might improve the prognosis of occupational hand dermatitis in metalworkers.

▶ Occupational hand dermatitis is a common problem that results in a high percentage of disability. The problem is generally multifactorial, with the inciting agent being a contact allergy or irritation in susceptible individuals, and may be exacerbated by concomitant infection. The best treatment is

TABLE 1.—Results of Patch Testing: The Most Common Relevant Allergic Reactions

Allergen	Male (no. tested: 58)	Female (no. tested: 6)
chromate	8	—
nickel	3	4
cobalt	4	1
formaldehyde	5	—
chloroacetamide	5	—
Bioban CS 1246	5	—
Bioban CS 1135	5	—
colophony	3	—
Bioban P1487	3	—

(Courtesy of Shah M, Lewis FM, Gawkrodger DJ: Prognosis of occupational hand dermatitis in metalworkers. *Contact Dermatitis* 34:27–30, Copyright 1996, Munksgaard International Publishers Ltd., Copenhagen.)

avoidance of the inciting agent, which is not easily possible. This study is basically a questionnaire survey of 64 patients with an 82% response rate. Positive patch testing results are listed in Table 1. A high prevalence of contact sensitivity is found in their group of metalworkers; however, irritant and endogenous factors were also important in the etiology of occupational hand dermatitis in their patients. The patch test results showed a wide range of allergens, thereby underlining the importance of testing to a full complement of oil constituents. The survey demonstrated a poor prognosis with hand dermatitis in metalworkers. Most remained symptomatic regardless of whether they continued to work with oils and metals. Unemployment or a change of jobs had little effect on the outcome.

R.K. Roenigk, M.D.

Suggested Reading

Meinke WB: The work of piano virtuosity: An ergonomic analysis. *Med Prob Perform Art* June:48–61, 1995.
▶ This paper makes for interesting reading and seemed to be an attempt to encompass a terribly complex problem by relatively simple means. It could serve as a first step or introduction to this impossibly complex field. I would prefer to see the authors, having introduced the complexity of the field, reduce piano playing to a single element or two and then do a true anatomical, physiological, and biomechanical anaylsis of one or two simple movements. These, in themselves, become very complex when one starts with the opposite cerebral cortex.

R.A. Chase, M.D.

Sakai N, Liv MC, Su F-C, et al: Motion analysis of the fingers and wrist of the pianist. *Med Probl Perform Art* 11:24–29, 1996.

Kihira M, Ryu J, Han JS, et al: Wrist motion analysis in violinists. *Med Probl Perform Art* 10:79–85, 1995.

Smutz WP, Bishop A, Niblock H, et al: Load on the right thumb of the oboist. *Med Probl Perform Art* September:94–99, 1995.

Batson G: Conscious use of the human body in movement: The peripheral neuroanatomic basis of the Alexander technique. *Med Probl Perform Art* March:3–11, 1996.

Das SK, Johnson MB, Cohly HHP: Catfish stings in Mississippi. *South Med J* 88:809–812, 1995.

16 Microsurgery

Evaluation of the Effectiveness of Sensory Reeducation Following Digital Replantation and Revascularization
Shieh S-J, Chiu H-Y, Lee J-W, et al (Natl Cheng-Kung Univ, Taiwan, Republic of China)
Microsurgery 16:578–582, 1995 16–1

Introduction.—Advancements in microsurgical techniques have allowed the reconstruction of amputated hand parts to become a routine procedure. Recovery of motor function has been emphasized in the medical literature. Poor sensory recovery, however, can adversely affect hand function. The use of a sensory reeducation program in effecting sensory recovery after digital replantation or revascularization was compared with a conventional rehabilitation program.

Methods.—Of 113 patients who had undergone replantation or revascularization of 174 digits, 12 were randomly assigned to a sensory reeducation program. Another 15 patients participated in a regular postoperative rehabilitation program. Baseline levels of a moving 2-point discrimination test and Semmes-Weinstein pressure threshold were recorded. The moving 2-point discrimination test was considered positive if 7 of 10 responses were correct. If the stimuli were not correctly identified, the patient was given a series of sensory reeducation exercises to perform. These exercises included moving-touch stimuli and object-identification by touch. Exercises were performed in 10–15 minute sessions, 2–3 times per day. Patients were given a disk-discriminator and objects to practice with at home. Semmes-Weinstein and moving 2-point discrimination tests were performed every 2 weeks to assess constant touch and functional sensory return.

Results.—Patients who underwent sensory reeducation had significantly better sensory recovery compared with patients who received regular rehabilitation. Use of sensory reeducation resulted in a mean moving 2-point discrimination of 4.5 ± 2.377 mm, compared with 7.591 ± 3.750 without sensory reeducation. The mean Semmes-Weinstein pressure threshold was 0.040 ± 0.032 g with sensory reeducation, compared with 0.306 ± 0.432 g without. These differences were statistically significant. Continuing improvement in the moving 2-point discrimination test was seen throughout the follow-up period (Fig 1). Factors such as age, digit involved, and level of injury did not have a significant effect on moving

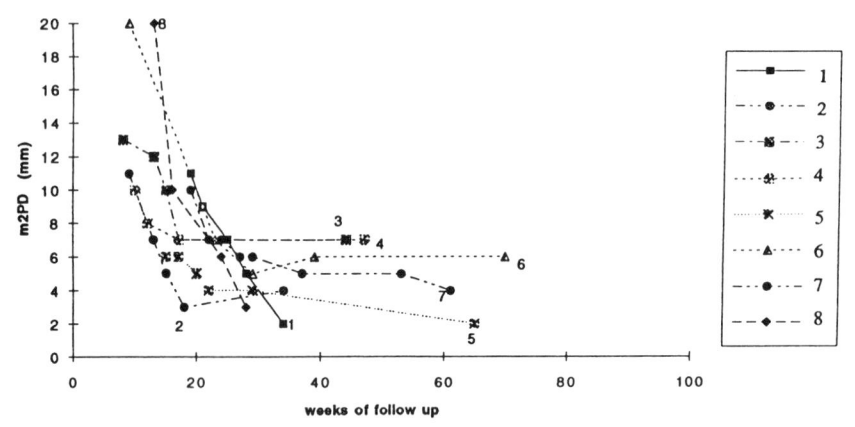

FIGURE 1.—Improvement of 2-point discrimination test ($m2PD$) after sensory reeducation (index finger). The numbers in the *insert* represent 8 revascularized or replanted index fingers with sensory reeducation (Courtesy of Shieh S-J, Chiu H-Y, Lee J-W, et al: Evaluation of the effectiveness of sensory reeducation following digital replantation and revascularization. *Microsurgery* 16:578–582, Copyright 1995. Reprinted by permission of John Wiley & Sons, Inc.)

2-point discrimination or Semmes-Weinstein tests. Both the mechanism of injury and the type of amputation has a significant effect on the moving 2-point discrimination test.

Conclusion.—Use of sensory reeducation significantly improved sensory recovery after replantation or revascularization of digits. Use of this technique as part of a rehabilitation program may aid in the restoration of satisfactory hand function.

▶ In spite of the importance of recovery of sensibility after nerve reconstruction, there still is little known about the effectiveness of sensory re-education to enhance sensory recovery. The study of Shieh et al. suggests that a course of sensory reeducation will improve the results of nerve reconstruction. The weakness of this report is that the study group was trained or "re-educated" with a discriminator and then tested with the same instrument to measure 2-point discrimination. A better test of outcome of sensory reeducation would be functional tests of object identification and hand use. The study, however, does provide the impetus for further investigation to determine potential merits of sensory rehabilitation.

S.E. Mackinnon, M.D.

Free Transplants of the Phalanges of the Foot in Deformities of the Hand [in Spanish]
Minguella J, Cabrera M (Hosp Sant Joan de Déu, Barcelona)
Rev Ortop Traum 40:120–125, 1995   16–2

Introduction.—Treatment of aphalangism or severe hypoplastic digits is controversial, as prostheses are cumbersome and do not provide sensibility, and toe-to-hand transfer is a major operation, with disappointing results in most cases.

Methods.—The results of 81 grafts from the proximal phalanx of a toe performed in 42 children were reviewed. The phalanx of the foot (usually from the third toe) was removed, preserving the periosteum and part of the capsule of the metatarsophalangeal joint. The capsular remnant was used to stabilize the toe to the head of the metacarpal and to suture the remains of flexor and extensor tendons in 34 cases.

Results.—There were complications in 6 (7.4%) phalanges out of a total of 81 grafts: 2 infections from the K wire, 1 dislocation of the phalanx on the metacarpal head, and 3 cases of skin necrosis from excessive pressure. No bone reabsorbtions were observed. The average growth of the transplanted phalanges was 1.5 mm in the revision performed at between 18 and 23 months, 2.3 mm at between 2 and 3 years, and 3 mm after more than 3 years.

▶ Only 42 toe bone grafts in 22 children (52% of the total) were reviewed here, because these were the only ones with enough follow-up to determine the growth of the transplanted phalanges. Superior growth was observed in the children in whom the surgery was done at an earlier age (between 18 and 23 months of age), with an average of 5.5 mm at the age of 9 years. The results are not fantastic, but this seems a reasonable treatment for reconstruction in children with empty digital soft-tissue sleeves. The 2 most important points for the survival of the bone physis are the removal of the phalanx with its periosteum and the performance of the procedure at the earliest possible age.

A. Lluch, M.D., Ph.D.

The Psychological Impact of Microvascular Free Toe Transfer for Children and Their Parents
Bradbury ET, Kay SPJ, Hewison J (St James's Univ Hosp, Leeds, England)
J Hand Surg (Br) 19B:689–695, 1994   16–3

Background.—Parents' reactions to congenital hand deformities are of primary importance in understanding the impact of such deformities. The parents' emotional state is rarely considered, however, in the preoperative assessment of the child. The preoperative psychological state of both parents and children was assessed, and factors that influence the psychological outcome of surgery were determined.

Methods.—Nine girls and 5 boys, aged 6 months to 13 years, were included. The 14 families were assessed before and 2 years after surgery. The parents underwent adjustment measurement, a detailed semi-structured interview, and measures of anxiety and depression. The children's assessment was based on behavior and social competence, social experience, self-consciousness about the hand, and their perceptions of their functional competence. Parents and children rated their satisfaction with the hand, and an independent professional panel rated function and appearance.

Findings.—Parental adjustment to the child's hand was an important independent variable in determining psychosocial outcome. The children of poorly adjusted parents had more social and psychological problems before surgery and increased behavioral problems after surgery. The parents of such children were less anxious and happier after the surgery. The children of well-adjusted parents had fewer problems before surgery and showed a slight, general improvement after surgery. The function and appearance of the operated hands were improved significantly in all children.

Conclusions.—It is important to identify vulnerable children who have congenital hand malformations to help them cope psychologically and benefit more fully from surgical treatment. Parents' responses seem to be extremely important. A multidisciplinary approach is necessary for the treatment of such patients to meet the needs of both the children and their families.

▶ This very interesting article looked critically at the impact of microvascular toe transfer on the parent and child. Several features stand out. Surgery performed too early was perhaps detrimental. A better time was between the ages of 3 and 7 years. The parents did not view the foot as "mutilated" by the surgery, even when hand function was only minimally improved. Even excellent surgery will not appreciably alter a child who has pre-existing problems of coping with his or her deformity.

V.R. Hentz, M.D.

Ring Avulsion Injuries: Microsurgical Management
Adani R, Castagnetti C, Busa R, et al (Univ of Modena, Italy)
J Reconstr Microsurg 12:189–194, 1996   16–4

Introduction.—The advent of microsurgery has altered the management of ring avulsion injuries, permitting early revascularization with generally satisfactory results. Several different classifications of these injuries have been proposed to help in deciding whether to amputate the finger or attempt microsurgical salvage. An experience with the microsurgical management of ring avulsion injuries is presented.

Patients.—The experience included 31 patients with ring injuries: 23 men and 8 women (mean age, 37 years). Surgery was performed in 23 patients, 15 of whom underwent microsurgical revascularization. According to Kay's classification, there were 10 class II, 3 class III, and 2 class IV injuries. All 15 patients underwent the usual procedures for attempted salvage: arteriolysis, direct vessel suture, and vein grafting. Seven patients also received a vessel transfer from the middle finger. In 5 patients, the ulnar digital artery of the middle finger was transferred to the ring finger, and in 4 patients, at least 1 vein was transferred from the dorsal aspect of the middle finger.

Outcomes.—Reconstruction was successful in 12 of 15 cases. At an average follow-up of 48 months, this group of patients had very good functional recovery, with a mean total active range of motion of 234 degrees and mean static 2-point discrimination (s2PD) of nearly 10 mm. The cosmetic results were also favorable.

Conclusions.—Good results can be achieved with microreconstructive surgery in patients with ring avulsion injuries. The authors believe that microsurgical treatment is indicated for all such injuries, except for those characterized by proximal amputation at the flexor superficialis tendon. Accordingly, they propose a new prognostic subclassification of Kay's class IV degloving and amputation lesions.

▶ The management of ring avulsion injuries, especially with fracture or joint injury, is controversial. In a classic article, Urbaniak et al[1] concluded: "Considerable judgment is involved when deciding whether to replant a completely amputated or degloved finger but generally we favor revision of the amputation." Adani and coauthors concluded that all ring avulsion injuries, with the exception of amputations proximal to the superficialis insertion, should be treated by microsurgical reconstruction. This conclusion is based on their technique of transferring an artery or vein from an adjacent finger to revascularize the avulsed digit rather than using traditional interposition vascular grafts. Their technique has the advantage of requiring a single anastomosis with a similar-caliber lumen, and they reported no morbid events in donors.

I have no doubt that this technique has merit and that it can be applied to many other situations.

However, given the expense of surgery, the time off from work, as well as the potential for morbid conditions (cold intolerance, loss of digital mobility, and sensibility), I am not convinced that Kay's class III and IV injuries are best served by revascularization or replantation. If amputation is done and esthetic considerations become an issue, ring ray resection results in a hand with acceptable appearance.

P.J. Stern, M.D.

Reference

1. Urbaniak JR, Evans JP, Bright DS: Microvascular management of ring avulsion injuries. *J Hand Surg* 6:25–30, 1981.

Microsurgical Composite Tissue Transplantation at Difficult Recipient Sites Facilitated by Preliminary Installation of Vein Grafts as Arteriovenous Loops

Ritter EF, Anthony JP, Levin LS, et al (Duke Univ, Durham NC; Univ of California, San Francisco)
J Reconstr Microsurg 12:231–240, 1996

Objective.—Vein grafting, sometimes necessary during microvascular surgery, has disadvantages that can result in higher failure rates in tissue transplantation. Use of a temporary looped arteriovenous fistula (AVF) during harvesting and positioning of the flap has been associated with improved results. A retrospective review of procedures using AVF construction, guidelines for construction, and indications for use were presented, and 2 cases were described.

Methods.—In 9 patients, fistulas were constructed and divided in 1 operation. In another 7 patients, the fistulas were constructed in 1 operation and divided in a later operation. Ten patients had acute fistulas and 7 had chronic fistulas. Six defects were located in the head and neck, 5 in the trunk, and 6 in the extremities. Arteriovenous fistulas were constructed of autologous saphenous veins in 18 cases and of an autologous cephalic vein in 1 case.

Case 1.—Woman, 43, operated on for a recurring meningioma after previous embolization and occlusion of her common carotid artery and resection and orbital exenteration, received an AVF between the carotid stump and the internal jugular vein. A rectus flap was set into the defect, and a microanastomosis was constructed from the divided loop.

Case 2.—Woman, 40, had radiation treatment after resection of a malignant fibrohistiocytoma of the right orbit and maxilla. An AVF was created between the external carotid artery and internal jugular vein, and a scapular osteofasciocutaneous flap was used to correct a defect created by a missing right temporalis muscle and the absence of the right zygotic arch and lateral orbital wall, orbital floor, and anterior maxilla. The flap was revascularized and survived.

Results.—Eight of nine 1-operation reconstructions were successful at follow-up. Two 2-operation reconstructions were patent at division 14 and 19 days later, and 6 were occluded.

Conclusion.—Atrioventricular fistulas should be created and divided. The flap should be harvested and placed in 1 procedure to avoid the high rates of thrombosis seen with the 2-operation method.

▶ It is often advantageous to create an AVF at the recipient site of a free flap. This creates added pedicle length beyond that allowed by the flap itself and thereby permits more rapid anastomoses and shorter ischemia time.

One team can harvest the vein graft (often just a long segment of the recipient vein) and anastomose it to the recipient artery, while a second team harvests the flap. Cut the resulting AVF in two and—voila!—2 long recipient vessels are ready for end-to-end anastomosis. In this interesting study, the authors examined what would happen if this 2-step approach were done in 2 different operations rather than as simultaneous parts of 1 procedure. Unfortunately, this appears to be too much of a good thing; the subsequent flaps are more likely to thrombose when the fistulae are given time to mature before division.

P.C. Amadio, M.D.

Cold-induced Vasospasm After Finger Replantation: Abnormal Sensory Regeneration and Sensitisation of Cold Nociceptors
Povlsen B (Univ Hosp, Linköping, Sweden)
Scand J Plast Reconstr Hand Surg 30:63–66, 1996   16–6

Introduction.—Cold-induced vasospasm, seen clinically as "white fingers," is a common problem in patients who have replanted digits. A prevalence of up to 100% has been reported. The reason for this complication is unknown, and there is no specific treatment. The postregenerative function of low-threshold mechanoreceptors could play a role in the development of secondary Raynaud's phenomenon after hand injuries. A series of patients who underwent digital replantation was studied to clarify the cause of cold-induced vasospasm.

Methods.—Seven patients whose replantations were performed more than 10 years previously were included to ensure sufficient time for sensory recovery. The circulatory effects of cold stimulation were studied in the replanted digit and in control fingers. The function of the low-threshold mechanoreceptors was assessed by measuring 2-point discrimination. Cold nociceptor thresholds were evaluated as well.

Results.—Six patients had problems with cold-induced vasospasm. All patients but 1 had evidence of vasospasm at 10°C and recovered cold nociception above 0°C. These patients had cold-induced pain at significantly higher temperatures in the replanted fingers than in the control fingers. The patients without cold nociception lacked low-threshold mechanoreceptor function, and the remaining patients had abnormal 2-point discrimination in the replanted finger.

Conclusions.—The occurrence of cold-induced vasospasm after finger replantation may be related to sensitization of cold nociceptors. This mechanism could account for the development of circulatory disturbances, even in patients who have nerve injuries only. Patients who have complete absence of functional low-threshold mechanoreceptors and cold nociception may be protected against cold-induced vasospasm.

▶ Pain on exposure to cold and associated vasospasm is estimated to affect 10% of the population of the United States and is common after severe nerve injury or replantation. The role of sensitized nociceptors in the etiology of cold intolerance is intriguing. The exact pathophysiology of the phenomenon, however, is still incompletely explained.

The use of completely amputated digits is an excellent model and could help elucidate the involved pathophysiology. Unfortunately, only 1 patient had good 2-point sensibility; interestingly, that patient had minimal vasospasm. This observation corresponds with the work of others and suggests that microvascular physiology approaches normal in patients who have good nerve return, as evidenced by the presence of 2-point discrimination less than 10 mm and/or intrinsic motor function. In patients who have incomplete nerve regeneration, cold-induced vasospasm may be based on the upregulation of α-adrenergic or other receptors in addition to or instead of stimulation of nociceptor discharges. Nevertheless, these observations confirm the presence of cold intolerance related to incomplete neural recovery.

L.A. Koman, M.D.

Suggested Reading

Guelinckx PJ, Sinsel NK: The "Eve" procedure: The transfer of vascularized seventh rib, fascia, cartilage, and serratus muscle to reconstruct difficult defects. *Plast Reconstr Surg* 97:527–535, 1996.
▶ Although this article presents a very nice experience in some commendable imaginative microsurgery, I have already been through the process of using composite grafts of rib and surrounding chest wall muscles and fascia. I have been completely disappointed in rib as a vascularized bone graft, more so in head and neck surgery than in extremity surgery. The donor sites with this rib graft are exceedingly painful, and the pain can last for 2–3 years. The harvest is extremely complex with risk of pneumothorax and neuromas from the intercostal nerves. I think that our armamentarium for vascularized bone grafting has much more to offer, with previously documented, large series, than this.

N.B. Meland, M.D.

Wei F-C, Ma H-S: Delayed sensory reeducation after toe-to-hand transfer. *Microsurgery* 16:583–585, 1995.
▶ The authors have demonstrated the ability and the importance of the sensory cortex in influencing recovery of 2-point discrimination after nerve reconstruction. Patients who are trained to discriminate between 1 and 2 points can learn this task. Whether this translates into improvement in object identification and functional recovery remains to be seen but is likely. The authors emphasize the importance of sensory rehabilitation, which continues to be under utilized in many clinical hand practices.

S.E. Mackinnon, M.D.

Lee KW, Chae IJ, Hahn SB: Thumb reconstruction with a free neurovascular wrap-around flap from the big toe: Long-term follow-up of thirty cases. *Microsurgery* 16:692–697, 1995.
▶ I favor the toe wrap-around flap for patients who have degloving injuries or intact osteo-articular columns, or for those concerned about the complete do-

nation of the entire great toe. This review adds further evidence to the excellent track record of the toe wrap-around flap.

C.H. Johnson, M.D.

Hallock GG: Liability of recipient vessels distal to the zone of injury when used for extremity free flaps. *J Reconstr Microsurg* 12:89–92, 1996.
▶ The concept of the "zone of injury" and the implications it carries regarding free-tissue transfer continue to undergo modification as experience is acquired. Although one would always prefer to use recipient vessels proximal to the zone of injury, circumstances sometimes dictate otherwise. In the event that failure to control the wound will lead to a loss of extremity, one should not hesitate to move distally. Although the move distally is usually undertaken for inflow considerations, care must be taken to ensure that the venous drainage will also be adequate. This is probably best done in the deep system. If the deep system proximally is involved because of being in "the zone," there is often enough collateralization to continue to adequately drain the extremity and flap. My own preference is to assess the recipient site distally for suitability before considering vein grafting as an alternative plan.

C.H. Johnson, M.D.

17 Vascular and Dystrophic Disorders

Hand Ischaemia Following Radial Artery Cannulation
Lee KSL, Miller JG, Laitung G (Royal Preston Hosp, Lancashire, England)
J Hand Surg (Br) 20B:493–495, 1995   17–1

Objective.—Radial artery catheterization is widely used for direct intra-arterial pressure monitoring in critically ill patients. Cannulation of the radial artery is sometimes followed by digital ischemia, which is most often caused by thrombotic occlusion of a dominant radial artery. Arterial thrombosis, however, is not the only possible cause of digital ischemia in this situation. A patient who had ischemia of the hand after radial artery cannulation was described, and the possible mechanisms of digital ischemia were reviewed.

> *Case Report.*—Man, 46, who had multiple sclerosis and a known urethral stricture was admitted with acute urinary retention. He went into septic shock, and a right subclavian central venous pressure monitoring line, a left radial arterial line, and a Swann Ganz catheter were inserted. The digits of the left hand became discolored 12 hours after admission, which was thought to have resulted from radial artery cannulation. The thumb was uninvolved; the radial artery was palpable up to the level of the anatomical snuff box and the ulnar artery to the level of Guyon's canal. The patient's condition precluded arteriography and thrombolysis. The patient did not respond to treatment for septicemic shock, and gangrene developed in the affected fingers. The patient died 7 days after admission to the ICU. At autopsy, the patient showed diffuse intracerebral hemorrhages consistent with disseminated intravascular coagulation. The radial and ulnar arteries and their superficial and deep palmar arches were patent. All the common digital arteries, however, were completely occluded (Fig 3).

Discussion.—Although radial artery thrombosis and occlusion are common complications of radial cannulation, irreversible digital ischemia is rare. Many factors may contribute to ischemia of the hand in critically ill

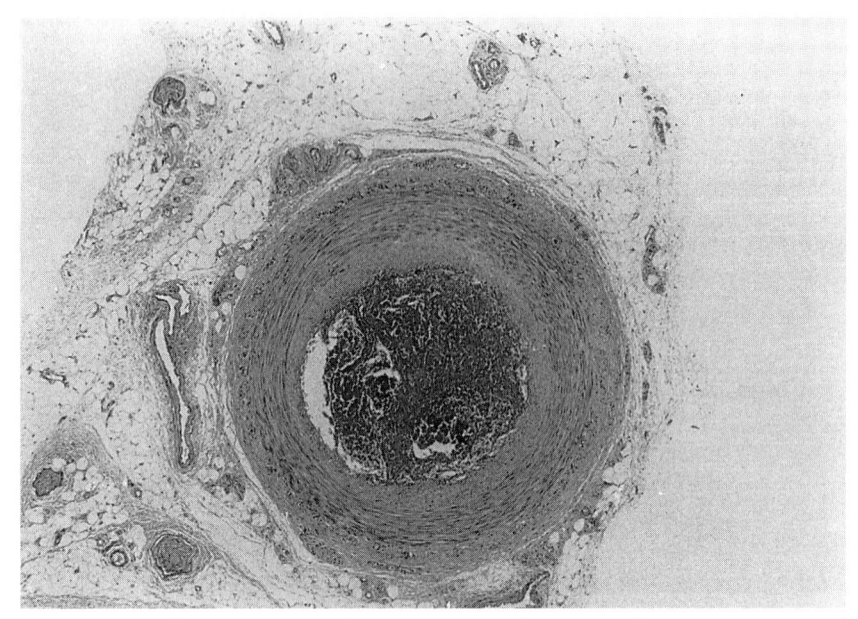

FIGURE 3.—Thrombosis in a digital artery. (Courtesy of Lee KL, Miller JG, Laitung G: Hand ischaemia following radial artery cannulation. *J Hand Surg (Br)* 20B:493–495, 1995.)

patients who have radial artery catheters; it does not necessarily result from the cannula alone. In this patient, systemic hypotension and disseminated intravascular coagulation probably played a role in the development of digital ischemic gangrene.

▶ Optimal management of digital ischemia associated with arterial cannulation is often complicated by associated critical medical problems. Early recognition of ischemic defects is crucial and should prompt rapid evaluation by experienced hand or vascular surgeons. If the catheter is patent, arteriography in the ICU can be achieved with the use of a low-pressure infusion of contrast below an inflated tourniquet and a portable x-ray machine. The tourniquet will not need to be up more than 5–10 minutes. At the same time, under tourniquet control, the extent of distal damage can be assessed by arteriography, and urokinase or other agents can be injected before the catheter is removed. The artery can be examined through a longitudinal incision under local anesthesia. The vessel can then be repaired or ligated depending on the clinical findings and other circumstances. Expert treatment of these problems, even under suboptimal conditions, is better than no treatment and may provide alternative management that is otherwise unavailable.

L.A. Koman, M.D.

Prognosis of Vibration Induced White Finger: A Follow Up Study
Petersen R, Andersen M, Mikkelsen S, et al (Univ of Copenhagen)
Occup Environ Med 52:110–115, 1995   17–2

Objective.—Because of uncertainty regarding the prognosis of vibration-induced white finger (VWF), which is a form of Raynaud's phenomenon caused by persistent exposure to vibration, 102 affected individuals were reevaluated 1–13 years after VWF had been diagnosed.

Methods.—The patients had worked in the metal or building industries or other trades and had used a variety of vibrating hand tools. The interval between the initial and follow-up assessments averaged 5 years. The patients were asked in detail about their work. They were also asked to sketch the areas affected in a drawing of the hands. Cold provocation testing was done with water at 8–12° C; a strain gauge plethysmograph was used to measure finger systolic pressure (FSP).

Findings.—The frequency of attacks had reportedly increased in 32% of patients, remained the same in 46%, and decreased in 22%. Attacks were significantly less frequent in those who had avoided high-vibration tools for 2 years or longer, in nonsmokers, and in those lacking other circulatory problems. The percent FSP increased, representing improvement, in nearly half the patients. Increased FSP correlated with age at initial assessment but not with recent exposure, smoking, other circulatory disorders, or the reported frequency of attacks.

Conclusion.—Patients who have moderate to severe VWF appear to have a good outlook as long as they avoid smoking and working with high-vibration hand tools and have no other circulatory disease.

▶ Post-traumatic Raynaud's phenomenon, in the absence of other causes and associated with the use of vibratory tools, has been termed VWF. Vibration white finger is a clinical entity of exclusion and has no pathognomonic sign, symptom, or test. Post-traumatic vasospastic or vaso-occlusive disease accounts for the digital findings and the concomitant Raynaud's phenomenon. In contradistinction to other reports, this article documents clinical improvement, including better digital perfusion after cold exposure, in a large group of patients who altered their traumatic exposure, avoided smoking, and did not have vascular disease.

L.A. Koman, M.D.

The Role of Bone Scintigraphy in Diagnosing Reflex Sympathetic Dystrophy
Lee GW, Weeks PM (Washington Univ, St Louis)
J Hand Surg (Am) 20A:458–463, 1995   17–3

Background.—Reflex sympathetic dystrophy (RSD) is a pain syndrome accompanied by functional loss and evidence of autonomic dysfunction. The syndrome can occur after trauma, surgery, or cerebrovas-

TABLE 1.—Calculation of Correlation Between 3-Phase Bone Scintigraphy and Reflex Sympathetic Dystrophy (*RSD*)

Bone Scan	Diagnosis Positive	Diagnosis Negative
Positive	True positive (a)	False positive (b)
Negative	False negative (c)	True negative (d)

Sensitivity = a/(a + c)
   The percentage of patients with clinical RSD that have positive scans for RSD.
Specificity = d/(b + d)
   The percentage of patients without clinical RSD that have negative scans for RSD.
Positive predictive value = a/(a + b)
   The likelihood that a patient has clinical RSD when the scan is positive.
Negative predictive value = d/(c + d)
   The likelihood that a patient will not have clinical RSD when the scan is negative.

(Courtesy of Lee GW, Weeks PM: The role of bone scintigraphy in diagnosing reflex sympathetic dystrophy. *J Hand Surg (Am)* 20A:458–463, 1995.)

cular accidents. Symptoms and clinical findings change over time, and 3 distinct stages of RSD have been identified. Diagnosis is often difficult, because there is no objective test for the syndrome. The validity of 3-phase bone scintigraphy (TPBS), a method that has gained acceptance during the past decade as an objective diagnostic test for RSD, was assessed, and the literature was reviewed.

Methods.—Bone scintigraphy to diagnose RSD is performed after IV administration of 20 mCi of Tc-99m labeled diphosphonate or polyphosphonate. The patient's upper extremities are scanned from the elbow to finger tips. The third phase of the study, 1.5–4 hours after injection, reflects tracer uptake within the bone. Although diffusely increased uptake in the affected areas is thought to confirm a diagnosis of RSD, other conditions yield similar findings. Nineteen articles relating bone scintigraphy with the diagnosis of RSD of the upper extremity were reviewed, and the degree of correlation between TPBS and RSD was expressed as sensitivity, specificity, and positive and negative predictive values (Table 1).

Results.—There was a wide variability in the sensitivity, specificity, and positive and negative predictive values when TPBS was used in the diagnosis of RSD of the hand (Table 3). Interobserver variability was considerable, even in the evaluation of scintigrams of patients known to have the syndrome. None of the studies used quantitative analysis to interpret periarticular uptake, and the performance of bone scintigraphy at various times after symptoms onset had an effect on findings.

Discussion.—Results of TPBS correlate best with the clinical diagnosis of RSD within the first 20–26 weeks of the onset of symptoms. After this time, the degree of correlation is poor. Clinical diagnosis by an experienced hand surgeon remains the most accurate method of diagnos-

TABLE 3.—Comparison of 3 Retrospective Studies and 1 Prospective Study Evaluating Usefulness of 3-Phase Bone Scintigraphy in Diagnosing Reflex Sympathetic Dystrophy

Author	Sensitivity (%)	Specificity (%)	Positive Predictive Value (%)	Negative Predictive Value (%)	No. of Static Scintigrams Examined	No. of Patients With RSD	Mean Age (years)	Average Duration of Symptoms (weeks)	No. of Positive Scintigrams
Kozin et al., groups 1,2,4,5	—	93	95	61	43	28	—	76	20
Kozin et al., group 1 only	83	NA	NA	NA	18	18	—	76	15
Mackinnon and Holder	96	98	88	99	145	23	43	28	22
Werner et al., groups 1,2*	50	92	67	84	63	16	38	84	8
Werner et al.,†	64	94	88	79	27	—	—	—	—
Werner et al.,‡	100	85	75	100	19	—	—	—	—
Pollock et al.	54	—	—	—	28	28	39	32	15

Note: Kozin's study group has been listed twice to show results when groups 1 and 2 are combined and when the more selective group 1 is analyzed alone. Mackinnon and Holder's group would be comparable to Kozin's group 1 criteria. Werner et al.'s data are broken down into 3 categories: *asterisk*, hand patients; *dagger*, hand patients with reflex sympathetic dystrophy less than 26 weeks; *double dagger*, hand patients older than 50 years of age.

Abbreviations: RSD, reflex sympathetic dystrophy; *dash*, data not available; NA, cannot be defined in this group.

(Courtesy of Lee GW, Weeks PM: The role of bone scintigraphy in diagnosing reflex sympathetic dystrophy. *J Hand Surg (Am)* 20A:458–463, 1995.)

ing RSD. Many patients who have clinical RSD will have a negative scan, whereas false positive scintigrams occur in asymptomatic patients.

▶ This is a very timely paper. The report by Mackinnon and Holder[1] in 1984 has been misinterpreted by many. The concept that a negative TPBS essentially rules out RSD may not be widespread but is accepted by many, and these same clinicians quote the 1984 article. The specificity of the examination, especially a positive third phase, is high, which means that a very high percentage of individuals without clinical RSD will have a negative scan. The sensitivity, however, is much less high, which means that many patients with clinical RSD will have a negative scan. Reflex sympathetic dystrophy remains a clinical diagnosis.

V.R. Hentz, M.D.

Reference

1. Mackinnon JE, Holder LE: The use of three-phase radionuclide bone scanning in the diagnosis of reflex sympathetic dystrophy. *J Hand Surg (Am)* 9A:556–563, 1984.

Suggested Reading

Isogai N, Fukunishi K, Kamiishi H: Patterns of thermoregulation associated with cold intolerance after digital replantation. *Microsurgery* 16:556–565, 1995.
▶ The authors advocate the use of thermography as a possible means of identifying patients who are more likely to suffer cold intolerance. The authors' conjecture that early intervention by sympathetic blockade or by digital sympathectomy might ameliorate suffering. In their patients, postoperative circulation correlated with sensory recovery. Others disagree.

V.R. Hentz, M.D.

Backman CO, Nyström Å, Backman C, et al: Cold induced vasospasm in replanted digits: A comparison between different methods of arterial reconstruction. *Scand J Plast Reconstr Hand Surg* 29:343–348, 1995.
▶ This is a continuation of previous work from Umea, Sweden, designed to provide a better understanding of the incidence, presentation, and mechanisms of cold intolerance after replantation of amputated digits. Although the causes remain poorly understood, this study recognized that the use of a long graft anastomosed to the radial artery at the wrist and then to the digital artery of the amputated thumb resulted in a reduced incidence of cold intolerance, indicating that cold-induced spasm was related to the replanted or grafted structures as opposed to a pre-existing tendency to spasm in the feeding vessel. Their work supports the notion that cold intolerance in patients who exhibit spasm in response to either a systemic or local cold challenge may really not improve with time.

V.R. Hentz, M.D.

Celli L, Mingione A, Maleti O, et al: Deep venous thrombosis of the upper limb (in Italian), in Gandolfi M (ed): *La Trombosi Venosa Profonda in Ortopedia e Traumatologia*. Rome, Antonio Delfino, 1995, pp 53–65.

▶ This paper provides a comprehensive overview of deep venous thrombosis of the upper limb. The crushing type of lesion of the upper limb; complex trauma; and fractures of the humerus, clavicle, and elbow might be related to this complication. The specific merit of the authors was to classify, in a meticulous fashion, all the possible predisposing anatomical factors. Therefore this paper might be useful for consultation when dealing with this infrequent complication. Unfortunately no personal series are presented and neither the problem of differential diagnosis with compartmental syndromes nor lymphatic obstructions are discussed.

A. Landi, M.D.

18 Research

Dispersion of Regenerating Axons Across Enclosed Neural Gaps
Brushart TM, Mathur V, Sood R, et al (Johns Hopkins Hosps, Baltimore, Md)
J Hand Surg (Am) 20A:557–564, 1995   18–1

Background.—Tubular prostheses in primates have been shown to support peripheral axon regeneration across gaps of up to 3 cm. The precision with which axons cross a gap and reinnervate the periphery, however, is debated. Continuous tracing of regenerated rat sciatic nerve axons with horseradish peroxidase–wheat germ agglutinin (HRP-WGA) was used to determine the dispersion of axons as they cross a gap. The effects of gap distance and fascicular orientation on this dispersion were also studied.

Methods and Findings.—Proximal and distal tibial and peroneal fascicles were oriented precisely around the longitudinal midplane of a silicon tube. Fascicular alignment was correct or reversed, and the gaps were 2 and 5 mm. The application of HRP-WGA to the distal peroneal fascicle was done after 6 weeks of regeneration to label the reinnervating axons continuously. The axons tended to grow straight across the tube. Dispersion increased as a factor of distance when correct fascicular alignment was maintained. When fascicular alignment was reversed, fascicular size, rather than identity, determined axonal dispersion.

Conclusions.—These data do not support the notion that neurotropic interactions promote "correct" fascicular reinnervation. Increased random reinnervation and functional disruption with larger gaps will result from progressive axonal dispersion and the absence of variables that promote fascicular specificity. When reconstructing a nerve that serves many functions, an enclosed gap is not an acceptable substitute for nerve graft.

▶ The results of this significant study contradict the notion that, given the opportunity, a regenerating axon knows best where it should grow. This idea has led to a sense that alignment of proximal and distal stumps is less important than providing an appropriate size gap between approximated nerve ends. Indeed, leaving a gap so that sprouting axons can make a choice will more than make up for misalignment. Good science compels us to take seriously the authors admonition that "an enclosed gap is not an acceptable substitute for nerve graft when reconstructing a nerve that serves multiple functions."

                                                                          V.R. Hentz, M.D.

Bioartificial Nerve Grafts: A Prototype
Lundborg G, Kanje M (Malmö Univ, Sweden; Lund Univ, Sweden)
Scand J Plast Reconstr Hand Surg 30:105–110, 1996   18–2

Introduction.—Tubes made of a variety of absorbable materials have been used successfully to bridge nerve gaps in both animals and humans. The tube technique has not been useful, however, for bridging extended gaps. A bioartificial nerve graft was developed that introduces synthetic filaments within a silicone tube to stabilize the fibrin matrix and support axonal growth between nerve stumps.

Methods.—In a basic model designed to set a baseline for a series of experimental studies, synthetic filaments were used to bridge a 10-mm gap in the continuity of rat sciatic nerve. After exposure of the sciatic nerve on the left side, a 5-mm segment was resected to produce a gap measuring 10 mm. The gap was treated with polyamide filaments introduced into a silicone tube in 8 animals (Fig 1). Eight additional rats received empty silicone tubes with no filaments inside; 8 controls had no conduit to bridge the nerve gap. The surgical area was examined 4 weeks later and the nerve segments classified as "response," indicating the presence of regenerating sensory axons, or "no response," indicating an absence of sensory axons.

Results.—In the filament group, multiple axons organized into minifascicles were noted in all cases between the synthetic filaments and in the space between the filaments and the silicone tube. Filaments were well incorporated in a loose connective tissue matrix containing numerous

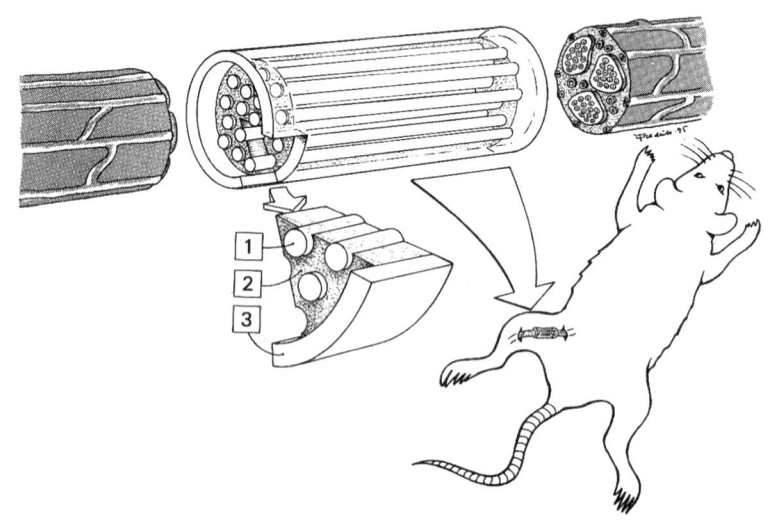

FIGURE 1.—Diagram of the bioartificial nerve graft. A number of polyamide (nylon) filaments (size ≈250 μm) are introduced into a silicone tube (inner diameter, 1.8 mm). This prototype was used to bridge a 10-mm gap in the continuity of the rat sciatic nerve. 1: Polyamide filament. 2: Space between filaments. 3: Silicone tube. (Courtesy of Lundborg G, Kanje M: Bioartificial nerve grafts: A prototype. *Scand J Plast Reconstr Hand Surg* 30:105–110, 1996.)

longitudinally oriented capillaries. Pinching of the nerve distal to the tube caused a response in 4 of 8 animals. In the empty tube group, the gap was bridged by a nervelike structure containing multiple minifascicles and numerous capillaries. All 8 animals exhibited response to the pinch test. Controls had no structure bridging the gap between proximal and distal nerve segments, and none responded to the pinch.

Conclusion.—In its present form, the prototype for a bioartificial nerve graft is inferior to an empty tube with respect to overgrowth of axons in a 10-mm gap. The finding that regeneration is supported by the filament-filled tubes offers a basis, however, for future development of a bridge for extended nerve gaps.

▶ A glimpse of the future, perhaps?

P.C. Amadio, M.D.

Effect of Motion on Digital Nerve Repair in a Fresh Cadaver Model
Malczewski MC, Zamboni WA, Haws MJ, et al (Southern Illinois Univ, Springfield; Univ of Nevada, Las Vegas; Univ of Tennessee, Memphis)
Plast Reconstr Surg 96:1672–1675, 1995   18–3

Purpose.—Isolated digital nerve injuries commonly occur at the level of the proximal interphalangeal joint. Treatment includes a tension-free epineurial repair using standard microsurgical technique. Previous reports, however, have provided only vague information about the postoperative management of these repairs; up to 3 weeks of postoperative immobilization is commonly recommended. The optimal postoperative motion regimen after digital nerve injuries was clarified in a cadaver study.

Methods.—In 1 fresh cadaver, 10 digital nerves at the level of the proximal interphalangeal joint or, in the case of the thumb, at the level of the midproximal phalanx were divided then repaired. After the digits were repeatedly taken through a full passive range of motion, the nerve repairs were reexamined. In 8 subsequent groups, intact nerve repairs underwent serial resection to identify the resection limits that would permit motion without disruption of the repair.

Findings.—Even with hyperextension up to a resection length of 2.5 mm, all repairs demonstrated resistance to disruption. When splinted in neutral position, the repairs were resistant to disruption up to a resection length of 5 mm. Not until the resection length reached 1 cm, with a range of motion including hyperextension, did all repairs become disrupted.

Conclusions.—Although drawn from a cadaver model, the findings provide objective data for use in designing postoperative motion and splinting protocols for patients who have various degrees of digital nerve injury. Early mobilization without finger splinting could be considered for sharp digital nerve injuries with resection lengths of 2.5 mm or less. For injuries with gaps of 5 mm, early full range of motion with a dorsal blocking splint may be considered. Postoperative immobilization appears to be indicated for injuries with gaps of 7.5 mm or greater.

▶ The goal of this study was to bring some scientific basis to the clinicians' postoperative practices after repair of lacerated digital nerves. Because it is strictly an acute experiment and because only disruption of the repair site constituted an unfavorable end point, it is difficult to judge the significance of the results. Still, we are probably overprotective in our management of the repaired digital nerve where there is no loss of substance.

V.R. Hentz, M.D.

Orientated Mats of Fibronectin as a Conduit Material for Use in Peripheral Nerve Repair
Whitworth IH, Brown RA, Doré C, et al (Queen Victoria Hosp, East Grinstead, England; Univ College Hosp, London; Northwick Park Hosp, Harrow, England)
J Hand Surg (Br) 20B:429–436, 1995
18–4

Introduction.—Fibronectin (Fn) mats are novel 3-dimensional fibrous materials made by aggregating purified plasma Fn under a unidirectional shear so that the fibers are aligned in parallel and suitable for promoting cell contact guidance. The ability of Fn-mat substrates to act as a solid guide for regenerating axons was assessed. In addition, axonal regeneration was compared within similar length grafts using isograft sciatic nerve or freeze-thawed muscle grafts.

Methods.—Axonal regeneration, Schwann cell behavior, and degree of inflammation were quantified by using immunohistochemical techniques and computerized image analysis. Fibronectin was used to bridge a 1-cm defect in the sciatic nerve in 30 rats. This approach was compared with autologous nerve grafts and freeze-thawed muscle grafts in 2 control groups of 30 rats each.

Results.—The nerve grafts supported the highest rate and amount of axonal regeneration in the first 10 days, but the Fn supported a significantly faster rate of growth and amount of axons than did the freeze-thawed muscle grafts. The large amount was achieved in the Fn group despite the lack of an initial depot of Schwann cells. Amounts of regenerating axons and Schwann cells were comparable in Fn and nerve grafts from day 15 onward. The nerve grafts had the lowest number of macrophages at all times, but the freeze-thawed muscle grafts had marginally higher levels only at days 15 and 60. The Fn-mats had higher levels at days 5, 10, and 15 but had levels comparable to those of nerve grafts by day 30.

Conclusion.—The oriented form of Fn is a suitable material for successful nerve repair and has potential for clinical use.

▶ Fibronectin mats have a parallel alignment suitable for promotion of cell contact guidance. This material may allow neurites and Schwann cells to grow in a milieu of nerve growth factors. Previous studies have shown different nerve cells rapidly attach to single strands of Fn.

In this study, it appears that axonal regeneration using Fn-mats was comparable to that with isograft sciatic nerve grafts and somewhat better than that with freeze-thawed muscle autografts.

E. Akelman, M.D.

Different Muscle Graft Denaturing Methods and Their Use for Nerve Repair
Whitworth IH, Doré C, Hall S, et al (Queen Victoria Hosp, East Grinstead, England; Northwick Park Hosp, London; Guy's Campus, London)
Br J Plast Surg 48:492–499, 1995
18–5

Background.—Freezing, then thawing, skeletal muscle disrupts muscle protein but leaves basement membranes intact. This tissue can then serve as a scaffold for axons and Schwann cells to bridge nerve defects. Two methods of denaturing muscle grafts, microwaving them, and immersing them in hot, hypo-osmolar water, were compared with nerve grafts and frozen-thawed muscle grafts for suitability as nerve graft material.

Methods.—In properly anesthetized adult rats, a 10-mm gap in the sciatic nerve was filled with 1 of 4 autologous grafts: a nerve graft; a frozen-thawed muscle graft; a microwaved muscle graft; or a muscle graft bathed in 60°C sterile water. At 5, 10, 15, 30, and 60 days after insertion, grafts were collected and examined for the rate and volume of axonal and Schwann cell penetration and for the degree of inflammation.

Results.—Shrinkage during denaturation varied among muscle grafts. Frozen-thawed tissue shrank to 42% of its pretreated length, and microwaved tissue shrank to only 89% of its pretreated length. The water-bathed tissue did not shrink. At days 5 and 10, the rate of axonal penetration was significantly higher for nerve grafts than for any type of muscle graft. The rate for microwaved and frozen-thawed muscle grafts was similar and significantly faster than water-bathed grafts. Regeneration across all muscle grafts was complete by day 15. The volume of regenerating neurons was initially highest in nerve grafts, but microwaved and frozen-thawed muscle grafts showed comparable axon volume by day 15. Water-bathed muscle grafts showed significantly less axonal volume for all 60 days. Proximal Schwann cell penetration of graft tissue was significantly more rapid for microwaved grafts than for frozen-thawed or water-bathed grafts until day 15, when Schwann cell penetration was complete in all muscle grafts. The degree of inflammation was lowest in the nerve grafts and frozen-thawed muscle grafts and significantly higher in the microwaved and water-bathed muscle grafts, especially the latter.

Conclusion.—Microwaving is a suitable technique for denaturing muscle to be used in nerve replacement over short gaps. It is comparable to freeze-thawing and superior to water-bathing.

▶ The authors have used a rat sciatic nerve model to investigate axonal regeneration in a gap space of 10 mm. They compare frozen-thawed muscle graft, microwaved muscle graft, 60°C (distilled water) warmed muscle graft, and reversed autologous nerve graft. The aim of the study was to determine whether axonal regeneration across a 10-mm gap could be enhanced by denaturing muscle grafts with methods other than freeze-thawing, which causes significant shrinkage of the original length of muscle.

The authors have concluded that autologous nerve grafts supported the highest rates and volumes of axonal regeneration until day 30, when the microwaved muscle grafts surpassed all other grafts based on axonal and Schwann cell immunostaining. The authors concluded that microwave heating may be suitable as an alternative denaturing method for bridging a nerve gap with a muscle graft and may have potential clinical use.

A significant advantage in this study is the low percentage of shrinkage (11%) of the original muscle induced by the microwave denaturing method compared with the frozen-thawed muscle graft (58%) and warmed muscle graft (0%). Although nerve grafts initially supported the highest levels of axonal regeneration, in the longer term both the frozen-thawed and microwave muscle grafts showed similar enhanced rates of regeneration.

A flaw in this study relates to the authors' use of S-100 protein antibody immunostaining as a specific marker for Schwann cells. S-100 immunoreactivity is not confined only to Schwann cells; it can also stain for neurofilament protein. Interestingly, the microwaved muscle grafts did contain high S-100 protein immunoreactivity compared with the other grafts, which is perhaps indicative of enhanced rates of regeneration, as suggested by the other results presented. The authors' conclusion that the clinical use of microwaved denatured muscle grafts to bridge a nerve gap appears well founded based on the data presented. Further studies in animal models to assess functional reinnervation should be performed, however, before consideration of human clinical trials.

M.A. Badalamente, Ph.D.

Electrophysiological, Morphological, and Morphometric Effects of Aging on Nerve Regeneration in Rats
Choi S-J, Harii K, Lee M-J, et al (Univ of Tokyo; Jichi Med School, Japan)
Scand J Plast Reconstr Hand Surg 29:133–140, 1995   18–6

Introduction.—In the structure and function of the peripheral nerves in normal animals, age-related changes, such as a decrease in the number of myelinated fibers, an increase in axonal degeneration, and a decrease in conduction velocity, have been found. Little is known about age-related effects on the process of nerve regeneration after injury. The effects of aging on the time course of nerve and muscle regeneration were assessed in rats from a functional and anatomical point of view.

Methods.—The right common peroneal nerves of 14 2-month-old and 14 10-month-old rats were transected and resutured to investigate the influence of age on the process of nerve regeneration. Measurements were taken of the motor nerve conduction velocity, latency, and amplitude of the evoked potential from the peroneus longus muscle at 4 and 8 weeks after the nerve repair. Measurements were also taken of the axon area, axon diameter, number of regenerated myelinated fibers, axon circumference, and myelin thickness. As a control, measurements were taken of the left common peroneal nerve and muscle.

Results.—Higher recovery rates were seen with the motor nerve conduction velocity, latency, and amplitude in 2-month old rats than in 10-month old rats, particularly at 4 weeks after the operation. Two-month-old rats also recovered more quickly in the morphometric study, axon area, axon diameter, and myelin thickness, particularly 4 weeks after the operation. In 2-month-old rats 8 weeks after the operation, myelin remnants were not found; however, they were seen in 10-month-old rats.

Conclusion.—A significantly greater recovery rate was seen in 2-month-old rats than in 10-month-old rats. The difference in the speed of Wallerian degeneration, axonal regeneration, and myelin regeneration seems to be the explanation. No changes were found in neuromuscular junctions or muscle fibers between the two age groups. Measurements of the isometric muscle contraction and sensory function by receptor quantitation and the walking track test may be necessary to confirm functional recovery.

▶ Just as there are well-recognized, age-related, physiologic and morphologic parameters of normal nerves, there are clearly age-related effects of nerve regeneration after injury and/or repair. This study supports several postulates including a more rapid rate of clearing away the debris of Wallerian degeneration as well as the processes of axonal growth and myelin maturation. In other words, preparing the ground for regeneration and the actual growth and maturation of axons are enhanced in the very young vs. the old. As the important proteins and their controlling genetic factors are identified and categorized further, it might be possible, with chemical manipulation, to fool old nerves into believing that they are young nerves.

V.R. Hentz, M.D.

Acute Stretching of Peripheral Nerves Inhibits Retrograde Axonal Transport
Tanoue M, Yamaga M, Ide J, et al (Kumamoto Univ, Japan)
J Hand Surg (Br) 21B:358–363, 1996   18–7

Introduction.—Changes in retrograde axonal transport have been shown to play an important role in the development of nerve abnormalities. There are no reports, however, of changes in retrograde axonal transport during stretching of the peripheral nerve, a subject of interest because of its relationship to compression nerve injuries. An experimental study used the conjugation of horseradish peroxidase with wheat germ agglutinin to determine the effect of stretching the peripheral nerve on retrograde axonal transport.

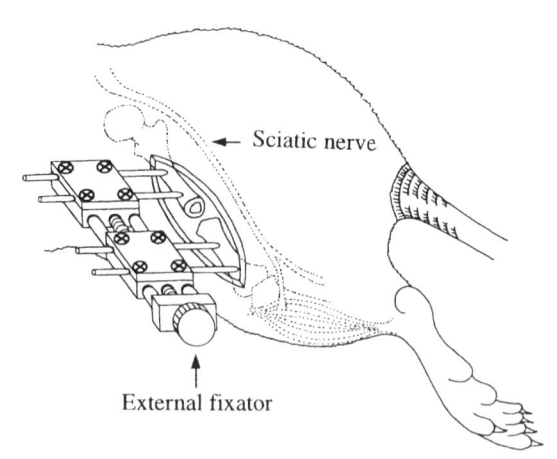

FIGURE 1.—Diagram of the method for indirectly stretching the rat sciatic nerve. (Courtesy of Tanoue M, Yamaga M, Ide J, et al: Acute stretching of peripheral nerves inhibits retrograde axonal transport. J Hand Surg (Br) 21B:358–363, 1996.)

Methods.—A unilateral external fixator was used to indirectly stretch the sciatic nerve (Fig 1) in adult male Wistar-derived strain rats. The model was used in 4 experiments. The first investigated the relationship between the amount of femoral lengthening and the percentage of elongation of the sciatic nerve. Left femurs in 20 rats were distracted at a rate of 10% per minute to the predetermined level. In 10 rats, the operated femur was distracted by 10% of the initial bone length; the remaining 10 rats had the operated femur distracted by 20% of the initial bone length. Other experiments determined the retrograde axonal transport index, nerve blood flow in the sciatic nerve, and histologic changes.

Results.—The mean percentage of elongation of the sciatic nerve was 6% for the 10% group and 11% for the 20% group. Most horseradish peroxidase–labelled motor neuron cells were located in the L4 segment on the control side and on the operated side. On the stretched side, these cells were significantly decreased compared with the control side (Fig 4B). In the 10% group and a sham group, numbers of horseradish peroxidase–labelled motor neuron cells did not differ between control and stretched sides. The retrograde axonal transport index was significantly decreased in the 20% group compared with the 10% group and the sham group; the latter 2 groups did not differ significantly from one another in retrograde axonal transport index. Measurements of nerve blood flow and histologic studies yielded similar results, with the 20% group differing significantly from the 10% and sham groups.

Discussion.—Acute stretching of the rat sciatic nerve led to an inhibition of retrograde axonal transport. The critical low limit that produces this effect lies between 6% and 11% strain. In the 20% group (11% strain), retrograde axonal transport and nerve blood flow decreased by a similar percentage (43% and 50%, respectively). Only nerves in the 20% group exhibited endoneurial edema.

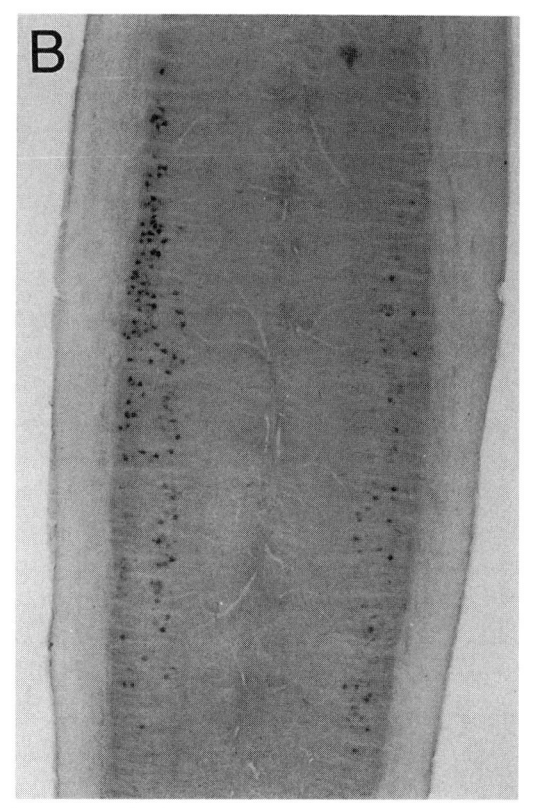

FIGURE 4B.—Photomicrograph of a 40-μm horizontal section of the rat spinal cord. Motor neurons were labelled by the retrograde transport of horseradish peroxidase–wheat germ agglutinin from the tibialis anterior muscle. These are typical spinal cords in the 20% group. The stretched side is on the right; original magnification, ×12.5. (Courtesy of Tanoue M, Yamaga M, Ide J, et al: Acute stretching of peripheral nerves inhibits retrograde axonal transport. *J Hand Surg (Br)* 21B:358–363, 1996.)

▶ This model may be useful in determining how to lengthen limbs (and nerves) more safely.

P.C. Amadio, M.D.

Free Radical Damage in Acute Nerve Compression
Ress AM, Babovic S, Angel MF, et al (Johns Hopkins Univ, Baltimore, Md)
Ann Plast Surg 34:388–395, 1995   18-8

Background.—The pathophysiology of acute peripheral nerve compression injury is not completely understood. Previous studies have shown that patients with diabetes have an increased susceptibility to chronic peripheral nerve compression. Whether increased oxidative activity and impaired cellular antioxidant defense mechanisms contribute to peripheral nerve injury in patients with diabetes was determined in a rat model after mechanical nerve compression.

Methods.—Experimental rats were assigned to 2 groups: the control group and a group in which diabetes was induced with streptozocin injection. Both groups were then assigned to 3 operative subgroups: sham operation, right sciatic nerve compression for 24 hours with silastic tubing, or 24-hour nerve compression followed by 1 hour of reperfusion. Some rats in the reperfusion subgroups were injected with deferoxamine mesylate or lazaroid U74389 during reperfusion. At the end of each experiment, blood flow to the nerve was assessed fluorometrically after fluorescein IV injection; nerve biopsy specimens were then obtained to evaluate levels of malonyldialdehyde (MDA) and enzyme activities.

Results.—Baseline fluorescein distribution was similar in the control and diabetic groups and was reduced by approximately 75% in compressed nerves in both groups. After reperfusion, fluorescein distribution returned to baseline levels in the nondiabetic nerves but to only 50% of the baseline levels in the diabetic nerves. Levels of MDA did not change significantly during compression but increased significantly after reperfusion: by 147% in nondiabetic nerve tissue and by 310% in diabetic nerve tissue. Levels of MDA were significantly reduced with deferoxamine or lazaroid U74389 treatment in diabetic rats but did not improve significantly in nondiabetic rats. Enzymes of the antioxidant defense system increased in both diabetic and normal rats during compression but decreased after reperfusion in diabetic rats and remained high or increased further in nondiabetic rats.

Conclusions.—Peripheral nerves in diabetic rats demonstrated greater expression of MDA, which is an indicator of free radical cell membrane damage, and demonstrated less antioxidant enzyme activity after reperfusion. These findings support the hypothesis that peripheral nerves can undergo ischemia and reperfusion injury mediated by free radicals.

▶ The authors convincingly demonstrate that production of free radicals occurs in association with acute nerve compression and suggest that damage by free-radical release may be responsible for some of the functional effects, thereby equating this to reperfusion injury seen in other ischemic or partially ischemic than reperfused tissues. Protecting tissues from the damage caused by release of noxious substances produced by cerebral occlusion and reperfusion is the subject of intense research. Perhaps we can protect our patients who have peripheral nerve injury by using free radical scavengers or antioxidants.

V.R. Hentz, M.D.

Work of Flexion After Tendon Repair With Various Suture Methods: A Human Cadaveric Study

Aoki M, Manske PR, Pruitt DL, et al (Washington Univ, St Louis)
J Hand Surg (Br) 20B:310–313, 1995   18–9

Background.—Flexor tendon repair is commonly followed by increased resistance to tendon gliding at the site of the repair. This may be a particular problem with techniques that use increased suture strands or suture material. The mechanical "work of flexion" (WOF) before and after 6 different techniques of tendon repair was determined in a cadaver study.

Methods.—Thirty-three flexor digitorum profundus tendons from 9 fresh-frozen cadaver hands were used. The tendons were attached to a

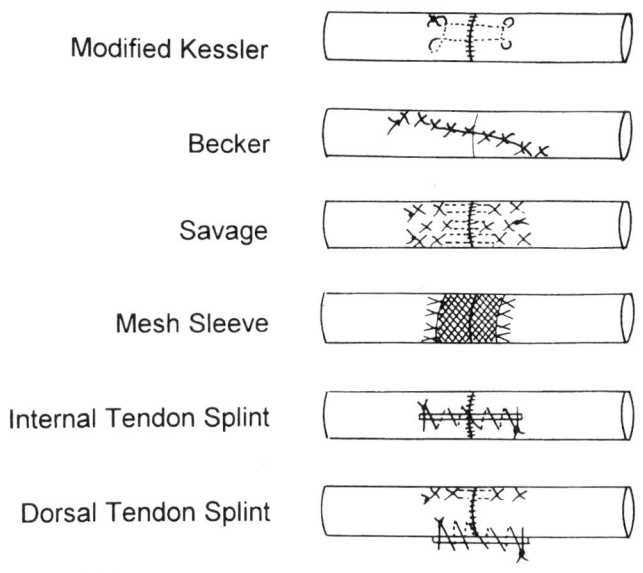

FIGURE 1.—*Modified Kessler* technique: A grasping suture with 4/0 Ethibond in which 1 knot is located outside tendon laceration site; there is a 2-strand suture across the repair site. *Becker* technique: A beveled suture using 6/0 Prolene. Running sutures are placed along each lateral margin of the tendon; there are 4 strands and 2 knots located outside the tendon repair site. *Savage* technique: Using 4/0 Ethibond, 3 individual interrupted sutures are placed with 2 knots proximal to the tendon repair site and 1 knot distal. This is thus a 6-strand suture. Each core suture has 3 grasps on each tendon end, and a 6/0 Prolene epitenon suture is placed circumferentially. External *mesh sleeve* technique: A woven polyester material with 12-mm lengths, 0.23 thickness is used. The sleeve is rolled around the lacerated tendon ends to fix the size of each profundus tendon and fixed to the proximal and distal tendons using 6/0 Prolene cross-stitch epitenon sutures. *Internal tendon splint* technique: A 1-cm horizontal slit is made transversely in each tendon end proximal and distal to the laceration site. A 5 × 18 × 0.22–mm Dacron splint is placed into this slit. Longitudinal sutures (4/0 Ethibond) placed along each lateral margin of the tendon close the 1-cm slit, and the splint is incorporated into the repair site. A 6/0 Prolene epitenon suture is placed circumferentially. *Dorsal tendon splint* technique: A 2-strand Savage-type core suture (4/0 Ethibond) is placed volarly aligning both tendon ends. A 5 × 18 × 0.22–mm Dacron splint is placed on the dorsal surface of tendon across laceration site and sutured to the tendon along each lateral margin. A 6/0 Prolene epitenon suture is placed circumferentially. (Courtesy of Aoki M, Manske PR, Pruitt DL, et al: Work of flexion after tendon repair with various suture methods: A human cadaveric study. *J Hand Surg (Br)* 20B:310–313, 1995.)

specially designed frame and mounted on a tensile testing machine. After baseline measurements of WOF were obtained, sharp lacerations were made in zone 2 of the tendon and repaired by the 2-strand Kessler, the lateral Becker, the 6-strand Savage, the internal and dorsal splint, or the external mesh sleeve techniques (Fig 1). The WOF measurements were repeated after the repair.

Results.—The Kessler and Becker procedures were associated with the lowest average increases in WOF, 4.8% and 6.5%, respectively. Greater increases in WOF were noted for the Savage repair (10.9%), the dorsal tendon splint (16.2%), and the internal tendon splint (19.3%). The greatest increase, 44.3%, occurred with the nylon mesh sleeve repair. The increase associated with the external mesh sleeve repair was significantly greater than that with all the other techniques.

Conclusions.—The results suggest that the WOF after tendon repair increases in direct proportion to amount of suture material used at the repair site. The Savage and tendon splint techniques appear to provide good initial tensile strength, while producing little increase in resistance to gliding. In vivo studies in animals are needed to examine the effects of soft tissue swelling, edema, and other factors involved in tissue healing.

▶ Numerous laboratory studies have shown us that the tensile strength of a flexor tendon repair increases as additional sutures are passed across the repair site. This study explores the adverse effects of adding suture material. The WOF was measured after 6 different repair types, with increasing amounts of suture material crossing the repair site. The techniques varied from the 2-strand modified Kessler up to a repair augmented by a mesh wrap. Their results demonstrated that the WOF increased proportionally with the amount of suture material used.

All too often, we are overzealous in applying laboratory findings to the clinical setting. This study serves as a reminder that we need to study all the ramifications of a new procedure before placing it into widespread clinical application. Hopefully, future studies will discover the ideal amount and placement of suture in flexor tendon repairs.

T. Kiefhaber, M.D.

Autogenous Flexor Tendon Grafts: Fibroblast Activity and Matrix Remodeling in Dogs
Abrahamsson S-O, Gelberman RH, Amiel D, et al (Massachusetts Gen Hosp, Boston; Univ of California, San Diego, La Jolla)
J Orthop Res 13:58–66, 1995   18–10

Background.—The use of extrasynovial tendons for autogenous donor flexor tendon grafts has yielded poor results. Recent research suggests that using intrasynovial donor tendons for transfer to an intrasynovial site yields better results. The repair characteristics of extrasynovial and intrasynovial donor tendons, when placed in an intrasynovial environment, were compared in a canine model.

Methods.—In 18 anesthetized dogs, the flexor digitorum profundus tendon (intrasynovial) from the fifth toe of the hindpaw was grafted to the digital sheath of the ipsilateral front second toe, and the peroneus longus tendon (extrasynovial) was grafted from the hindlimb to the digital sheath of the front fifth toe. Surgery was followed by early controlled passive mobilization. On postoperative days 10, 21, and 42, the tendon grafts were harvested, as were control tendon segments from the contralateral hindlimbs. In vitro measurement of collagen matrix synthesis, DNA synthesis, collagen and protein content, and collagen cross-link formation was performed.

Results.—At each harvest interval, extrasynovial tendon grafts showed more adhesions than did the intrasynovial tendon grafts. Extrasynovial tendon grafts showed significantly greater DNA synthesis and greater synthesis of proteoglycan, collagen, and noncollagen protein than did either control tendons or intrasynovial tendon grafts. Intrasynovial tendon grafts showed significantly greater synthesis of DNA and collagen than did controls, although to a lesser degree than for extrasynovial tendon grafts. Reducible collagen cross-link concentrations were generally higher in extrasynovial tendon grafts than in intrasynovial tendon grafts and control tendons; in some cases, the difference was significant.

Conclusion.—These findings suggest that greater tissue injury occurs when extrasynovial tendon grafts are placed intrasynovially than when intrasynovial tendon grafts are used.

▶ In this landmark study, the authors investigate important biochemical events related to tendon grafts of extrasynovial or intrasynovial origin in a dog model. The data have significant clinical implications regarding autogenous donor flexor tendon grafts used to replace injured flexor tendons. The authors cite that, in the clinical setting, autogeneous grafts have consistently been of extrasynovial origin, the results of which have met with limited success.

The data show that tendon grafts of extrasynovial origin showed greater rates of DNA synthesis and increased levels of proteoglycan, collagen synthesis, noncollagen protein synthesis, and Schiff base covalent collagen cross-links. The implication that extrasynovial tendon grafts may have more pronounced fibrous adhesions than intrasynovial tendon grafts is well founded. The data presented by the authors may form a foundation on which future flexor tendon surgery using intrasynovial grafts may be tested for clinical efficacy compared with the use of extrasynovial grafts.

M.A. Badalamente, Ph.D.

Effects of Laser Versus Scalpel Tenolysis in the Rabbit Flexor Tendon
Constantinescu MA, Greenwald DP, Amarante MTJ, et al (Massachusetts Gen Hosp, Boston; Harvard Med School, Boston; Tampa Gen Hosp, Fla; et al)
Plast Reconstr Surg 97:595–601, 1996   18–11

Background.—The outcome of repair of lacerated flexor tendons is often unsatisfactory. Peritendinous adhesions can form, which increase friction, restrict gliding, and prevent active motion of the digit. This can remain a problem even after careful tenolysis. Other surgical fields have reported significantly lower adhesion formation when surgical lasers are used. Decreased peritendoneal adhesions would improve the functional outcome of tenolysis.

Study.—The benefits of lasers over the scalpel in maintaining tendon gliding after tenolysis were evaluated. Whether thermal adhesion ablation with lasers weakens tenolyzed tendons was also studied.

Methods.—In phase I, a model for creating and analyzing tendon adhesions was tested. In phase II, the effectiveness of scalpel tenolysis, holmium:YAG [yttrium-argon-garnet] laser tenolysis, and CO_2 laser tenolysis was tested. In phase I, bilateral standardized crush abrasion injuries were induced in the hind leg plantar flexor tendons of rabbits. After 4 weeks of immobilization, peritendoneal adhesions were evaluated biomechanically. In phase II, the same standardized tendon trauma was

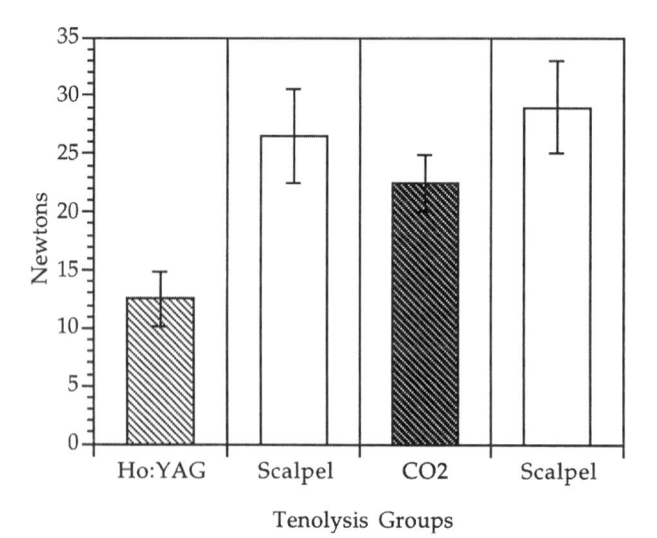

FIGURE 2.—Mean maximal force (± SEM) required for tendon extraction 1 week after tenolysis. Holmium:YAG [yttrium-argon-garnet] laser-tenolyzed tendons required significantly less force than did their intraindividual scalpel-tenolyzed controls. (Courtesy of Constantinescu MA, Greenwald DP, Amarante MTJ, et al: Effects of laser versus scalpel tenolysis in the rabbit flexor tendon. *Plast Reconstr Surg* 97:595–601, 1996.)

induced in 6 groups of rabbits. After 4 weeks, either holmium:YAG laser tenolysis or CO_2 laser tenolysis was performed in one foot. In the other foot, scalpel lysis was performed as a control.

Results.—In phase I, a significantly higher maximal force was needed to extract the adherent tendons from the foot compared to control tendons. In phase II, significantly less force was needed to extract the treated tendons 1 and 2 weeks after holmium:YAG laser tenolysis compared with CO_2 laser tenolysis and scalpel tenolysis (Fig 2). At 4 weeks, these differences were no longer significant. Breaking strength of extracted tendons did not differ among the study groups.

Conclusions.—Early after tenolysis, the holmium:YAG laser produced results superior to those seen with CO_2 laser and scalpel. Holmium:YAG laser tenolysis resulted in easier tendon gliding. This laser did not affect tendon strength. Use of the holmium:YAG laser may cause better hemostasis, less charring, and less postoperative swelling; these may be some factors responsible for the better outcome.

▶ This is potentially interesting work, but the lack of detail on technique limits our ability to draw conclusions. For example, was hemostasis obtained in each group before closure? The laser coagulates as it cuts, but a scalpel does not: for the treatments to be compared, hemostasis should be obtained before closure. Postoperative management after tenolysis is also unclear. The authors say postoperative care was as described in phase I, which would be immobilization in hyperextension. That is certainly not a clinically relevant program after tenolysis, when motion, motion, motion is the rule. Thus, although a very expensive knife (the Ho:YAG laser) may be less traumatic after tenolysis, I believe that additional information is needed before one should accept the results of this study as justification for a change in clinical practice.

P.C. Amadio, M.D.

***In Vivo* Inflammatory Response to Silicone Elastomer Particulate Debris**
Naidu SH, Beredjiklian P, Adler L, et al (Pennsylvania State Univ, Hershey; Univ of Pennsylvania, Philadelphia; VA Hosp, Philadelphia)
J Hand Surg (Am) 21A:496–500, 1996   18–12

Background.—The inflammatory response that results from breakdown of silicone elastomer particles has not been quantified. Tissue-cellular response to implanted materials may vary, however, according to the size of the particulate material. One study found that polymethylmethacrylate (PMMA) in particles induced a much larger and thicker interface membrane between bone and cement than the bulk form of PMMA. An animal model was used to study the inflammatory response to 3 different types of particles.

Methods.—The 3 types of particles were Silastic silicone elastomer (Dow Corning), PMMA (bone cement), and monosodium urate particles

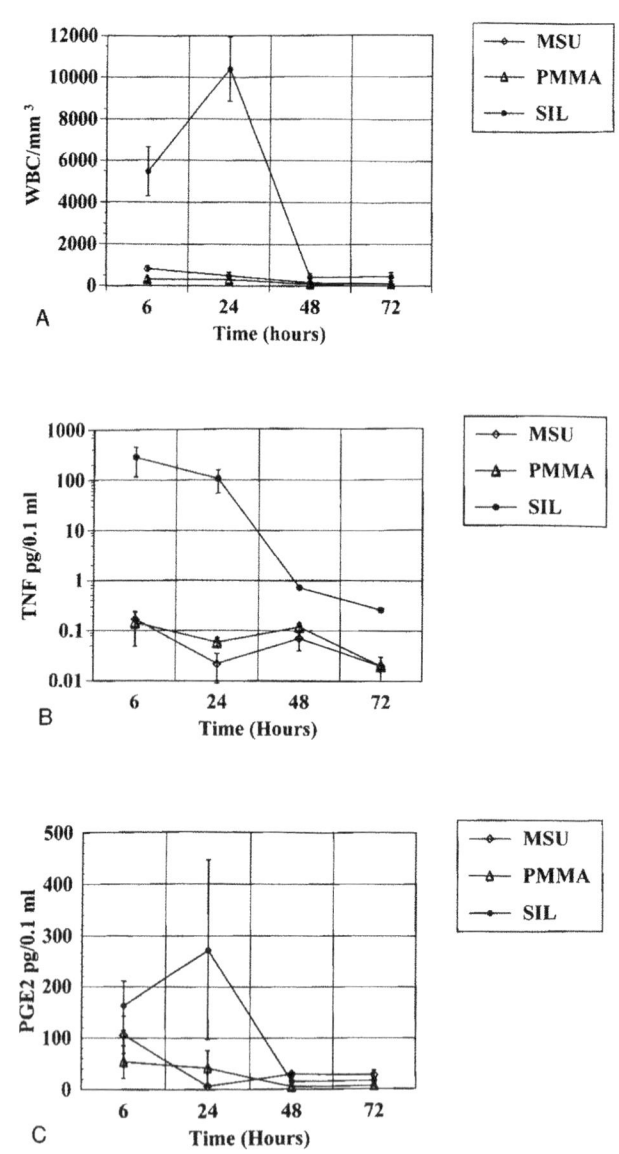

FIGURE 2.—Temporal profile of inflammatory mediators. **A,** the white blood cell counts are significantly higher in the silicone group at 6 hours and 24 hours ($P < 0.0001$) after injection. **B,** tumor necrosis is significantly higher in the silicone group at 6 hours ($P < 0.021$) and 24 hours ($P < 0.006$) after injection. The graph is plotted on a logarithmic scale. **C,** prostaglandin E_2 is significantly higher in the Silastic silicone group at 24 hours ($P < 0.039$) after injection. *Abbreviations: MSU,* monosodium urate; *PMMA,* polymethylmethacrylate; *SIL,* silicone; *WBC,* white blood cell count; *TNF,* tumor necrosis factor; *PGE_2,* prostaglandin E_2. (Courtesy of Naidu SH, Beredjiklian P, Adler L, et al: In vivo inflammatory response to silicone elastomer particulate debris. *J Hand Surg (Am)* 21A:496–500, 1996.)

(MSU). Five milliliters of various suspensions of PMMA, silicone, and MSU were drawn into 10-mL syringes using 16-gauge needles. The suspensions were injected into a rat subcutaneous air pouch lined with synovial membranelike cells. This model was selected because it contains cell populations analogous to the membrane surrounding failed prostheses. Exudate retrieved from the air pouch at 6, 24, 48, and 72 hours after injection was examined for white blood cell count, tumor necrosis factor (TNF), and prostaglandin E_2 (PGE_2).

Results.—Silastic silicone particles of < 1.2 µm were injected at one tenth the concentration of either PMMA or MSU. The PMMA particles were smaller than 10 µm, and the MSU particles were smaller than 1.2 µm. White blood cell counts and levels of TNF in the exudate were highest for the silicone group at 6 and 24 hours after injection; PGE_2 was significantly higher in this group at 24 hours (Fig 2).

Discussion.—Previous studies have shown PMMA to be minimally inflammatory in the rat model, and MSU also failed to cause significant inflammation. In contrast, silicone elastomer particles equivalent in size to those of PMMA and MSU led to acute inflammation, indicating that the inflammatory response is particle-specific. Particle shape and particulate microstructure were not examined, but these factors may also play a role in the inflammatory response.

▶ Literature on immune humeral and cellular responses to "noncytotoxic" materials that have, nevertheless, become clinical problems remains relatively sparse. There has been a limited amount of good basic science in this problem area in which patients with implants (such as silicone, polyethylene, steel, and titanium) believed "biologically inert" are now known to be associated with bone destruction in late-term follow-up. This problem (noted in the literature for 2 decades) was reported initially but not understood. About 10 years ago, the concept of "microparticulate-induced inflammation" began to be accepted.

It seems, in summary, that materials that are otherwise not cytotoxic and inflammatory—foreign particles that produce an end-stage fibrous response of scar envelopment ("pseudocapsule/pseudojoint") when macroparticulate—become recognized as (for lack of a better term) "dangerous invaders" which incite a significant inflammatory response when presented to the same cells at sizes ≤ 50–100 micrometers. In the musculoskeletal system, generation of these microparticles occurs under compression and bearing and shear loads. The inflammatory response produces "giant osteolytic lesions," "bone cysts," [sic] and similar osteoblastic bone resorption and symptomatic inflammation, which leads to the need for revision surgery with implant removal and appropriate salvage.

This particular study reviews the specific response—in an accepted experimental model—to silicone and urate microparticles. That materials induce atom- and molecule-specific reactions is not news in physiology and should not come as a surprise (even to surgeons). The care and work that went into this report is laudable, and it represents another piece of useful information explaining how and why failing implants (i.e., those used in locations where they are subjected to physiologic forces for which they have not been tested and/or cannot withstand) produce unwanted and sometimes disastrous clinical outcomes.

C.A. Peimer, M.D.

Suggested Reading

McAllister RMR, Urban LA, Dray A, et al: Comparison of the sensory threshold in healthy human volunteers with the sensory nerve response of the rat *in vitro* hindlimb skin and saphenous nerve preparation on cutaneous electrical stimulation. *J Hand Surg (Br)* 20B:437–443, 1995.
▶ This interesting article seeks to determine what we as clinicians are actually doing when we tap along the course of a repaired nerve to detect the presence of regenerating axons. Perhaps it may be possible to use stimulation thresholds as a measure of expected regeneration.

V.R. Hentz, M.D.

Lolley RD, Bose WJ, Bastian F, et al: Vein, silastic, and polyglycolic acid fine mesh: A comparative study in peripheral nerve repair. *Ann Plast Surg* 35:266–271, 1995.
▶ The authors demonstrate the lack of benefit of wrapping a repaired nerve in a rat sciatic nerve transsection model. So many rats, so little progress!

V.R. Hentz, M.D.

Abrahamsson S-O: Exposure to air during surgery inhibits cellular activity in flexor tendons. *J Hand Surg (Br)* 21B:299–302, 1996.
▶ The title says it all. Keep those tissues moist!

P.C. Amadio, M.D.

Subject Index*

A

Abductor
  mediana pollicis of thumb
    metacarpophalangeal joint, 96: 22
  pollicis longus arthroplasty, suspension,
    in basal joint arthrosis, 95: 259
Abscess
  upper extremity, from injection drug
    abuse, 95: 83
Abuse
  drug, injection, causing upper extremity
    abscesses, 95: 83
  substance, and carpal tunnel syndrome,
    96: 141
Accessory nerve
  neurotization in infants with brachial
    plexus birth palsy, 96: 250
Acetylcholinesterase
  staining for, in evaluation of ulnar nerve
    grafts in brachial plexus lesions,
    95: 108
Actin
  expression, α-smooth muscle,
    correlation with contraction in
    Dupuytren's disease fibroblasts,
    97: 304
Actinomycotic
  mycetoma of hand, 96: 307
Active motion (see under Motion)
Activity(ies)
  of daily living tests for hand function
    assessment, 95: 34
  low-force, high-frequency
    carpal tunnel syndrome and, 95: 252
    creep strain of flexor tendons during,
      measurement of, 96: 19
Acufex bone anchors, 96: 47
Adactyly
  congenital, advances in microsurgical
    reconstruction of, 96: 319
  pathomorphology and treatment of,
    95: 303
Adductor
  muscles, thumb, force-generating
    capacity in parallel and
    perpendicular plane of adduction,
    96: 31
  pollicis muscle, Botulinum A
    chemodenervation in cerebral
    palsied hand, 95: 229
Adhesions
  flexor tendon, MRI of, 97: 96

Adolescent
  athletes, gymnast's wrist in, 96: 225
  camptodactyly, results of nonoperative
    treatment, 96: 314
  epiphysiodesis of distal end of radius in,
    post-traumatic, progressive
    lengthening in, 97: 324
  tetraplegia in
    C5, reliability of percutaneous
      intramuscular electrodes for upper
      extremity functional neuromuscular
      stimulation in, 96: 256
    neuromuscular stimulation in,
      functional, grasp and release
      abilities after, 97: 246
Aesthesiometry
  results in hand-arm vibration syndrome,
    95: 237
Affective
  disorders and carpal tunnel syndrome,
    96: 141
Afferent fiber
  large and small, function deficits in
    carpal tunnel syndrome, 96: 144
Age
  carpal tunnel syndrome and, 96: 136
    in U.S., 96: 157
  digital nerve repair and, primary,
    results, 96: 117
  effect on distal latency comparisons in
    carpal tunnel syndrome, 96: 134
  radius fracture and, distal, 95: 164
  -related wear patterns of articular
    cartilage and triangular
    fibrocartilage complex of wrist,
    96: 3
Agee endoscopic carpal tunnel release
  topographical landmarks used to
    improve outcome, 96: 167
  vs. open release, 95: 146
Aging
  electrophysiological, morphological, and
    morphometric effects on nerve
    regeneration (in rat), 97: 366
Air
  exposure during surgery, effect on flexor
    tendon cellular activity, 97: 378
Airbag
  -related upper extremity injuries, 96: 67
Algodystrophy
  after Colles' fracture, and tightness of
    casts, 96: 360

---

* All entries refer to the year and page number(s) for data appearing in this and previous editions of the YEAR BOOK.

Algorithm
  for wrist pain, chronic, 96: 179
Alkaloids
  Vinca, extravasation
    at dorsum of hand, treatment of, 95: 279
    management and surgical treatment, 95: 280
Allen's test
  in evaluation of collateral circulation to hand, 96: 37
Allograft
  (See also Transplantation)
  replacement of elbow, massive, 96: 248
Allotransplant (see Allograft)
Alphanumeric keyboard work
  investigation of applied forces in, 95: 254
Alveolar
  rhabdomyosarcoma, combined modality therapy for, 96: 297
Amputated
  digit, temporary ectopic implantation for salvage of, 97: 67
  fingertip, treatment of, 97: 76
Amputating
  hand injury and left-hand dominance, 97: 22
Amputation
  below-elbow, for giant cell tumors of distal radius, 95: 282
  finger
    elongation of metacarpal bones for treatment of, 96: 58
    four-finger, toe transfer combined with wrap-around flap for, 96: 349
    rolling belt injury causing, in children, 96: 83
  fingertip, volar-oblique, long-term results of neurovascular island flap for, 97: 73
  hand, for soft tissue sarcoma, 96: 293
  in hand, somatosensory system responsiveness after, 96: 126
  thumb-tip, dorso-ulnar flap for, 95: 73
  upper extremity, major, prosthetic usage in, 97: 337
Amyloid
  deposits and carpal tunnel syndrome in patients undergoing continuous ambulatory peritoneal dialysis, 97: 123
Analgesia
  axillary catheter, in distraction elbow arthroplasty, 95: 222
  postoperative, comparison of continuous brachial plexus infusion of butorphanol, mepivacaine and mepivacaine-butorphanol mixtures for, 97: 31
Anastomosis
  end-to-side, sensory and motor collateral sprouting induced from intact peripheral nerve by (in rat), 96: 366
  hypoglossal-facial, permanent motor hyperinnervation of whisker-pad muscles after (in rat), 95: 327
  Martin-Gruber, 95: 15
  telescoping, in vein grafting for venous defects (in rat), 95: 317
  of thoracic nerve, medial, to musculocutaneous nerve, functional recovery of elbow flexion by, 95: 117
Anatomical
  basis
    of Carlos Zaidemberg's vascularized graft, 97: 17
    for use of retrograde-flow neurocutaneous island flaps in forearm, 96: 70
  guidelines for proper placement of internal fixation for radial head and neck fractures, 97: 233
  results five years after remanipulated Colles' fractures, 97: 200
  study
    of innervation and vascular supply of nail bed and matrix, 97: 5
    of Kirschner wire fixation through snuff box, percutaneous, 96: 186
    of ulnar parametacarpal flap, 97: 78
Anatomy
  arterial, of thumb, 95: 1
  arthroscopic, of lateral elbow, 96: 245
  of brachioradialis forearm flap, 96: 354
  carpal bone, measured by computer analysis of 3D reconstruction of CT images, 97: 152
  clinical
    of chiasma tendinum in fingers, 95: 7
    of forearm interosseous arteries, 96: 21
  collateral ligament
    elbow joint, lateral, 97: 16
    ulnar, origin and insertion, 95: 219
  of de Quervain's disease, 97: 273
  flexor synovial sheath, of little finger, 97: 19
  functional, of fifth carpometacarpal joint, 95: 14
  of innervation of wrist joint, 95: 174

Subject Index / 381

interosseous nerve, posterior, 95: 8
neuroanatomy in elbow arthroscopy, 97: 239
radial nerve, sensory, 96: 120
retinacular ligament of index finger, oblique, 95: 16
scapholunate interosseous ligament, gross and histologic, 97: 158
scapholunate ligament, 95: 157
scaphotriquetral ligament, 95: 167
of wrist arthroscopy portals, 96: 184
Anesthesia
  digital, through flexor tendon sheath at palmar level, 95: 33
  of finger, transthecal vs. traditional digital block for, 96: 44
  for hand surgery for epidermolysis bullosa, 97: 35
  regional, intraarterial, for hand surgery, radial vs. brachial artery injections for, 96: 42
Angioleiomyomas
  of hand, 97: 301
Angular
  malunion, correction osteotomies of phalanges and metacarpals for, 95: 55
Anomaly (see Deformity)
Antibiotics
  after brachial artery injuries, penetrating, 96: 345
  for mycetoma of hand, 96: 308
Antiblastic
  drug extravasation
    at dorsum of hand, treatment, 95: 279
    management and surgical treatment, 95: 280
Anticoagulated blood
  ex vivo perfusion, effect on ischemia/reperfusion injury (in rat), 95: 338
Antifungal
  pulse therapy for onychomycosis, 97: 70
Antigen
  HLA
    reflex sympathetic dystrophy and, 96: 357
    in wrist tenosynovitis and humeral epicondylitis, 97: 293
Anti-inflammatory agents
  nonsteroidal
    in carpal tunnel syndrome, early mild, 95: 132
    in carpal tunnel syndrome in primary care, 95: 134
    for rupture of long finger flexor pulleys in climbers, 95: 90
Antitumor
  drugs, extravasation of
    at dorsum of hand, treatment, 95: 279
    management and surgical treatment, 95: 280
Anxiety
  disorders and carpal tunnel syndrome, 96: 141
AO compression
  arthrodesis of wrist in posttraumatic arthritis, 95: 274
AO distractor
  small, ulnar shortening using, 97: 224
A-O fixator
  miniexternal, for comminuted intraarticular radial fractures, 96: 214
AO miniplate
  fixation of radius head fracture, late results, 97: 231
AO miniscrew
  fixation of radius head fracture, late results, 97: 231
AO/ASIF wrist arthrodesis
  complications after, 96: 192
A1
  pulley in rheumatoid flexor tenosynovectomy, 95: 276
Aortic
  Y-chambers, selective nerve regeneration in (in rat), 95: 329
Aphalangism
  congenital, toe phalangeal grafts in, 95: 295
Aponeurosis
  pulley, palmar, mechanical analysis of, 97: 11
Applied forces
  in alphanumeric keyboard work, investigation of, 95: 254
Arborization
  normal, of deep branch of ulnar nerve into interossei and lumbricals, 96: 27
Arm
  (See also Extremity, upper)
  flap (see Flap, arm)
  fractures, open, in children, 97: 321
  hand-arm vibration
    platers and truck assemblers exposed to, impaired nerve conduction in carpal tunnel of, 96: 264
    syndrome, sensorineural objective tests in, 95: 236

position, effect on effectiveness of
    perivascular axillary nerve block,
    96: 43
tumors, primary malignant,
    resection-replantation for, 96: 296
upper, tourniquet tolerance, vs. forearm
    tourniquet tolerance, 95: 26
vibration energy absorption in, 95: 322
Arterialized
  tendocutaneous venous flap for dorsal
    finger reconstruction, 96: 84
Arteriorrhaphy
  lateral, in penetrating brachial artery
    injuries, 96: 345
Arteriovenous
  fistula
    acquired, in children, 96: 364
    creation for hemodialysis, neurologic
      and ischemic complications in
      upper extremities after, 96: 362
    loops, vein grafts installed as, in
      microsurgical composite tissue
      transplantation at difficult recipient
      sites, 97: 348
  malformations, congenital, embolization
    therapy for, 95: 292
Artery(ies)
  anatomy of thumb, 95: 1
  brachial
    injuries of, penetrating, 96: 345
    vs. radial artery injections for
      intraarterial regional anesthesia for
      hand surgery, 96: 42
  digital, reverse flap
    innervated, through bilateral
      neurorrhaphy for pulp defects,
      95: 83
    island, for fingertip injuries, 95: 71
  injuries in open arm fractures, in
    children, 97: 322
  interosseous, forearm, clinical anatomy
    of, 96: 21
  metacarpal, flap, second dorsal
    with double pivot points, 97: 83
    neurovascular island, clinical
      applications, 97: 86
  radial (see Radial, artery)
  radial styloid process, anatomy of,
    97: 17
  reconstruction methods for cold-induced
    vasospasm after digital
    replantation, 97: 358
  of thumb metacarpophalangeal joint,
    96: 22
  ulnar (see Ulnar, artery)
Arthritis
  of adjacent joints after AO/ASIF wrist
    arthrodesis, 96: 194

basal joint, trapeziectomy with ligament
    reconstruction and tendon
    interposition arthroplasty for,
    97: 281
capitolunate, proximal row carpectomy
    contraindicated in, 96: 204
carpometacarpal joint
  first, comparison of two arthroplasty
    techniques for, 97: 282
  of thumb, arthroplasty for, stabilized
    resection, 96: 281
  of thumb, prosthesis for, GUEPAR
    total trapeziometacarpal, 95: 258
degenerative
  (See also Osteoarthritis)
  posttraumatic, of carpometacarpal
    joint of small finger, silicone
    implant arthroplasty for, 96: 290
inflammatory, systemic, flexible implant
    resection arthroplasty of proximal
    interphalangeal joint in, 96: 274
juvenile chronic, of elbow, short-term
    complications of lateral approach
    for non-constrained elbow
    replacement for, 97: 237
osteoarthritis (see Osteoarthritis)
outcome measures, translation and
    validation into Spanish, 97: 36
painful, of wrist, Meuli cementless wrist
    prosthesis for, first experience with,
    95: 274
periscaphoid
  scaphoid nonunion with, long-term
    results after proximal row
    carpectomy for, 96: 203
  scapholunate dissociation with,
    long-term results after proximal
    row carpectomy for, 96: 203
posttraumatic
  arthrodesis in, wrist, 95: 274
  arthroplasty in, proximal
    interphalangeal joint silicone
    replacement, clinical results using
    anterior approach, 96: 276
  degenerative, of carpometacarpal
    joint of small finger, silicone
    implant arthroplasty for, 96: 290
  of sesamoid bones in finger joints,
    96: 1
  wrist, revision total wrist arthroplasty
    for, 95: 275
psoriatic
  sesamoid bone enlargement in, 96: 1
  wrist, Meuli cementless wrist
    prosthesis for, 95: 274
radioscaphoid, scaphoid excision and
    capitolunate arthrodesis for,
    95: 185

rheumatoid (see Rheumatoid arthritis)
scaphotrapeziotrapezoid, isolated
  idiopathic, results of
  scaphotrapeziotrapezoid fusion for,
  97: 279
trapeziometacarpal, stabilized resection
  arthroplasty by anterior approach
  in, 97: 283, 295
Arthrodesis
  capitolunate
    for radioscaphoid arthritis, 95: 185
    for scapholunate advanced collapse of
      wrist, 97: 192
  carpal, partial, for scapholunate
    diastasis in distal radius fractures,
    95: 190
  carpometacarpal
    flexor carpi radialis tendinitis after,
      results of operative treatment,
      96: 111
    small finger, for posttraumatic
      degenerative arthritis, 96: 290
  four-corner, for scapholunate advanced
    collapse wrist, 97: 186
  interphalangeal joint
    distal, tension-band wire vs. Herbert
      screw in, 97: 60
    of thumb, in spinal cord injury,
      97: 245
  metacarpophalangeal joint of thumb, in
    Charcot-Marie-Tooth disease,
    97: 248
  midcarpal, 97: 192
  for osteoarthritis of carpometacarpal
    joint of thumb, revision procedures
    for complication of, 95: 261
  radiocapitohamate, in posttraumatic
    arthritis, 95: 274
  radiocarpal
    partial, for scapholunate diastasis in
      distal radius fractures, 95: 190
    after resection of distal radius for
      giant cell tumor, 95: 282
  radiolunate
    in Kienböck's disease, 95: 192
    for Madelung's deformity, 95: 299
    malunion, distal radial intraarticular,
      97: 173
    radiological evolution of rheumatoid
      wrist after, 96: 267
    for ulnar translation, traumatic, 96: 3
  radioulnar, distal, for Madelung's
    deformity, 95: 299
  radius bone graft for, distal anterior,
    97: 59
  in rheumatoid arthritis using absorbable
    screws and rods, 97: 295

scaphocapitate, for Kienböck's disease,
  97: 182
scaphoid-trapezium-trapezoid
  for arthritis, isolated idiopathic,
    results of, 97: 279
  combined with Caffinière arthroplasty
    for pantrapezial osteoarthritis,
    95: 262
  follow-up after, long-term, 95: 187
  in Kienböck's disease, preoperative
    factors and outcome after, 95: 180
  for scapholunate diastasis in distal
    radius fractures, 95: 190
sesamoid, for hyperextension of thumb
  metacarpophalangeal joint, 96: 53
trapeziometacarpal joint, power staple
  fixation in, 95: 263
triquetrohamate, for midcarpal
  instability, 97: 169
wrist
  AO/ASIF, complications after,
    96: 192
  in arthritis, posttraumatic, 95: 274
  limited, outcome assessment after,
    95: 187
  secondary, after brachial plexus
    injuries, 96: 251
Arthrography
  CT, in preoperative evaluation of ulnar
    collateral ligament, 95: 217
  of ligament tears or perforations in
    diagnosis of wrist pain, 96: 187
  wrist
    contralateral, asymptomatic, for
      symmetric ligamentous defects,
      97: 191
    contralateral, asymptomatic, in
      patients with unilateral wrist pain,
      96: 188
    for ligament integrity in young
      asymptomatic adults, 97: 190
    in pain, chronic, 95: 161
    three-compartment, 97: 37
    three-compartment,
      noncommunicating defects on,
      correlation with site of wrist pain,
      95: 162
Arthrogryposis
  multiplex congenita, early corrective
    surgery of wrist and elbow in,
    95: 290
Arthroplasty
  abductor pollicis longus suspension, in
    basal joint arthrosis, 95: 259
  basal joint of thumb, 96: 282

Caffinière, combined with scapho-trapezio-trapezoid arthrodesis in pantrapezial osteoarthritis, 95: 262
elbow
  complications in, late, 97: 242
  distraction, axillary catheter analgesia in, 95: 222
  interposition, in rheumatoid arthritis, 97: 243
  non-constrained, short-term complications of lateral approach for, 97: 237
  total, failed, salvage of, 97: 236
  total, fixation strength of ulnar component of, 97: 238
flexor carpis radialis sling, for osteoarthrosis of thumb base, 95: 257
hemiresection interposition
  matched, of distal radioulnar joint, 97: 216
  for subluxation of distal ulna, chronic posttraumatic dorsal, 95: 205
interphalangeal joint, proximal
  implant arthroplasty, flexible resection, in systemic inflammatory arthritis, 96: 274
  implant arthroplasty, lateral stability of, 96: 368
  silicone replacement type, clinical results using anterior approach, 96: 276
metacarpophalangeal joint, based on osseointegration concept, 95: 264
Outerbridge-Kashiwagi's method, for elbow osteoarthritis, 97: 234
radiocarpal joint, flexible implant, titanium grommet in, 97: 289
resection
  of radioulnar joint, distal, pronator quadratus interposition transfer as adjunct to, 97: 214
  stabilized, 96: 281
  stabilized, by anterior approach, in trapeziometacarpal arthritis, 97: 283, 295
Silastic implant
  of carpal scaphoid, 96: 200
  for osteoarthritis of carpometacarpal joint of thumb, revision procedures for complications of, 95: 261
silicone implant, for posttraumatic degenerative arthritis of carpometacarpal joint of small finger, 96: 290
stabilized, of fifth metacarpal, 96: 61
Swanson
  for rheumatoid metacarpophalangeal joints, motion after, 95: 266
Silastic, long-term results in rheumatoid wrist, 95: 270
techniques for first carpometacarpal joint arthritis, comparison of, 97: 282
tendon, for trapeziometacarpal arthrosis, 96: 285
tendon interposition
  for basal joint arthritis, 97: 281
  for basal joint arthrosis, radiographic assessment of trapezial space before and after, 97: 280
wrist, total
  revision, 95: 275
  uncemented, 96: 287
  Volz, long-term outcome of, 95: 272
Arthroscopy
  of additional lesions associated with distal radial fractures, 97: 206
  anatomy of lateral elbow, 96: 245
  débridement of triangular fibrocartilage complex tears by, clinical results of, 97: 223
  elbow, neuroanatomy in, 97: 239
  in intercarpal ligament injuries, for categorization, 95: 157
  ligament tears treated by, acute complete thumb metacarpophalangeal ulnar collateral, 97: 48
  repair of radial-sided lesions of fibrocartilage complex, 96: 238
  resection
    of ganglion of wrist, dorsal, 96: 195
    of triangular fibrocartilage complex, partial, 95: 206
  scapholunate and lunotriquetral injuries of wrist managed by, partial, 97: 170
  sign of longstanding triquetrolunate ligament rupture, frayed ulnotriquetral and ulnolunate ligaments as, 96: 206
  trampoline test, 96: 231
  triangular fibrocartilage complex repair via, in wrist injuries, 97: 226
  valgus instability test of elbow, evaluation of, 97: 30
  wrist
    in carpal instability diagnosis, 95: 159
    extensor pollicis longus rupture after, late, 96: 194
    indications and clinical applications, 96: 183
    in pain, chronic, 95: 161, 163

palmar approaches/portals for, 96: 194
portals, anatomic study, 96: 184
value of, 97: 21
vs. cinearthrography, triple-injection, 97: 193
Arthrosis
 basal joint
  arthroplasty in, abductor pollicis longus suspension, 95: 259
  radiographic assessment of trapezial space before and after ligament reconstruction and tendon interposition arthroplasty, 97: 280
 scaphoid-trapezium-trapezoid, isolated, long-term follow-up of scaphoid-trapezium-trapezoid arthrodesis in, 95: 189
 trapeziometacarpal, tendon arthroplasty for, 96: 285
Arthrotomy
 in wrist pain evaluation, chronic, 95: 161
Articular
 (*See also* Intraarticular)
 cartilage of wrist, wear patterns of, 96: 3
 disk
  of triangular fibrocartilage complex, strains in, 95: 208
  of wrist, healing of (in dog), 95: 209
 fracture
  metacarpal base, first, direct osteosynthesis *vs.* closed pinning of, 97: 66
  radius, distal, compression flexion type, proposed classification for, 96: 208
  wrist, carpal tunnel pressures in, 96: 217
 inclination, relative, of distal radioulnar joint, radiographic study, 97: 208
Aseptic
 necrosis of lunate, vascular bundle implantation into bone for, 97: 179
Ashworth-Blatt type implant
 for posttraumatic degenerative arthritis of carpometacarpal joint of small finger, 96: 290
Athletes
 adolescent, gymnast's wrist in, 96: 225
 scaphoid fracture in
  midthird, alternative management of, 96: 199
  stable, acute, internal fixation of, 97: 172
 ulnar nerve transfer in, anterior subcutaneous, 95: 141

wheelchair, upper extremity peripheral nerve entrapments among, 95: 309
Atrophy
 first web space, free fat autotransplantation for cosmetic treatment of, 97: 87
Autograft
 ligament, from foot, for reconstruction of scapholunate interosseous ligament, 97: 164
 nerve, old degenerated and fresh, comparison of passage of regenerating axons through (in rat), 95: 325
Automobile
 assembly line workers
  characteristics of forearm-hand exposure in relation to symptoms among, 97: 272
  self-reported physical exposure and musculoskeletal symptoms of forearm-hand among, 97: 328
 workers, carpal tunnel syndrome in, current perception threshold testing as screening procedure for, 96: 260
Automotive
 airbag-related upper extremity injuries, 96: 67
Autonomic
 denervation and reflex sympathetic dystrophy, 96: 355
Autotransplantation
 free fat, for cosmetic treatment of first web space atrophy, 97: 87
Avulsion
 brachial plexus root, neurotizations by means of cervical plexus for, 95: 106
 brachial plexus (*see* Brachial plexus, avulsion)
 fractures
  hand, tension band fixation of, clinical results, 96: 48
  metacarpophalangeal joint of thumb, tension wire fixation of, 96: 49
  triquetral bone, volar aspect, 97: 187
 injuries
  morbidity of pedicled groin flap for, 95: 78
  ring, microsurgical management of, 97: 346
  nerve root, endoscopic diagnosis and possible treatment in management of brachial plexus injuries (in goat), 96: 121
 traumatic, of triangular fibrocartilage complex at its ulnar insertion new reattachment technique, 96: 230

reinsertion and hemiepiphyseal
 osteotomy at distal ulna for,
 97: 222
Axes
 of rotation of thumb interphalangeal
  and metacarpophalangeal joints,
  97: 6
Axial
 congenital deformities in upper limb,
  nosology of, 95: 300
Axillary
 catheter analgesia in distraction elbow
  arthroplasty, 95: 222
 dissection, prior ipsilateral, in breast
  cancer patient, elective hand
  surgery in, 96: 295
 nerve block, perivascular, effect of arm
  position on effectiveness of, 96: 43
Axonal
 transport, retrograde, effect of acute
  stretching of peripheral nerves on
  (in rat), 97: 367
Axons
 regenerating
  comparison of passage through old
   degenerated and fresh nerve
   autografts (n rat), 95: 325
  dispersion across enclosed neural
   gaps, 97: 361

B

Backhand
 stroke, wrist kinematics in tennis
  players performing, 96: 334
Ballottement test
 in wrist pain evaluation, 96: 181
Bandage
 plaster bandage immobilization after
  closed reduction of volar
  dislocation of distal radioulnar
  joint, 96: 233
Basal
 joint of thumb
  arthritis, trapeziectomy with ligament
   reconstruction and tendon
   interposition arthroplasty for,
   97: 281
  arthroplasty of, 96: 282
  arthrosis, abductor pollicis longus
   suspension arthroplasty in, 95: 259
  arthrosis, radiographic assessment of
   trapezial space before and after
   ligament reconstruction and tendon
   interposition arthroplasty, 97: 280
  osteoarthrosis, osteotomy of first
   metacarpal for, 97: 285

Baseball
 players, preoperative evaluation of ulnar
  collateral ligament by MRI and CT
  arthrography in, 95: 217
Basic fibroblast growth factor
 modulation of formation of molded
  vascularized bone graft in vivo (in
  rat), 96: 382
Bauth
 classification of thumb hypoplasia,
  97: 315
 type II hypoplastic thumb, transposition
  of third metatarsus for
  reconstruction of, 97: 317
Beck revascularization technique
 in Kienböck's disease, early stage 3,
  96: 201
Becker
 repair with crisscrossing superficial
  sutures, new augmented,
  mechanical analysis of (in rabbit),
  96: 378
 suture techniques, modified #1 and #2,
  mechanical analysis of (in rabbit),
  96: 378
 tendon repair, lateral, work of flexion
  after, 97: 372
 tenorrhaphy, augmented, vs. modified
  Kessler, dynamic mechanical
  analysis (in monkey), 96: 98
Bedeschi procedure
 early-staged, for radial club hand,
  95: 300
Belt
 rolling, injuries, in children, 96: 83
Bennett's fracture
 treatment, 96: 54
Betamethasone
 injection/splinting for carpal tunnel
  syndrome, reexamination of,
  96: 148
Bi-articular
 chain, massless, graphic analysis of
  biomechanics of, 97: 7
Biaxial prosthesis
 in wrist arthroplasty, revision total,
  95: 275
Biceps
 brachii rerouting for paralytic
  supination contracture of forearm
  due to traumatic paraplegia,
  95: 223
 muscle recovery in brachial plexus
  reconstruction, maximizing
  technique, 95: 105
 tendon
  distal, repair with suture anchors and
   anterior approach, 97: 229

rupture, MRI of, 95: 104
Bier's block
   change of injection site, 97: 34
Bilhaut procedure
   for duplicated thumb, 95: 287
   modified, for thumb polydactyly,
      long-term results, 97: 319
Bilhaut-Cloquet procedure, 96: 313
Billericay controlled active-motion flexor
   tendon mobilization regimen,
   96: 106
Bioartificial
   nerve graft, 97: 362
Biochemical
   changes after carpal tunnel release,
      96: 168
Biomechanical
   abnormalities in musicians with
      occupational cramp/focal dystonia,
      95: 306
   alterations in carpal arch and hand
      muscles after carpal tunnel release,
      97: 14
   analysis
      of arthrodesis of distal
         interphalangeal joint with
         tension-band wire vs. Herbert
         screw, 97: 60
      of epitenon, 96: 91
      of external fixation of distal radius,
         95: 200
      of flexor-tendon grafts, autogenous
         (in dog), 95: 332
      of metacarpal osteotomy, extension,
         for trapeziometacarpal
         osteoarthritis, 97: 277
      of plate fixation, dorsal, in proximal
         phalangeal fractures, 95: 49
      of radial wedge osteotomy in
         Kienböck's disease, 95: 182
      of scapholunate ligament sectioning,
         97: 155
      of strains in articular disk of
         triangular fibrocartilage complex,
         95: 208
      of suture methods for flexor tendon
         repair, in vitro, 95: 331
      of usefulness of valgus stress testing
         in injuries of ulnar collateral
         ligament of thumb
         metacarpophalangeal joint, 95: 41
   characteristics of suture techniques in
      extensor zone IV, 97: 93
   design of wrist motors, 97: 8
   evaluation (see analysis above)
   investigation of radial instability of
      metacarpophalangeal joint of
      thumb, 96: 11
   motions and forces in high-profile vs.
      low-profile dynamic splinting,
      96: 326
   properties, tendon, effect on wrist
      muscle specialization, 97: 9
   stability of titanium bone fixation
      systems in metacarpal fractures,
      97: 18
   study (see analysis above)
Biomechanics
   of bi-articular chain, massless, graphic
      analysis of, 97: 7
   special issue on, 97: 1
   of thumb flexor pulley system, 95: 2
Birth
   palsy, brachial plexus (see Brachial
      plexus, palsy, birth)
Bite
   dog, causing penetrating brachial artery
      injuries, 96: 345
   wound, infected clench-fist human, in
      area of metacarpophalangeal joints,
      treatment of, 97: 54
BIZCAD
   in osteotomy for deformity of radius,
      95: 197
Block
   axillary nerve, perivascular, effect of
      arm position on effectiveness of,
      96: 43
   Bier's, change of injection site, 97: 34
   digital nerve, transthecal vs. traditional,
      for anesthesia of finger, 96: 44
   muscle afferent, in writer's cramp,
      97: 334
   regional IV, combined with
      corticosteroid for reflex
      sympathetic dystrophy after distal
      radius fractures, 96: 220
   silicone, in nubbin-digits hand, 95: 303
Blood
   anticoagulated, ex vivo perfusion, effect
      on ischemia/reperfusion injury (in
      rat), 95: 338
   flow
      after digital replantation, at 12 years,
         96: 348
      finger skin, after microvascular repair
         of ulnar artery at wrist, laser
         Doppler imaging of, 96: 364
   supply, extrinsic, of ulnar nerve at
      elbow, 95: 4
Body
   mass index related to diagnosis of
      carpal tunnel syndrome, 96: 135
Bone
   anchor, Mitek, in thumb ulnar collateral
      ligament ruptures, 97: 50

carpal
   anatomy, measured by computer analysis of 3D reconstruction of CT images, 97: 152
   kinematics, during full range of joint movement, 95: 170
   cortical, effect on strength of osteopenic distal radius, 95: 201
   cysts after Swanson silicone finger joint implants, 97: 287
   formation, heterotrophic, in Swanson silicone finger joint implants, 97: 287
   graft (see Graft, bone)
   growth after replantation in children, 96: 346
   imaging (see Imaging, bone)
   implantation of vascular bundle into, for aseptic necrosis of lunate, 97: 179
   metacarpal, elongation for treatment of finger amputations, 96: 58
   mineral phase, skeletal repair by in situ formation of, 96: 365
   one-bone forearm, clinical results of, 97: 58
   resorption around Swanson silicone finger joint implants, 97: 287
   scan (see Imaging, bone)
   sesamoid (see Sesamoid)
   suture anchors in hand surgery, 96: 47
   trabecular, effect on strength of osteopenic distal radius, 95: 201
Botox (see Botulinum toxin)
Botulinum toxin
   chemodenervation for cerebral palsied hands, 95: 229
   in focal dystonia of hand, 95: 308, 309
Boutonnière deformity
   potential, central slip tenodesis test for early diagnosis, 95: 36
Bowing
   of ulna after treatment of chronic post-traumatic dislocation of radial head, in children, 95: 58
Brachial artery
   injuries, penetrating, 96: 345
   vs. radial artery injections for intraarterial regional anesthesia for hand surgery, 96: 42
Brachial plexopathy
   in infants after traumatic delivery, MRI of, 95: 224
Brachial plexus
   avulsion
      complete, double free-muscle transfer to restore prehension after, 97: 106

contralateral C7 root transfer with vascularized nerve grafting for (in rat), 95: 339
   elbow flexion restoration after, spinal accessory neurotization for, 97: 105
   gunshot wound, low-velocity, 96: 121
   infusion, continuous, of butorphanol vs. mepivacaine vs. mepivacaine-butorphanol mixtures for postoperative analgesia, 97: 31
injuries
   complete, restoration of hand sensibility after, 97: 103
   elbow flexion restoration after spinal accessory neurotization for, 97: 105
   management, endoscopic diagnosis and possible treatment of nerve root avulsions in (in goat), 96: 121
   muscle transplantation for, functioning free, 96: 253
   secondary surgery after, 96: 250
   tendon transposition across two joints in, 95: 108
   traumatic, MRI in diagnosis of, 95: 226
lesions
   enzymhistochemical evaluation of ulnar nerve grafts in, 95: 107
   spinal nerve root injuries in, 96: 252
palsy
   birth (see below)
   obstetrical (see palsy, birth below)
palsy, birth
   accessory nerve neurotization in infant with, 96: 250
   forearm rotation deformities due to, severe, surgical radioulnar osteoclasis for, 96: 67
   lower, discussion of, 96: 249
   natural history of, 95: 228
   prognostic value of concurrent clavicular fractures in newborns with, 96: 126
reconstruction
   phrenic nerve used in, 97: 104
   technique for maximizing biceps recovery in, 95: 105
root avulsions, neurotizations by means of cervical plexus for, 95: 106
Brachioradialis
   forearm flap, anatomy and clinical application, 96: 354
Brachysyndactyly
   congenital, morbidity of pedicled groin flap for, 95: 78

Bracing
  functional fracture, in metacarpal fractures, 95: 59
  of ulnar shaft fracture, stable, 95: 66
Braided
  plantaris tendon as extensor tendon graft, 96: 89
Breast
  cancer patient with prior ipsilateral axillary dissection, elective hand surgery in, 96: 295
Brown technique
  of endoscopic carpal tunnel release, results of, 95: 147
Bullet
  wounds causing penetrating brachial artery injuries, 96: 345
Bunnell around bone method
  for finger pulley reconstruction after closed traumatic rupture, 96: 98
Bunnell suture
  modified
    in extensor zone IV, biomechanical characteristics of, 97: 93
    in flexor tendon repair, evaluation of, 97: 95
Burn(s)
  extremity, upper, expanded polytetrafluoroethylene gloves for care of, 96: 79
  hand
    coverage with narrow pedicled intercostal cutaneous perforator flap, 95: 314
    edema after, chronic, effect of mechanical compression on, 96: 79
    skin graft take in, optimizing, in children, 95: 79
  palmar pediatric, study of, 96: 81
Burned
  skin, previously, use in local fasciocutaneous flaps for upper extremity reconstruction, 96: 80
Burton and Pelligrini technique
  of trapeziectomy and ligament reconstruction for osteoarthrosis of thumb base, 95: 257
Butorphanol
  vs. mepivacaine vs. mepivacaine-butorphanol mixtures in continuous brachial plexus infusion for postoperative analgesia, 97: 31
Bypass
  extensor tendon transfer, 97: 102

C

Caffinière arthroplasty
  combined with scapho-trapezio-trapezoid arthrodesis in pantrapezial osteoarthritis, 95: 262
Calcaneocuboid
  ligament autograft for reconstruction of scapholunate interosseous ligament, 97: 165
Camptodactyly
  classification and results of nonoperative treatment, 96: 314
Cancer
  breast, elective hand surgery in cancer patient with prior ipsilateral axillary dissection, 96: 295
Cannulation
  radial artery, hand ischemia after, 97: 353
Capillary
  microscopy in reflex sympathetic dystrophy due to autonomic denervation, 96: 355
Capitate
  resection, partial, proximal row carpectomy with, 97: 183
Capitolunate
  arthritis, proximal row carpectomy contraindicated in, 96: 204
  arthrodesis
    for radioscaphoid arthritis, 95: 185
    for scapholunate advanced collapse of wrist, 97: 192
Capsular
  contracture, elbow, surgical release, in children, 96: 242
  defects on wrist arthrography, lack of correlation between site of wrist pain and, 95: 162
  injuries of thumb metacarpophalangeal joint, dorsoradial, isolated injuries to, 97: 51
  tissues of proximal interphalangeal joint, 95: 9
Capsulodesis
  dorsal, for dynamic scapholunate instability, results of, 97: 163
Carbon dioxide
  laser tenolysis in flexor tendon (in rabbit), 97: 374
Carcinoma
  of hand, recurrent squamous cell, in immunosuppressed patients, treatment of, 96: 294
Care
  guidelines for nail disorders, 97: 87

primary, carpal tunnel syndrome in, 95: 134
Carpal
(See also Wrist)
alignment changes after radial osteotomy for Kienböck's disease, 95: 181
arch, biomechanical alterations after carpal tunnel release, 97: 14
bone
anatomy measured by computer analysis of 3D reconstruction of CT images, 97: 152
kinematics, during full range of joint movement, 95: 170
boss, 20-year review of operative management, 97: 188
canal, median nerve displacement through, 96: 26
-compression test in diagnosis of carpal tunnel syndrome, 96: 142
fusion, partial, for scapholunate diastasis in distal radius fractures, 95: 190
height
measurement of, 96: 7
ratio, alternative method for determination of, 95: 166
instability
diagnosis, wrist arthroscopy in, 95: 159
with scapholunate dissociation, new operation for, 97: 167
scapholunate pseudoarthrosis and, 97: 171
ligament(s)
injury, avulsion fracture of volar aspect of triquetral bone as sign of, 97: 187
interosseous, tears, with intraarticular distal radial fractures, 97: 204
lengthening during full range of joint movement, 95: 170
palmar, defects, resurfacing with retinaculum flexorum flap, 95: 269
palmar, tensions in, 95: 172
transverse, endoscopic release in palmar-dorsal direction, 96: 174
volar, MRI of, 95: 168
malalignment after intra-articular fractures of distal radius, in workers, 96: 220
row, distal, traumatic dislocations of, 96: 208
scaphoid, Silastic implant arthroplasty of, 96: 200
Carpal tunnel
decompression (see release below)

lumbrical muscle incursion into effect on carpal tunnel pressure, 96: 155
during finger flexion, 96: 17
median nerve decompression in endoscopic, 96: 175
for palmar space infections, 96: 308
nerve conduction measurements at, predictive value of, 95: 127
of platers and truck assemblers exposed to hand-arm vibration, impaired nerve conduction in, 96: 264
pressure
dynamics, relation to pressure dynamics of flexor compartment of forearm, 96: 153
effect of lumbrical muscle incursion within carpal tunnel on, 96: 155
increase after externally applied forces to palm, 96: 161
lowest, and wrist position, 97: 130
normal, vs. pressures in articular wrist fractures, 96: 217
in radius fractures, distal, 96: 216
in wrist fractures, articular, 96: 217
release
for bilateral carpal tunnel syndrome, 96: 161
biochemical changes after, 96: 168
biomechanical alterations in carpal arch and hand muscles after, 97: 14
in breast cancer patient with prior ipsilateral axillary dissection, 96: 295
in Charcot-Marie-Tooth disease, 97: 248
emergent, for acute median neuropathy after wrist trauma, 95: 109
endoscopic (see below)
grip strength after, 95: 120
mobilization after, early, 96: 158
myofascial manipulative, 95: 129
open, double incision, 96: 162
open, minimal excision, vs. two-portal endoscopic, 97: 118
open, twin incision, 95: 121
open, vs. endoscopic, 97: 113; 95: 145, l46
outcome, and electrodiagnostic testing, 97: 137
outcome, assessment of, 97: 120
outcome, in diabetics, 96: 131
outcome, in workers' compensation, 97: 125
outcome, in workers' compensation, Washington State, 95: 233

outcome, preliminary scoring system
for assessing, 96: 129
palmar sensory latency changes in
response to, 96: 149
in patients exposed to vibration from
handheld tools, 95: 235
results, 95: 155
results, long-term, 97: 126; 95: 123
for scapholunate advanced collapse,
asymptomatic, 95: 185
secondary, 95: 119
secondary, subjective and employment
outcome after, 95: 144
sensory recovery after, 95: 144
sequelae of, 97: 128
subfascial, complications after,
95: 155
symptoms, functional status, and
neuromuscular impairment after,
97: 122
two-portal subcutaneous,
morphologic changes after, 96: 175
using limited direct vision, 96: 172
release, endoscopic, 97: 148
Agee, topographical landmarks used
to improve outcome, 96: 167
bilateral, *vs.* open release, 96: 161
Brown technique, results of, 95: 147
cadaveric, 95: 153
Chow technique, results of, 95: 149
Chow technique, transbursal and
extrabursal, 97: 114
in community-based series, 95: 152
complete, 97: 115
complications and surgical
experience, 96: 171
early experience with, 95: 151
morphologic changes after, 96: 175
palmar uniportal extrabursal,
96: 165
risk and complications in, 96: 174
significance of incomplete release of
distal portion of flexor retinaculum
in, 96: 174
single-portal, 97: 117
two-portal, sensory disturbances after,
96: 164
two-portal *vs.* minimal incision open,
97: 118
ulnar neurovascular bundle at wrist
in, 95: 148
vs. open, 97: 113; 95: 145, 146
screening tests, and temperature effects
on vibrotactile sensitivity threshold
measurements, 97: 136
surgery *(see release above)*
syndrome
bilateral, surgery for, 96: 161

in CAPD patients, 97: 123
clinicopathologic study of, 96: 127
correlation of MRI, clinical,
electrodiagnostic, and
intraoperative findings in, 97: 139
CT in, tridimensional, 96: 148
diabetes mellitus and, 96: 303
diagnosis, body mass index related to,
96: 135
diagnosis, carpal-compression test in,
96: 142
diagnosis, comparison of traditional
electrodiagnostic studies,
electroneurometry, and vibrometry
in, 97: 133
diagnosis, nerve conduction studies
in, correlation with clinical signs,
96: 152
diagnosis, sensitivity of various tests
for, 96: 161
diagnostic criteria of, 95: 233
distal latency comparisons in, and
age, 96: 134
early mild, iontophoresis, wrist
splinting and antiinflammatory
medication in, 95: 132
fiber function deficits in, small and
large afferent, 96: 144
flexor retinaculum in, explant culture,
immunofluorescence and electron
microscopic study of, 97: 140
idiopathic, comparison to
vibration-damaged hands, 95: 239
in industrial setting, vibrometry
testing *vs.* sensory nerve conduction
measures in screening for, 96: 338
in industrial workers, current
perception threshold testing as
screening procedure for, 96: 260
in industrial workers, Japanese *vs.*
American, 95: 242
intracarpal canal pressure recordings
in, serial overnight, 95: 138
lifestyle correlates of, 96: 159
low-force high-frequency activities
and, 95: 252
management, conservative, 96: 147
median nerve circulation in, MRI
evaluation of, 95: 135
median nerve motion in, restricted,
97: 131
nerve conduction studies in, effect of
provocative exercise maneuver on,
95: 255
nerve conduction studies in, relation
between needle electromyography
and, 96: 137
in officer workers, 95: 244

patients, prevalence of psychopathology in, 96: 141
prednisone in, 97: 132
in primary care, 95: 134
psychomotor deficits and, functional, 95: 128
pyridoxine in, 95: 131
recurrent, surgical management of, 95: 124
recurrent, synovialis flap plasty for, 95: 125
relation to repetitive movements at work, 96: 258
release (see Carpal tunnel, release above)
reoperation for, outcome, 97: 124
retrograde changes in, and forearm mixed nerve conduction velocity, 96: 145
self-reported, prevalence and work-relatedness of, in U.S. workers, 96: 265
self-reported, prevalence in U.S., 96: 157
Semmes-Weinstein monofilament thresholds in, abnormal, decision making in detection of, 96: 39
sensory deficits associated with, gap detection tactility test for, 97: 24
severe, anterior interosseous nerve latency in diagnosis of, 96: 338
severity, responsiveness of self-reported and objective measures of, 96: 132
severity of symptoms and functional status in, self-administered questionnaire for, 95: 21
sleep-related disorders in, 97: 148
splinting for, search for optimal angle, 96: 146
treatment, surgical, electrical studies as prognostic factor in, 96: 133
undetected, in fibromyalgia syndrome patients, 96: 151
workers' compensation recipients with, validity of self-reported health measures, 97: 127
in workplace, surveillance for, 95: 248
in workplace, surveillance for, using hand diagrams, 96: 138
topology during dynamic stress situations of wrist, 96: 23
Carpectomy
proximal row
in arthrogryposis multiplex congenita, 95: 290

in Kienböck's disease, advanced, 96: 204
with partial capitate resection, 97: 183
results after, long-term, 96: 203
for scapholunate advanced collapse wrist, 97: 186
Carpometacarpal joint
arthrodesis, flexor carpi radialis tendinitis after, results of operative treatment, 96: 111
fifth
anatomy of, functional, 95: 14
arthritis, posttraumatic degenerative, silicone implant arthroplasty for, 96: 290
first, arthritis of, comparison of two arthroplasty techniques for, 97: 282
thumb
arthritis, arthroplasty for, stabilized resection, 96: 281
arthritis, GUEPAR total trapeziometacarpal prosthesis for, 95: 258
contact areas in, 97: 3
osteoarthritis, revision procedures for complications of surgery for, 95: 261
Cartilage
articular, of wrist, wear patterns of, 96: 3
transfer in Eve procedure, 97: 350
Cartilaginous
exostosis, multiple, classification system for, in children, 97: 326
Cast
above-elbow, for Galeazzi-equivalent wrist injuries, in children, 95: 61
immobilization for Colles' fracture, ulnar wrist pain after, 95: 195
plaster
for metacarpal base fracture, first, 96: 54
short arm, for distal pediatric forearm fractures, 95: 63
vs. Galveston metacarpal brace, 95: 59
playing, for midthird scaphoid fracture, in athlete, 96: 200
for radial fractures, isolated distal, in children, 95: 202
tightness and algodystrophy after Colles' fracture, 96: 360
Catheter
axillary, analgesia, in distraction elbow arthroplasty, 95: 222

placement for measurement of forearm
compartment pressures, cadaveric
and radiologic assessment of,
96: 380
Cefazolin
after brachial artery injuries,
penetrating, 96: 345
Cell
giant cell tumor of distal radius,
97: 297
treatment of, 95: 281
loss in sensory ganglia after peripheral
nerve injury, 96: 384
Schwann cell-derived neurotrophic
factor, partial purification
characterization of, 95: 324
T cell-mediated response in Dupuytren's
disease, 95: 285
Cellular
activity, flexor tendon, effect of air
exposure during surgery on,
97: 378
Central slip
repaired, early active short arc motion
for, 96: 100
tenodesis test for early diagnosis of
potential boutonnière deformities,
95: 36
Centrode
analysis in study of kinematics of distal
radioulnar joint in rheumatoid
arthritis, 97: 19
Cerclage
fixation for fracture-dislocation of
proximal interphalangeal joint,
97: 42
Cerebral palsy
hand, Botulinum A chemodenervation
of, 95: 229
hyperextension of thumb
metacarpophalangeal joint in,
sesamoid arthrodesis for, 96: 53
Cervical
plexus, neurotizations by means of, for
brachial plexus root avulsions,
95: 106
spinal cord injury, shoulder-hand
syndrome in, 96: 256
spinal nerve root, C7
sensory endings, distribution and
clinical significance, 95: 339
transfer, contralateral, with
vascularized nerve grafting for
brachial plexus root avulsion (in
rat), 95: 339
Charcot-Marie-Tooth disease
treatment of upper limb in, 97: 248

Chemodenervation
Botulinum A, for cerebral palsied
hands, 95: 229
Chemotherapy
agents, extravasation of
at dorsum of hand, treatment,
95: 279
management and surgical treatment,
95: 280
for sarcomas of hand and foot, 96: 297
Chiasma
tendinum in fingers, clinical anatomy of,
95: 7
Children
adolescent (see Adolescent)
arteriovenous fistula in, acquired,
96: 364
arthritis in
elbow, chronic, short-term
complications of lateral approach
for non-constrained elbow
replacement for, 97: 237
rheumatoid, flexible implant resection
arthroplasty of proximal
interphalangeal joint in, 96: 275
arthrogryposis multiplex congenita in,
early corrective surgery of wrist
and elbow in, 95: 290
Botulinum A chemodenervation for
cerebral palsied hands in, 95: 229
brachial plexus root avulsions in,
neurotizations by means of cervical
plexus for, 95: 107
burns in
hand, optimizing skin graft take in,
95: 79
palmar, study of, 96: 81
cartilaginous exostosis in, multiple,
classification system for, 97: 326
clubhand deformity in, radial, due to
osteomyelitis, 96: 63
decision making by, in pediatric hand
surgery, 96: 315
digital nerve repair in, secondary, results
of, 95: 115
Dupuytren's disease in, 97: 323
elbow capsular contracture in, surgical
release of, 96: 242
epidermolysis bullosa in
anesthesia for hand surgery in,
97: 35
surgical treatment of contracture and
syndactyly in, 95: 291
fibrous proliferations in, 97: 300
finger joint repair with ipsilateral
osteochondral grafting, 95: 53
flexor tendon injuries in, 96: 85

forearm rotation deformities in, severe, surgical radioulnar osteoclasis for, 96: 65
fracture in
 arm, open, 97: 321
 forearm, short arm plaster cast for, 95: 63
 humerus, supracondylar, 95: 219
 radius, distal, entrapment of pronator quadratus in, 96: 229
 radius, distal, isolated, management of, 95: 202
 radius, distal, severely displaced, percutaneous Kirschner wire pinning for, 97: 322
hand deformities in, free transplants of phalanges of foot in, 97: 345
hand surgery in, decision making by parents and children in, 96: 315
hemiplegia in, spastic, functional outcome of upper limb tendon transfer for, 95: 231
infant (see Infant; Infantile)
osteochondromata in, multiple hereditary, and forearm deformities and problems, 95: 288
radius head dislocation in, chronic post-traumatic, treatment of, 95: 56
radius head dislocation in, "isolated" traumatic, 96: 243
replantation in
 bone growth after, 96: 346
 limb, 96: 353
 limb, upper, results of, 96: 351
revascularization in upper extremity in, results, 96: 351
rolling belt injuries in, 96: 83
thumb contracture in, acquired flexion, 97: 325
thumb reconstruction in, heterodigital neurovascular island flap in, 96: 69
toe phalangeal grafts in
 for congenital hand anomalies, 95: 294
 in symbrachydactyly, 95: 294
toe transfer in, microvascular free, psychological impact of, 97: 345
ulnar physeal arrest in, traumatic, after distal forearm fractures, 97: 320
wrist injuries in, Galeazzi-equivalent, 95: 61
Chitin
 fingertip cap of, for fingertip injuries, 96: 73

Chondral
 fractures of proximal pole of scaphoid with distal radial fractures, arthroscopic diagnosis and minimally invasive treatment of, 97: 206
Chow technique of endoscopic carpal tunnel release
 early experience with, 95: 151
 results of, 95: 149
 transbursal and extrabursal, 97: 114
 two-portal, sensory disturbances after, 96: 164
 vs. open release, 95: 146
CHOX-1 and *CHOX-4*
 syndecan and axial congenital deformities of upper limb, 95: 301
Cigarette
 smoking, and microvascular tissue transfers, 95: 320
Cinearthrography
 triple-injection, of wrist, vs. arthroscopy, 97: 193
Cinematography
 MRI, in diagnosis of triangular fibrocartilage complex lesions, 96: 233
Circulation
 collateral, to hand, noninvasive evaluation of, 96: 37
 median nerve, in carpal tunnel syndrome, MRI of, 95: 135
Clam-digger splint
 after flexible intramedullary nailing of metacarpal fractures, 97: 45
Clavicle
 fractures
  concurrent in newborns with obstetric brachial plexus palsy, prognostic value of, 96: 126
  open, in children, 97: 321
Claw finger
 correction methods, evaluation using finger dynamography, 95: 230
Climbers
 flexor pulley rupture in, subcutaneous long finger, 95: 90
Clindamycin
 irrigation with, local, for palmar space infections, 96: 308
Clinicopathologic
 study of carpal tunnel syndrome, 96: 127
Club
 hand, radial, 95: 299
  acquired, due to osteomyelitis, 96: 62

CO_2
  laser tenolysis in flexor tendon (in rabbit), 97: 374
Cognitive
  capacities after nerve repair, correlation with functional sensibility, 96: 118
Cold
  hypersensitivity to, after bipedicle digital advancement island flaps, 96: 78
  -induced discomfort 12 years after digital replantation, 96: 348
  -induced vasospasm after digital replantation (see Vasospasm, cold-induced)
  intolerance
    after digital replantation, thermoregulation patterns in, 97: 358
    after Hueston flap for fingertip skin loss, 95: 76
    after thumb reconstruction with heterodigital neurovascular island flap, 96: 69
  nociceptors, sensitization of, and cold-induced vasospasm after finger replantation, 97: 349
  stress testing, isolated, for microvascular response associated with reflex sympathetic dystrophy of hand and wrist, 95: 27
Collagen
  degeneration in carpal tunnel syndrome, 96: 127
Collateral circulation
  to hand, noninvasive evaluation of, 96: 37
Collateral ligament
  excision, total, for contractures of proximal interphalangeal joint, 95: 67
  lateral, of elbow joint, anatomy and kinematics of, 97: 16
  reconstruction in metacarpal synostosis, 95: 291
  ulnar
    anatomy of origin and insertion of, 95: 219
    of metacarpophalangeal joint of thumb, acute complete tears of, arthroscopic treatment, 97: 48
    of metacarpophalangeal joint of thumb, chronic instability, ligament replacement for, 95: 68
    of metacarpophalangeal joint of thumb, injuries of, 95: 41
    preoperative evaluation by MRI and CT arthrography, 95: 217
    tears, MRI of, 95: 42
    tears, ultrasound differentiation of displaced and nondisplaced, 96: 33
  thumb, dislocated, ultrasound diagnosis of, 97: 28
  thumb, injured, sonography of, 96: 35
  thumb, ruptures, Mitek bone anchor for, 97: 50
Collateral sprouting
  sensory and motor, induced from intact peripheral nerve by end-to-side anastomosis (in rat), 96: 366
Colles' fracture (see Fracture, Colles')
Combustion
  injuries, morbidity of pedicled groin flap for, 95: 78
Compartment
  pressure
    in carpal tunnel in distal radius fractures, 96: 216
    forearm, measurement, cadaveric and radiologic assessment of catheter placement for, 96: 380
  sixth dorsal, release of, 96: 110
Compensable
  upper extremity cumulative trauma disorders, cost of, 96: 257
Compensation
  workers' (see Workers, compensation)
Compliance
  impact on rehabilitation of mallet finger, 95: 98
Compression
  arthrodesis, AO, of wrist in posttraumatic arthritis, 95: 274
  carpal-compression test in diagnosis of carpal tunnel syndrome, 96: 142
  device in precision oblique osteotomy for shortening of ulnar, 95: 174
  -extension fractures of distal radius, posterior plate osteosynthesis in treatment of, 96: 211
  flexion articular fractures of distal end of radius, proposed classification for, 96: 208
  glove
    for palmar burns, in children, 96: 82
    vs. splintage for closed metacarpal fracture, 96: 57
  injuries, morbidity of pedicled groin flap for, 95: 78
  mechanical, effect on chronic hand edema after burn injury, 96: 79
  nerve (see Nerve, compression)
  screws in fracture-dislocations of proximal interphalangeal joint, 97: 40

syndrome, thoracic outlet, orthosis in, 96: 330
Computed tomography
arthrography in preoperative evaluation of ulnar collateral ligament, 95: 217
of digital pulley rupture, 97: 99
images, carpal bone anatomy measured by computer analysis of 3D reconstructions of, 97: 152
longitudinal, of scaphoid, 97: 37
three-dimensional, role in carpal tunnel syndrome, 96: 148
Computer
analysis of 3D reconstruction of CT images, carpal bone anatomy measured by, 97: 152
-assisted 3-D modelling in osteotomy for radius deformity, 95: 197
-controlled mechanostimulator in assessing recovery after carpal tunnel release, 95: 144
keyboard (see Keyboard)
mouse use
cumulative trauma disorders of upper extremity and, 97: 260
variation in upper limb posture and movement during word processing with, 96: 265
Conduit
material in peripheral nerve repair, orientated mats of fibronectin as (in rat), 97: 364
Congenital
deformities
arteriovenous, embolization therapy for, 95: 292
axial, in upper limb, nosology of, 95: 300
hand, classification of, position of symbrachydactyly in, 96: 317
hand, toe phalangeal grafts in, 95: 294
Connective tissue
disease, mixed, flexible implant resection arthroplasty of proximal interphalangeal joint in, 96: 275
Connexus
intertendineus at metacarpophalangeal joint of little finger in musicians, treatment of radial subluxation of, 95: 102
Contact
areas in thumb carpometacarpal joint, 97: 3
stresses, effect of displaced intra-articular distal radial fractures on, 97: 211

Contraction
in Dupuytren's disease fibroblasts, correlation with α-smooth muscle actin expression, 97: 304
Contracture
Dupuytren's
dermofasciectomy for, long-term follow-up, 96: 309
neurovascular displacement in hands with, 96: 305
skin defects in, distally-based hand flap for resurfacing, 96: 309
transforming growth factor-β role in, 96: 381
treatment, TEC device in, 95: 282
work-related, 97: 305
elbow capsular, surgical release, in children, 96: 242
in epidermolysis bullosa, surgical treatment, in children, 95: 291
flexion, of thumb, acquired, in children, 97: 325
interphalangeal joint, proximal, total collateral ligament excision for, 95: 67
scar
morbidity of pedicled groin flap for, 95: 78
after thumb reconstruction with heterodigital neurovascular island flap, 96: 69
supination, paralytic, of forearm, due to traumatic tetraplegia, rerouting of biceps brachii for, 95: 223
Volkmann's, free muscle transfer in, 95: 311
follow-up studies, 95: 312
web space, first, and hand function, 95: 5
Contrast material
MRI reflex sympathetic dystrophy findings before and after infusion of, 96: 361
Cooling
surface, effectiveness in reducing heat injury, 95: 335
Coordination
of index finger movements, 95: 10
Corpuscles
Meissner's, in nail bed and matrix, 97: 5
Cortex
remodeling of hand representation in, determination by timing of tactile stimulation, 97: 18
Cortical
bone and strength in osteopenic distal radius, 95: 201

Corticosteroid
  combined with regional IV block for reflex sympathetic dystrophy after distal radius fractures, 96: 220
  injections
    in carpal tunnel syndrome combined with splinting, reexamination of, 96: 147
    in De Quervain's disease, 96: 273
    in trigger finger, 97: 264
  ointment, topical, for extravasation of antitumor agents, 95: 280
    at dorsum of hand, 95: 279
Cosmetic
  treatment of first web space atrophy, free fat autotransplantation for, 97: 87
Cost
  of cumulative trauma disorders of upper extremity, compensable, 96: 257
  economic, of musculoskeletal conditions, 97: 327
  -effectiveness analysis of diagnostic management of suspected scaphoid fracture, 96: 196
  of Silastic foam dressings after skin graft in children's hand burns, 95: 80
Cowen's distraction apparatus
  for phalanx lengthening for shortened fingers after trauma, 95: 67
Cramp
  musician's
    botulinum toxin in, 95: 308
    occupational, and biomechanical abnormalities, 95: 306
  typist's, botulinum toxin in, 95: 308
  writer's
    botulinum toxin in, 95: 308, 309
    tonic vibration reflex and muscle afferent block in, 97: 334
Creep strain
  of flexor tendons during low-force high-frequency activities, measurement of, 96: 19
Crossed intrinsic transfer
  for rheumatoid metacarpophalangeal joints, motion after, 95: 266
Crush
  load, magnitude and duration, effect on functional recovery of peripheral nerve (in rat), 95: 110
Cryosurgery
  /curettage for giant cell tumor of distal radius, 97: 297
CT (*see* Computed tomography)
Cubital
  fossa, management of extravasation of antitumor agents in, 95: 280
  tunnel
    decompression, operative techniques for, intraneural ulnar pressure changes related to, 96: 161
    surgery, range of motion after, early *vs.* late, 97: 145
    syndrome, nonoperative management of, 95: 139
    syndrome, treatment, relevance of extrinsic blood supply of ulnar nerve at elbow in, 95: 4
    syndrome, ulnar nerve in, anterior submuscular transposition of, 97: 146
    syndrome after Outerbridge-Kashiwagi's method of arthroplasty for elbow osteoarthritis, 97: 235
    ulnar nerve in, intraneural topography facilitates anterior transposition, 96: 29
Culture
  explant, of flexor retinaculum in carpal tunnel syndrome, 97: 140
Cumulative trauma disorders
  control of, active surveillance for, 95: 245
  how to assess the risks, 97: 258
  in music students, 97: 331
  outcome study for work survivability, 97: 261
  upper extremity
    compensable, cost of, 96: 257
    computer mouse use and, 97: 260
    medical screening of office workers for, 95: 244
  in workers performing repetitive tasks, detection of, 96: 265
Curettage
  for giant cell tumors of distal radius, 97: 297; 95: 282
Current perception threshold testing
  as screening procedure for carpal tunnel syndrome in industrial workers, 96: 260
Cutaneous
  (*See also* Skin)
  mycoses, efficacy and tolerability of Lamisil in, 97: 68
  neuralgia, medial antebrachial, after anterior submuscular transposition of ulnar nerve for cubital tunnel syndrome, 97: 147

Cyclic
 tensile loading, effect on water content and solute diffusion in flexor tendons (in dog), 96: 372
Cyst
 bone, after Swanson silicone finger joint implants, 97: 287
 mucous, of distal interphalangeal joints, 96: 269
 radius bone graft for, distal anterior, 97: 59

D

Dacron
 tendon splints in tendon repair, 96: 376
Dahllite
 in skeletal repair, 96: 365
Daily living
 activities of, for hand function assessment, 95: 34
Dancing
 -related distal radius fractures, 96: 222
Darrach procedure
 modified, for painful distal radioulnar joint, 97: 217
 radioulnar convergence after, dynamic, 97: 218
Débridement
 aggressive, before primary extensor tendon reconstruction in dorsal hand defects requiring free flaps, 95: 97
 arthroscopic, of triangular fibrocartilage complex tears, clinical results of, 97: 223
 of mycetoma of hand, 96: 308
 of osteocytes for fingernail deformities secondary to ganglions of distal interphalangeal joint, 97: 294
 of palmar space infections, 96: 308
Decision
 making
  in detecting abnormal Semmes-Weinstein monofilament thresholds in carpal tunnel syndrome, 96: 39
  by parents and children in pediatric hand surgery, 96: 315
Decompression
 cubital tunnel, operative techniques for, intraneural ulnar pressure changes related to, 96: 161
 of flexor carpi radialis tunnel for tendinitis, results of, 96: 111
 lunate, for Kienböck's disease, preoperative factors and outcome after, 95: 180

median nerve
 in carpal tunnel, for palmar space infections, 96: 308
 endoscopic, in carpal tunnel, 96: 175
 radial nerve, in radial tunnel syndrome, review of, 97: 142
Deformity(ies)
 arteriovenous, congenital, embolization therapy for, 95: 292
 axial, congenital, in upper limb, nosology of, 95: 300
 boutonnière, potential, central slip tenodesis test for early diagnosis, 95: 36
 in Dupuytren's disease, assessment of, 97: 312
forearm
 osteochondromas causing, multiple, hereditary, in children, 95: 288
 rotational, severe, surgical radioulnar osteoclasis for, 96: 65
hand
 congenital, classification of, position of symbrachydactyly in, 96: 317
 congenital, toe phalangeal grafts in, 95: 294
 transplants of phalanges of foot in, free, 97: 345
 hypoplastic thumb associated with, 97: 315
 intestinal, and thumb duplication, 97: 316
 Kirner's, case report and review of literature, 96: 321
Madelung
 new therapeutic approach to, 95: 298
 surgical technique, 95: 296
nail
 nontraumatic, classification and diagnosis of, 97: 87
 secondary to ganglions of distal interphalangeal joint, treatment of, 97: 294
 radius, osteotomy for, 95: 197
 Wassel type IV, management and new classification, 97: 318
Degenerative
 arthritis
  (See also Osteoarthritis)
  posttraumatic, of carpometacarpal joint of small finger, silicone implant arthroplasty for, 96: 290
 changes of trapeziometacarpal joint, radiologic assessment of, 97: 275
 triangular fibrocartilage complex perforations, arthroscopic partial resection for, 95: 206

Degloving
  injuries of hand and fingers, 96: 347
Delivery
  traumatic, brachial plexopathy in infant after, MRI of, 95: 224
Denaturating
  methods, muscle graft, for nerve repair (in rat), 97: 365
Denervation
  autonomic, and reflex sympathetic dystrophy, 96: 355
  of wrist, Wilhelm's technique, 95: 174
de Quervain's disease
  anatomy of, 97: 273
  treatment of, 96: 273
  Wartenberg's disease and, 95: 143
  Wartenberg's syndrome and, 97: 267
  of wrist, MRI features in, 97: 265
Derma-Durometer
  for skin hardness in fingertip, 96: 41
Dermatitis
  hand, occupational, in metalworkers, prognosis of, 97: 340
Dermofasciectomy
  for Dupuytren's contracture, long-term follow-up, 96: 309
  in Dupuytren's disease, in children, 97: 324
Desmoid
  tumor of ulna and neurofibromatosis, 97: 312
Dexamethasone
  injection in early mild carpal tunnel syndrome, 95: 132
Diabetes mellitus
  carpal tunnel release outcome in, 96: 131
  Dupuytren's disease, carpal tunnel syndrome, and trigger finger in, 96: 303
Diagnostix 2048 scanner
  for digitizing conventional wrist x-rays, 96: 38
Diagrams
  hand, workplace surveillance for carpal tunnel syndrome using, 96: 138
Dialysis
  peritoneal, continuous ambulatory, carpal tunnel syndrome in patients undergoing, 97: 123
  vascular access for, upper extremity, neurologic and ischemic complications of, 96: 362
Diastasis
  scapholunate, in distal radius fractures, pathomechanics and treatment options, 95: 190

Digit
  (See also Finger; Thumb; Toe)
  amputated, temporary ectopic implantation for salvage of, 97: 67
  fibromas, infantile, 97: 299
  fractures, prospective study of, 97: 65
  hypoplasia, congenital, toe phalangeal grafts in, 95: 295
  nubbin-digits hand, pathomorphology and treatment of, 95: 303
  prostheses, benefits and use of, 97: 335
  pulley rupture, CT of, 97: 99
  reconstruction, flap in
    dorsometacarpal, reverse, 96: 342
    V-Y advancement, dorsal, 95: 69
  replantation (see Replantation, digit)
  revascularization, effectiveness of sensory reeducation after, 97: 343
Digital
  anesthesia through flexor tendon sheath at palmar level, 95: 33
  artery flap, reverse
    innervated, through bilateral neurorrhaphy for pulp defects, 95: 83
    island, for fingertip injuries, 95: 71
  electroneurometer (see Electroneurometer)
  flap, bipedicle advancement island, long-term evaluation of sensory sequelae of, 96: 78
  nerve
    block, transthecal vs. traditional, for anesthesia of finger, 96: 44
    conduction velocity as sensitive indication of peripheral neuropathy in vibration syndrome, 96: 261
    defects, vein conduits with interposition of nerve tissue for, 96: 124
    divided, on one side of finger, unrepaired, 95: 116
    injuries, outcome, 97: 111
    injuries, repair of, primary, results, 96: 117
    injuries, segmental, posterior interosseous nerve as graft for, 95: 8
    repair, after rolling belt injuries, in children, 96: 83
    repair, effect of motion on, 97: 363
    repair, primary, clinical assessment results after, 95: 38
    repair, secondary, 95: 115
    repair, unilateral, interpreting results of, 95: 113

traction, dynamic, for unstable comminuted intra-articular fracture-dislocations of proximal interphalangeal joint, 97: 40
Digitalized
  conventional wrist x-rays, monitor findings of, 96: 38
Disability
  work, and work-related upper extremity disorders, 97: 262
Discrimination
  two-point (see Two-point discrimination)
Disk
  articular
    of triangular fibrocartilage complex, strains in, 95: 208
    of wrist, healing of (in dog), 95: 209
Disk-Criminator
  establishment of reliability with, 95: 16
Dislocation
  carpal row, distal traumatic, 96: 208
  elbow, airbag-related, 96: 68
  of extensor pollicis longus, ulnar, 95: 68
  fracture- (see Fracture, -dislocation)
  implant, Silastic, after arthroplasty of carpal scaphoid, 96: 201
  ligament, ulnar collateral, of thumb, sonography of, 97: 28; 96: 35
  partial (see Subluxation)
  perilunate, 95: 175
  phalanx of foot on metacarpal head, after free transplants of phalanges of foot in hand deformities, 97: 345
  radioulnar joint, distal
    ulna styloid fracture and triangular fibrocartilage complex injury with, 95: 207
    volar type, 96: 233
  radius head
    "isolated" traumatic, 96: 243
    post-traumatic, chronic, treatment, in children, 95: 56
  sesamoid bone in metacarpophalangeal joint of thumb, 96: 1
Disruption
  separation, effect of wrist position on extensor mechanism after, 96: 112
Dissociation
  scapholunate
    new operation for, 97: 167
    with periscaphoid arthritis, long-term results after proximal row carpectomy for, 96: 203

Distal
  site of compression, effect on neural regeneration (in rat), 95: 321
Distraction
  apparatus, Cowen's, for phalanx lengthening for shortened fingers after trauma, 95: 67
  device in treatment of infected clench-fist human bite wounds in area of metacarpophalangeal joints, 97: 55
  lengthening, preoperative, for radial longitudinal deficiency, 97: 326
  Matev continuous, in thumb reconstruction, 96: 60
Diurnal
  changes in carpal tunnel pressure in carpal tunnel syndrome, 95: 138
Dog
  bites causing penetrating brachial artery injuries, 96: 345
Dominance
  left-hand, and hand trauma, 97: 22
Donor
  site deficit of osteocutaneous radial forearm flap, 95: 313
Doppler
  flowmetry, laser
    in evaluation of collateral circulation to hand, 96: 37
    in reflex sympathetic dystrophy, 96: 356
    in reflex sympathetic dystrophy due to autonomic denervation, 96: 355
    vs. thermometry in postoperative monitoring of replantations, 96: 352
  imaging, laser, of finger skin blood flow after microvascular repair of ulnar artery at wrist, 96: 364
  ultrasound, color, in assessment of patency rates after radial and ulnar artery repairs, 95: 319
Dorsal
  compartment, sixth, release of, 96: 110
  gliding and functional spaces in metacarpophalangeal region, 96: 31
Dorsometacarpal
  flap, reverse, in digits and web-space reconstruction, 96: 342
Dorsoradial capsule
  of thumb metacarpophalangeal joint, isolated injuries to, 97: 51
Dorso-ulnar
  thumb flap, 95: 73

Subject Index / 401

Double-grasping suture
  in flexor tendon repair, evaluation of, 97: 95
Doxorubicin
  extravasation of
    at dorsum of hand, treatment of, 95: 279
    management and surgical treatment, 95: 280
Drainage
  wound, for palmar space infections, 96: 308
Dressings
  Silastic foam, after skin grafts in pediatric hand burns, 95: 80
Drilling
  through phalanges, heat recordings at tips of Kirschner wires during, 96: 383
Drug(s)
  abuse, injection, causing upper extremity abscesses, 95: 83
  antiblastic, extravasation of
    at dorsum of hand, treatment, 95: 279
    management and surgical treatment, 95: 280
  anti-inflammatory (see Anti-inflammatory agents)
  antitumor, extravasation of
    at dorsum of hand, treatment, 95: 279
    management and surgical treatment, 95: 280
Duplication of thumb (see Thumb, duplication)
Dupuytren's contracture (see Contracture, Dupuytren's)
Dupuytren's disease
  capsular tissues of proximal interphalangeal joint in, 95: 9
  in children, 97: 323
  contracture of (see Contracture, Dupuytren's)
  deformity in, assessment of, 97: 312
  diabetes mellitus and, 96: 303
  epithelioid sarcoma masquerading as, 96: 298
  fasciotomy for, needle, 95: 284
  fibroblasts, contraction in, correlation with α-smooth muscle actin expression, 97: 304
  follow-up, long-term, 96: 306
  interphalangeal joint in, flexed proximal, skeletal traction for, 96: 301
  open palm technique for, modified, 97: 302

T cell-mediated response in, 95: 285
Dynamic
  components, hand glove splint for attachment of, 96: 338
Dynamography
  finger
    in evaluation of claw finger correction methods, 95: 230
    in functional evaluation of hand, 95: 230
Dynamometer (see Jamar dynamometer)
Dynamometry
  identification of low-effort patients through, 97: 22
Dysesthesia
  distal, after modified open palm technique for Dupuytren's disease, 97: 304
Dysplasia
  finger, with metacarpal base defect, treatment of, 96: 322
Dystonia
  focal
    hand, botulinum toxin in, 95: 309
    hand, botulinum toxin in, long-term, 95: 308
    hand, sensory dysfunction associated with, 97: 272
    in instrumentalists, treatment outcomes, 97: 330
    in musicians, and biomechanical abnormalities, 95: 306
Dystrophy
  reflex sympathetic (see Reflex, sympathetic dystrophy)

E

Echography
  in gamekeeper's thumb, 95: 44
Economic
  cost of musculoskeletal conditions, 97: 327
Edema
  in carpal tunnel syndrome, 96: 127
  hand, chronic, after burn injury, effect of mechanical compression on, 96: 79
Elbow
  allograft replacement of, massive, 96: 248
  arthroplasty (see Arthroplasty, elbow)
  arthroscopy, neuroanatomy in, 97: 239
  below-elbow amputation for giant cell tumors of distal radius, 95: 282
  capsular contracture, surgical release, in children, 96: 242
  dislocation, airbag-related, 96: 68

extension in tetraplegics, single-stage reconstruction of, 96: 254
flexion
  functional recovery by anastomosing medial thoracic nerve to musculocutaneous nerve, 95: 117
  restoration after avulsion injuries of brachial plexus, spinal accessory neurotization for, 97: 105
  restoration with intercostal nerve transfers, 96: 122
joint, lateral collateral ligament of, anatomy and kinematics of, 97: 16
lateral, arthroscopic anatomy of, 96: 245
osteoarthritis, Outerbridge-Kashiwagi's method of arthroplasty for, 97: 234
pain, lateral, and extensor carpi radialis brevis muscle relation to posterior interosseous nerve, 96: 246
range of motion, functional, 96: 239
replacement (see Arthroplasty, elbow)
soft tissue coverage, reverse lateral arm flap in, 95: 316
surgery, early corrective, in arthrogryposis multiplex congenita, 95: 290
tennis
  correlation of MRI, surgical, and histopathologic findings, 97: 270
  extensor release for, lateral, long-term follow-up, 95: 215
  persistent, low-energy extracorporeal shock wave therapy for, 97: 268
  wrist kinematics in expert vs. novice tennis players performing backhand stroke and, 96: 334
ulnar nerve at, extrinsic blood supply of, 95: 4
valgus instability test of, arthroscopic, evaluation of, 97: 30
Elderly
  carpal tunnel syndrome in, distal latencies in, 96: 134
Electrical
  shock, effectiveness of surface cooling in reducing heat injury after, 95: 335
  stimulation
    cutaneous, sensory nerve response in saphenous nerve on (in rat), 97: 378
    functional, after tendon transfers for hand function restoration in spinal cord injury, 97: 245
    nerve, direct, for chronic peripheral nerve pain, 96: 358
  studies as prognostic factor in surgical treatment of carpal tunnel syndrome, 96: 133
Electrodes
  percutaneous intramuscular, reliability for upper extremity functional neuromuscular stimulation in adolescents with C5 tetraplegia, 96: 256
Electrodiagnostic
  findings in carpal tunnel syndrome, correlation with MRI, clinical, and intraoperative findings, 97: 139
  studies in carpal tunnel syndrome diagnosis, vs. electroneurometry and vibrometry, 97: 133
  testing in carpal tunnel syndrome and carpal tunnel release outcome, 97: 137
Electromyography
  botulinum toxin injections guided by, in focal hand dystonia, 95: 308
  dynamic, for phasic relationships of intrinsic and extrinsic thumb musculature, 97: 252
  needle, in carpal tunnel syndrome, relation to nerve conduction studies, 96: 137
Electron
  microscopic study of flexor retinaculum in carpal tunnel syndrome, 97: 140
Electroneurometer
  for measures of median nerve sensory latency
    reliability of, 95: 19
    vs. standard nerve conduction studies, 95: 20
Electroneurometry
  in carpal tunnel syndrome diagnosis, vs. traditional electrodiagnostic studies and vibrometry, 97: 133
Electrophysiological
  effects of aging on nerve regeneration (in rat), 97: 366
  results of bipedicle digital advancement island flaps, 96: 78
Elongation
  (See also Lengthening)
  of metacarpal bones for treatment of finger amputations, 96: 58
  treatment, continuous, by TEC device, for Dupuytren's contracture, 95: 282
Embolization
  therapy for congenital arteriovenous malformations, 95: 292
Emergency room
  Kirschner wire placement in, 97: 65

Employees
  managerial/professional, median sensory
    distal amplitude and latency in,
    95: 250
Employment
  outcome after secondary carpal tunnel
    surgery, 95: 144
Endoscopic
  carpal tunnel release (see Carpal tunnel,
    release, endoscopic)
  diagnosis and possible treatment of
    nerve root avulsions in
    management of brachial plexus
    injuries (in goat), 96: 121
  median nerve decompression in carpal
    tunnel, 96: 175
  retrieval of severed flexor tendons,
    96: 89
Energy
  vibration, absorption in hand and arm,
    95: 322
Entrapment
  nerve
    peripheral, upper extremity, among
      wheelchair athletes, 95: 309
    radial, superficial branch, 95: 143
    after radius fractures, distal, 96: 218
    of pronator quadratus in pediatric distal
      radius fractures, 96: 229
Enzymhistochemical
  evaluation of ulnar nerve grafts in
    brachial plexus injuries, 95: 107
Epicondyle
  humeral medial, fracture, treatment of,
    97: 243
Epicondylectomy
  medial, for cubital tunnel syndrome,
    early vs. late range of motion after,
    97: 145
Epicondylitis
  humeral, rheumatoid factor and HLA
    antigens in, 97: 293
  lateral (see Elbow, tennis)
Epidermal
  growth factor, role in Dupuytren's
    contracture, 96: 381
Epidermolysis bullosa
  contracture and syndactyly with,
    surgical treatment, in children,
    95: 291
  hand surgery for, anesthesia for, 97: 35
Epigastric
  vein defects, vein grafting with
    telescopic anastomotic technique
    for (in rat), 95: 317

Epineurium
  polydioxanone ribbons sutured to, in
    relief of tension in nerve repair,
    95: 112
  suture, secondary, for digital nerve
    repair, 95: 115
Epiphysiodesis
  post-traumatic, of distal end of radius,
    progressive lengthening in, 97: 324
Epiphysis
  double, in hand, 95: 295
Epitenon
  biomechanical and clinical evaluation
    of, 96: 91
  -first technique in augmented Becker
    tenorrhaphy (in monkey), 96: 99
  stitch, running peripheral, mechanical
    analysis of (in rabbit), 96: 378
Epithelioid
  sarcoma masquerading as Dupuytren's
    disease, 96: 298
Ergonomic
  analysis of piano virtuoso's work,
    97: 341; 96: 333
Ethanol
  in embolization therapy of congenital
    arteriovenous malformations,
    95: 293
  injections in writer's cramp, 97: 334
Eve procedure, 97: 350
Ewald elbow prosthesis
  unconstrained, lateral approach,
    short-term complications of,
    97: 238
Ewing's sarcoma
  combined modality therapy for, 96: 297
Excision
  of carcinoma of hand, recurrent
    squamous cell, in
    immunosuppressed patients,
    96: 294
  of fibromas, infantile digital, 97: 299
  lunate, simple, in advanced Kienböck's
    disease, 96: 205
  of osteochondromata, multiple
    hereditary, in children, 95: 289
  for radioulnar synostosis, traumatic,
    and postoperative low-dose
    irradiation, 96: 247
  radius, en bloc, for giant cell tumor,
    97: 297
  of sarcoma, soft tissue, 96: 293
  scaphoid, in radioscaphoid arthritis,
    95: 185
  trapezium, for osteoarthritis at thumb
    base, 96: 284
  ulna, distal, in rheumatoid arthritis,
    97: 290

wide, and full-thickness skin grafts for mucous cysts of distal interphalangeal joints, 96: 269
Exercise
devices, rubber band, for children after flexor tendon injuries, 96: 85
for mallet finger injuries, compliance with, 95: 99
maneuver, provocative, effect on nerve conduction studies in carpal tunnel syndrome, 95: 255
Exostosis
cartilaginous, multiple, classification system for, in children, 97: 326
Expansion
tissue, for complete syndactyly of first web, 96: 311
Extension
-compression fractures of distal radius, posterior plate osteosynthesis in treatment of, 96: 211
passive flexion-active extension for postoperative mobilization of flexor tendon repairs, 96: 102
splint for mallet finger injuries, compliance with, 95: 99
wrist, after Kapandji procedure for posttraumatic distal radioulnar joint problems, 95: 204
Extensor
carpi radialis brevis, relation to posterior interosseous nerve, 96: 16, 246
carpi ulnaris
subluxation and stenosing tenosynovitis of, 97: 273
transfer of extensor pollicis brevis to, in Charcot-Marie-Tooth disease, 97: 248–249
digiti minimi
quinti transposition for metacarpal synostosis, 95: 291
transfer in prevention of recurrent ulnar drift, 95: 277
indicis transfer in Charcot-Marie-Tooth disease, 97: 249
lateral, release for tennis elbow, long-term follow-up, 95: 215
mechanism after disruption separation, effect of wrist position on, 96: 112
pollicis brevis, transfer to extensor carpi ulnaris in Charcot-Marie-Tooth disease, 97: 248–249
pollicis longus
opposition by, restoration of, 96: 86
rupture, late, after wrist arthroscopy, 96: 194
ulnar dislocation of, 95: 68

tendon
graft, braided plantaris tendon as, 96: 89
in hand, flexor tendon transfer to, 96: 87
lacerations, zones II and III, early controlled motion with dynamic *vs.* static splinting for, 96: 107
reconstruction, primary, in dorsal hand defects requiring free flaps, 95: 96
rupture at musculotendinous junction, traumatic, 97: 101
transfer, bypass, 97: 102
wrist, commercial orthoses, 96: 338
zone IV, biomechanical characteristics of suture techniques in, 97: 93
Extracorporeal
shock wave therapy, low-energy, for persistent tennis elbow, 97: 268
Extradigital
glomus tumor, 97: 302
Extravasation
of antitumor drugs
at dorsum of hand, treatment, 95: 279
management and surgical treatment, 95: 280
Extremity
flaps, free, liability of recipient vessels distal to zone of injury when used for, 97: 351
replantation, in children, 96: 353
upper
(*See also* Arm)
abscesses from injection drug abuse, 95: 83
airbag-related injuries, 96: 67
amputations, major, prosthetic usage in, 97: 337
burns, gloves for, expanded polytetrafluoroethylene gloves, 96: 79
in Charcot-Marie-Tooth disease, treatment of, 97: 248
deformities, axial congenital, nosology of, 95: 300
disorders, cumulative trauma (*see* Cumulative trauma disorder, upper extremity)
disorders, soft tissue, classification systems of, 97: 255
disorders, soft tissue, relation to repetitive movements at work, 96: 258
disorders, work-related, and work disability, 97: 262

functional neuromuscular stimulation in adolescents with C5 tetraplegia, reliability of percutaneous intramuscular electrodes for, 96: 256
growth prediction, straight-line graphs for, 95: 301
injuries, severe, emergency free tissue transfer for, 96: 72
nerve entrapments, peripheral, among wheelchair athletes, 95: 309
neuromas, subjective outcome after surgical management, 96: 125
pain, persistent, in sewing machine operators, 95: 241
posture and movement variations during word processing with and without mouse use, 96: 265
reconstruction, flaps in, local fasciocutaneous, use of previously burned skin in, 96: 80
reconstruction, microvascular, with rectus abdominis muscle, 96: 340
replantation in, results, in children, 96: 351
revascularization, results, in children, 96: 351
tendinitis, in music students, 97: 331
tendon transfers, in spastic hemiplegia, functional outcome, in children, 95: 231
thrombosis of, deep venous, 97: 358
vascular access for dialysis, neurologic and ischemic complications of, 96: 362

F

Facial
-hypoglossal anastomosis, permanent motor hyperinnervation of whisker-pad muscles after (in rat), 95: 327
Falls
flexor-pronator origin ruptures due to, after anterior submuscular transposition of ulnar nerve for cubital tunnel syndrome, 97: 147
Farm
rolling belt injuries on, in children, 96: 83
Fascia
forearm flap, retrograde radial, 97: 85
transfer in Eve procedure, 97: 350

Fascicular
constriction, hourglass-like, within main trunk of median nerve in spontaneous interior interosseous nerve palsy, 97: 143
graft for secondary digital nerve repair, 95: 115
suturing for secondary digital nerve repair, 95: 115
Fasciocutaneous
flaps, local, for upper extremity reconstruction, use of previously burned skin in, 96: 80
Fasciotomy
needle, for Dupuytren's disease, 95: 284
Fat
autotransplantation, free, for cosmetic treatment of first web space atrophy, 97: 87
Fatigability
of hand muscle, effect of short-term immobilization on, 96: 20
Feet (see Foot)
Fiber
afferent, large and small, function deficits in carpal tunnel syndrome, 96: 144
Fibroblast
activity and matrix remodeling after autogenous flexor tendon grafts (in dog), 97: 372
Dupuytren's disease, contraction in, correlation with α-smooth muscle actin expression, 97: 304
growth factor, basic, modulation of formation of molded vascularized bone graft in vivo (in rat), 96: 382
Fibrocartilage
complex
lesions with distal radius fracture, arthroscopic diagnosis and minimally invasive treatment of, 97: 206
triangular (see Triangular fibrocartilage complex)
in interphalangeal joint, proximal, 95: 9
Fibroma
infantile digital, 97: 299
Fibromyalgia
syndrome
carpal tunnel syndrome and, undetected, 96: 151
tautology and, 95: 255

Fibronectin
  mats, orientated, as conduit material in peripheral nerve repair (in rat), 97: 364
Fibrous
  histiocytoma, malignant, of hand, treatment, 96: 293
  proliferations of infancy and childhood, 97: 300
Fibula
  graft (see Graft, fibular)
Figure-of-8 suture
  in extensor zone IV, biomechanical characteristics of, 97: 93
Finger
  (See also Digit)
  amputation (see Amputation, finger)
  anesthesia of, transthecal vs. traditional digital block for, 96: 44
  chiasma tendinum in, clinical anatomy of, 95: 7
  claw, correction methods, evaluation using finger dynamography, 95: 230
  dynamography
    in evaluation of claw finger correction methods, 95: 230
    in functional evaluation of hand, 95: 230
  dysplasia with metacarpal base defect, treatment of, 96: 322
  flexion, lumbrical muscle incursion into carpal tunnel during, 96: 17
  flexors, extrinsic, activity during mobilization in Kleinert splint, 97: 91
  index
    motion, effect of ulnar nerve lesion on, 97: 37
    movements, coordination of, 95: 10
    oblique retinacular ligament of, anatomy of, 95: 16
  injuries, degloving, 96: 347
  joint
    forces in pianists, 95: 11
    implants, Swanson silicone, long-term complications of, 97: 287
    repair, ipsilateral osteochondral graft for, 95: 53
  little (see small below)
  long, subcutaneous flexor pulley rupture, in climbers, 95: 90
  losses, repair with toe transfers, 95: 320
  mallet
    injuries, impact of compliance on rehabilitation, 95: 98
    surgery for, reassessment, 95: 97
  nail (see Nail)
  reconstruction
    dorsal, arterialized tendocutaneous venous flap for, 96: 84
    sensory, radial thenar innervated flap for, 97: 112
  shortened, after trauma, phalanx lengthening for, 95: 67
  skin blood flow after microvascular repair of ulnar artery at wrist, laser Doppler imaging of, 96: 364
  small
    carpometacarpal joint of, anatomy of, functional, 95: 14
    carpometacarpal joint of, arthritis of, posttraumatic degenerative, silicone implant arthroplasty for, 96: 290
    flexor synovial sheath, anatomy of, 97: 19
    metacarpophalangeal joint, radial subluxation of connexus intertendineus at, treatment of, 95: 102
  tendon
    forces in pianists, 95: 11
    injury, acute, MRI of, 97: 29
  tip (see Fingertip below)
  trigger (see Trigger finger)
  ulnar deviation of, congenital unilateral muscle hyperplasia of hand with, 96: 321
  vibration-induced white, prognosis of, 97: 355
Fingertip
  amputated, treatment of, 97: 76
  amputation, volar-oblique, long-term results of neurovascular island flap for, 97: 73
  cap for fingertip injuries, 96: 73
  injuries
    flap for, reversed digital artery island, 95: 71
    treatment for, simple and efficient, 96: 73
  reconstruction, syndactylic toe transfer for, 96: 321
  skin
    hardness related to pressure perception and two-point discrimination in, 96: 41
    loss, Hueston flap for, 95: 75
Fist
  infected clench-fist human bite wounds in area of metacarpophalangeal joints, treatment of, 97: 54
Fistula
  arteriovenous
    acquired, in children, 96: 364

creation for hemodialysis, neurologic
and ischemic complications in
upper extremities after, 96: 362
Fixation
  cerclage, for fracture-dislocation of
    proximal interphalangeal joint,
    97: 42
  device, hinged, for fractures of proximal
    interphalangeal joint, 97: 64
  external
    combined with internal fixation, for
      severe AO-C3 distal radius
      fracture, 97: 193
    dynamic device, for fractures of base
      of middle phalanx, 97: 64
    posterior approach, for supracondylar
      fractures of humerus, in children,
      95: 219
    of radius, distal, biomechanical study
      of, 95: 200
    of radius fracture, distal, comminuted
      intraarticular, results of, 96: 214
    of radius fracture, distal, unstable, vs.
      pins and plaster, 97: 212
    trapeziolunate, for scaphoid fracture,
      96: 197
  of hand fractures, open, recovery of
    motion and complications after,
    95: 50
  internal
    combined with external fixation, for
      severe AO-C3 distal radius
      fracture, 97: 193
    of forearm fractures, airbag-related,
      96: 68
    of Galeazzi fracture-dislocation, distal
      radioulnar joint function after,
      95: 213
    of metacarpal fracture, oblique,
      97: 47
    of perilunate dislocations and
      fracture-dislocations, 95: 176
    of radius fracture, distal, 97: 198
    of radius fracture, distal, with
      scapholunate diastasis, 95: 190
    of radius fracture, head, anatomic
      guidelines for proper placement of,
      97: 233
    of radius fracture, head, late results,
      97: 231
    of radius fracture, neck, anatomic
      guidelines for proper placement of,
      97: 233
    of scaphoid fractures, acute stable, in
      athletes, 97: 172
  Kapandji vs. trans-styloid, of distal
    radius fracture, 97: 196
  Kirschner wire (see Kirschner wire,
    fixation)
  miniscrew
    AO, of radius head fracture, late
      results, 97: 231
    for phalanx fracture, proximal, distal
      unicondylar, 95: 47
  plate (see Plate, fixation)
  staple, power, in trapeziometacarpal
    arthrodesis, 95: 263
  strength of ulnar component of total
    elbow replacement, 97: 238
  systems, titanium, in metacarpal
    fractures, biomechanical stability
    of, 97: 18
  tension band, of avulsion fractures of
    hand, clinical results, 96: 48
  tension wire, of avulsion fractures of
    thumb metacarpophalangeal joint,
    96: 49
  trans-styloid vs. Kapandji, of distal
    radius fracture, 97: 196
Fixator
  A-O miniexternal, for comminuted
    intraarticular distal radial fractures,
    96: 214
  external
    dynamic, unilateral, in
      fracture-dislocations of proximal
      interphalangeal joint, 97: 40
    for metacarpal base fractures, first,
      recent, 96: 54
    mono-segmental, radio-radial, for
      extra-articular fractures of distal
      radius in young adults, 96: 229
Flap
  advancement
    bipedicle digital island, long-term
      evaluation of sensory sequelae of,
      96: 78
    dorsal V-Y, in digital reconstruction,
      95: 69
  arm, lateral
    combined with dorsal forearm flap,
      97: 87
    lateral arm/proximal forearm, 95: 82
    reverse, in soft tissue coverage of
      elbow, 95: 316
  coverage
    after degloving injuries of hand and
      fingers, 96: 347
    after fibroma excision, infantile
      digital, 97: 299
  digital artery, reverse
    innervated, through bilateral
      neurorrhaphy for pulp defects,
      95: 83
    island, for fingertip injuries, 95: 71

dorsometacarpal, reverse, in digits and web-space reconstruction, 96: 342
fasciocutaneous, local, for upper extremity reconstruction, use of previously burned skin in, 96: 80
forearm
  brachioradialis, anatomy and clinical application, 96: 354
  combined dorsal forearm and lateral arm, 97: 87
  lateral arm/proximal forearm, 95: 82
  posterior interosseous reverse, 95: 77
  radial, osteocutaneous, donor site deficit of, 95: 313
  radial, retrograde fascial, 97: 85
  retrograde-flow neurocutaneous island, 96: 70
  transposition, for soft tissue coverage of elbow, 95: 317
free, dorsal hand defects requiring, primary extensor tendon reconstruction in, 95: 96
groin, pedicled, morbidity of, 95: 78
hand, distally-based, for resurfacing skin defects in Dupuytren's contracture, 96: 309
Hueston, for fingertip skin loss, 95: 75
interosseous, posterior, in primary repair of hand injuries, 95: 82
metacarpal artery, second dorsal with double pivot points, 97: 83
neurovascular island, clinical applications, 97: 86
musculocutaneous, latissimus dorsi, without muscle, 97: 81
nail, short-pedicle vascularized, 97: 71
neurocutaneous, retrograde-flow island, in forearm, 96: 70
neurovascular
  island, for volar-oblique fingertip amputations, long-term results, 97: 73
  island, heterodigital, in thumb reconstruction, with and without nerve reconnection, 96: 69
  wrap-around, free, from big toe, in thumb reconstruction, long-term follow-up, 97: 350
parametacarpal, ulnar, anatomical study and clinical application, 97: 78
phalangeal, direct and reversed flow proximal island, 96: 76
procedures for radiation injuries of hand, 95: 81
pulp, in thumb duplication, 97: 317
radial thenar, innervated, for sensory reconstruction of fingers, 97: 112
retinaculum extensorum, for dorsal wrist ganglion, 95: 268
retinaculum flexorum, resurfacing palmar defects of carpal ligaments with, 95: 269
rotation, for thumb polydactyly, long-term results, 97: 319
second web bilobed island, for thumb reconstruction, 97: 87
skin, narrow pedicled intercostal perforator, for burned hand coverage, 95: 314
synovialis flap plasty for recurrent carpal tunnel syndrome, 95: 125
tendinocutaneous free, transfer for skin-tendon defect of dorsum of hand, 96: 74
thumb, dorso-ulnar, 95: 73
transposition, localized, for pediatric hand burns, Silastic foam dressings after, 95: 80
ulnar artery, free, 95: 320
venous
  arterialized tendocutaneous, for dorsal finger reconstruction, 96: 84
  for covering skin defects of hand, 96: 341
wrap-around, toe-to-finger transfer combined with, 96: 349
Flexion
  articular fractures, compression, of distal end of radius, proposed classification for, 96: 208
  contracture of thumb, acquired, in children, 97: 325
  elbow (see Elbow, flexion)
  finger, lumbrical muscle incursion into carpal tunnel during, 96: 17
  passive flexion-active extension for postoperative mobilization of flexor tendon repairs, 96: 102
  work of, after tendon repair with various suture methods, 97: 371
  wrist, after Kapandji procedure for posttraumatic distal radioulnar joint problems, 95: 204
Flexor
  apparatus, thumb, restoration of function, oblique and one adjacent flexor tendon pulley required for, 97: 102
  carpi radialis
    sling arthroplasty for osteoarthrosis of thumb base, 95: 257
    tendinitis, results of operative treatment, 96: 111

compartment of forearm, pressure dynamics of, and pressure dynamics of carpal tunnel, 96: 153
digitorum profundus tendon rupture, intratendinous, in zones II and III, 97: 101
extrinsic finger, activity during mobilization in Kleinert splint, 97: 91
plantaris, braided, as extensor tendon graft, 96: 89
pollicis longus repair, late secondary, masquerading as primary trauma, 96: 115
-pronator origin ruptures caused by falls after anterior submuscular transposition of ulnar nerve for cubital tunnel syndrome, 97: 147
pulley
  finger, long, subcutaneous rupture in climbers, 95: 90
  finger, rupture of, closed traumatic, 96: 97
  oblique and one adjacent, required for restoration of function of thumb flexor apparatus, 97: 102
  system, in hands, efficiency of, 97: 10
  system, thumb, biomechanics of, 95: 2
retinaculum
  in carpal tunnel syndrome, explant culture, immunofluorescence and electron microscopic study of, 97: 140
  distal portion, significance of incomplete release in endoscopic carpal tunnel surgery, 96: 174
  function after carpal tunnel release, 97: 14
  surface of distal radius, modified approach to, 97: 154
synovial sheath anatomy of little finger, 97: 19
tendon *(see below)*
tenosynovectomy in rheumatoid arthritis
  A1 pulley in, 95: 276
  finger mobility after, short- and long-term analysis of, 95: 267
tenosynovitis in diabetics, 96: 303
Flexor tendon
  cellular activity, effect of air exposure during surgery on, 97: 378
  chiasm region, clinical anatomy of, 95: 7
  graft, autogenous
    biomechanical and morphological study (in dog), 95: 332

(in rat), 97: 372
injuries
  in children, 96: 85
  in zone I, ultrasound in management of, 95: 88
measurement of creep strain during low-force high-frequency activities, 96: 19
mesovascularized island, 95: 86
mobilization regimen, Billericay controlled active-motion, 96: 106
repair
  acute, mobilized by controlled active motion regimen, rupture rate of, 96: 105
  epitenon-first technique, 96: 91
  mobilization after, early active, 95: 93
  mobilization after, with "passive flexion-active extension" and "controlled active motion" techniques, 96: 102
  in perfect safety, 96: 95
  after rolling belt injuries, in children, 96: 83
  strength of, in vitro, 97: 12
  suture in, caliber, evaluation of, 97: 94
  suture in, double loop locking, early active mobilization after, 97: 89
  suture in, methods, in vitro biomechanical analysis of, 95: 331
  suture in, methods, work of flexion after, 97: 371
  in zone 2C, 95: 85
  in zone II, effects of delayed therapeutic intervention after, 96: 92
  in zone II, gap formation after, 95: 104
  in zone II, rate of recovery after, 95: 104
repaired, effects of suture knots on tensile strength of (in dog), 96: 115
rupture
  MRI of, 97: 97
  after needle fasciotomy for Dupuytren's disease, 95: 285
  in rheumatoid arthritis, retinaculum flexorum flap in, 95: 269
  zone II, MRI of, 97: 95
severed, endoscopic retrieval of, 96: 89
sheath at palmar level, digital anesthesia through, 95: 33
splints in tendon repair, 96: 376
tenolysis
  laser *vs.* scalpel (in rabbit), 97: 374
  in zone 2, 96: 96

transfer to extensor tendon, in hand, 96: 87
water content and solute diffusion in, effect of cyclic and static tensile loading on (in dog), 96: 372
Flexorplasty
  secondary Steindler, after brachial plexus injuries, 96: 251
Floating radius
  in bipolar fracture-dislocation of forearm, 95: 65
Flowmetry
  laser Doppler (see Doppler, flowmetry, laser)
Fluconazole
  for mycetoma, 96: 308
Foam
  dressings, Silastic, after skin grafts in pediatric hand burns, 95: 80
Foot
  autografts from, for reconstruction of scapholunate interosseous ligament, 97: 164
  flap from, tendocutaneous free, for skin-tendon defect of dorsum of hand, 96: 74
  onychomycoses of, efficacy and tolerability of Lamisil in, 97: 68
  phalanges transplants, free, in hand deformities, 97: 345
  sarcoma of, combined modality therapy, 96: 297
Football
  -related distal radius fractures, 96: 222
Force(s)
  application to healing tendon, 95: 92
  applied
    in alphanumeric keyboard work, investigation of, 95: 254
    externally, to palm, increase in carpal tunnel pressure after, 96: 161
  biomechanical, in high-profile vs. low-profile dynamic splinting, 96: 326
  finger joint and tendon, in pianists, 95: 11
  -generating capacity of thumb adductor muscles on parallel and perpendicular plane of adduction, 96: 31
  transmission through wrist, normal, 96: 370
Forearm
  arteries, interosseous, clinical anatomy of, 96: 21
  communications between median nerve and ulnar nerve in, 95: 15
  compartment pressure measurement, cadaveric and radiologic assessment of catheter placement for, 96: 380
  contracture, paralytic supination, due to traumatic tetraplegia, rerouting of biceps brachii for, 95: 223
  deformities and hereditary multiple osteochondromas, in children, 95: 288
  exposure characteristics in relation to symptoms among automobile assembly line workers, 97: 272
  extravasation of antitumor agents in, management of, 95: 280
  flap (see Flap, forearm)
  flexor compartment, pressure dynamics of, and pressure dynamics of carpal tunnel, 96: 153
  fracture (see Fracture, forearm)
  fracture-dislocation, bipolar, floating radius in, 95: 65
  injuries, grip lock, in male gymnasts, 97: 332
  median nerve repair in, tubular, 96: 126
  mixed nerve conduction velocity and retrograde changes in carpal tunnel syndrome, 96: 145
  musculoskeletal symptoms among automobile assembly line workers, and self-reported physical exposure, 97: 328
  one-bone, clinical results of, 97: 58
  problems in children with multiple hereditary osteochondromata, 95: 288
  pseudarthrosis, congenital, vascularized fibular graft for, 95: 319
  rotation
    deformity, severe, surgical radioulnar osteoclasis for, 96: 65
    effect of dorsally angulated distal radius fractures on, 97: 210
    after Kapandji procedure for posttraumatic distal radioulnar joint problems, 95: 204
    stability, role of interosseous membrane and triangular fibrocartilage complex in, 95: 333
    in supination in above-elbow cast for Galeazzi-equivalent wrist injuries, in children, 95: 61
  tourniquet tolerance, vs. upper arm tourniquet tolerance, 95: 26
Foreign body
  in hand, sensitivity and specificity of ultrasound in diagnosis of, 97: 26

Subject Index / 411

reaction to silicone particles after
 Silastic implant arthroplasty of
 carpal scaphoid, 96: 201
Fossa
 cubital, management of extravasation of
 antitumor agents in, 95: 280
Fossil
 evidence for early hominid tool use,
 96: 30
Fracture
 arm, open, in children, 97: 321
 clavicle
  concurrent in newborns with obstetric
  brachial plexus palsy, prognostic
  value of, 96: 126
  open, in children, 97: 321
 Colles'
  algodystrophy after, and tightness of
  cast, 96: 360
  function ten years after, 95: 194
  malunited, 96: 227
  osteosynthesis in treatment of,
  posterior plate, 96: 211
  remanipulated, anatomical and
  functional results five years after,
  97: 200
  secondary displacement in, prediction
  of, 96: 229
  wrist pain after, ulnar, 95: 195
 digit, prospective study of, 97: 65
 -dislocation
  forearm, bipolar, floating radius in,
  95: 65
  Galeazzi, distal radioulnar joint
  function after open reduction and
  internal plate fixation of, 95: 213
  hand, pins and rubbers traction
  system for, 95: 51
  interphalangeal joint, proximal,
  cerclage fixation for, 97: 42
  interphalangeal joint, proximal,
  dorsal, percutaneous Kirschner wire
  pinning of, 95: 45
  interphalangeal joint, proximal,
  severe, surgical treatment of,
  97: 39
  interphalangeal joint, proximal,
  unstable comminuted
  intra-articular, dynamic digital
  traction for, 97: 40
  metacarpal, fifth, old, stabilized
  arthroplasty for, 96: 61
  perilunate, 95: 175
 forearm
  distal, short arm plaster cast for, in
  children, 95: 63
  distal, traumatic ulnar physeal arrest
  after, in children, 97: 320

 malunited, operative treatment of,
 97: 65
 Galeazzi, distal radioulnar joint after,
 96: 238
 Galeazzi-equivalent, in children, 95: 61
 hand
  avulsion, tension band fixation of,
  clinical results, 96: 48
  open, recovery of active motion and
  of complications, 95: 50
 humerus
  medial epicondyle, treatment of,
  97: 243
  open, in children, 97: 321
  supracondylar, 96: 248
  supracondylar, in children, 95: 219
  supracondylar and transcondylar,
  double tension band osteosynthesis
  in, 96: 239
 implant, Swanson silicone finger joint,
 97: 288
 interphalangeal joint, proximal, hinged
 device for, 97: 64
 intraarticular, comminuted, pins and
 rubbers traction system for, 95: 51
 mallet, avulsion, tension band fixation
 of, clinical results, 96: 48
 metacarpal
  bracing in, functional fracture, 95: 59
  closed, initial treatment of, 96: 57
  fifth, base, airbag-related, 96: 68
  fifth, distal displaced, reduction and
  intra-medullary osteosynthesis of,
  95: 68
  first, base, articular fracture, direct
  osteosynthesis vs. closed pinning in,
  97: 66
  first, base, recent fractures, 96: 54
  malunion, correction osteotomy for,
  95: 55
  nailing for, flexible intramedullary,
  97: 45
  oblique, internal fixation of, 97: 47
  plate in, minicondylar, 97: 65
  titanium bone fixation systems in,
  comparative biomechanical stability
  of, 97: 18
 metacarpophalangeal joint of thumb,
 avulsion type, tension wire fixation
 of, 96: 49
 phalanx
  base, middle, dynamic external
  fixation device for, 97: 64
  fracture (see Fracture, phalanx)
  plate in, minicondylar, 97: 65
  proximal, biomechanical analysis of
  dorsal plate fixation in, 95: 49

proximal, distal unicondylar fracture,
  95: 46
"puncher's," scaphoid fracture as,
  95: 193
radius
  airbag-related, 96: 68
  distal (see below)
  at donor site of osteocutaneous radial
    forearm flap, 95: 313–314
  head, 95: 216
  head, fixation of, internal, anatomic
    guidelines for proper placement of,
    97: 233
  head, fixation of, internal, late results,
    97: 231
  head, replacement with metal
    prosthesis, 95: 221
  head, resection for, 95: 221
  neck, fixation of, internal, anatomic
    guidelines for proper placement of,
    97: 233
  open, in children, 97: 321
  open, osteomyelitis causing radial
    clubhand after, in boys, 96: 63
radius, distal
  additional lesions with, arthroscopic
    diagnosis and minimally invasive
    treatment of, 97: 206
  AO-C3, severe, results of combined
    internal and external fixation for,
    97: 193
  carpal tunnel pressure in, 96: 216
  classification of, 97: 213
  compression-extension, posterior
    plate osteosynthesis in treatment of,
    96: 211
  compression flexion articular type,
    proposed classification for, 96: 208
  displaced, severely, percutaneous
    Kirschner wire pinning for, in
    children, 97: 322
  dorsally angulated, effect on distal
    radioulnar joint congruency and
    forearm rotation, 97: 210
  entrapment of pronator quadratus in,
    in children, 96: 229
  epidemiology of, 95: 164
  extra-articular, in young adults,
    96: 229
  fixation of, internal, 97: 198
  fixation of, trans-styloid vs. Kapandji,
    97: 196
  healed, x-ray film measurements of,
    97: 207
  intraarticular, carpal malalignment
    after, in workers, 96: 220
  intraarticular, comminuted, external
    fixation results in, 96: 214
  intraarticular, displaced, effect on
    contact stresses, 97: 211
  intraarticular, intracarpal soft tissue
    lesions with, 97: 204
  isolated, management, in children,
    95: 202
  malunited, early vs. late
    reconstruction for, 97: 198
  nerve entrapment and reflex
    sympathetic dystrophy after,
    96: 218
  osteotomy after, ulnar shortening,
    95: 199
  palmar, predicting palmar radiocarpal
    ligament disruption in, 95: 204
  scapholunate diastasis in,
    pathomechanics and treatment
    options, 95: 190
  in sports, epidemiology and outcome,
    96: 222
  tendinitis after, flexor carpi radialis,
    results of operative treatment,
    96: 111
  unstable, osteosynthesis for,
    in-the-socket, 97: 194
  unstable, pins and plaster vs. external
    fixation of, 97: 212
  unstable, redisplaced, comparison of
    four treatments, 97: 201
scaphoid
  chondral fracture of proximal pole,
    with distal radial fractures,
    arthroscopic diagnosis and
    minimally invasive treatment of,
    97: 206
  diagnosis by day 4 bone scan,
    97: 175
  epidemiology of, 95: 164
  fixation of, internal, with Herbert
    screw, 95: 62
  fixation of, trapeziolunate external,
    96: 197
  midthird, alternative management, in
    athlete, 96: 199
  nonunion (see Nonunion, scaphoid)
  as "puncher's fracture", 95: 193
  radiography of, digitalized
    conventional, 96: 38
  stable, acute, internal fixation, in
    athletes, 97: 172
  suspected, choosing strategy for
    diagnostic management of, 96: 196
  suspected, radiographs and bone
    scintigraphy in, 95: 193
  tendinitis after, flexor carpi radialis,
    results of operative treatment,
    96: 111
  tuberosity, nonunion of, 95: 193

scapula, open, in children, 97: 321
sesamoid
  finger joint, 96: 1
  of thumb, 97: 66
thumb, gamekeeper's, displaced, clinical results of tension band fixation of, 96: 48
triquetral, avulsion fracture on volar aspect, 97: 187
ulna
  airbag-related, 96: 68
  open, in children, 97: 321
  shaft, stable, bracing of, 95: 66
  styloid, with distal radioulnar joint dislocation, 95: 207
  wrist, articular, carpal tunnel pressure in, 96: 217
Francobal prosthesis
  in pantrapezial osteoarthritis, 95: 262
Free radical
  damage in acute nerve compression (in rat), 97: 369
Function
  ten years after Colles' fracture, 95: 194
Functional
  neuromuscular stimulation in adolescents with C5 tetraplegia, reliability of percutaneous intramuscular electrodes for, 96: 256
  results five years after remanipulated Colles' fractures, 97: 200
  sensibility restitution correlated with specific cognitive capacities after nerve repair, 96: 118
  spaces, dorsal, in metacarpophalangeal region, 96: 31
  status after carpal tunnel release, 97: 122

G

Gadolinium
  -enhanced MRI of median nerve circulation in carpal tunnel syndrome, 95: 135
Gadopentetate dimeglumine
  MRI in reflex sympathetic dystrophy, 96: 361
Galeazzi
  -equivalent injuries of wrist, in children, 95: 61
  fracture, distal radioulnar joint after, 96: 238
  fracture-dislocations, open reduction and internal plate fixation of, distal radioulnar joint function after, 95: 213

Galveston metacarpal brace
  vs. plaster-of-paris bandage, 95: 59
Gamekeeper's thumb
  acute, quantitative outcome of surgical repair, 96: 50
  echography in, 95: 44
  fracture of, displaced, clinical results of tension band fixation of, 96: 48
  MRI of, 95: 42
  splint for, 97: 53
Ganglia
  interphalangeal joint, distal, treatment of fingernail deformities secondary to, 97: 294
  sensory, cell loss in, after peripheral nerve injury (in cat), 96: 384
  upper limb, related to repetitive movements at work, 96: 258
  wrist
    anterior, 96: 309
    dorsal, arthroscopic resection of, 96: 195
    dorsal, retinaculum extensorum flap for, 95: 268
    intraosseous, 96: 299
Gap
  detection tactility test for sensory deficits associated with carpal tunnel syndrome, 97: 24
  formation after flexor tendon repair in zone II, 95: 104
Gelberman classification
  in zone 1 flexor tendon injuries, 95: 89
Gender
  female, as risk factor for carpal tunnel syndrome, 96: 136, 157
  radius fracture and, distal, 95: 164
Gene
  CHOX-1 and CHOX-4, and axial congenital deformities of upper limb, 95: 301
Genetic
  factors in nosology of axial congenital deformities in upper limb, 95: 300
  predisposition to reflex sympathetic dystrophy, in caucasian women, 96: 357
Geometry
  abnormal, of distal radioulnar joint, 96: 234
Giant cell
  tumor of distal radius, 97: 297
  treatment of, 95: 281
Gliding
  spaces, dorsal, in metacarpophalangeal region, 96: 31
Glomus
  tumor

extradigital, 97: 302
subungual, MRI of, 96: 291
Glove
  compression
    for palmar burns, in children, 96: 82
    vs. splintage, for closed metacarpal fracture, 96: 57
  polytetrafluoroethylene, expanded, for care of upper extremity burns, 96: 79
  splint, hand, for attachment of dynamic components, 96: 338
Goldberg-Lindblom vibrameter, 95: 240
Goniometer
  for hand function assessment, 95: 34
Gracilis
  muscle
    transfer, free neurovascular, secondary, after brachial plexus injuries, 96: 251
    transfer in Volkmann's contracture, 95: 311
    transfer in Volkmann's contracture, follow-up studies, 95: 312
    transplantation, free, for hand reconstruction, 96: 353
Graft
  allograft
    (See also Transplantation)
    replacement of elbow, massive, 96: 248
  autograft
    ligament, from foot, for reconstruction of scapholunate interosseous ligament, 97: 164
    nerve, old degenerated and fresh, comparison of passage of regenerating axons through (in rat), 95: 325
  bone
    cancellous, from distal radius, in fracture-dislocations of proximal interphalangeal joint, 97: 39
    delayed primary, in open hand fractures, 95: 51
    intercalary, in radiocarpal arthrodesis after resection of distal radius for giant cell tumor, 95: 282
    in metacarpal synostosis, 95: 291
    in nubbin-digits hand, 95: 303
    radius, distal anterior, in hand and wrist surgery, 97: 59
    for scaphoid nonunion, 96: 207
    for scaphoid nonunion, with vascular bundle implantation, 97: 176
    vascularized, molded, in vivo growth factor modulation of formation of (in rat), 96: 382

fascicular, for secondary digital nerve repair, 95: 115
fibular
  proximal, autologous, for reconstruction of distal radius for giant cell tumor, 95: 282
  in reconstruction of distal radius after resection for giant cell tumor, 95: 282
  vascularized, for congenital pseudoarthrosis of forearm, 95: 319
flap (see Flap)
interosseous nerve as source of, posterior, 95: 8
muscle, denaturating methods in nerve repair (in rat), 97: 365
nerve
  bioartificial, 97: 362
  morphology, relation to extent of neurotization (in rabbit), 95: 328
  motor recovery after, technique to quantitate, 97: 112
  ulnar, in brachial plexus lesions, enzymhistochemical evaluation of, 95: 107
  vascularized, with contralateral C7 root transfer, for brachial plexus root avulsion (in rat), 95: 339
osteochondral, ipsilateral, for finger joint repair, 95: 53
phalangeal, toe
  in congenital hand deformities, 95: 294
  in symbrachydactyly reconstruction, 95: 294
skin
  for carcinoma of hand, recurrent squamous cell, in immunosuppressed patients, 96: 294
  full-thickness, after wide excision for mucous cysts of distal interphalangeal joints, 96: 269
  full-thickness, for rolling belt injuries, in children, 96: 83
  optimizing take in children's hand burns, 95: 79
tendon
  extensor, braided plantaris tendon as, 96: 89
  flexor, autogenous, biomechanical and morphological study (in dog), 95: 332
  flexor, autogenous (in dog), 97: 372
  for scapholunate diastasis in distal radius fractures, 95: 190
vein

arteriovenous loops installed as, in
microsurgical composite tissue
transplantation at difficult recipient
sites, 97: 348
inside-out, effect on nerve
regeneration (in rat), 95: 324
with telescoping anastomotic
technique, for venous defects (in
rat), 95: 317
Graner's technique
of Kienböck's disease treatment,
95: 178
Graph
straight-line, for prediction of growth of
upper extremities, 95: 301
Graphic
analysis of biomechanics of massless
bi-articular chain, 97: 7
Grasp
abilities with functional neuromuscular
stimulation in adolescents with
tetraplegia, 97: 246
Grip
effort, submaximal, sensitivity of Jamar
dynamometer in detecting, 97: 263
exertions, sincere and feigned,
consistency with repeated testing,
95: 24
lock injuries to forearm in male
gymnasts, 97: 332
strength
after carpal tunnel decompression,
95: 120
in hand-arm vibration syndrome,
95: 237
after Kapandji procedure for
posttraumatic distal radioulnar
joint problems, 95: 204
testing reliability, 96: 46
wrist deviation and, 96: 194
ulnar variance change with, 95: 16
weakness after carpal tunnel release,
97: 14
Groin
flap, pedicled, morbidity of, 95: 78
Grommet
titanium, in flexible implant
arthroplasty of radiocarpal joint,
97: 289
Growth
factor
epidermal, role in Dupuytren's
contracture, 96: 381
modulation of formation of molded
vascularized bone graft in vivo (in
rat), 96: 382
transforming growth factor-β, role in
Dupuytren's contracture, 96: 381

of upper extremities, straight-line
graphs for prediction of, 95: 301
GUEPAR total trapezometacarpal
prosthesis
for carpometacarpal arthritis of thumb,
95: 258
Gunshot wound
low-velocity, of brachial plexus,
96: 121
Guyon's canal
ulnar nerve and ulnar artery variations
in, 96: 24
Gymnast
male, grip lock injuries to forearm in,
97: 332
wrist
in athletes, adolescent, 96: 225
in females, 96: 223

H

Hall-effect displacement transducer
for radioulnar ligament motion during
supination and pronation, distal,
95: 211
Halsted
peripheral suture technique, modified,
mechanical analysis of (in rabbit),
96: 378
tendon repair, in vitro strength of,
97: 12
Hamate
hook position in Agee endoscopic
carpal tunnel release, technique for
estimating, 96: 168
Hand
amputation for soft tissue sarcoma,
96: 293
amputation in, somatosensory system
responsiveness after, 96: 126
angioleiomyomas of, 97: 301
anomalies
congenital, classification of, position
of symbrachydactyly in, 96: 317
congenital, toe phalangeal grafts in,
95: 294
transplants of phalanges of foot for,
free, 97: 345
-arm vibration
platers and truck assemblers exposed
to, impaired nerve conduction in
carpal tunnel of, 96: 264
syndrome, sensorineural objective
tests in, 95: 236
bones of, sesamoid, pathology of, 96: 1
burns (see under Burns)

carcinoma, recurrent squamous cell, in immunosuppressed patients, treatment, 96: 294
cerebral palsied, Botulinum A chemodenervation of, 95: 229
circulation to, collateral, noninvasive evaluation of, 96: 37
club, radial, 95: 299
  acquired, due to osteomyelitis, 96: 62
deformities (see Hand, anomalies above)
dermatitis, occupational, in metalworkers, prognosis of, 97: 340
diagrams, workplace surveillance for carpal tunnel syndrome using, 96: 138
dorsum
  defects, requiring free flaps, primary extensor tendon reconstruction in, 95: 96
  extravasation of antiblastic drugs at, treatment of, 95: 279, 280
  reconstruction of, immediate vs. staged, 97: 80
  skin-tendon defect of, tendinocutaneous free flap transfer for, 96: 74
dystonia, focal (see Dystonia, focal, hand)
edema, chronic, after burn injury, effect of mechanical compression on, 96: 79
epiphysis in, double, 95: 295
exposure characteristics in relation to symptoms among automobile assembly line workers, 97: 272
foreign bodies in, sensitivity and specificity of ultrasound in diagnosis of, 97: 26
fracture
  avulsion, tension band fixation of, clinical results, 96: 48
  open, recovery of active motion and of complications, 95: 50
function
  evaluation, finger dynamography in, 95: 230
  restoration in spinal cord injury, tendon transfers and functional electrical stimulation for, 97: 245
  test, Sollerman, 97: 250
  tests, surgeon's selection of, 95: 34
  web space contracture and, first, 95: 5
glove splint for attachment of dynamic components, 96: 338
grasp neuroprosthesis, closed-loop, automated tuning of, 95: 310

happy, of Schoenberg, 95: 310
-held tools, vibration from, carpal tunnel release in patients exposed to, 95: 235
injuries
  compression, morbidity of pedicled groin flap for, 95: 78
  degloving, 96: 347
  left-hand dominance and, 97: 22
  nerve, somatosensory system responsiveness after, 96: 126
  physeal and periphyseal, 95: 67
  radiation-induced, surgical treatment of, 95: 81
  reconstruction of, serratus anterior free-muscle transplant for, 95: 319
  repair of, primary, posterior interosseous flap in, 95: 82
  rolling belt, in children, 96: 83
ischemia after radial artery cannulation, 97: 353
left, dominance, and hand trauma, 97: 22
muscle(s)
  biomechanical alterations after carpal tunnel release, 97: 14
  hyperplasia of, congenital unilateral, with ulnar deviation of fingers, 96: 321
  strength and fatigability, effect of short-term immobilization on, 96: 20
musculoskeletal symptoms among automobile assembly line workers, and self-reported physical exposure, 97: 328
mutilations, second toe-to-finger transfer in, 96: 344
mycetoma, case report and review of, 96: 307
nubbin-digits, pathomorphology and treatment of, 95: 303
Otto Bock System Electric, comparison with voluntary-opening split hook, 96: 323, 324
problems, performance-related, in music students, 97: 331
radiographs in rheumatoid arthritis, quantitative analysis of, 97: 294
reflex sympathetic dystrophy, microvascular response patterns associated with, 95: 27
rehabilitation, compliance with, 96: 331
representation in cortex, remodeling determined by timing of tactile stimulation, 97: 18
sarcoma

soft tissue, treatment, 96: 292
therapy, combined modality, 96: 297
sensibility
  establishment of reliability in
    evaluation of, 95: 17
  restoration after complete brachial
    plexus injury, 97: 103
shoulder-hand syndrome in cervical
  spinal cord injury, 96: 256
skin defects, venous flaps for covering,
  96: 341
surgery
  anesthesia for, intraarterial regional,
    radial vs. brachial artery injections
    for, 96: 42
  bone suture anchors in, 96: 47
  elective, in breast cancer patient with
    prior ipsilateral axillary dissection,
    96: 295
  for epidermolysis bullosa, anesthesia
    for, 97: 35
  pediatric, decision making by parents
    and children in, 96: 315
  radius bone graft in, distal anterior,
    97: 59
  x-rays during, risk of radiation
    exposure from, 96: 336
  toe-to-hand transplantation, pulp plasty
    after, 97: 77
  vibration damaged, neurophysiological
    investigation of, 95: 239
  vibration energy absorption in, 95: 322
Happy hand
  of Schoenberg, 95: 310
Healing
  of articular disk of wrist (in dog),
    95: 209
  tendon, application of forces to, 95: 92
Health
  beliefs and compliance with hand
    rehabilitation, 96: 331
Heat
  injury, effectiveness of surface cooling in
    reducing, 95: 335
  recordings at tips of Kirschner wires
    during drilling through phalanges,
    96: 383
Hematogenous
  infection, deep, after lateral approach
    for non-constrained elbow
    replacement, 97: 237
Hematoma
  subcutaneous, after anterior
    submuscular transposition of ulnar
    nerve for cubital tunnel syndrome,
    97: 147

Hemiepiphyseal
  osteotomy at distal ulna for traumatic
    avulsion of triangular fibrocartilage
    complex at its ulnar insertion,
    97: 222
  stapling of distal radius in children with
    multiple hereditary
    osteochondromata, 95: 289
Hemiplegia
  spastic, functional outcome of upper
    limb tendon transfer for, in
    children, 95: 231
Hemodialysis
  vascular access for, upper extremity,
    neurologic and ischemic
    complications of, 96: 362
Herbert screw
  fixation
    of radius head fracture, late results,
      97: 231
    of scaphoid fracture, acute stable, in
      athlete, 97: 172
    of scaphoid fracture, midthird, in
      athlete, 96: 200
  for scaphoid injuries, dorsal approach,
    95: 62
  vs. tension-band wire in distal
    interphalangeal joint arthrodesis,
    97: 60
Herbert-Whipple screw
  cannulated, in radius head fracture,
    97: 232
Hinged device
  for fractures of proximal
    interphalangeal joint, 97: 64
Histiocytoma
  of hand, malignant fibrous, treatment,
    96: 293
Histologic
  anatomy of scapholunate interosseous
    ligament, 97: 158
  study of nerve endings in nail bed and
    matrix, 97: 5
Histopathologic
  findings in tennis elbow, correlation
    with MRI and surgical findings,
    97: 270
HLAs
  reflex sympathetic dystrophy and,
    96: 357
  in wrist tenosynovitis and humeral
    epicondylitis, 97: 293
Holmium: YAG
  laser tenolysis in flexor tendon (in
    rabbit), 97: 374
Holt-Oram syndrome
  hypoplastic thumb and, 97: 315

Hominid
  tool use, early, fossil evidence for, 96: 30
Hook
  split, voluntary-opening, comparison of three myoelectrically controlled prehensors and, 96: 323
Hori revascularization technique
  in Kienböck's disease, early stage 3, 96: 201
Hosmer NU-VA Synergetic Prehensor
  comparison with voluntary-opening split hook, 96: 324, 325
Hueston flap
  for fingertip skin loss, 95: 75
Hui-Linscheid ligamentoplasty
  stabilization of distal radioulnar joint by, 97: 227
Humerus
  epicondylitis, rheumatoid factor and HLA antigens in, 97: 293
  fracture (see Fracture, humerus)
Hyperesthesia
  after bipedicle digital advancement island flaps, 96: 78
  after carpal tunnel release, two-portal endoscopic, 96: 164
Hyperextension
  injuries of metacarpophalangeal joint of thumb, 96: 51
  of thumb metacarpophalangeal joint, sesamoid arthrodesis for, 96: 53
Hyperinnervation
  motor, of whisker-pad muscles, permanent, after hypoglossal-facial anastomosis (in rat), 95: 327
Hypermobility
  joint, among musicians, benefits and disadvantages of, 95: 307
Hyperplasia
  muscle, congenital unilateral, with ulnar deviation of fingers, 96: 321
  synovial, in carpal tunnel syndrome, 96: 127
Hypertrophic
  scarring after triradiate incision for dorsal approach to wrist, 97: 149
Hyphecan
  for fingertip injuries, 96: 73
Hypoglossal
  -facial anastomosis, permanent motor hyperinnervation of whisker-pad muscles after (in rat), 95: 327
Hypoplasia
  digital, congenital, toe phalangeal grafts in, 95: 295
  thumb

Bauth type III, transposition of third metatarsus for reconstruction of, 97: 317
  patient characteristics, 97: 315
Hypoxia
  chronic, in carpal tunnel syndrome, 95: 136

I

Ibuprofen
  in carpal tunnel syndrome, early mild, 95: 132
Imaging
  bone
    day 4, accuracy in diagnosing scaphoid fracture, 97: 175
    of ganglia of wrist, intraosseous, 96: 300
    in reflex sympathetic dystrophy diagnosis, 97: 355
    of scaphoid fracture, suspected, 96: 196; 95: 193
    technetium, for microvascular response associated with reflex sympathetic dystrophy of hand and wrist, 95: 27
    three-phase, in reflex sympathetic dystrophy, 95: 28
    three-phase, in reflex sympathetic dystrophy, segmental, 95: 30
  Doppler, laser, of finger skin blood flow after microvascular repair of ulnar artery at wrist, 96: 364
  magnetic resonance (see Magnetic resonance imaging)
Immobilization
  cast, for Colles' fracture, ulnar wrist pain after, 95: 195
  plaster bandage, after closed reduction of volar dislocation of distal radioulnar joint, 96: 233
  plaster (see Cast, plaster)
  short-term, effect on strength and fatigability of hand muscle, 96: 20
  splint (see Splint)
Immunofluorescence
  microscopic study of flexor retinaculum in carpal tunnel syndrome, 97: 140
Immunosuppressed patients
  carcinoma of hand in, recurrent squamous cell, treatment of, 96: 294
Implant
  arthroplasty
    flexible, of radiocarpal joint, titanium grommet in, 97: 289

Subject Index / 419

flexible resection, of proximal
  interphalangeal joint, in systemic
  inflammatory arthritis, 96: 274
interphalangeal joint, proximal,
  lateral stability of, 96: 368
Silastic, of carpal scaphoid, 96: 200
Ashworth-Blatt type, for posttraumatic
  degenerative arthritis of
  carpometacarpal joint of small
  finger, 96: 290
finger joint, Swanson silicone, long-term
  complications of, 97: 287
Meuli wrist prosthesis III, correctly
  implanted, 96: 288
Silastic (see Silastic, implant)
silicone (see under Silicone)
temporary ectopic, for salvage of
  amputated digits, 97: 67
Incision
  double incision open technique for
    carpal tunnel release, 96: 162
  triradiate, for dorsal approach to wrist,
    97: 149
  twin, in open carpal tunnel release,
    95: 121
Index finger (see Finger, index)
Industry
  newspaper, acute surveillance for
    control of cumulative trauma
    disorders in, 95: 245
  setting, carpal tunnel syndrome
    screening in, vibrometry testing vs.
    sensory nerve conduction measures
    in, 96: 338
  workers
    carpal tunnel syndrome in, current
      perception threshold testing as
      screening procedure for, 96: 260
    Japanese vs. American, slowing of
      sensory conduction of median
      nerve and carpal tunnel syndrome
      in, 95: 242
    median sensory distal amplitude and
      latency in, 95: 250
Infant
  brachial plexopathy in, after traumatic
    delivery, MRI of, 95: 224
  with brachial plexus birth palsy,
    accessory nerve neurotization in,
    96: 250
  fibrous proliferations in, 97: 300
Infantile
  camptodactyly, isolated, results of
    nonoperative treatment, 96: 314
  digital fibromas, 97: 299

Infection
  from bite wound, clench-fist human, in
    area of metacarpophalangeal joints,
    treatment of, 97: 54
  hematogenous, deep, after lateral
    approach for non-constrained
    elbow replacement, 97: 237
  from K wire after free transplants of
    phalanges of foot in hand
    deformities, 97: 345
  palmar space, treatment and results,
    96: 308
  after trapezio-lunate external fixation
    for scaphoid fractures, 96: 199
  after wrist arthrodesis, AO/ASIF,
    96: 194
Inflammation
  in carpal tunnel syndrome, 96: 127
Inflammatory
  arthritis, systemic, flexible implant
    resection arthroplasty of proximal
    interphalangeal joint in, 96: 274
  response to silicone elastomer
    particulate debris (in rat), 97: 375
Infrared
  thermometry in reflex sympathetic
    dystrophy, 96: 356
Injection
  injuries, high-pressure, morbidity of
    pedicled groin flap for, 95: 78
  site for Bier's block, change of, 97: 34
Injuries
  (See also Trauma)
  arterial, in open arm fractures, in
    children, 97: 322
  brachial plexus (see Brachial plexus,
    injuries)
  carpal ligament, avulsion fracture of
    volar aspect of triquetral bone as
    sign of, 97: 187
  degloving, of hand and fingers, 96: 347
  digital nerve (see Digital, nerve, injuries)
  fingertip
    flap for, reversed digital artery island,
      95: 71
    treatment for, simple and efficient,
      96: 73
  flexor tendon
    in children, 96: 85
    in zone I, ultrasound in management
      of, 95: 88
  grip lock, to forearm, in male gymnasts,
    97: 332
  heat, effectiveness of surface cooling in
    reducing, 95: 335
  hyperextension, of metacarpophalangeal
    joint of thumb, 96: 51

injection, high-pressure, morbidity of pedicled groin flap for, 95: 78
intercarpal ligament, arthroscopic categorization of, 95: 157
isolated, to dorsoradial capsule of thumb metacarpophalangeal joint, 97: 51
lunotriquetral, partial, of wrist, arthroscopic management of, 97: 170
mallet finger, impact of compliance on rehabilitation, 95: 98
median nerve, measuring outcome in, 95: 23
nerve, in open arm fractures, in children, 97: 322
penetrating, of brachial artery, 96: 345
peripheral nerve
  cell loss in sensory ganglia after (in cat), 96: 384
  consequences of, paradoxical clinical, 97: 112
radiation-induced, of hand, surgical treatment of, 95: 81
ring avulsion, microsurgical management of, 97: 346
scaphoid, internal fixation with Herbert screw through dorsal approach, 95: 62
scapholunate, partial, of wrist, arthroscopic management of, 97: 170
scapho-trapezio-trapezoid ligament, isolated, diagnosis and treatment, 95: 192
spinal cord
  cervical, shoulder-hand syndrome in, 96: 256
  hand function restoration after, tendon transfers and functional electrical stimulation for, 97: 245
spinal nerve root, in brachial plexus lesions, 96: 252
strain, repetitive, of tendinitis and focal hand dystonia, sensory dysfunction associated with, 97: 272
ulnar collateral ligament
  sonography of, 96: 35
  of thumb metacarpophalangeal joint, 95: 41
ulnar nerve, secondary microsurgical repair results, 95: 114
wrist (see Wrist, injuries)
zone of, liability of recipient vessels distal to, when used for extremity free flaps, 97: 351

Innervated flap
  radial thenar, for sensory reconstruction of fingers, 97: 112
Innervation
  density of lumbrical muscles, 95: 13
  of nail bed and matrix, anatomical study of, 97: 5
  of wrist joint, anatomic study of, 95: 174
Inside Job device
  in endoscopic carpal tunnel release, 95: 152
Instron testing
  in injuries of ulnar collateral ligament of thumb metacarpophalangeal joint, 95: 41
Instrumentalists
  treatment outcome in, 97: 330
Intercarpal
  ligament injuries, arthroscopic categorization of, 95: 157
Intercostal
  cutaneous perforator flap, narrow pedicled, for burned hand coverage, 95: 314
  nerve
    in restoration of hand sensibility after complete brachial plexus injury, 97: 103
    transfer, elbow flexion restoration with, 96: 122
Interosseous
  arteries, forearm, clinical anatomy of, 96: 21
  flap, posterior
    in hand injury repair, primary, 95: 82
    reverse forearm, 95: 77
  ligament of wrist, scapholunate, MR appearances, 96: 205
  membrane, role in forearm stability, 95: 333
  muscles
    first dorsal, effect of short-term immobilization on strength and fatigability of, 96: 20
    normal arborization of deep branch of ulnar nerve into, 96: 27
  nerve
    anterior, latency in diagnosis of severe carpal tunnel syndrome, 96: 338
    anterior, palsy, spontaneous, with hourglass-like fascicular constriction within main trunk of median nerve, 97: 143
    posterior, as graft source, 95: 8
    posterior, relation to extensor carpi radialis brevis muscle, 96: 16, 246

Interphalangeal joint
  distal
    arthrodesis, tension-band wire vs.
      Herbert screw in, 97: 60
    cysts of, mucous, 96: 269
    fibroma in, infantile, 97: 299
    ganglions of, treatment of fingernail
      deformities secondary to, 97: 294
  proximal
    arthroplasty (see Arthroplasty,
      interphalangeal joint, proximal)
    capsular tissues of, 95: 9
    contracture, collateral ligament
      excision for, total, 95: 67
    fibroma in, infantile, 97: 299
    flexed, in Dupuytren's disease,
      skeletal traction for, 96: 301
    fracture, hinged device for, 97: 64
    fracture-dislocation (see Fracture,
      -dislocation, interphalangeal joint,
      proximal)
    replacement, lateral stability of,
      96: 368
  thumb
    arthrodesis, in spinal cord injury,
      97: 245
    axes of rotation of, 97: 6
Interposition
  of nerve tissue for peripheral nerve
    defects, vein conduits with,
    96: 123
Intestinal
  malformations and thumb duplication,
    97: 316
Intraarterial
  regional anesthesia for hand surgery,
    radial vs. brachial artery injections
    for, 96: 42
Intraarticular
  fracture
    comminuted, pins and rubbers
      traction system for, 95: 51
    radius, distal (see Fracture, radius,
      distal, intraarticular)
    malunion, distal radial, radiolunate
      arthrodesis for, 97: 173
Intracarpal
  canal pressure recordings, serial
    overnight, in carpal tunnel
    syndrome, 95: 138
  soft tissue lesions with intra-articular
    fractures of distal radius, 97: 204
Intramedullary
  nailing, flexible, for metacarpal
    fractures, 97: 45
  osteosynthesis of displaced fracture of
    distal fifth metacarpal, 95: 68

Intramuscular
  electrodes, percutaneous, reliability for
    upper extremity functional
    neuromuscular stimulation in
    adolescents with C5 tetraplegia,
    96: 256
Intraneural
  topography of ulnar nerve in cubital
    tunnel facilitates anterior
    transposition, 96: 29
  ulnar nerve pressure changes related to
    operative techniques for cubital
    tunnel decompression, 96: 161
Intraosseous
  ganglia of wrist, 96: 299
Intrinsic
  transfer, crossed, for rheumatoid
    metacarpophalangeal joint, motion
    after, 95: 266
Iontophoresis
  in carpal tunnel syndrome, early mild,
    95: 132
Irradiation (see Radiation)
Irrigation
  local, with clindamycin, for palmar
    space infections, 96: 308
Ischemia
  decrease after ex vivo perfusion with
    anticoagulated blood (in rat),
    95: 338
  hand, after radial artery cannulation,
    97: 353
Ischemic
  complications of upper extremity
    vascular access for dialysis,
    96: 362
  contracture, Volkmann's, free muscle
    transfer in, 95: 311
    follow-up studies, 95: 312
Iselin procedure
  for recent fractures of first metacarpal
    base, 96: 54
Itraconazole
  for mycetoma of hand, 96: 308
  in mycoses, cutaneous and ungual,
    97: 69
  pulse therapy for onychomycosis,
    97: 70

J

Jamar dynamometer
  consistency of sincere and feigned grip
    exertions with repeated testing,
    95: 24
  for hand function assessment, 95: 34
  sensitivity in detecting submaximal grip
    effort, 97: 263

Japanese
  industrial workers, slowing of sensory
    conduction of median nerve and
    carpal tunnel syndrome in, 95: 242
Jebsen Hand Function Test, 95: 34
Job
  modification
    for carpal tunnel syndrome in
      primary care, 95: 135
    for cubital tunnel syndrome, 95: 140
Joint
  basal (see Basal, joint)
  carpometacarpal (see Carpometacarpal
    joint)
  finger (see Finger, joint)
  hypermobility among musicians,
    benefits and disadvantages of,
    95: 307
  interphalangeal (see Interphalangeal
    joint)
  laxity, influence on scaphoid kinematics,
    97: 160
  metacarpophalangeal (see
    Metacarpophalangeal joint)
  motion, limited, in diabetics, 96: 303
  movement, full range, carpal bone
    kinematics and ligament
    lengthening during, 95: 170
  radiocarpal, flexible implant
    arthroplasty, titanium grommet in,
    97: 289
  radioulnar (see Radioulnar, joint)
  tendon transposition across two joints
    in brachial nerve injuries, 95: 108
  thumb (see Thumb, joint)
  trapeziometacarpal (see
    Trapeziometacarpal)
  wrist (see Wrist, joint)
Juvenile (see Children)

K

Kapandji fixation
  of radius fracture, distal, 97: 196
Kapandji procedure
  for Madelung's deformity, 95: 299
  for post-traumatic problems of distal
    radioulnar joint, 95: 204
Kelikian operation
  for thumb duplication, 97: 316
Kessler suture
  modified
    in extensor zone IV, biomechanical
      characteristics of, 97: 93
    in flexor tendon repair, evaluation of,
      97: 95
  technique

core stitch, mechanical analysis of (in
  rabbit), 96: 378
for flexor tendon repair, in vitro
  biomechanical analysis of, 95: 331
modified, mechanical analysis of (in
  rabbit), 96: 378
two-strand, in tendon repair, work of
  flexion after, 97: 372
Kessler tenorrhaphy
  modified, vs. augmented Becker,
    dynamic mechanical analysis (in
    monkey), 96: 98
Kessler-Mason-Allen suture
  modified, for flexor tendon injuries, in
    children, 96: 85
Key
  pinch, single-stage reconstruction in
    tetraplegics, 96: 254
Keyboard
  computer
    operators, risk of upper limb soft
      tissue disorders in, 96: 258
    use, measurement of creep strain of
      flexor tendons during, 96: 19
  work, alphanumeric, investigation of
    applied forces in, 95: 254
Kidney
  transplantation, treatment of recurrent
    squamous cell carcinoma of hand
    after, 96: 294
Kienböck's disease
  advanced
    carpectomy in, proximal row,
      96: 204
    lunate excision in, simple, 96: 205
  arthrodesis in
    radiolunate, 95: 192
    scaphocapitate, 97: 182
  carpectomy in, proximal row, long-term
    results, 96: 203
  early stage 3, treatment of, 96: 201
  fusion in (see arthrodesis in above)
  lunate decompression for, preoperative
    factors and outcome after, 95: 180
  osteotomy for, radial
    carpal alignment changes after,
      95: 181
    wedge, biomechanical analysis of,
      95: 182
  pisiform transposition in, pedicled,
    95: 177
  treatment, Graner's technique, 95: 178
  ulnar lengthening and radial recession
    procedures for, long-term
    follow-up, 97: 180
Killian nasal speculum
  lighted, for direct vision in carpal tunnel
    release, 96: 172

Kinematics
  carpal bone, during full range of joint
    movement, 95: 170
  of collateral ligament of elbow joint,
    lateral, 97: 16
  of radioulnar joint, distal, in
    rheumatoid arthritis, 97: 19
  scaphoid
    influence of joint laxity on, 97: 160
    role of scaphoid-trapezio-trapezoid
      ligament complex on, 96: 207
  wrist
    during pitching, 97: 157
    in tennis players performing
      backhand stroke, 96: 334
Kirner's deformity
  case report and review of literature,
    96: 321
Kirschner wire(s)
  fixation
    of metacarpal fracture, airbag-related,
      96: 68
    of metacarpal fractures, oblique,
      97: 47
    multiple, of distal unicondylar
      fractures of proximal phalanx,
      95: 47
    percutaneous, through snuff box,
      96: 186
    of radius fracture, distal, comparative
      study, 97: 198
    of scaphoid nonunion after
      implantation of vascular bundle
      and bone grafting, 97: 176
  heat recordings at tips during drilling
    through phalanges, 96: 383
  in humerus fractures, supracondylar, in
    children, 95: 220
  infection from, after free transplants of
    phalanges of foot in hand
    deformities, 97: 345
  in mallet finger, 95: 98
  percutaneous
    in interphalangeal joint
      fracture-dislocation, proximal,
      dorsal fracture, 95: 45
    in radial fractures, distal, isolated, in
      children, 95: 202
    in radial fractures, distal, severely
      displaced, in children, 97: 322
    in radioulnar joint dislocation, volar
      distal, 96: 233
  in pins and rubbers traction system for
    comminuted intraarticular fractures
    and fracture-dislocations in hand,
    95: 51
  placement in emergency room, 97: 65

Kleinert finger flexor pulley reconstruction
  after closed traumatic rupture, 96: 98
Kleinert splint
  activity of extrinsic finger flexors during
    mobilization in, 97: 91
Klumpke's birth palsy
  discussion of, 96: 249
Knife
  wounds causing penetrating brachial
    artery injuries, 96: 345
Knots
  suture, effect on tensile strength of
    repaired flexor tendons (in dog),
    96: 115
K-wire (see Kirschner wire)

L

Laboratory
  findings in reflex sympathetic dystrophy,
    96: 356
Laborers
  heavy, carpal malalignment after
    intra-articular fractures of distal
    radius in, 96: 220
Lacerations
  extensor tendon, zones III and IV, early
    controlled motion with dynamic
    splinting vs. static splinting for,
    96: 107
  flap for, pedicled groin, morbidity of,
    95: 78
Lag
  screw
    fixation of oblique metacarpal
      fractures, 97: 47
    in precision oblique osteotomy for
      shortening of ulna, 95: 174
Lamisil
  efficacy and tolerability of, 97: 68
Laparotomy
  after brachial artery injuries,
    penetrating, 96: 345
Laser
  Doppler
    flowmetry (see Doppler, flowmetry,
      laser)
    imaging of finger skin blood flow
      after microvascular repair of ulnar
      artery at wrist, 96: 364
  tenolysis in flexor tendon (in rabbit),
    97: 374
Latency
  distal, comparisons in carpal tunnel
    syndrome, and age, 96: 134
  sensory (see Sensory, latency)

Latissimus dorsi
  muscle transfer in Volkmann's
    contracture, 95: 311
  musculocutaneous flap without muscle,
    97: 81
  translocation, secondary, after brachial
    plexus injuries, 96: 251
Lee 4-strand suture method
  for flexor tendon repair, in vitro
    biomechanical analysis of, 95: 331
Left-hand dominance
  hand trauma and, 97: 22
Legal
  implications of Silastic foam dressings
    for children's hand burns, 95: 81
Leiomyosarcoma
  hand, treatment, 96: 293
Lengthening
  (See also Elongation)
  distraction, preoperative, for radial
    longitudinal deficiency, 97: 326
  phalanx, for shortened fingers after
    trauma, 95: 67
  radius, progressive, in post-traumatic
    epiphysiodesis of distal end of
    radius, 97: 324
  ulna
    in Kienböck's disease, long-term
      follow-up, 97: 180
    in osteochondromata, multiple
      hereditary, in children, 95: 289
Lidocaine
  /dexamethasone in early, mild carpal
    tunnel syndrome, 95: 132
  injections
    radial vs. brachial artery, for
      intraarterial regional anesthesia for
      hand surgery, 96: 42
    in writer's cramp, 97: 334
  in percutaneous release of trigger finger,
    95: 101
  /steroid injection in De Quervain's
    disease, 96: 273
Lifestyle
  correlates of carpal tunnel syndrome,
    96: 159
Ligament(s)
  autograft from foot for reconstruction
    of scapholunate interosseous
    ligament, 97: 164
  carpal (see Carpal, ligament)
  collateral (see Collateral ligament)
  dorsal, of triangular fibrocartilage
    complex, reconstruction of,
    96: 231
  intercarpal, injuries, arthroscopic
    categorization of, 95: 157
  lunotriquetral (see Lunotriquetral,
    ligament)
  radiolunate
    MRI of, 95: 168
    tensions in, 95: 173
  radiolunotriquetral, MRI of, 95: 168
  radioulnar, distal, motion during
    supination and pronation, 95: 211
  reconstruction
    for basal joint arthritis, 97: 281
    for basal joint arthrosis, radiographic
      assessment of trapezial space before
      and after, 97: 280
    -tendon interposition arthroplasty of
      basal joint of thumb, 96: 282
    -tendon interposition for
      osteoarthritis of thumb base,
      96: 285
    for thumb base osteoarthrosis,
      95: 257
  replacement for chronic instability of
    ulnar collateral ligament of
    metacarpophalangeal joint of
    thumb, 95: 68
  retinacular, oblique, of index finger,
    anatomy of, 95: 16
  scapholunate (see Scapholunate,
    ligament)
  scapho-trapezio-trapezoid
    complex, role on scaphoid
      kinematics, 96: 207
    injury of, isolated, diagnosis and
      treatment, 95: 192
  scaphotriquetral, palmar, 96: 177
    anatomy of, 95: 167
    tears or perforations, relevance in
      diagnosis of wrist pain, 96: 187
  triquetrolunate, rupture, longstanding,
    frayed ulnotriquetral and
    ulnolunate ligaments as
    arthroscopic sign of, 96: 206
  triquetroscaphoid, MRI of, 95: 168
  ulnolunate (see Ulnolunate, ligament)
  ulnotriquetral
    frayed, as arthroscopic sign of
      longstanding triquetrolunate
      ligament rupture, 96: 206
    MRI of, 95: 168
  wrist (see Wrist, ligaments)
Ligamentoplasty
  Hui-Linscheid, stabilization of distal
    radioulnar joint by, 97: 227
Lighted Killian nasal speculum
  for direct vision in carpal tunnel release,
    96: 172

Limb (see Extremity)
Littler technique
  for raising heterodigital neurovascular island flap in thumb reconstruction, 96: 69
Living
  daily, activities of, for hand function assessment, 95: 34
Lloyd-Roberts and Bucknill technique
  for treatment of chronic post-traumatic dislocation of radial head, in children, 95: 57
Load
  crush, magnitude and duration, effect on functional recovery of peripheral nerve (in rat), 95: 110
Loading
  tensile, cyclic and static, effect on water content and solute diffusion in flexor tendons (in dog), 96: 372
Loupe
  magnification in free tissue transfer, 96: 339
Low-effort patients
  identification through dynamometry, 97: 22
Lumbrical
  muscle(s)
    arborization of deep branch of ulnar nerve into, normal, 96: 27
    construction of, functional, 95: 13
    incursion into carpal tunnel during finger flexion, 96: 17
    incursion within carpal tunnel, effect on carpal tunnel pressure, 96: 155
Lunate
  aseptic necrosis, vascular bundle implantation into bone for, 97: 179
  decompression for Kienböck's disease, preoperative factors and outcome after, 95: 180
  excision, simple, in advanced Kienböck's disease, 96: 205
  height reconstruction and core revascularization in early stage 3 Kienböck's disease, 96: 201
  implants, Silastic, 95: 193
  morphology, prediction with routine x-rays, 96: 5
  prosthesis, failed, long-term results of proximal row carpectomy for, 96: 203
Lundborg vibrogram, 95: 240
Lunotriquetral
  injuries of wrist, partial, arthroscopic management of, 97: 170
  ligament

defects, incomplete, on wrist arthrography, lack of correlation between site of wrist pain and, 95: 162
MRI of, 95: 174
tears, evaluation by arthrography, arthroscopy, and arthrotomy, 95: 161
test in wrist pain evaluation, 96: 181
Lupus
  erythematosus, systemic, flexible implant resection arthroplasty of proximal interphalangeal joint in, 96: 275
Luxation (see Dislocation)
Lymphadenopathy
  after Swanson silicone finger joint implants, 97: 287
Lymphoma
  non-Hodgkin's, due to Swanson silicone finger joint implants, 97: 287

M

Machine
  operators, risk of upper limb soft tissue disorders in, 96: 258
  sewing, persistent neck and upper limb pain in operators of, 95: 241
Macroscopic
  study of flexor synovial sheath anatomy of little finger, 97: 19
Madelung deformity
  new therapeutic approach to, 95: 298
  surgical technique, 95: 296
Magnetic resonance imaging
  of biceps tendon rupture, 95: 104
  of brachial plexopathy in infant after traumatic delivery, 95: 224
  of brachial plexus injury, 95: 226
  of carpal ligaments, volar, 95: 168
  in carpal tunnel syndrome
    correlation with clinical, electrodiagnostic, and intraoperative findings, 97: 139
    for median nerve circulation, 95: 135
    after myofascial manipulative release, 95: 129
  cinematography in diagnosis of triangular fibrocartilage complex lesions, 96: 233
  coronal 3D gradient-recalled-echo, normal appearance of triangular fibrocartilage complex on, 96: 12
  in de Quervain's tenosynovitis of wrist, 97: 265
  of flexor pulley rupture, traumatic, 96: 97

of flexor tendon rupture, 97: 97
  zone II, 97: 95
of gamekeeper thumb, 95: 42
of ganglia of wrist, intraosseous,
  96: 300
of lunotriquetral ligament, 95: 174
of radioulnar joint geometry, distal,
  96: 234
in reflex sympathetic dystrophy,
  96: 361
of scapholunate interosseous ligament
  of wrist, 96: 205
of scaphotriquetral ligament, 95: 167
of Stener lesion, 97: 37
of subungual glomus tumors, 96: 291
of tendon injury in finger, acute, 97: 29
in tennis elbow, correlation with
  surgical and histopathologic
  findings, 97: 270
of ulnar collateral ligament,
  preoperative, 95: 217
of wrist
  gymnast's, in adolescents, 96: 225
  ligaments, palmar, 96: 177
Magnification
  loupe, in free tissue transfer, 96: 339
Malformation (*see* Deformity)
Mallet
  finger
    injuries, impact of compliance on
      rehabilitation, 95: 98
    surgery for, reassessment, 95: 97
  fracture, avulsion, tension band fixation
    of, clinical results, 96: 48
Malunion
  Colles' fracture, 96: 227
  forearm fracture, operative treatment
    of, 97: 65
  metacarpal, correction osteotomy for,
    95: 55
  phalangeal, rotational and angular
    osteotomy for, 95: 55
  phalanges, post-traumatic, corrective
    osteotomy for, 97: 43
  radial intraarticular, distal, radiolunate
    arthrodesis for, 97: 173
  of radius fractures, distal, early *vs.* late
    reconstruction for, 97: 198
  of radius fractures, distal, sports-related,
    96: 222
Managerial employees
  median sensory distal amplitude and
    latency in, 95: 250
Mandible
  defects, osteocutaneous radial forearm
    flap for, and flap donor site deficits,
    95: 313

Martin-Gruber anastomosis, 95: 15
Matev continuous distraction
  in thumb reconstruction, 96: 60
Mattress suture
  in extensor zone IV, biomechanical
    characteristics of, 97: 93
Meat
  processing plant workers, wrist
    tenosynovitis and psychomotor
    capacity in, 95: 252
Mechanical
  analysis
    dynamic, of augmented Becker *vs.*
      modified Kessler tenorrhaphy (in
      monkey), 96: 98
    of palmar aponeuroses pulley, 97: 11
    of tendon suture techniques (in
      rabbit), 96: 378
  compression, effect on chronic hand
    edema after burn injury, 96: 79
Mechanostimulator
  computer-controlled, in assessing
    recovery after carpal tunnel release,
    95: 144
Median nerve
  circulation in carpal tunnel syndrome,
    MRI of, 95: 135
  compression after fractures of distal
    radius, incidence of, 96: 219
  decompression
    in carpal tunnel for palmar space
      infections, 96: 308
    endoscopic, in carpal tunnel, 96: 175
  defects, vein conduits with interposition
    of nerve tissue for, 96: 124
  displacement through carpal canal,
    96: 26
  impairment and wrist squareness,
    97: 134
  injuries, measuring outcome in, 95: 23
  lesion at wrist, benign and minor, value
    of special motor and sensory tests
    for diagnosis, 97: 147
  motion, restricted, in carpal tunnel
    syndrome, 97: 131
  neurolysis, internal, for recurrent carpal
    tunnel syndrome, 95: 124
  repair
    functional sensibility and cognitive
      capacities after, 96: 118
    tubular, in forearm, 96: 126
  sensory conduction, in Japanese *vs.*
    American industry, 95: 242
  sensory distal amplitude, 95: 250
  sensory latency (*see* Sensory, latency,
    median nerve)

transection, complete, combined with
complete ulnar nerve transection,
two-point discrimination tests *vs.*
functional sensory recovery in,
95: 117
trunk, main, hourglass-like fascicular
constriction in, spontaneous
anterior interosseous nerve palsy
with, 97: 143
/ulnar nerve in forearm,
communications between, 95: 15
Median neuropathy
acute, after wrist trauma, 95: 109
Medical
-legal implications of Silastic foam
dressings for children's hand burns,
95: 81
screening for upper extremity
cumulative trauma disorders in
office workers, 95: 244
Meissner's corpuscles
in nail bed and matrix, 97: 5
Membrane
interosseous, role in forearm stability,
95: 333
Mepivacaine
for digital anesthesia through flexor
tendon sheath at palmar level,
95: 33
in perivascular axillary nerve block,
effect of arm position on
effectiveness of, 96: 43
vs. butorphanol *vs.*
mepivacaine-butorphanol mixtures
in continuous brachial plexus
infusion for postoperative
analgesia, 97: 31
Mesh
reinforced sutures in tendon transfers,
early active mobilization after,
97: 108
sleeve technique of tendon repair, work
of flexion after, 97: 372
vein, silastic, and polyglycolic acid fine
mesh, comparative study, 97: 378
Mesovascularized
island flexor tendon, 95: 86
Metacarpal
artery flap, second dorsal
with double pivot points, 97: 83
neurovascular island, clinical
applications, 97: 86
base defect, finger dysplasia with,
treatment of, 96: 322
bones, elongation for treatment of
finger amputations, 96: 58
fifth, stabilized arthroplasty of, 96: 61

first, osteotomy, for osteoarthrosis of
basal joints of thumb, 97: 285
fracture (*see* Fracture, metacarpal)
head, parrot operation for extensive
bone loss of, 96: 59
osteotomy, extension, for
trapeziometacarpal osteoarthritis,
97: 277
synostosis, treatment of, 95: 290
Metacarpophalangeal joint
arthroplasty based on osseointegration
concept, 95: 264
bite wounds in area of, infected
clench-fist human, treatment of,
97: 54
little finger, radial subluxation of
connexus intertendineus at, in
musicians, treatment of, 95: 102
motion lag after AO/ASIF wrist
arthrodesis, 96: 194
reconstruction in rheumatoid disease,
motion after, 95: 266
region, dorsal gliding and functional
spaces in, 96: 31
thumb
artery of, 96: 22
axes of rotation of, 97: 6
collateral ligament of, ulnar,
arthroscopic treatment of acute
complete tears of, 97: 48
collateral ligament of, ulnar, ligament
replacement for chronic instability
of, 95: 68
dorsoradial capsule, isolated injuries
to, 97: 51
fracture, avulsion, tension wire
fixation of, 96: 49
fusion in Charcot-Marie-Tooth
disease, 97: 248
hyperextension, sesamoid arthrodesis
for, 96: 53
hyperextension injuries of, 96: 51
radial instability of, 96: 11
sesamoid bone in, arthritis of,
posttraumatic, 96: 1
sesamoid bone in, dislocation of,
96: 1
thumb duplication at, management and
new classification, 97: 318
Metal
prosthesis in radial head fracture,
95: 221
workers, prognosis of occupational
hand dermatitis in, 97: 340
Metatarsal
ligament autograft for reconstruction of
scapholunate interosseous ligament,
97: 165

Metatarsus
  third, transposition for reconstruction of Bauth type III hypoplastic thumb, 97: 317
Methylmethacrylate
  packing after curettage for giant cell tumors of radius, 95: 282
Meuli wrist prosthesis
  cementless, first experience with, 95: 273
  III implant, correctly implanted, 96: 288
Microangiopathy
  Dupuytren's disease and diabetes mellitus, 96: 303
Microscopy
  capillary, in reflex sympathetic dystrophy due to autonomic denervation, 96: 355
  electron, of flexor retinaculum in carpal tunnel syndrome, 97: 140
  immunofluorescence, of flexor retinaculum in carpal tunnel syndrome, 97: 140
Microsurgical
  management of ring avulsion injuries, 97: 346
  reconstruction of congenital adactylous hand, advances in, 96: 319
  repair, secondary
    of radial nerve, 95: 116
    of ulnar nerve injuries, results, 95: 114
Microvascular
  reconstruction of upper extremity with rectus abdominis muscle, 96: 340
  repair of ulnar artery at wrist, laser Doppler imaging of finger skin blood flow after, 96: 364
  response patterns associated with reflex sympathetic dystrophy of hand and wrist, 95: 27
  tissue transfers and smoking, 95: 320
  toe-to-hand transfer, pediatric, decision-making by parents and children in, 96: 315
Midcarpal
  arthrodesis, 97: 192
  instability, triquetrohamate arthrodesis for, 97: 169
Mineral
  phase of bone, skeletal repair by in situ formation of, 96: 365
Minicondylar
  plate in metacarpal and phalangeal fractures, 97: 65
Mini-image intensifier
  in hand fractures, open, 95: 51

Miniplate
  fixation, AO, of radius head fracture, late results, 97: 231
Miniscrew
  fixation
    AO, of radius head fracture, late results, 97: 231
    of phalanx fracture, proximal distal unicondylar, 95: 47
Minnesota Multiphasic Personality Inventory
  before direct electrical nerve stimulation for chronic peripheral nerve pain, 96: 358
Mitek
  bone anchor, in thumb ulnar collateral ligament ruptures, 97: 50
  suture anchors in distal biceps tendon repair, 97: 229
Mobilization
  active, early
    after flexor tendon repair with double loop locking suture, 97: 89
    after tendon transfers using mesh reinforced suture techniques, 97: 108
  in Kleinert splint, activity of extrinsic finger flexors during, 97: 91
  postoperative
    early, after carpal tunnel release, 96: 158
    early, after carpal tunnel release for recurrent carpal tunnel syndrome, 95: 124
  of flexor tendon repairs with "passive flexion-active extension" vs. "controlled active motion" techniques, 96: 102
Model
  Health Belief, as adapted for hand rehabilitation, 96: 332
  for student practice, flexor tendon repair in perfect safety, 96: 95
  working, for control of cumulative trauma disorders in newspaper industry, 95: 245
Modelling
  computer-assisted 3-dimensional, in osteotomy for radius deformity, 95: 197
Molecular
  factors in nosology of axial congenital deformities of upper limb, 95: 300
Monitor
  findings of digitalized conventional wrist x-rays, 96: 38

Subject Index / 429

Monitoring
  postoperative, of replantations, laser Doppler flowmetry vs. thermometry in, 96: 352
Monofilament
  thresholds, abnormal Semmes-Weinstein, in carpal tunnel syndrome, decision making in detecting, 96: 39
Monosodium
  urate particulate debris, inflammatory response to (in rat), 97: 375
Morbidity
  of pedicled groin flap, 95: 78
Morphological
  effects of aging on nerve regeneration (in rat), 97: 366
  study of autogenous flexor-tendon grafts (in dog), 95: 332
Morphology
  lunate, prediction with routine x-rays, 96: 5
Morphometric
  effects of aging on nerve regeneration (in rat), 97: 366
Morrey-Coonrad elbow
  in salvage of failed total elbow arthroplasty, 97: 236
Motion(s)
  active
    controlled, for mobilization after acute flexor tendon repair, effect on rupture rate, 96: 105
    controlled, for postoperative mobilization of flexor tendon repairs, 96: 102
    early, after flexor tendon repairs, 95: 93
    recovery after open hand fractures, 95: 50
    in tendon healing, 95: 92
  biomechanical, in high-profile vs. low-profile dynamic splinting, 96: 326
  controlled, early, with dynamic vs. static splinting for zones III and IV extensor tendon lacerations, 96: 107
  effect on digital nerve repair, 97: 363
  after flexor tenosynovectomy in rheumatoid arthritis, 95: 267
  index finger, effect of ulnar nerve lesion on, 97: 37
  median nerve, restricted, in carpal tunnel syndrome, 97: 131
  after metacarpophalangeal joint reconstruction in rheumatoid disease, 95: 266
  -preserving procedures for scapholunate advanced collapse wrist, 97: 186
  radioulnar ligament, distal, during supination and pronation, 95: 211
  range of
    after cubital tunnel surgery, 97: 145
    functional, of elbow, 96: 239
    short arc, early active, for repaired central slip, 96: 100
Motor
  collateral sprouting induced from intact peripheral nerve by end-to-side anastomosis (in rat), 96: 366
  hyperinnervation of whisker-pad muscles, permanent, after hypoglossal-facial anastomosis (in rat), 95: 327
  recovery after nerve grafting, technique to quantitate, 97: 112
  tests, special, value for diagnosis of benign and minor median nerve lesion at wrist, 97: 147
Mouse
  use
    cumulative trauma disorders of upper extremity and, 97: 260
    variation in upper limb posture and movement during word processing with, 96: 265
Movements
  index finger, coordination of, 95: 10
  repetitive, at work, relation to upper limb soft tissue disorders, 96: 258
  upper limb, variation during word processing with and without mouse use, 96: 265
MRI (see Magnetic resonance imaging)
Mucous
  cysts of distal interphalangeal joints, 96: 269
Muscle(s)
  adductor
    pollicis, Botulinum A chemodenervation in cerebral palsied hand, 95: 229
    thumb, force-generating capacity in parallel and perpendicular plane of adduction, 96: 31
  afferent block in writer's cramp, 97: 334
  biceps, technique for maximizing recovery in brachial plexus reconstruction, 95: 105
  extensor (see under Extensor)
  gracilis (see Gracilis, muscle)
  graft denaturating methods in nerve repair (in rat), 97: 365
  hand

biomechanical alterations after carpal tunnel release, 97: 14
hyperplasia of, congenital unilateral, with ulnar deviation of fingers, 96: 321
strength and fatigability, effect of short-term immobilization on, 96: 20
interosseous
arborization of deep branch of ulnar nerve into, normal, 96: 27
first dorsal, effect of short-term immobilization on strength and fatigability of, 96: 20
latissimus dorsi, transfer in Volkmann's contracture, 95: 311
lumbrical (see Lumbrical, muscle)
neuromuscular (see Neuromuscular)
overuse syndrome in music students, 97: 331
rectus abdominis, microvascular reconstruction of upper extremity with, 96: 340
serratus, transfer in Eve procedure, 97: 350
α-smooth muscle actin expression correlated with contraction in Dupuytren's disease fibroblasts, 97: 304
transfer
free, double, to restore prehension after complete brachial plexus avulsion, 97: 106
free, in Volkmann's ischemic contracture, 95: 311
free, in Volkmann's ischemic contracture, follow-up studies, 95: 312
free, serratus anterior, for reconstruction of injured hand, 95: 319
latissimus dorsi, in Volkmann's contracture, 95: 311
serratus, secondary, after brachial plexus injuries, 96: 251
transplantation, free functioning, for brachial plexus injury, 96: 253
whisker-pad, permanent motor hyperinnervation after hypoglossal-facial anastomosis (n rat), 95: 327
wrist, specialization, effect of tendon biomechanical properties on, 97: 9
Musculature
thumb, intrinsic and extrinsic, phasic relationships of, 97: 252

Musculocutaneous
flap, latissimus dorsi, without muscle, 97: 81
nerve, anastomosis of medial thoracic nerve to, functional recovery of elbow flexion by, 95: 117
Musculoskeletal
conditions, economic cost and social and psychological impact of, 97: 327
problems, generic, and carpal tunnel syndrome, 96: 159
symptoms
of forearm-hand among automobile assembly line workers, and self-reported physical exposure, 97: 328
in instrumentalists, treatment outcome, 97: 330
Musculotendinous
junction, traumatic rupture of extensor tendons at, 97: 101
Music
students, performance-related hand problems in, 97: 331
teachers, risk of upper limb soft tissue disorders in, 96: 258
Musicians
cramp
botulinum toxin in, 95: 308
occupational, and biomechanical abnormalities, 95: 306
dystonia in, focal, and biomechanical abnormalities, 95: 306
joint hypermobility among, benefits and disadvantages of, 95: 307
radial subluxation of connexus intertendineus at metacarpophalangeal joint of little finger in, treatment of, 95: 102
Mutilations
hand, second toe-to-finger transfer in, 96: 344
Mycetoma
hand, case report and review of, 96: 307
Mycoses
cutaneous and ungual, efficacy and tolerability of Lamisil in, 97: 68
Myoelectric
controlled prehensors, three, comparison with voluntary opening split hook, 96: 323
prosthesis, long-term follow-up, 95: 305
Myofascial
carpal tunnel release, 95: 129

Myxoid
 changes in carpal tunnel syndrome, 96: 127

N

Nail
 bed and matrix, anatomical study of innervation and vascular supply of, 97: 5
 deformities
  nontraumatic, classification and differential diagnosis of, 97: 87
  secondary to ganglions of distal interphalangeal joint, treatment of, 97: 294
 disorders, guidelines for care of, 97: 87
 flap, short-pedicle vascularized, 97: 71
 plasty for duplicated thumb, 95: 287
 prosthesis, osseointegrated, 97: 75
 toe, onychomycosis, antifungal pulse therapy for, 97: 70
Nailing
 intramedullary, flexible, for metacarpal fractures, 97: 45
Nasal
 speculum, lighted Killian, for direct vision in carpal tunnel release, 96: 172
Neck
 pain, persistent, in sewing machine operators, 95: 241
 soft tissue disorders, classification systems of, 97: 255
Necrobiosis
 of collagen in carpal tunnel syndrome, 96: 127
Necrosis
 aseptic, of lunate, vascular bundle implantation into bone for, 97: 179
 partial, in pedicled groin flap, 95: 78
 skin, after free transplants of phalanges of foot in hand deformities, 97: 345
Needle
 electromyography in carpal tunnel syndrome, relation to nerve conduction studies, 96: 137
 fasciotomy for Dupuytren's disease, 95: 284
 19-gauge, for percutaneous release of trigger finger, 96: 114
Neo-tendon
 generation using synthetic polymers seeded with tenocytes, 96: 374
Nerve
 accessory, neurotization in infants with brachial plexus birth palsy, 96: 250
 autograft, old degenerated and fresh, comparison of passage of regenerating axons through (in rat), 95: 325
 axillary, perivascular block, effect of arm position on effectiveness of, 96: 43
 compression
  acute, free radical damage in (in rat), 97: 369
  distal, effect on neural regeneration (in rat), 95: 321
  syndromes in instrumentalists, treatment outcomes, 97: 330
 conduction
  impaired, in carpal tunnel of platers and truck assemblers exposed to hand-arm vibration, 96: 264
  measurements at carpal tunnel, predictive value of, 95: 127
  measures, sensory, vs. vibrometry testing in screening for carpal tunnel syndrome in industrial setting, 96: 338
  studies in carpal tunnel syndrome, effect of provocative exercise maneuver on, 95: 255
  studies in carpal tunnel syndrome, in diagnosis, correlation with clinical signs, 96: 152
  studies in carpal tunnel syndrome, relation between needle electromyography and, 96: 137
  studies vs. digital electroneurometer for measurement of median nerve sensory latency, 95: 20
  velocity, digital, as sensitive indication of peripheral neuropathy in vibration syndrome, 96: 261
  velocity, mixed forearm, and retrograde changes in carpal tunnel syndrome, 96: 145
 digital (see Digital, nerve)
 endings in nail bed and matrix, histologic study of, 97: 5
 entrapment after fractures of distal radius, 96: 218
 fibers in angioleiomyomas of hand, 97: 301
 graft (see Graft, nerve)
 injuries
  in arm fractures, open, in children, 97: 322
  in hand, somatosensory responsiveness after, 96: 126
 intercostal

in restoration of hand sensibility after
  complete brachial plexus injury,
  97: 103
 transfer, elbow flexion restoration
  with, 96: 122
interosseous (see Interosseous, nerve)
median (see Median nerve)
musculocutaneous, anastomosis of
  medial thoracic nerve to, functional
  recovery of elbow flexion by,
  95: 117
peripheral (see Peripheral nerve)
phrenic, use in brachial plexus
  reconstruction, 97: 104
radial (see Radial, nerve)
reconnection, heterodigital
  neurovascular island flap in thumb
  reconstruction with and without,
  96: 69
regeneration (in rat)
 aging effects on, electrophysiological,
  morphological, and morphometric,
  97: 366
 effect of distal site of compression on,
  95: 321
 effect of inside-out vein graft on,
  95: 324
 selective, in aortic Y-chambers,
  95: 329
repair
 functional sensibility and cognitive
  capacities after, 96: 118
 muscle graft denaturating methods
  for (in rat), 97: 365
 relief of tension in, 95: 112
root
 avulsions, endoscopic diagnosis and
  possible treatment, in management
  of brachial plexus injuries (in goat),
  96: 121
 spinal (see Spinal, nerve root)
sensory, response in saphenous nerve on
  cutaneous electrical stimulation (in
  rat), 97: 378
spiral, formation in Dupuytren's
  contracture, 96: 305
stimulation, direct electrical, for chronic
  peripheral nerve pain, 96: 358
supply, original, recovery after
  hypoglossal-facial anastomosis,
  permanent motor hyperinnervation
  of whisker-pad muscles after (in
  rat), 95: 327
supraclavicular, in restoration of hand
  sensibility after complete brachial
  plexus injury, 97: 103

thoracic, medial, anastomosis to
  musculocutaneous nerve, functional
  recovery of elbow flexion by,
  95: 117
tissue, interposition and vein conduits
  for peripheral nerve defects,
  96: 123
ulnar (see Ulnar, nerve)
Neural
 gaps, enclosed, dispersion of
  regenerating axons across, 97: 361
Neuralgia
 cutaneous, medial antebrachial, after
  anterior submuscular transposition
  of ulnar nerve for cubital tunnel
  syndrome, 97: 147
Neuritis
 ulnar, at elbow, anterior subcutaneous
  ulnar nerve transfer for, in athlete,
  95: 141
Neuroanatomy
 in elbow arthroscopy, 97: 239
Neurocutaneous
 flap, retrograde-flow island, in forearm,
  96: 70
Neurofibromatosis
 desmoid tumor of ulna and, 97: 312
Neurologic
 complications of upper extremity
  vascular access for dialysis,
  96: 362
Neurolysis
 interfascicular, in spontaneous anterior
  interosseous nerve palsy with
  hourglass-like fascicular
  constriction within main trunk of
  median nerve, 97: 143
 internal, median nerve, for recurrent
  carpal tunnel syndrome, 95: 124
Neuroma
 upper extremity, subjective outcome
  after surgical management, 96: 125
Neurometer
 CPT device in screening for carpal
  tunnel syndrome in industrial
  workers, 96: 260
 electroneurometer for measures of
  median nerve sensory latency
  reliability of, 95: 19
  vs. standard nerve conduction studies,
  95: 20
Neuromuscular
 impairment after carpal tunnel release,
  97: 122
 stimulation, functional, in adolescents
  with tetraplegia

C5, reliability of percutaneous
  intramuscular electrodes for,
  96: 256
  grasp and release abilities after,
    97: 246
Neuropathy
  diabetic peripheral, and outcome of
    carpal tunnel release, 96: 131
  median, acute, after wrist trauma,
    95: 109
  peripheral, in vibration syndrome,
    digital nerve conduction velocity as
    sensitive indication of, 96: 261
  ulnar, after median sternotomy, 95: 142
Neurophysiological
  investigation of hands damaged by
    vibration, 95: 239
Neuroprosthesis
  closed-loop hand grasp, automated
    tuning of, 95: 310
Neurorrhaphy
  bilateral, innervated reverse digital
    artery flap through, for pulp
    defects, 95: 83
Neurotization
  accessory nerve, in infants with brachial
    plexus birth palsy, 96: 250
  extent of, related to nerve graft
    morphology (in rabbit), 95: 328
  by means of cervical plexus for brachial
    plexus root avulsions, 95: 106
  phrenic nerve, for brachial plexus
    reconstruction, 97: 104
  spinal accessory, for elbow flexion
    restoration after avulsion injuries of
    brachial plexus, 97: 105
Neurotrophic factor
  Schwann cell-derived, partial
    purification characterization of,
    95: 324
Neurovascular
  bundle, ulnar, at wrist, in endoscopic
    carpal tunnel release, 96: 148
  displacement in hands with Dupuytren's
    contracture, predictors of, 96: 305
  flap, island
    for fingertip amputations,
      volar-oblique, long-term results,
      97: 73
    heterodigital, in thumb
      reconstruction, 96: 69
  metacarpal artery, second dorsal,
    clinical applications, 97: 86
  gracilis transfer, free, secondary, after
    brachial plexus injuries, 96: 251

Newspaper
  industry, active surveillance for control
    of cumulative trauma disorders in,
    95: 245
Nonsteroidal anti-inflammatory agents
  (see Anti-inflammatory agents,
  nonsteroidal)
Nonunion
  of arthrodesis,
    scaphoid-trapezium-trapezoid,
    95: 189
  after one-bone forearm construction,
    97: 59
  scaphoid
    Herbert screw fixation through dorsal
      approach for, 95: 62
    periscaphoid arthritis with, long-term
      results after proximal row
      carpectomy for, 96: 203
    radius bone graft for, distal anterior,
      97: 59
    revascularization of proximal pole
      with implantation of vascular
      bundle and bone grafting for,
      97: 176
  after scaphoid tuberosity fracture,
    95: 193
  treatment by open reduction, bone
    graft, and staple function, 96: 207
Nosology
  of axial congenital deformities in upper
    limb, 95: 300
Nubbin-digits hand
  pathomorphology and treatment of,
    95: 303

O

Obsessive-compulsive disorder
  carpal tunnel syndrome and, 96: 141
Obstetrical
  brachial plexus palsy (see Brachial
    plexus, palsy, birth)
Occupation
  median nerve dysfunction and, 95: 250
Occupational
  carpal tunnel syndrome, workers'
    compensation and surgery
    outcomes, 97: 125
  cramp in musicians, and biomechanical
    abnormalities, 95: 306
  hand dermatitis in metalworkers,
    prognosis of, 97: 340
  radiation injuries of hand, surgical
    treatment of, 95: 81

Office workers
  medical screening for upper extremity cumulative trauma disorders in, 95: 244
Olympus ureteroscope
  flexible, for retrieval of severed flexor tendons, 96: 89
Onychomycosis
  antifungal pulse therapy for, 97: 70
  feet, efficacy and tolerability of Lamisil in, 97: 68
Opponensplasty
  secondary, after brachial plexus injuries, 96: 251
Opposition
  by extensor pollicis longus, restoration of, 96: 86
Orthoplast
  splint, custom-made, and betamethasone injection for carpal tunnel syndrome, reexamination of, 96: 148
Orthosis
  in thoracic outlet syndrome, 96: 330
  wrist extensor, commercial, 96: 338
Osseointegrated
  prosthesis
    nail, 97: 75
    thumb, 97: 62
Osseointegration
  concept, metacarpophalangeal joint arthroplasty based on, 95: 264
Osteoarthritis
  (See also Arthritis, degenerative)
  arthroplasty in, proximal interphalangeal joint silicone replacement, clinical results using anterior approach, 96: 276
  carpometacarpal joint of thumb, revision procedures for complications of surgery for, 95: 261
  elbow, Outerbridge-Kashiwagi's method of arthroplasty for, 97: 234
  pantrapezial, scapho-trapezio-trapezoid arthrodesis combined with Caffinière arthroplasty for, 95: 262
  radioulnar joint, distal, Sauvé-Kapandji procedure for, 97: 225
  scapho-trapezio-trapezoid, and static dorsal intercalated segment instability, 96: 207
  thumb base, excision of trapezium for, 96: 284
  trapeziometacarpal, extension metacarpal osteotomy for, 97: 277
  wrist, asymptomatic scapholunate advanced collapse in, 95: 184

Osteoarthrosis
  basal joints of thumb, osteotomy of first metacarpal for, 97: 285
  of thumb base, trapeziectomy and ligament reconstruction for, 95: 257
Osteochondral
  graft, ipsilateral, for finger joint repair, 95: 53
Osteochondromas
  multiple, hereditary, forearm deformities and problems in children with, 95: 288
Osteoclasis
  radioulnar, surgical, for severe forearm rotation deformities, 96: 65
Osteocutaneous
  radial forearm flap, donor site deficit of, 95: 313
Osteocytes
  débridement of, for fingernail deformities secondary to ganglions of distal interphalangeal joint, 97: 294
Osteomyelitis
  clubhand deformity due to, acquired radial, 96: 62
Osteopenic
  radius, distal, effect of cortical and trabecular bone on strength of, 95: 201
Osteosynthesis
  direct, for first metacarpal base fractures, 96: 54
  intraarticular fractures, vs. closed pinning in, 97: 66
  in-the-socket, for unstable distal radius fracture, 97: 194
  intra-medullary, of displaced fracture of distal fifth metacarpal, 95: 68
  posterior plate, in treatment of compression-extension fractures of distal radius, 96: 211
  procedures after rolling belt injuries, in children, 96: 83
  tension band, double, in supra- and transcondylar humeral fractures, 96: 239
Osteotomy
  correction
    for malunion of phalanges, post-traumatic, 97: 43
    of phalanges and metacarpals for rotational and angular malunion, 95: 55

hemiepiphyseal, at distal ulna for traumatic avulsion of triangular fibrocartilage complex at its ulnar insertion, 97: 222
metacarpal
  extension, for trapeziometacarpal osteoarthritis, 97: 277
  first, for osteoarthrosis of basal joints of thumb, 97: 285
  in metacarpal synostosis, 95: 291
radial
  for Kienböck's disease, changes in carpal alignment after, 95: 181
  in Madelung's deformity, 95: 297, 299
  wedge, for Kienböck's disease, biomechanical analysis of, 95: 182
  in radial head dislocation, chronic post-traumatic, in children, 95: 56
  for radius deformity, 95: 197
ulnar shortening
  oblique, by single saw cut, 97: 56
  oblique, precision, 95: 173
  after radius fracture, distal, 95: 199
  for traumatic avulsion of triangular fibrocartilage complex, reattachment of TFCC after, 96: 230
Otto Bock System Electric Greifer prehensor
  comparison with voluntary-opening split hook, 96: 324
Otto Bock System Electric Hand
  comparison with voluntary-opening split hook, 96: 323, 324
Outerbridge-Kashiwagi's method of arthroplasty for elbow osteoarthritis, 97: 234
Oximetry
  pulse, in evaluation of collateral circulation to hand, 96: 37

P

Packing
  methylmethacrylate, after curettage for giant cell tumors of radius, 95: 282
Pain
  after carpal tunnel syndrome reoperation, 95: 125
  elbow, lateral, and extensor carpi radialis brevis muscle relation to posterior interosseous nerve, 96: 246
  limb, upper, persistent, in sewing machine operators, 95: 241
  neck, persistent, in sewing machine operators, 95: 241

nerve, chronic peripheral, direct electrical nerve stimulation for, 96: 358
radioulnar joint, distal
  arthroplasty for, matched hemiresection interposition, 97: 216
  Darrach procedure for, modified, 97: 217
score, patient's, for hand function assessment, 95: 34
treatment and research, importance of placebo effects in, 95: 32
Wheelchair User's Shoulder Pain Index, reliability and validity of, 97: 337
wrist
  chronic, arthroscopy of, 95: 163
  chronic, diagnosis, traction radiography in, 96: 191
  chronic, diagnostic approach, 96: 179
  chronic, evaluation by arthrography, arthroscopy, and arthrotomy, 95: 161
  chronic, MRI-cinematography of triangular fibrocartilage complex in, 96: 233
  diagnosis, relevance of ligament tears or perforations in, 96: 187
  evaluation, clinical provocative tests in, 96: 181
  site, correlation with noncommunicating defects on wrist arthrography, 95: 162
  transient, after AO/ASIF wrist arthrodesis, 96: 194
  ulnar, after Colles' fracture, 95: 195
  unilateral, arthrography of contralateral, asymptomatic wrist in patients with, 96: 188
Palm
  technique, modified open, for Dupuytren's disease, 97: 302
Palmar
  aponeurosis pulley, mechanical analysis of, 97: 11
  approaches/portals for wrist arthroscopy, 96: 194
  burns, pediatric, 96: 81
  defects of carpal ligaments, resurfacing with retinaculum flexorum flap, 95: 269
  -dorsal direction, endoscopic release of transverse carpal ligament in, 96: 174
  forces, externally applied, causing increase in carpal tunnel pressure, 96: 161

level, digital anesthesia through flexor tendon sheath at, 95: 33
ligament tensions in wrist, 95: 172
radiocarpal ligament disruption, prediction in distal radial fractures, 95: 203
scaphotriquetral ligament, anatomy of, 95: 167
sensory latency changes in response to carpal tunnel release, 96: 149
space infections, treatment and results, 96: 308
tilt, effect on determination of radial shortening, 96: 9
uniportal extrabursal endoscopic carpal tunnel release, 96: 165
wrist ligaments, clinical relevance of, 96: 177

Palmaris
longus interposition arthroplasty for first carpometacarpal joint arthritis, 97: 282

Palsy
brachial plexus (see Brachial plexus, palsy)
cerebral
hand, Botulinum A chemodenervation of, 95: 229
hyperextension of thumb metacarpophalangeal joint in, sesamoid arthrodesis for, 96: 53
interosseous nerve, spontaneous anterior, with hourglass-like fascicular constriction within main trunk of median nerve, 97: 143
ulnar nerve, after lateral approach for non-constrained elbow replacement, 97: 237

Pantrapezial
osteoarthritis, scapho-trapezio-trapezoid arthrodesis combined with Caffinière arthroplasty for, 95: 262

Paralytic
supination contracture of forearm due to traumatic tetraplegia, rerouting of biceps brachii for, 95: 223

Parametacarpal
flap, ulnar, anatomical study and clinical application, 97: 78

Paranoid
personality disorders and carpal tunnel syndrome, 96: 141

Parents
decision making by, in pediatric hand surgery, 96: 315
psychological impact of microvascular free toe transfer in children, 97: 345

Paresthesia
after restoration of hand sensibility after complete brachial plexus injury, 97: 103
transient, after AO/ASIF wrist arthrodesis, 96: 194

Parrot operation
discussion of, 96: 59

Pathomechanics
of scapholunate diastasis in distal radial fractures, 95: 190

Pectoralis major
muscle transfer in Volkmann's contracture, follow-up studies, 95: 312

Pediatric patients (see Children)

Penicillin
for mycetoma of hand, 96: 308

Perception
threshold testing, current, as screening procedure for carpal tunnel syndrome in industrial workers, 96: 260

Percutaneous
intramuscular electrodes, reliability for upper extremity functional neuromuscular stimulation in adolescents with C5 tetraplegia, 96: 256
Kirschner wire (see under Kirschner wire)
release of trigger finger, 95: 101
safety and efficacy of, 96: 114

Performance
-related hand problems in music students, 97: 331

Perilunate
dislocations and fracture-dislocations, 95: 175

Perinatal
brachial plexus root avulsions, neurotizations by means of cervical plexus for, 95: 107

Periostitis
sesamoid bone, 96: 1

Peripheral nerve
defects, vein conduits with interposition of nerve tissue for, 96: 123
entrapments, upper extremity, among wheelchair athletes, 95: 309
functional recovery, effect of magnitude and duration of crush load on (in rat), 95: 110
injury
cell loss in sensory ganglia after (in cat), 96: 384
consequences of, paradoxical clinical, 97: 112

intact, sensory and motor collateral sprouting induced from, by end-to-side anastomosis (in rat), 96: 366
pain, chronic, direct electrical nerve stimulation for, 96: 358
repair, orientated mats of fibronectin as conduit material in (in rat), 97: 364
stretching, acute, effect on retrograde axonal transport (in rat), 97: 367

Peripheral neuropathy
in vibration syndrome, digital nerve conduction velocity as sensitive indication of, 96: 261

Periphyseal
injuries of hand, 95: 67

Periscaphoid
arthritis
scaphoid nonunion with, long-term results after proximal row carpectomy for, 96: 203
scapholunate dissociation with, long-term results after proximal row carpectomy for, 96: 203

Peritoneal
dialysis, continuous ambulatory, carpal tunnel syndrome in patients undergoing, 97: 123

Perivascular
axillary nerve block, effect of arm position on effectiveness of, 96: 43

Personality
disorders and carpal tunnel syndrome, 96: 141

Phalanx
base, lateral, avulsion fractures of, clinical results of tension band fixation of, 96: 48
drilling through, heat recordings at tips of Kirschner wires during, 96: 383
flaps, direct and reversed flow proximal island, 96: 76
foot, free transplants in hand deformities, 97: 345
fracture (see Fracture, phalanx)
lengthening for shortened fingers after trauma, 95: 67
malunion, posttraumatic, corrective osteotomy for, 97: 43
toe, graft
in congenital hand deformities, 95: 294
in symbrachydactyly reconstruction, 95: 294

Phalen's sign
in carpal tunnel syndrome diagnosis in primary care, 95: 134

Pharmacodynamic
investigation of pulse therapy with itraconazole for onychomycosis, 97: 70

Pharmacokinetic
investigation of pulse therapy with itraconazole for onychomycosis, 97: 70

Pharmacologic
agents (see Drugs)

Phasic
relationships of intrinsic and extrinsic thumb musculature, 97: 252

Phrenic nerve
use in brachial plexus reconstruction, 97: 104

Physeal
arrest, traumatic ulnar, after distal forearm fracture, in children, 97: 320

Physical
exposure, self-reported, and musculoskeletal symptoms of forearm-hand among automobile assembly line workers, 97: 328
therapy after subcutaneous long finger flexor pulley rupture, in climbers, 95: 90

Physis
injuries of hand, 95: 67
radial, stress changes, in female gymnasts, 96: 223

Pianists
finger joint and tendon forces in, 95: 11

Piano
virtuosity, work of, 97: 341; 96: 333

Pin
fixation of unstable distal radial fractures, 97: 212
pins and rubbers traction system for comminuted intraarticular fractures and fracture-dislocations, 95: 51
Steinmann, in metacarpal fractures, 97: 46

Pinch
key, single-stage reconstruction in tetraplegics, 96: 254
strength, effect of wrist deviation on, 96: 194

Pinning
closed, vs. direct osteosynthesis in articular fractures of base of first metacarpal, 97: 66

Pipster
in correction of flexed proximal interphalangeal joint in Dupuytren's disease, 96: 301

Pisiform
  transposition, pedicled, in Kienböck's disease, 95: 177
Pitching
  wrist kinematics during, 97: 157
Placebo
  effects, importance in pain treatment and research, 95: 32
Plantaris tendon
  braided, as extensor tendon graft, 96: 89
Plaster
  bandage immobilization after closed reduction of volar dislocation of distal radioulnar joint, 96: 233
  cast (see Cast, plaster)
  fixation of unstable distal radial fractures, 97: 212
Plate
  fixation
    dorsal, of proximal phalangeal fractures, biomechanical analysis of, 95: 49
    internal, of Galeazzi fracture-dislocations, distal radioulnar joint function after, 95: 213
    T-plate, for distal radius fracture, 97: 198
    minicondylar, in metacarpal and phalangeal fractures, 97: 65
  osteosynthesis, posterior, in treatment of compression-extension fractures of distal radius, 96: 211
Platers
  exposed to hand-arm vibration, impaired nerve conduction in carpal tunnel of, 96: 264
Plating
  dorsal, with lag screws, in oblique metacarpal fractures, 97: 47
Playing cast
  for scaphoid fracture, midthird, in athlete, 96: 200
Plethysmography
  in evaluation of collateral circulation to hand, 96: 37
Plexopathy
  brachial, in infants after traumatic delivery, MRI of, 95: 224
Polyarthritis
  chronic, wrist, Meuli cementless wrist prosthesis for, 95: 274
Polydactyly
  thumb, long-term results of surgical treatment, 97: 319

Polydioxanone
  ribbons, resorbable, for relief of tension in nerve repair, 95: 112
Polyglycolic
  acid fine mesh, comparison to vein and silastic mesh, 97: 378
Polyglycolide
  rod fixation of distal radius fracture, comparative study, 97: 198
Polylactide
  rod fixation of distal radius fracture, comparative study, 97: 198
Polymers
  synthetic, seeded with tenocytes, generation of neo-tendon using, 96: 374
Polymethylmethacrylate
  particulate debris, inflammatory response to (in rat), 97: 375
Polytetrafluoroethylene
  gloves, expanded, for care of upper extremity burns, 96: 79
Polyvinyl
  alcohol particles in embolization therapy of congenital arteriovenous malformations, 95: 293
Postoperative
  analgesia, comparison of continuous brachial plexus infusion of butorphanol, mepivacaine and mepivacaine-butorphanol mixtures for, 97: 31
  mobilization (see Mobilization, postoperative)
  monitoring of replantations, laser Doppler flowmetry vs. thermometry in, 96: 352
Postures
  upper limb, variation during word processing with and without mouse use, 96: 265
Power
  staple fixation in trapeziometacarpal arthrodesis, 95: 263
Prednisone
  in carpal tunnel syndrome, 97: 132
Prehension
  restoration after complete brachial plexus avulsion, double free-muscle transfer for, 97: 106
Prehensors
  myoelectrically controlled, three, comparison with voluntary opening split hook, 96: 323
Pressure
  carpal tunnel (see Carpal tunnel, pressure)

compartment, forearm, cadaveric and radiologic assessment of catheter placement for measurement of, 96: 380
dynamics of carpal tunnel and flexor compartment of forearm, 96: 153
intracarpal canal, in carpal tunnel syndrome, overnight serial recordings, 95: 138
perception, relation to skin hardness and two-point discrimination in fingertip, 96: 41
-Specified Sensory Device for pressure perception in fingertip, 96: 41
transmission through normal wrist, 96: 370
Primary care
carpal tunnel syndrome in, 95: 134
Professional
employees, median sensory distal amplitude and latency in, 95: 250
Pronation
plasty, secondary, after brachial plexus injuries, 96: 251
radioulnar ligament motion during, distal, 95: 211
stabilizing mechanism of distal radioulnar joint during, 97: 220
Pronator
quadratus
entrapment in pediatric distal radius fractures, recognition and treatment of, 96: 229
interposition transfer as adjunct to resection arthroplasty of distal radioulnar joint, 97: 214
Prosthesis
biaxial, in revision total wrist arthroplasty, 95: 275
digital, benefits and use of, 97: 335
Francobal, in pantrapezial osteoarthritis, 95: 262
lunate, failed, long-term results of proximal row carpectomy for, 96: 203
metal, in radial head fracture, 95: 221
Meuli cementless wrist, first experience with, 95: 273
myoelectric, long-term follow-up, 95: 305
nail, osseointegrated, 97: 75
neuroprosthesis, closed loop hand grasp, automated tuning of, 95: 310
thumb, osseointegrated, 97: 62
trapezometacarpal, GUEPAR total, for carpometacarpal arthritis of thumb, 95: 258

usage in major upper extremity amputations, 97: 337
Provocative
tests, clinical, used in evaluating wrist pain, 96: 181
Proximalization
connexus intertendineus, for radial subluxation at metacarpophalangeal joint of little finger in musicians, 95: 102
Pseudarthrosis
after capitolunate arthrodesis for radioscaphoid arthritis, 95: 186
forearm, congenital, vascularized fibular graft for, 95: 319
after Graner's technique of Kienböck's disease treatment, 95: 179
scaphoid, results of anatomical staple for, 97: 178
scapholunate, and carpal instability, 97: 171
Pseudomeningocele
traumatic, in infants with brachial plexopathy, MRI of, 95: 224
Psoriatic
arthritis
sesamoid bone enlargement in, 96: 1
of wrist, Meuli cementless wrist prosthesis in, 95: 274
Psychological
impact
of musculoskeletal conditions, 97: 327
of toe transfer, microvascular free, for children and their parents, 97: 345
Psychomotor
capacity and wrist tenosynovitis, 95: 251
deficits, functional, and carpal tunnel syndrome, 95: 128
Psychopathology
prevalence in carpal tunnel syndrome patients, 96: 141
PTFE
gloves, expanded, for care of upper extremity burns, 96: 79
Pulley
A1, in rheumatoid flexor in tenosynovectomy, 95: 276
aponeurosis, palmar, mechanical analysis of, 97: 11
digital, rupture, CT of, 97: 99
flexor (see Flexor, pulley)
Pulp
defects, innervated reverse digital artery flap through bilateral neurorrhaphy for, 95: 83
flaps in thumb duplication, 97: 317

plasty after toe-to-hand transplantation, 97: 77
Pulse
  oximetry in evaluation of collateral circulation to hand, 96: 37
"Puncher's fracture"
  scaphoid fracture as, 95: 193
Pyridoxine
  in carpal tunnel syndrome, 95: 131

Q

Questionnaire
  self-administered, in carpal tunnel syndrome
    for severity of symptoms and functional status, 95: 21
    in workplace surveillance, 95: 248
Quick Pressure Monitor System
  for carpal tunnel pressures in articular fractures of wrist, 96: 217

R

Race
  carpal tunnel syndrome and, in U.S., 96: 157
Radial
  artery
    cannulation, hand ischemia after, 97: 353
    repairs, patency rates assessed with color Doppler ultrasound, 95: 319
    vs. brachial artery injections, for intraarterial regional anesthesia for hand surgery, 96: 42
  club hand, 95: 299
    acquired, due to osteomyelitis, 96: 62
  forearm flap, retrograde fascial, 97: 85
  instability of metacarpophalangeal joint of thumb, 96: 11
  nerve
    decompressions in radial tunnel syndrome, 97: 142
    microsurgical repair, secondary, results of, 95: 116
    sensory, anatomic study, 96: 120
    superficial, defects, vein conduits with interposition of nerve tissue for, 96: 124
    superficial branch, entrapment of, 95: 143
  physis, stress changes, in female gymnasts, 96: 223
  sesamoid, radiographic techniques for visualization of, 96: 53
  -sided lesions of fibrocartilage complex, arthroscopic repair of, 96: 238

styloid process artery, anatomy of, 97: 17
subluxation of connexus intertendineus at metacarpophalangeal joint of little finger in musicians, treatment of, 95: 102
thenar flap, innervated, for sensory reconstruction of fingers, 97: 112
tunnel
  release, outcome, 97: 147
  syndrome, 96: 16
  syndrome, radial nerve decompressions in, 97: 142
Radiation
  diagnostic (see Radiography)
  exposure during operative x-ray screening in hand surgery, risk from, 96: 336
  hand injuries, surgical treatment of, 95: 81
  therapy
    for radioulnar synostosis, traumatic, 96: 247
    for sarcomas of hand and foot, 96: 297
Radiocapitohamate
  arthrodesis in posttraumatic arthritis, 95: 274
Radiocarpal
  arthrodesis
    partial, for scapholunate diastasis in distal radius fractures, 95: 190
    after resection of distal radius for giant cell tumor, 95: 282
  joint arthroplasty, flexible implant, titanium grommet in, 97: 289
  ligament, palmar, disruption in distal radial fractures, prediction of, 95: 204
Radiography
  of articular inclination, relative, of distal radioulnar joint, 97: 208
  assessment of trapezial space before and after ligament reconstruction and tendon interposition arthroplasty for basal joint arthrosis, 97: 280
  film measurements of healed distal radius fractures, 97: 207
  follow-up, long-term, after ulnar lengthening and radial recession procedures for Kienböck's disease, 97: 180
  of ganglia of wrist, intraosseous, 96: 299
  of hand in rheumatoid arthritis, quantitative analysis of, 97: 294
  operative, in hand surgery, risk of radiation exposure from, 96: 336

routine, prediction of lunate
  morphology with, 96: 5
of scaphoid fracture, suspected,
  96: 196; 95: 193
techniques for visualization of radial
  sesamoid, 96: 53
traction, in diagnosis of chronic wrist
  pain, 96: 191
of wrist
  digitalized conventional, monitor
    findings of, 96: 38
  gymnast's, adolescent, 96: 225
  pathologic, is normal contralateral
    wrist best reference for? 97: 151
Radiological
  assessment
    of catheter placement for
      measurement of forearm
      compartment pressures, 96: 380
    of trapeziometacarpal joint
      degenerative changes, 97: 275
    evaluation of long-term effects of
      resection of distal ulna in
      rheumatoid arthritis, 96: 270
    evolution of rheumatoid wrist after
      radiolunate arthrodesis, 96: 267
    screening criteria in wrist instability,
      96: 190
Radiolunate
  arthrodesis (see Arthrodesis,
    radiolunate)
  ligament
    MRI of, 95: 168
    tensions in, 95: 173
Radiolunotriquetral
  ligament, MRI of, 95: 168
Radionuclide
  probes for tissue damage, 95: 38
Radioscaphocapitate
  ligament tensions, 95: 173
Radioscaphoid
  arthritis, scaphoid excision and
    capitolunate arthrodesis for,
    95: 185
  ligament, MRI of, 95: 168
Radioscapholunate
  ligament, MRI of, 95: 168
Radiotherapy
  for radioulnar synostosis, traumatic,
    96: 247
  for sarcomas of hand and foot, 96: 297
Radioulnar
  arthrodesis, distal, for Madelung's
    deformity, 95: 299
  convergence, dynamic, after Darrach
    procedure, 97: 218
  joint, distal

arthroplasty of, matched
  hemiresection interposition,
  97: 216
arthroplasty of, resection, pronator
  quadratus interposition transfer as
  adjunct to, 97: 214
articular inclination of, relative,
  radiographic study, 97: 208
congruency, effect of dorsally
  angulated distal radius fractures on,
  97: 210
dislocation, volar type, 96: 233
dislocation, with ulna styloid fracture
  and triangular fibrocartilage
  complex injury, 95: 207
function after Galeazzi
  fracture-dislocations treated by
  open reduction and internal plate
  fixation, 95: 213
after Galeazzi's fracture, 96: 238
geometry of, abnormal, 96: 234
instability, treatment of acute injuries
  of triangular fibrocartilage complex
  associated with, 96: 237
osteoarthritis, Sauvé-Kapandji
  procedure for, 97: 225
painful, modified Darrach procedure
  for, 97: 217
post-traumatic disorders, Kapandji
  procedure for, 95: 204
in rheumatoid arthritis, kinematics of,
  97: 19
stabilization by Hui-Linscheid
  ligamentoplasty, 97: 227
stabilizing mechanism during
  pronation and supination, 97: 220
ligament, distal, motion during
  supination and pronation, 95: 211
osteoclasis, surgical, for severe forearm
  rotation deformities, 96: 65
synostosis (see Synostosis, radioulnar)
Radius
  bone graft, distal anterior, in hand and
    wrist surgery, 97: 59
  deformity, osteotomy for, 95: 197
  distal
    fixation of, external, biomechanical
      study of, 95: 200
    flexor surface, modified approach to,
      97: 154
    graft from, cancellous, in
      fracture-dislocations of proximal
      interphalangeal joint, 97: 39
    osteopenic, strength, effect of cortical
      and trabecular bone on, 95: 201
    resection for giant cell tumors,
      95: 282

stapling of, hemiepiphyseal, in
children with multiple hereditary
osteochondromata, 95: 289
tumor of, giant cell, 97: 297
tumor of, giant cell, treatment,
95: 281
floating, in bipolar forearm
fracture-dislocation, 95: 65
fracture (see Fracture, radius)
head
dislocation, "isolated" traumatic,
96: 243
dislocation, post-traumatic, chronic,
treatment, in children, 95: 56
subluxation after treatment of chronic
post-traumatic dislocation of radial
head, in children, 95: 58
lengthening, progressive, in
post-traumatic epiphysiodesis of
distal end of radius, 97: 324
longitudinal deficiency, preoperative
distraction lengthening for, 97: 326
malunion, distal intraarticular,
radiolunate arthrodesis for, 97: 173
osteotomy (see Osteotomy, radial)
recession procedures for Kienböck's
disease, long-term follow-up,
97: 180
shortening
for Kienböck's disease, preoperative
factors and outcome after, 95: 180
reliability of different methods of
determination of, 96: 9
Range of motion
after cubital tunnel surgery, 97: 145
functional, of elbow, 96: 239
Reattachment
technique, new, after traumatic avulsion
of triangular fibrocartilage complex
at its ulnar insertion, 96: 230
Reconstruction
arterial, for cold-induced vasospasm
after digital replantation, 97: 358
brachial plexus
phrenic nerve used in, 97: 104
technique for maximizing biceps
recovery in, 95: 105
digital, flap in
dorsometacarpal, reverse, 96: 342
V-Y advancement, dorsal, 95: 69
extensor tendon, primary, in dorsal
hand defects requiring free flaps,
95: 96
extremity, upper, local fasciocutaneous
flaps in, use of previously burned
skin in, 96: 80
finger

dorsal, arterialized tendocutaneous
venous flap for, 96: 84
sensory, radial thenar innervated flap
for, 97: 112
fingertip, syndactylic toe transfer for,
96: 321
hand
dorsum, immediate vs. staged
reconstruction, 97: 80
gracilis muscle transplantation for,
free, 96: 353
serratus anterior free muscle transfer
for, 95: 319
height, of lunate, in early stage 3
Kienböck's disease, 96: 201
ligament (see under Ligament,
reconstruction)
of malunited distal radius fractures,
early vs. late, 97: 198
metacarpophalangeal joint, in
rheumatoid disease, motion after,
95: 266
microsurgical, of congenital adactylous
hand, advances in, 96: 319
microvascular, of upper extremity with
rectus abdominis muscle, 96: 340
sensory, of fingers, radial thenar
innervated flap for, 97: 112
single-stage, of key pinch and extension
of elbow in tetraplegics, 96: 254
symbrachydactyly, toe phalangeal grafts
for, 95: 294
thumb (see Thumb, reconstruction)
web space, reverse dorsometacarpal flap
in, 96: 342
Recordings
heat, at tips of Kirschner wires during
drilling through phalanges, 96: 383
of intracarpal canal pressure in carpal
tunnel syndrome, serial overnight,
95: 138
Rectus
abdominis muscle, microvascular
reconstruction of upper extremity
with, 96: 340
Reduction
closed
of Colles' fracture, ulnar wrist pain
after, 95: 195
of forearm fracture, distal, in
children, short arm plaster cast
after, 95: 63
of metacarpal base fractures, first,
recent, 96: 54
of radioulnar joint dislocation, volar
distal, 96: 233
of metacarpal fracture, displaced distal
fifth, 95: 68

Subject Index / 443

open
  of forearm fractures, airbag-related, 96: 68
  of Galeazzi fracture-dislocation, distal radioulnar joint function after, 95: 213
  of humerus fracture, supracondylar, in children, 95: 219
  of perilunate dislocations and fracture-dislocations, 95: 176
  of radial fractures, distal, with scapholunate diastasis, 95: 190
  of radial head dislocation, chronic post-traumatic, in children, 95: 56
  for scaphoid nonunion, 96: 207
Reeducation
  sensory
    delayed, after toe-to-hand transfer, 97: 350
    after digital replantation and revascularization, 97: 343
Reflex
  sympathetic dystrophy
    after arthrodesis, scapho-trapezio-trapezoid, combined with Caffinière arthroplasty for pantrapezial osteoarthritis, 95: 262
    autonomic denervation and, 96: 355
    bone scintigraphy in, three-phase, 95: 28
    after cubital tunnel surgery with anterior submuscular transposition of ulnar nerve, 97: 147
    diagnosis, bone scintigraphy in, 97: 355
    after Dupuytren's disease treatment with modified open palm technique, 97: 304
    after fractures of distal radius, 96: 218
    of hand and wrist, microvascular response patterns associated with, 95: 27
    laboratory findings in, 96: 356
    MRI findings, 96: 361
    segmental, clinical and scintigraphic criteria, 95: 30
    signs and symptoms of, 95: 38
    sympathectomy for, factors affecting outcome, 96: 364
    in women, caucasian, 96: 357
    tonic vibration, in writer's cramp, 97: 334
Regeneration
  nerve (see Nerve, regeneration)
Rehabilitation
  hand, compliance with, 96: 331
  of mallet finger, impact of compliance on, 95: 98
Release
  abilities with functional neuromuscular stimulation in adolescents with tetraplegia, 97: 246
Reliability
  of electroneurometer measures of distal sensory latency of median nerve, 95: 19
  in evaluation of hand sensibility, establishment of, 95: 17
Remanipulation
  of Colles' fracture, anatomical and functional results five years after, 97: 200
Remodeling
  of hand representation in cortex determined by timing of tactile stimulation, 97: 18
Reperfusion
  injury, effect of ex vivo perfusion with anticoagulated blood on (in rat), 95: 338
Repetitive
  movements at work, relation to upper limb soft tissue disorders, 96: 258
  tasks, detection of cumulative trauma disorders in workers performing, 96: 265
Replantation
  bone growth in children after, 96: 346
  after degloving injuries of hand and fingers, 96: 347
  digit
    cold intolerance after, and thermoregulation patterns, 97: 358
    natural history of, 96: 348
    after rolling belt injury, in children, 96: 83
    sensory reeducation after, 97: 343
    vasospasm after, cold-induced (see Vasospasm, cold-induced, after digital replantation)
  ischemia/reperfusion injury in, effect of ex vivo perfusion with anticoagulated blood on (in rat), 95: 338
  limb, in children, 96: 353
    upper, results, 96: 351
  monitoring of, postoperative, laser Doppler flowmetry vs. thermometry in, 96: 352
  after resection for primary malignant tumors of arm, 96: 296
Research
  pain, importance of placebo effects in, 95: 32

Resection
-replantation for primary malignant tumors of arm, 96: 296
Resurfacing
of palmar defects of carpal ligaments with retinaculum flexorum flap, 95: 269
Retinacular
ligament, oblique, of index finger, anatomy of, 95: 16
Retinaculum
extensorum flap for dorsal wrist ganglion, 95: 268
flexorum flap, resurfacing palmar defects of carpal ligaments with, 95: 269
Return to work
after carpal tunnel release, open vs. endoscopic, 97: 113
Revascularization
after degloving injuries of hand and fingers, 96: 347
digital, sensory reeducation after, 97: 343
of lunate, core, in early stage 3 Kienböck's disease, 96: 201
procedures after rolling belt injuries, in children, 96: 83
of proximal pole for scaphoid nonunion with implantation of vascular bundle and bone grafting, 97: 176
upper extremity, results, in children, 96: 351
Rhabdomyosarcoma
alveolar, combined modality therapy for, 96: 297
hand, treatment, 96: 293
Rheumatoid arthritis
arthrodesis using absorbable screws and rods in, 97: 295
capsular tissues of proximal interphalangeal joint in, 95: 9
elbow, arthroplasty for
interposition, 97: 243
non-constrained, short-term complications of lateral approach, 97: 237
flexor tendon rupture in, retinaculum flexorum flap in, 95: 269
hand radiographs in, quantitative analysis of, 97: 294
interphalangeal joint in, proximal, flexible implant resection arthroplasty of, 96: 275
juvenile, flexible implant resection arthroplasty of proximal interphalangeal joint in, 96: 275
metacarpophalangeal joint reconstruction in, motion after, 95: 266
radiocarpal joint, titanium grommet in flexible implant arthroplasty for, 97: 289
radioulnar joint in, distal, kinematics of, 97: 19
sesamoid bone, 96: 1
tenosynovectomy in, flexor
A1 pulley in, 95: 276
finger mobility after, short- and long-term analysis of, 95: 267
ulna excision in, distal, 97: 290
ulna resection in, distal, radiological evaluation of long-term effects of, 96: 270
wrist
arthroplasty in, revision total, 95: 275
arthroplasty in, Swanson, 95: 270
arthroplasty in, Volz total wrist, long-term outcome, 95: 272
classification of, new, 96: 268
radiological evolution after radiolunate arthrodesis, 96: 267
Rheumatoid factor
in wrist tenosynovitis and humeral epicondylitis, 97: 293
Rib
vascularized seventh, transfer in Eve procedure, 97: 350
Ribbons
resorbable polydioxanone, for tension relief in nerve repair, 95: 112
Rigid-body spring-modeling program
for evaluation of force and pressure transmission through normal wrist, 96: 371
Ring
avulsion injuries, microsurgical management of, 97: 346
protection, for subcutaneous rupture of long finger flexor pulleys in climbers, 95: 90
Rod
absorbable, use in arthrodesis in rheumatoid arthritis, 97: 295
fixation, polylactide and polyglycolide, of distal radius fracture, comparative study, 97: 198
Rolando fracture
treatment, 96: 54
Rolling belt
injuries, in children, 96: 83
Rotation
axes of, of thumb interphalangeal and metacarpophalangeal joints, 97: 6

deformity of forearm, severe, surgical
    radioulnar osteoclasis for, 96: 65
forearm (see Forearm, rotation)
Rotational
  malunion, correction osteotomies of
    phalanges and metacarpals for,
    95: 55
Rubber
  band exercise devices for children after
    flexor tendon injuries, 96: 85
  pins and rubbers traction system for
    comminuted intraarticular fractures
    and fracture-dislocation, 95: 51
Rugby
  -related distal radius fractures, 96: 222
Rupture
  biceps tendon
    distal, repair with suture anchors and
      anterior approach, 97: 229
    MRI of, 95: 104
  extensor pollicis longus, late, after wrist
    arthroscopy, 96: 194
  extensor tendons at musculotendinous
    junction, traumatic, 97: 101
  flexor digitorum tendon, intratendinous,
    in zones II and III, 97: 101
  flexor pulley, finger
    closed traumatic, 96: 97
    long finger, subcutaneous rupture, in
      climbers, 95: 90
  flexor tendon (see Flexor tendon;
    rupture)
  flexor-pronator origin, caused by falls,
    after anterior submuscular
    transposition of ulnar nerve for
    cubital tunnel syndrome, 97: 147
  ligament
    collateral, ulnar, displaced and
      nondisplaced, ultrasound
      differentiation of, 96: 33
    collateral, ulnar, thumb, treatment
      with Mitek bone anchor, 97: 50
    collateral, ulnar, thumb
      metacarpophalangeal, arthroscopic
      treatment of, 97: 48
    relevance in diagnosis of wrist pain,
      96: 187
    scapholunate, with distal radius
      fracture, arthroscopic diagnosis and
      minimally invasive treatment of,
      97: 206
    triquetrolunate, longstanding, frayed
      ulnotriquetral and ulnolunate
      ligaments as arthroscopic sign of,
      96: 206
    ulnar collateral, MRI of, 95: 42
  pulley, digital, CT of, 97: 99

rate of acute flexor tendon repairs
  mobilized by controlled active
  motion regimen, 96: 105
triangular fibrocartilage complex
  arthrographic evaluation of, 95: 161
  arthroscopic debridement of, clinical
    results, 97: 223

S

Saline
  infiltration for extravasation of
    antitumor agents, 95: 280
  at dorsum of hand, 95: 279
Saphenous
  nerve, sensory nerve response on
    cutaneous electrical stimulation (in
    rat), 97: 378
Sarcoma
  epithelioid, masquerading as
    Dupuytren's disease, 96: 298
  of hand and foot, combined modality
    therapy, 96: 297
  soft tissue
    arm, resection-replantation for,
      96: 296
    hand, treatment of, 96: 292
    hand and foot, combined modality
      therapy for, 96: 297
Sauvé-Kapandji procedure
  for osteoarthritis of distal radioulnar
    joint, 97: 225
Savage
  suture technique, 4-strand, for flexor
    tendon repair, in vitro
    biomechanical analysis of, 95: 331
  tendon repair
    six-strand, work of flexion after,
      97: 372
    strength of, in vitro, 97: 12
Saw
  cut, single, oblique ulnar shortening
    osteotomy by, 97: 56
Scalpel
  tenolysis in flexor tendon (in rabbit),
    97: 374
Scanning (see Imaging)
Scaphocapitate
  arthrodesis for Kienböck's disease,
    97: 182
Scaphoid
  carpal, Silastic implant arthroplasty of,
    96: 200
  CT of, longitudinal, 97: 37
  excision in radioscaphoid arthritis,
    95: 185
  fracture (see Fracture, scaphoid)

injuries, internal fixation with Herbert screw through dorsal approach, 95: 62
kinematics
  influence of joint laxity on, 97: 160
  role of scaphoid-trapezio-trapezoid ligament complex on, 96: 207
nonunion (see Nonunion, scaphoid)
pseudarthrosis, results of anatomical staple for, 97: 178
shift test
  in uninjured wrist, 96: 182
  in wrist pain evaluation, 96: 181
Silastic implants of, 95: 193
Scaphoidectomy
  for scapholunate advanced collapse of wrist, 97: 192
Scapholunate
  advanced collapse wrist
    motion-preserving procedures for, 97: 186
    scaphoidectomy and capitolunate arthrodesis for, 97: 192
  collapse, advanced asymptomatic, 95: 184
  diastasis in distal radius fractures, pathomechanics and treatment options, 95: 190
  dissociation
    new operation for, 97: 167
    with periscaphoid arthritis, long-term results after proximal row carpectomy for, 96: 203
  injuries of wrist, partial, arthroscopic management of, 97: 170
  instability
    chronic, scaphoid-trapezium-trapezoid arthrodesis in, long-term follow-up, 95: 189
    dynamic, results of operative treatment with dorsal capsulodesis, 97: 163
  ligament
    anatomy of, 95: 157
    defects, incomplete, on wrist arthrography, lack of correlation between site of wrist pain and, 95: 162
    interosseous, anatomy of, gross and histologic, 97: 158
    interosseous, of wrist, MR appearances, 96: 205
    interosseous, reconstruction of, autografts from foot for, 97: 164
    rupture with distal radius fracture, arthroscopic diagnosis and minimally invasive treatment of, 97: 206

sectioning, biomechanical study of, 97: 155
tears, evaluation by arthrography, arthroscopy, and arthrotomy, 95: 161
pseudarthrosis and carpal instability, 97: 171
Scapho-trapezio-trapezoid
  arthrodesis (see Arthrodesis, scaphoid-trapezium-trapezoid)
  arthrosis, isolated, long-term follow-up of scaphoid-trapezium-trapezoid arthrodesis in, 95: 189
  ligament
    complex, role on scaphoid kinematics, 96: 207
    injury, isolated, diagnosis and treatment, 95: 192
    osteoarthritis and static dorsal intercalated segment instability, 96: 207
Scaphotriquetral
  ligament, palmar, 96: 177
  anatomy of, 95: 167
Scapula
  fracture, open, in children, 97: 321
Scar
  contracture
    morbidity of pedicled groin flap for, 95: 78
    after thumb reconstruction with heterodigital neurovascular island flap, 96: 69
    hypertrophic, after triradiate incision for dorsal approach to wrist, 97: 149
    symptomatic, after anterior submuscular transposition of ulnar nerve for cubital tunnel syndrome, 97: 147
  tenderness after carpal tunnel release, effect of open twin incision technique on, 95: 121
Schoenberg
  happy hand of, 95: 310
Schwann cell
  -derived neurotrophic factor, partial purification characterization of, 95: 324
Sciatic
  nerve graft, bioartificial (in rat), 97: 362
Scintigraphy (see Imaging)
Screw
  absorbable, use in arthrodesis in rheumatoid arthritis, 97: 295
  compression, in fracture-dislocations of proximal interphalangeal joint, 97: 40

Herbert (see Herbert screw)
Herbert-Whipple cannulated, in radius head fracture, 97: 232
lag
　in fixation of oblique metacarpal fractures, 97: 47
　in precision oblique osteotomy for shortening of ulna, 95: 174
miniscrew fixation
　AO, of radius head fracture, late results, 97: 231
　of phalanx fracture, proximal distal unicondylar, 95: 47
Self-reported
　health measures, validity of, from workers' compensation recipients with carpal tunnel syndrome, 97: 127
　physical exposure and musculoskeletal symptoms of forearm-hand among automobile assembly line workers, 97: 328
Semitendinosus
　muscle transfer, in Volkmann's contracture, follow-up studies, 95: 312
Semmes-Weinstein monofilament
　test, establishment of reliability with, 95: 16
　thresholds, abnormal, in carpal tunnel syndrome, decision making in detection of, 96: 39
Sensation
　abnormal, after endoscopic carpal tunnel release, 96: 171
Sensibility
　functional, restitution after nerve repair, correlation with specific cognitive capacities, 96: 118
　hand
　　establishment of reliability in evaluation of, 95: 17
　　restoration after complete brachial plexus injury, 97: 103
　　testing, 95: 38
　　tests, measuring outcome in median nerve injuries, 95: 23
Sensitivity
　threshold measurements, vibrotactile, temperature effects on, implications for carpal tunnel screening tests, 97: 136
Sensorineural
　objective tests in hand-arm vibration syndrome, 95: 236

Sensory
　collateral sprouting induced from intact peripheral nerve by end-to-side anastomosis (in rat), 96: 366
　conduction, median nerve, in Japanese vs. American industry, 95: 242
　deficits associated with carpal tunnel syndrome, gap detection tactility test for, 97: 24
　distal amplitude, median, 95: 250
　disturbances after two-portal endoscopic carpal tunnel release, 96: 164
　dysfunction associated with repetitive strain injuries of tendinitis and focal hand dystonia, 97: 272
　endings of C7 nerve root, distribution and clinical significance, 95: 339
　ganglia, cell loss in, after peripheral nerve injury (in cat), 96: 384
　latency, median nerve
　　distal, 95: 250
　　measures of, electroneurometer for, reliability of, 95: 19
　　measures of, electroneurometer for, vs. standard nerve conduction studies, 95: 20
　latency, palmar, changes in response to carpal tunnel release, 96: 149
　nerve
　　conduction measures vs. vibrometry testing in screening for carpal tunnel syndrome in industrial setting, 96: 338
　　radial, anatomic study, 96: 120
　　response in saphenous nerve on cutaneous electrical stimulation (in rat), 97: 378
　reconstruction of fingers, radial thenar innervated flap for, 97: 112
　recovery
　　after carpal tunnel release, 95: 144
　　functional, vs. two-point discrimination tests in both median and ulnar nerve complete transections, 95: 117
　reeducation
　　delayed, after toe-to-hand transfer, 97: 350
　　after digital replantation and revascularization, 97: 343
　regeneration, abnormal, and cold-induced vasospasm after finger replantation, 97: 349
　sequelae of bipedicle digital advancement island flaps, 96: 78

tests, special, value for diagnosis of benign and minor median nerve lesion at wrist, 97: 147
Separation
　disruption, effect of wrist position on extensor mechanism after, 96: 112
Serratus muscle
　transfer
　　anterior free, for reconstruction of injured hand, 95: 319
　　in Eve procedure, 97: 350
　　pedicled, secondary, after brachial plexus injuries, 96: 251
Sesamoid
　arthrodesis for hyperextension of thumb metacarpophalangeal joint, 96: 53
　bones
　　of hand, pathology of, 96: 1
　　of thumb, fractures of, 97: 66
　　radial, radiographic techniques for visualization of, 96: 53
Severed
　flexor tendon, endoscopic retrieval of, 96: 89
Sewing machine
　operators, persistent neck and upper limb pain in, 95: 241
Sex (see Gender)
Shock
　electric, effectiveness of surface cooling in reducing heat injury after, 95: 335
　wave therapy, low-energy extracorporeal, for persistent tennis elbow, 97: 268
Short arc motion
　early active, for repaired central slip, 96: 100
Shortened finger
　after trauma, phalanx lengthening for, 95: 67
Shortening
　radius
　　for Kienböck's disease, preoperative factors and outcome after, 95: 180
　　reliability of different methods of determination of, 96: 9
　ulna
　　osteotomy for (see Osteotomy, ulnar shortening)
　　using AO small distractor, 97: 224
Shoulder
　-hand syndrome in cervical spinal cord injury, 96: 256
　Pain Index, Wheelchair User's, reliability and validity of, 97: 337

Silastic
　foam dressings after skin grafts in pediatric hand burns, 95: 80
　implant
　　arthroplasty of carpal scaphoid, 96: 200
　　arthroplasty of carpometacarpal joint of thumb, revision procedures for complications of, 95: 261
　　of scaphoid and lunate, 95: 193
　mesh, comparison to vein and polyglycolic acid fine mesh, 97: 378
　silicone elastomer particulate debris, inflammatory response to (in rat), 97: 375
Silfverskiold tendon repair
　strength of, in vitro, 97: 12
Silicone
　arthroplasty
　　of carpometacarpal joint of small finger for posttraumatic degenerative arthritis, 96: 290
　　of interphalangeal joint, proximal, clinical results using anterior approach, 96: 276
　block in nubbin-digits hand, 95: 303
　elastomer particulate debris, inflammatory response to (in rat), 97: 375
　finger joint implants, Swanson, long-term complications of, 97: 287
　-hinge proximal interphalangeal joint implant, failure of, 96: 369
　scaphoid replacement for radioscaphoid arthritis, 95: 186
　spacer in metacarpophalangeal joint arthroplasty, 95: 265
Sixth dorsal compartment
　release of, 96: 110
Skeletal
　musculoskeletal (see Musculoskeletal)
　repair by in situ formation of mineral phase of bone, 96: 365
　traction for flexed proximal interphalangeal joint in Dupuytren's disease, 96: 301
Skiing
　-related distal radius fractures, 96: 222
Skin
　(See also Cutaneous)
　blood flow, finger, after microvascular repair of ulnar artery at wrist, laser Doppler imaging of, 96: 364
　burned, previously, use in local fasciocutaneous flaps for upper extremity reconstruction, 96: 80

defects
  in Dupuytren's contracture,
    distally-based hand flap for
    resurfacing, 96: 309
  of hand, venous flap for covering,
    96: 341
flap, narrow pedicled intercostal
  perforator, for burned hand
  coverage, 95: 324
graft (see Graft, skin)
hardness, and pressure perception and
  two-point discrimination in
  fingertip, 96: 41
loss, fingertip, Hueston flap for, 95: 75
necrosis after free transplants of
  phalanges of foot in hand
  deformities, 97: 345
-tendon defect of dorsum of hand,
  tendinocutaneous free flap transfer
  for, 96: 74
Sleep
  -related disorders in carpal tunnel
    syndrome, 97: 148
Slip
  central
    repaired, early active short arc
      motion for, 96: 100
    tenodesis test for early diagnosis of
      potential boutonnière deformities,
      95: 36
Smith's fractures
  classification for, proposed, 96: 208
Smoking
  microvascular tissue transfers and,
    95: 320
Smooth muscle
  α-, actin expression, correlation with
    contraction in Dupuytren's disease
    fibroblasts, 97: 304
Snuff box
  percutaneous Kirschner wire fixation
    through, 96: 186
Soccer
  -related distal radius fractures, 96: 222
Social
  impact of musculoskeletal conditions,
    97: 327
Sodium
  tetradecyl sulfate in embolization
    therapy of congenital arteriovenous
    malformations, 95: 293
Soft tissue
  coverage of elbow, reverse lateral arm
    flap in, 95: 316
  disorders
    of neck and upper limb, classification
      systems of, 97: 255

upper limb, relation to repetitive
  movements at work, 96: 258
lesions, intracarpal, with intra-articular
  fractures of distal radius, 97: 204
sarcoma (see Sarcoma, soft tissue)
Sollerman hand function test, 97: 250
Solute
  diffusion in flexor tendons, effect of
    cyclic and static tensile loading on
    (in dog), 96: 372
Somatosensory
  system responsiveness after nerve injury
    and amputation in hand, 96: 126
Souquet modification
  of Hueston flap for fingertip skin loss,
    95: 76
Souter-Strathclyde total elbow
  arthroplasties
  fixation strength of ulnar component of,
    97: 238
Spastic
  hemiplegia in children, functional
    outcome of upper limb tendon
    transfer for, 95: 231
Speculum
  nasal, lighted Killian, for direct vision in
    carpal tunnel release, 96: 172
Spinal
  accessory neurotization for elbow
    flexion restoration after avulsion
    injuries of brachial plexus, 97: 105
  cord injury
    cervical, shoulder-hand syndrome in,
      96: 256
    hand function restoration after,
      tendon transfers and functional
      electrical stimulation for, 97: 245
  nerve root
    C7, sensory endings, distribution and
      clinical significance, 95: 339
    C7, transfer, contralateral, with
      vascularized nerve grafting for
      brachial plexus root avulsion (in
      rat), 95: 339
    injuries in brachial plexus lesions,
      96: 252
Spiral
  nerve formation in Dupuytren's
    contracture, 96: 305
Splint
  clam-digger, after flexible intramedullary
    nailing of metacarpal fractures,
    97: 45
  in De Quervain's disease, 96: 273
  extension, for mallet finger injuries,
    compliance with, 95: 99
  flexor tendon, in tendon repair, 96: 376
  for gamekeeper's thumb, 97: 53

hand glove, for attachment of dynamic
  components, 96: 338
Kleinert, activity of extrinsic finger
  flexors during mobilization in,
  97: 91
padded, for cubital tunnel syndrome,
  95: 140
tendon, internal and dorsal, in tendon
  repair, work of flexion after,
  97: 372
thermoplastic
  after extensor tendon laceration
    repair, 96: 107
  after flexor tendon repair, acute,
    96: 105
  after flexor tendon repair with double
    loop locking suture technique,
    97: 89
  vs. compression glove for closed
    metacarpal fracture, 96: 57
wrist, in carpal tunnel syndrome
  design of, 97: 130
  early mild, 95: 132
  in primary care, 95: 134
Splinting
  for camptodactyly, results of, 96: 314
  after carpal tunnel release, 96: 158
  for carpal tunnel syndrome
    combined with steroid injections,
      reexamination of, 96: 147
    search for optimal angle, 96: 146
  dynamic
    high- vs. low-profile, biomechanical
      motions and forces involved in,
      96: 326
    vs. static, for zones III and IV
      extensor tendon lacerations, early
      controlled motion with, 96: 107
Sports
  radius fractures in, distal, epidemiology
    and outcome, 96: 222
Spring
  balance test of strength for hand
    function assessment, 95: 34
Squamous cell carcinoma
  of hand, recurrent, in
    immunosuppressed patients,
    treatment, 96: 294
Stability
  forearm, role of interosseous membrane
    and triangular fibrocartilage
    complex in, 95: 333
  lateral, of proximal interphalangeal
    joint replacement, 96: 368
Staining
  for acetylcholinesterase in evaluation of
    ulnar nerve grafts in brachial
    plexus lesions, 95: 108

Stainless steel
  plate and screw fixation of proximal
    phalangeal fractures, 95: 49
  wire in mallet finger surgery, 95: 98
Staple
  anatomical, for scaphoid pseudarthrosis,
    results of, 97: 178
  fixation, power, in trapeziometacarpal
    arthrodesis, 95: 263
  function in treatment of scaphoid
    nonunion, 96: 207
Stapling
  hemiepiphyseal, of distal radius in
    children with multiple hereditary
    osteochondromata, 95: 289
Static
  tensile loading, effect on water content
    and solute diffusion in flexor
    tendons (in dog), 96: 372
Steel
  stainless
    plate and screw fixation of proximal
      phalangeal fractures, 95: 49
    wire, in mallet finger surgery, 95: 98
Steindler flexorplasty
  secondary, after brachial plexus injuries,
    96: 251
Steinmann pin
  in metacarpal fractures, 97: 46
Stener lesion
  MRI of, 97: 37
Stenosing
  tenosynovitis of extensor carpi ulnaris,
    97: 273
Stereophotogrammetry
  for contact areas in thumb
    carpometacarpal joint, 97: 3
Sternotomy
  median, ulnar neuropathy after, 95: 142
Steroid (see Corticosteroid)
Straight-line graphs
  for prediction of growth of upper
    extremities, 95: 301
Strain
  in articular disk of triangular
    fibrocartilage complex, 95: 208
  creep, of flexor tendons during
    low-force high-frequency activities,
    measurement of, 96: 19
  injuries, repetitive, of tendinitis and
    focal hand dystonia, sensory
    dysfunction associated with,
    97: 272
Strength
  fixation, of ulnar component of total
    elbow replacement, 97: 238
  grip (see Grip, strength)

of hand muscle, effect of short-term
    immobilization on, 96: 20
pinch, effect of wrist deviation on,
    96: 194
spring balance test, for hand function
    assessment, 95: 34
tensile, of repaired flexor tendons, effect
    of suture knots on (in dog),
    96: 115
in vitro, of flexor tendon repairs,
    97: 12
Stress
  changes of radial physis in female
    gymnasts, 96: 223
  distribution analysis in malunited
    Colles' fracture, 96: 227
  situations of wrist, dynamic, topology
    of carpal tunnel during, 96: 23
  test, positive ulnocarpal, 97: 162
  testing
    cold, isolated, for microvascular
      response associated with reflex
      sympathetic dystrophy of hand and
      wrist, 95: 27
    valgus, in injuries of ulnar collateral
      ligament of thumb
      metacarpophalangeal joint, 95: 41
Stretching
  passive, after splinting for
    camptodactyly, results of, 96: 314
Strickland formula
  role in management of zone 1 flexor
    tendon injuries, 95: 88
Stroke
  backhand, wrist kinematics in expert vs.
    novice tennis players performing,
    96: 334
Student
  music, performance-related hand
    problems in, 97: 331
  practice model, flexor tendon repair in
    perfect safety, 96: 95
Styloid
  fracture, ulnar, with distal radioulnar
    joint dislocation, 95: 207
Subcutaneous
  hematoma after anterior submuscular
    transposition of ulnar nerve for
    cubital tunnel syndrome, 97: 147
  rupture of long finger flexor pulleys, in
    climbers, 95: 90
  ulnar nerve transfer, anterior, in athlete,
    95: 141
Subfascial
  carpal tunnel release, complications
    after, 95: 155
  ulnar nerve transfer, subcutaneous, in
    athlete, 95: 141

Subluxation
  of extensor carpi ulnaris, 97: 273
  radial, of connexus intertendineus at
    metacarpophalangeal joint of little
    finger in musicians, treatment of,
    95: 102
  radial head, after treatment of chronic
    post-traumatic dislocation of radial
    head, in children, 95: 58
  ulna, distal, chronic post-traumatic
    dorsal, hemiresection-interposition
    arthroplasty for, 95: 205
Submuscular
  transposition, anterior, of ulnar nerve
    for cubital tunnel syndrome,
    97: 146
Substance
  abuse and carpal tunnel syndrome,
    96: 141
Subungual
  glomus tumors, MRI of, 96: 291
Sudomotor
  changes in reflex sympathetic dystrophy,
    96: 356
Supination
  contracture of forearm, paralytic, due to
    traumatic tetraplegia, rerouting of
    biceps brachii for, 95: 223
  radioulnar ligament motion during,
    distal, 95: 211
  stabilizing mechanism of distal
    radioulnar joint during, 97: 220
Supraclavicular
  nerve in restoration of hand sensibility
    after complete brachial plexus
    injury, 97: 103
Supracondylar
  humerus fracture (see Fracture,
    humerus, supracondylar)
Surface
  cooling, effectiveness in reducing heat
    injury, 95: 335
Surgery
  hand (see Hand, surgery)
  microsurgery (see Microsurgical)
Suture
  anchors
    in biceps tendon repair, distal,
      97: 229
    bone, in hand surgery, 96: 47
  caliber in flexor tendon repair,
    evaluation of, 97: 94
  epineurial, secondary, for digital nerve
    repair, 95: 115
  Kessler (see Kessler suture)
  Kessler-Mason-Allen, modified, for
    flexor tendon injuries, in children,
    96: 85

knots, effect on tensile strength of repaired flexor tendons (in dog), 96: 115
locking, double loop, flexor tendon repair with, early active mobilization after, 97: 89
mesh reinforced, in tendon transfers, early active mobilization after, 97: 108
methods in tendon repair, work of flexion after, 97: 371
techniques
  epitenon-first, in flexor tendon repair, 96: 91
  in extensor zone IV, biomechanical characteristics of, 97: 93
  tendon, mechanical analysis of (in rabbit), 96: 378
tendon repair
  double and multiple looped, 96: 115
  flexor tendon, in vitro biomechanical analysis of methods, 95: 331
  Tsuge, in zone 2C flexor tendon repair, 95: 85
Suturing
  fascicular, for secondary digital nerve repair, 95: 115
Swanson
  arthroplasty
    for rheumatoid metacarpophalangeal joints, motion after, 95: 266
    Silastic, long-term results in rheumatoid wrist, 95: 270
  silicone finger joint implants, long-term complications of, 97: 287
Symbrachydactyly
  position in classification of congenital hand anomalies, 96: 317
  reconstruction, toe phalanx graft in, 95: 294
Sympathectomy
  for reflex sympathetic dystrophy, factors affecting outcome, 96: 364
Sympathetic
  dystrophy, reflex (see Reflex, sympathetic dystrophy)
Syndactylic
  toe transfer for fingertip reconstruction, 96: 321
Syndactyly
  complete, of first web, tissue expansion for, 96: 311
  correction without skin grafting, 97: 325
  in epidermolysis bullosa, surgical treatment, in children, 95: 291

Syndecan
  axial congenital deformities of upper limb and, 95: 301
Synostosis
  metacarpal, treatment of, 95: 290
  radioulnar
    congenital, causing severe forearm rotation deformities, surgical radioulnar osteoclasis for, 96: 67
    traumatic, excision and postoperative low-dose irradiation for, 96: 247
    after treatment of chronic post-traumatic dislocation of radial head, in children, 95: 58
Synovial
  hyperplasia in carpal tunnel syndrome, 96: 127
  sarcoma of hand, treatment, 96: 293
  sheath, flexor, of little finger, anatomy of, 97: 19
Synovialis
  flap plasty for recurrent carpal tunnel syndrome, 95: 125
Synovitis
  particulate, after Swanson silicone finger joint implants, 97: 287
Synthetic
  polymers seeded with tenocytes, generation of neo-tendon using, 96: 374
  surfaces, sports-related distal radius fractures on, 96: 222

T

Tactile
  stimulation, remodeling of hand representation in cortex determined by timing of, 97: 18
Tactility
  test, gap detection, for sensory deficits associated with carpal tunnel syndrome, 97: 24
Tajima
  suture technique for flexor tendon repair, in vitro biomechanical analysis of, 95: 331
  tendon repair, in vitro strength of, 97: 12
Tarsometatarsal
  ligament autograft for reconstruction of scapholunate interosseous ligament, 97: 165
T cell
  -mediated response in Dupuytren's disease, 95: 285

Subject Index / 453

Teachers
  music, risk of upper limb soft tissue disorders in, 96: 258
Tear (*see* Rupture)
TEC device
  for Dupuytren's contracture, 95: 282
Technetium
  bone scan for microvascular response associated with reflex sympathetic dystrophy of hand and wrist, 95: 27
Telescoping anastomosis
  in vein grafting for venous defects (in rat), 95: 317
Temperature
  effects on vibrotactile sensitivity threshold measurements, implications for carpal tunnel screening tests, 97: 136
  neutral zone threshold measurement in hand-arm vibration syndrome, 95: 237
Tendinitis
  flexor carpi radialis, results of operative treatment, 96: 111
  repetitive strain injuries of, sensory dysfunction associated with, 97: 272
  upper extremity, in music students, 97: 331
Tendocutaneous
  flap
    free, transfer for skin-tendon defect of dorsum of hand, 96: 74
    venous, arterialized, for dorsal finger reconstruction, 96: 84
Tendolysis (*see* Tenolysis)
Tendon
  arthroplasty
    interposition, for basal joint arthritis, 97: 281
    interposition, for basal joint arthrosis, radiographic assessment of trapezial space before and after, 97: 280
    for trapeziometacarpal arthrosis, 96: 285
    two-tendon, for first carpometacarpal joint arthritis, 97: 282
  biceps
    distal, repair with suture anchors and anterior approach, 97: 229
    rupture, MRI of, 95: 104
  extensor (*see under* Extensor)
  finger, forces in pianists, 95: 11
  flexor (*see* Flexor tendon)
  graft for scapholunate diastasis in distal radius fractures, 95: 190
  healing, application of forces to, 95: 92
  injury, acute, in finger, MRI of, 97: 29
  interposition-ligament reconstruction arthroplasty of basal joint of thumb, 96: 282
    for osteoarthritis of thumb base, 96: 285
  plantaris, braided, as extensor tendon graft, 96: 89
  repair
    flexor tendon splints in, 96: 376
    suture, double and multiple looped, 96: 115
    suture methods, work of flexion after, 97: 371
  -skin defect of dorsum of hand, tendinocutaneous free flap transfer for, 96: 74
  suture techniques, mechanical analysis of (in rabbit), 96: 378
  synchronization, side-to-side, for hand function restoration in spinal cord injury, 97: 245
  transfer
    biomechanical design of wrist motors and, 97: 8
    extensor digiti minimi, in prevention of recurrent ulnar drift, 95: 277
    flexor to extensor, in hand, 96: 87
    for hand function restoration in spinal cord injury, 97: 245
    secondary, after brachial plexus injuries, 96: 251
    simultaneous, in single-stage reconstruction of key pinch and extension of elbow in tetraplegics, 96: 255
    suture techniques in, mesh reinforced, early active mobilization after, 97: 108
    upper limb, in children with spastic hemiplegia, functional outcome, 95: 231
    to wrist in arthrogryposis multiplex congenita, 95: 290
  transposition across two joints in brachial nerve injuries, 95: 108
  triceps
    division in supracondylar fractures of humerus, in children, 95: 220
    slip in ligament reconstruction for chronic post-traumatic radial head dislocation, in children, 95: 56
  wrist, biomechanical properties enhance wrist muscle specialization, 97: 9
Tennis
  elbow (*see* Elbow, tennis)

players performing backhand stroke, wrist kinematics in, 96: 334
Tenocytes
  synthetic polymers seeded with, generation of neo-tendon using, 96: 374
Tenodesis
  test, central slip, for early diagnosis of potential boutonniére deformities, 95: 36
  wrist, secondary, after brachial plexus injuries, 96: 251
Tenography
  in diagnosis of traumatic rupture of finger flexor pulleys, 96: 97
Tenolysis
  flexor tendon
    laser vs. scalpel (in rabbit), 97: 374
    in zone 2, 96: 96
  for flexor tendon injuries, in children, 96: 86
Tenorrhaphy
  techniques, augmented Becker vs. modified Kessler, dynamic mechanical analysis (in monkey), 96: 98
Tenosynovectomy
  flexor, in rheumatoid arthritis
    A1 pulley in, 95: 276
    finger mobility after, short- and long-term analysis of, 95: 267
Tenosynovitis
  de Quervain's (see de Quervain's disease)
  flexor, in diabetics, 96: 303
  stenosing, of extensor carpi ulnaris, 97: 273
  wrist
    psychomotor capacity and, 95: 251
    rheumatoid factor and HLA antigens in, 97: 293
Tenovaginitis
  of sixth dorsal compartment, decompression for, 96: 110
Tensile
  loading, cyclic and static, effect on water content and solute diffusion in flexor tendons (in dog), 96: 372
  strength of repaired flexor tendons, effect of suture knots on (in dog), 96: 115
Tension
  band
    fixation of avulsion fractures of hand, clinical results, 96: 48
    osteosynthesis, double, in supra- and transcondylar humeral fractures, 96: 239

wire, vs. Herbert screw in distal interphalangeal joint arthrodesis, 97: 60
relief in nerve repair, 95: 112
wire fixation of avulsion fractures of thumb metacarpophalangeal joint, 96: 49
Terbinafine
  efficacy and tolerability of, 97: 68
Tetraplegia
  in adolescent, grasp and release abilities after functional neuromuscular stimulation in, 97: 246
  C5, in adolescents, reliability of percutaneous intramuscular electrodes for upper extremity functional neuromuscular stimulation in, 96: 256
  key pinch and extension of elbow in, single-stage reconstruction of, 96: 254
  Sollerman hand function test in, 97: 250
  traumatic, rerouting of biceps brachii for paralytic supination contracture in forearm due to, 95: 223
Therapeutic
  intervention, delayed, effects after zone II flexor tendon repair, 96: 92
Thermal
  thresholds, abnormal, in carpal tunnel syndrome, 96: 144
Thermometry
  infrared, in reflex sympathetic dystrophy, 96: 356
  vs. laser Doppler flowmetry in postoperative monitoring of replantations, 96: 352
Thermoplastic
  splint
    custom-made volar cock-up type, for carpal tunnel syndrome, in search of optimal angle, 96: 146
    after extensor tendon laceration repair, 96: 107
    after flexor tendon repairs, acute, 96: 105
Thermoregulation
  patterns in cold intolerance after digital replantation, 97: 358
Thoracic
  nerve, medial, anastomosis to musculocutaneous nerve, functional recovery of elbow flexion by, 95: 117
  outlet syndrome, orthosis in, 96: 330

Threshold
  testing, current perception, as screening procedure for carpal tunnel syndrome in industrial workers, 96: 260
Thrombosis
  deep venous, of upper limb, 97: 358
Thumb
  adductor muscles, force-generating capacity in parallel and perpendicular plane of adduction, 96: 31
  anatomy, arterial, 95: 1
  base
    osteoarthritis, excision of trapezium for, 96: 284
    osteoarthrosis, trapeziectomy and ligament reconstruction for, 95: 257
  bone, sesamoid, fracture of, 97: 66
  digital nerve repair, secondary, results of, 95: 115
  duplication
    at metacarpophalangeal joint, management and new classification, 97: 318
    nail plasty for, 95: 287
    retrospective review, 20-year, 96: 321
    surgical complications, 96: 312
    surgical treatment of, 97: 316
  flap, dorso-ulnar, 95: 73
  flexion contracture, acquired, in children, 97: 325
  flexor
    apparatus, restoration of function, oblique and one adjacent flexor tendon pulley required for, 97: 102
    pulley system, biomechanics of, 95: 2
  gamekeeper's (see Gamekeeper's thumb)
  hypoplasia
    Bauth type III, transposition of third metatarsus for reconstruction of, 97: 317
    patient characteristics, 97: 315
  joint
    basal (see Basal, joint of thumb)
    carpometacarpal (see Carpometacarpal joint, thumb)
    interphalangeal, arthrodesis, in spinal cord injury, 97: 245
    interphalangeal, axes of rotation of, 97: 6
    metacarpophalangeal (see Metacarpophalangeal joint, thumb)
  ligament, ulnar collateral (see Collateral ligament, ulnar, thumb)
  musculature, intrinsic and extrinsic, phasic relationships of, 97: 252
  polydactyly, long-term results of surgical treatment, 97: 319
  prosthesis, osseointegrated, 97: 62
  reconstruction
    flap for, heterodigital neurovascular island, with and without nerve reconnection, 96: 69
    flap for, second web bilobed island, 97: 87
    with free neurovascular wrap-around flap from big toe, long-term follow-up, 97: 350
    for hypoplastic thumb, Bauth type III, transposition of third metatarsus for, 97: 317
    Matev continuous distraction in, 96: 60
  trigger
    congenital, 97: 325
    corticosteroid injection in, 97: 264
Tinel's sign
  in carpal tunnel syndrome diagnosis in primary care, 95: 134
Tingling
  sensation, uncomfortable, after two-portal endoscopic carpal tunnel release, 96: 164
Tissue
  capsular, of proximal interphalangeal joint, 95: 9
  connective tissue disease, mixed, flexible implant resection arthroplasty of proximal interphalangeal joint in, 96: 275
  damage, radionuclide probes for, 95: 38
  expansion for complete syndactyly of first web, 96: 311
  nerve, interposition and vein conduits for peripheral nerve defects, 96: 123
  soft (see Soft tissue)
  transfer
    free, emergency, for severe upper extremity injuries, 96: 72
    free, for radiation injuries of hand, 95: 81
    free, with aid of loupe magnification, 96: 339
    microvascular, and smoking, 95: 320
  transplantation, microsurgical composite, at difficult recipient sites, vein grafts installed as arteriovenous loops in, 97: 348
Titanium
  fixation systems in metacarpal fractures, biomechanical stability of, 97: 18
  fixtures in metacarpophalangeal joint arthroplasty, 95: 265

grommet in flexible implant
arthroplasty of radiocarpal joint,
97: 289
in osseointegrated nail prosthesis,
97: 75
plate fixation of proximal phalangeal
fractures, 95: 49
Toe
(See also Digit)
big, free neurovascular wrap-around
flap from, in thumb reconstruction,
long-term follow-up, 97: 350
nail onychomycosis, antifungal pulse
therapy for, 97: 70
phalangeal graft
in congenital hand deformities,
95: 294
in symbrachydactyly reconstruction,
95: 294
transfer
combined with wrap-around flap,
96: 349
to hand, delayed sensory reeducation
after, 97: 350
to hand, pulp plasty after, 97: 77
microvascular, pediatric,
decision-making by parents and
children in, 96: 315
microvascular free, psychological
impact for children and their
parents, 97: 345
for repair of finger losses, 95: 320
second toe-to-finger, in hand
mutilations, 96: 344
syndactylic, for fingertip
reconstruction, 96: 321
Tomography
computed (see Computed tomography)
Tonic
vibration reflex in writer's cramp,
97: 334
Tools
handheld, vibration from, carpal tunnel
release in patients exposed to,
95: 235
use of, early hominid, fossil evidence
for, 96: 30
Topographical
landmarks, use to improve outcome of
Agee endoscopic carpal tunnel
release, 96: 167
Topography
intraneural, of ulnar nerve in cubital
tunnel facilitates anterior
transposition, 96: 29
Topology
of carpal tunnel during dynamic stress
situations of wrist, 96: 23

Tourniquet
arm, upper, tolerance, vs. forearm
tourniquet tolerance, 95: 26
forearm vs. upper arm, tolerance,
95: 26
Toxin
botulinum
chemodenervation for cerebral palsied
hands, 95: 229
in focal dystonia of hand, 95: 308,
309
T-plate
fixation of distal radius fracture,
comparative study, 97: 198
Trabecular
bone, and strength in osteopenic distal
radius, 95: 201
Traction
digital, dynamic, for unstable
comminuted intra-articular
fracture-dislocations of proximal
interphalangeal joint, 97: 40
radiography in diagnosis of chronic
wrist pain, 96: 191
skeletal, for flexed proximal
interphalangeal joint in
Dupuytren's disease, 96: 301
system, pins and rubbers, for
comminuted intraarticular fractures
and fracture-dislocations in hand,
95: 51
Trampoline
test, arthroscopic, 96: 231
Transducer
Hall-effect displacement, for distal
radioulnar ligament motion during
supination and pronation, 95: 211
Transfer
crossed intrinsic, for rheumatoid
metacarpophalangeal joints, motion
after, 95: 266
muscle (see Muscle, transfer)
nerve
intercostal, elbow flexion restoration
with, 96: 122
root, contralateral C7, with
vascularized nerve grafting for
brachial plexus root avulsion (in
rat), 95: 339
ulnar, anterior subcutaneous, in
athlete, 95: 141
pronator quadratus interposition, as
adjunct to resection arthroplasty of
distal radioulnar joint, 97: 214
tendon
(See also Tendon, transfer)
extensor, bypass, 97: 102
tissue (see Tissue, transfer)

toe (see Toe, transfer)
triceps-to-radius, for elbow flexion in arthrogryposis multiplex congenita, 95: 290
Transforming growth factor-β
  modulation of formation of molded vascularized bone graft in vivo (in rat), 96: 382
  role in Dupuytren's contracture, 96: 381
Translation
  ulnar (see Ulnar, translation)
Transplantation
  (See also Allograft)
  autotransplantation, free fat, for cosmetic treatment of first web space atrophy, 97: 87
  kidney, treatment of recurrent squamous cell carcinoma of hand after, 96: 294
  of metatarsus, third, for reconstruction of Bauth type III hypoplastic thumb, 97: 317
  muscle
    (See also Muscle, transfer)
    functioning free, for brachial plexus injury, 96: 253
    gracilis, free, for hand reconstruction, 96: 353
    phalanges of foot, free, in hand deformities, 97: 345
  tissue, microsurgical composite, at difficult recipient sites, vein grafts installed as arteriovenous loops in, 97: 348
  toe-to-hand, pulp plasty after, 97: 77
Transposition
  extensor digiti minimi quinti, for metacarpal synostosis, 95: 291
  pisiform, pedicled, in Kienböck's disease, 95: 177
Transthecal
  vs. traditional digital block for anesthesia of finger, 96: 44
Trapezial
  space before and after ligament reconstruction and tendon interposition arthroplasty for basal joint arthrosis, radiographic assessment of, 97: 280
Trapeziectomy
  with ligament reconstruction and tendon interposition arthroplasty for basal joint arthritis, 97: 281
  for osteoarthritis of carpometacarpal joint of thumb, revision procedures for complications of, 95: 261
  for osteoarthrosis, thumb base, 95: 257

Trapeziolunate
  external fixation for scaphoid fractures, 96: 197
Trapeziometacarpal
  arthritis, stabilized resection arthroplasty by anterior approach in, 97: 283, 295
  arthrosis, tendon arthroplasty for, 96: 285
  joint
    arthrodesis, power staple fixation in, 95: 263
    degenerative changes, radiologic assessment of, 97: 275
    osteoarthritis, extension metacarpal osteotomy for, 97: 277
  prosthesis, GUEPAR total, in carpometacarpal arthritis of thumb, 95: 258
Trapezium
  (See also Scapho-trapezio-trapezoid)
  excision for osteoarthritis at thumb base, 96: 284
Trapezius
  transfer, secondary, after brachial plexus injuries, 96: 251
Trapezoid (see Scapho-trapezio-trapezoid)
Trauma
  (See also Injuries)
  arthritis after
    (See also Arthritis, posttraumatic)
    degenerative, of carpometacarpal joint of small finger, silicone implant arthroplasty for, 96: 290
  avulsion of triangular fibrocartilage complex at its ulnar insertion due to
    new reattachment technique, 96: 230
    reinsertion and hemiepiphyseal osteotomy at distal ulna for, 97: 222
  blunt, causing flexor carpi radialis tendinitis, results of operative treatment, 96: 111
  brachial plexus, MRI in diagnosis of, 95: 226
  carpal row dislocations due to, distal, 96: 208
  closed, causing finger flexor pulley rupture, 96: 97
  cumulative (see Cumulative trauma disorders)
  delivery, brachial plexopathy in infants after, MRI of, 95: 224
  epiphysiodesis of distal end of radius after, progressive lengthening in, 97: 324

extensor tendon rupture at musculotendinous junction, 97: 101
extremity, upper
   airbag-related, 96: 67
   severe, emergency free tissue transfer for, 96: 72
finger shortening after, phalanx lengthening for, 95: 67
phalanges malunion after, corrective osteotomy for, 97: 43
primary, late secondary repair of flexor pollicis longus masquerading as, 96: 115
radioulnar joint, distal, disorders after, Kapandji procedure for, 95: 204
radioulnar synostosis due to, excision and postoperative low-dose irradiation for, 96: 247
radius head dislocation due to
   chronic, treatment, in children, 95: 56
   "isolated", 96: 243
rolling belt, in children, 96: 83
tetraplegia after, rerouting of biceps brachii for paralytic supination contracture of forearm due to, 95: 223
triangular fibrocartilage complex (see Triangular fibrocartilage complex, injuries)
ulna subluxation after, distal, hemiresection-interposition arthroplasty for, 95: 205
ulnar physeal arrest due to, after distal forearm fracture, in children, 97: 320
ulnar translation due to, radiolunate arthrodesis for, 96: 3
Triangular fibrocartilage complex
   appearance on coronal 3D gradient-recalled-echo MR images, normal, 96: 12
   avulsion, traumatic, at its ulnar insertion
      new reattachment technique, 96: 230
      reinsertion and hemiepiphyseal osteotomy at distal ulna for, 97: 222
   injuries
      acute, with distal radioulnar joint instability, treatment of, 96: 237
      arthroscopic partial resection after, 95: 206
      laboratory model, 97: 225
      with radial fractures, intraarticular distal, 97: 204
      with radioulnar joint dislocation, distal, 95: 207
   lesions
      diagnosis, MRI-cinematography in, 96: 233
      radial-sided, arthroscopic repair, 96: 238
   ligament of, dorsal, reconstruction, 96: 231
   perforations, incomplete, on wrist arthrography, lack of correlation between site of wrist pain and, 95: 162
   resection of, arthroscopic partial, 95: 206
   role in forearm stability, 95: 333
   strains in articular disk of, 95: 208
   tears
      arthrographic evaluation of, 95: 161
      arthroscopic debridement of, clinical results, 97: 223
   wear patterns of, 96: 3
   in wrist injuries, techniques of arthroscopic repair of, 97: 226
Triaxial elbow
   in salvage of failed total elbow arthroplasty, 97: 236
Triceps
   tendon
      division in supracondylar fractures of humerus, in children, 95: 220
      slip in ligament reconstruction for chronic post-traumatic radial head dislocation, in children, 95: 56
      -to-radius transfer for elbow flexion in arthrogryposis multiplex congenita, 95: 290
Trigger finger
   corticosteroid injections in, 97: 264
   diabetes mellitus and, 96: 303
   release, percutaneous, 95: 101
   safety and efficacy of, 96: 114
Trigger thumb
   congenital, 97: 325
Triquetral
   bone avulsion fracture, volar aspect, 97: 187
Triquetrohamate
   arthrodesis for midcarpal instability, 97: 169
Triquetrolunate
   ligament rupture, longstanding, frayed ulnotriquetral and ulnolunate ligaments as arthroscopic sign of, 96: 206
Triquetroscaphoid
   ligament, MRI of, 95: 168

Triradiate
    skin incision for dorsal approach to wrist, 97: 149
Truck
    assemblers exposed to hand-arm vibration, impaired nerve conduction in carpal tunnel of, 96: 264
Tsuge suture
    in flexor tendon repair
        biomechanical analysis of, in vitro, 95: 331
    in zone 2C, 95: 85
Tubiana staging system
    in Dupuytren's disease, 96: 306
Tubular
    repair of median nerve in forearm, 96: 126
Tumor
    arm, primary malignant, resection-replantation for, 96: 296
    desmoid, of ulna, and neurofibromatosis, 97: 312
    giant cell, of distal radius, 97: 297
        treatment of, 95: 281
    glomus
        extradigital, 97: 302
        subungual, MRI of, 96: 291
Tuning
    automated, of closed-loop hand grasp neuroprosthesis, 95: 310
Turf
    synthetic, sports-related distal radius fractures on, 96: 222
Two-dimensional
    study in posteroanterior plane of force and pressure transmission through normal wrist, 96: 370
Two-point discrimination
    in fingertip, and skin hardness and pressure perception, 96: 41
    testing
        before digital nerve repair, unilateral, 95: 113
        vs. functional sensory recovery in both median and ulnar nerve complete transections, 95: 117
        in workplace surveillance for carpal tunnel syndrome, 95: 248
Typist's cramp
    botulinum toxin in, 95: 308

U

Ulna
    bowing after treatment of chronic post-traumatic dislocation of radial head, in children, 95: 58
    distal
        excision in rheumatoid arthritis, 97: 290
        osteotomy at, hemiepiphyseal, for traumatic avulsion of triangular fibrocartilage complex at its ulnar insertion, 97: 222
        resection in rheumatoid arthritis, radiological evaluation of long-term effects of, 96: 270
        subluxation, chronic post-traumatic dorsal, hemiresection-interposition arthroplasty for, 95: 205
    fracture (see Fracture, ulna)
    lengthening
        in Kienböck's disease, long-term follow-up, 97: 180
        in osteochondromata, multiple hereditary, in children, 95: 289
    osteotomy, shortening (see Osteotomy, ulnar shortening)
    proximal, unstable, after Kapandji procedure for posttraumatic distal radioulnar joint problems, 95: 204
    shortening
        osteotomy (see Osteotomy, ulnar shortening)
        using AO small distractor, 97: 224
    straightening, surgical, in children with multiple hereditary osteochondromata, 95: 289
    tilt, effect on determination of radial shortening, 96: 9
    tumor, desmoid, and neurofibromatosis, 97: 312
    variance
        change with grip, 95: 16
        in gymnasts, female, 96: 223
Ulnar
    artery
        flap, free, 95: 320
        microvascular repair at wrist, laser Doppler imaging of finger skin blood flow after, 96: 364
        repair, patency rates assessed with color Doppler ultrasound, 95: 319
        variations in Guyon's canal, 96: 24
    bow sign in diagnosis of "isolated" traumatic radial head dislocation, 96: 244
    collateral ligament (see Collateral ligament, ulnar)
    component of total elbow replacement, fixation strength of, 97: 238
    deviation of fingers, congenital unilateral muscle hyperplasia of hand with, 96: 321

dislocation of extensor pollicis longus,
    95: 68
drift, recurrent, extensor digiti minimi
    tendon transfer in prevention of,
    95: 277
impaction syndrome, ulnar shortening
    using AO small distractor for,
    97: 224
insertion, traumatic avulsion of
    triangular fibrocartilage complex at
    new technique of reattachment,
    96: 230
    reinsertion and hemiepiphyseal
    osteotomy at distal ulna for,
    97: 222
nerve
    compression, incidence after fractures
        of distal radius, 96: 219
    in cubital tunnel, intraneural
        topography facilitates anterior
        transposition, 96: 29
    deep branch, normal arborization
        into interossei and lumbricals,
        96: 27
    defects, vein conduits with
        interposition of nerve tissue for,
        96: 124
    at elbow, extrinsic blood supply of,
        95: 4
    in forearm, communications between
        median nerve and, 95: 15
    grafts in brachial plexus lesions,
        enzymhistochemical evaluation of,
        95: 107
    injury, secondary microsurgical repair
        results, 95: 114
    lesion, effect on motion of index
        finger, 97: 37
    palsy after lateral approach for
        non-constrained elbow
        replacement, 97: 237
    pressure, intraneural, changes related
        to operative techniques for cubital
        tunnel decompression, 96: 161
    repair, functional sensibility and
        cognitive capacities after, 96: 118
    transection, complete, combined with
        median nerve complete transection,
        two-point discrimination tests *vs.*
        functional sensory recovery in,
        95: 117
    transfer, anterior subcutaneous, in
        athlete, 95: 141
    transposition, anterior submuscular,
        in cubital tunnel syndrome,
        97: 146
    variations in Guyon's canal, 96: 24

neuropathy after median sternotomy,
    95: 142
neurovascular bundle at wrist, in
    endoscopic carpal tunnel release,
    95: 148
parametacarpal flap, anatomical study
    and clinical application, 97: 78
physeal arrest, traumatic, after distal
    forearm fracture, in children,
    97: 320
translation
    instability, pathomechanics of,
        extrinsic wrist ligaments in, 96: 1
    measurement of, 96: 7
    wrist pain after Colles' fracture,
        95: 195
Ulnocarpal
    stress test, positive, 97: 162
Ulnolunate
    ligament
        frayed, as arthroscopic sign of
            longstanding triquetrolunate
            ligament rupture, 96: 206
        MRI of, 95: 168
        tensions, 95: 173
Ulnomesicotriquetral
    dorsal glide test in wrist pain
        evaluation, 96: 181
Ulnotriquetral
    ligament
        frayed, as arthroscopic sign of
            longstanding triquetrolunate
            ligament rupture, 96: 206
        MRI of, 95: 168
Ultrasound
    differentiation of displaced and
        nondisplaced ulnar collateral
        ligament tears, 96: 33
    Doppler, color, in assessment of patency
        rates after radial and ulnar artery
        repairs, 95: 319
    in flexor tendon injury management,
        zone 1, 95: 88
    sensitivity and specificity in diagnosis of
        foreign bodies in hand, 97: 26
    of ulnar collateral ligament of thumb
        dislocated, 97: 28
        injured, 96: 35
Ungual
    mycoses, efficacy and tolerability of
        Lamisil in, 97: 68
Unicondylar
    fracture, distal, of proximal phalanx,
        95: 46
Ureteroscope
    Olympus, flexible, for retrieval of
        severed flexor tendons, 96: 89

V

Valgus
  instability test of elbow, arthroscopic, evaluation of, 97: 30
  stress testing in injuries of ulnar collateral ligament of thumb metacarpophalangeal joint, 95: 41
Vascular
  access, upper extremity, for dialysis, neurologic and ischemic complications of, 96: 362
  bundle implantation
    into bone for aseptic necrosis of lunate, 97: 179
    with bone grafting, for scaphoid nonunion, 97: 176
  microvascular (see Microvascular)
  neurovascular (see Neurovascular)
  supply of nail bed and matrix, anatomical study of, 97: 5
Vascularized
  flap
    nail, short-pedicle, 97: 71
    for radiation injuries to hand, 95: 81
  graft
    bone, molded, in vivo growth factor modulation of formation of (in rat), 96: 382
    Carlos Zaidemberg's, anatomical basis of, 97: 17
    fibular, for congenital pseudoarthrosis of forearm, 95: 319
    nerve, with contralateral C7 root transfer, for brachial plexus root avulsion (in rat), 95: 339
Vasomotor
  changes in reflex sympathetic dystrophy, 96: 356
Vasospasm
  cold-induced, after digital replantation
    abnormal sensory regeneration and sensitization of cold nociceptors and, 97: 349
    arterial reconstruction methods in, 97: 358
    no improvement with time, 96: 347
Vein
  arteriovenous (see Arteriovenous)
  conduits with interposition of nerve tissue for peripheral nerve defects, 96: 123
  flap
    arterialized tendocutaneous, for dorsal finger reconstruction, 96: 84
    for covering skin defects of hand, 96: 341
  graft (see Graft, vein)
  mesh, comparison to silastic and polyglycolic acid fine mesh, 97: 378
  thrombosis, deep, of upper limb, 97: 358
Venorrhaphy
  in brachial artery injuries, penetrating, 96: 345
Vessels
  (See also Vascular)
  recipient, distal to zone of injury, liability when used for extremity free flaps, 97: 351
Vibrameter
  Goldberg-Lindblom, 95: 240
Vibration
  energy, absorption in hand and arm, 95: 322
  hand, and work-related Dupuytren's contracture, 97: 305
  hand-arm
    platers and truck assemblers exposed to, impaired nerve conduction in carpal tunnel of, 96: 264
    syndrome, sensorineural objective tests in, 95: 236
  from handheld tools, carpal tunnel release in patients exposed to, 95: 235
  hands damaged by, neurophysiological investigation of, 95: 239
  -induced white finger, prognosis of, 97: 355
  reflex, tonic, in writer's cramp, 97: 334
  syndrome, peripheral neuropathy in, digital nerve conduction velocity as sensitive indication of, 96: 261
Vibratron II fixed-frequency varying-amplitude device
  establishment of reliability with, 95: 16
Vibrogram
  Lundborg, 95: 240
Vibrometry
  in carpal tunnel syndrome diagnosis, vs. traditional electrodiagnostic studies and elcctroneurometry, 97: 133
  testing vs. sensory nerve conduction measures in screening for carpal tunnel syndrome in industrial setting, 96: 338
  in workplace surveillance for carpal tunnel syndrome, 95: 248
Vibrotactile
  sensitivity threshold measurements, temperature effects on, implications for carpal tunnel screening tests, 97: 136

Vigorimeter
  for hand function assessment, 95: 34
Vinca alkaloids
  extravasation
    at dorsum of hand, treatment of, 95: 279
    management and surgical treatment, 95: 280
Vision
  limited direct, in carpal tunnel release, 96: 172
Vitallium
  plate and screw fixation of proximal phalangeal fractures, 95: 49
  radial head prosthesis after radial head fracture, 95: 221
Volar
  carpal ligaments, MRI of, 95: 168
  dislocation of distal radioulnar joint, 96: 233
Volkmann's contracture
  muscle transfer in, free, 95: 311
  follow-up studies, 95: 312
Volz total wrist arthroplasty
  long-term outcome of, 95: 272
V-Y advancement flap
  dorsal, in digital reconstruction, 95: 69

W

Wartenberg's syndrome
  case reports, 95: 143
  de Quervain's disease and, 97: 267
Wassel type IV deformity
  management and new classification, 97: 318
Water
  content in flexor tendons, effect of cyclic and static tensile loading on (in dog), 96: 372
Wear
  patterns of articular cartilage and triangular fibrocartilaginous complex of wrist, 96: 3
Web
  first, tissue expansion for complete syndactyly of, 96: 311
  plasty, first, for thumb polydactyly, long-term results, 97: 319
  space
    first, atrophy, free fat autotransplantation for cosmetic treatment of, 97: 87
    first, contracture, and hand function, 95: 5
    reconstruction, reverse dorsometacarpal flap in, 96: 342

Wheelchair
  athletes, upper extremity peripheral nerve entrapments among, 95: 309
  User's Shoulder Pain Index, reliability and validity of, 97: 337
Whisker-pad
  muscles, permanent motor hyperinnervation after hypoglossal-facial anastomosis (in rat), 95: 327
White finger
  vibration-induced, prognosis of, 97: 355
Wilhelm's technique
  for denervation of wrist joint, 95: 174
Wire
  implant in mallet finger, 95: 98
  K- (see Kirschner wire)
  Kirschner (see Kirschner wire)
  tension band, vs. Herbert screw in distal interphalangeal joint arthrodesis, 97: 60
  tension wire fixation of avulsion fractures at thumb metacarpophalangeal joint, 96: 49
Women
  carpal tunnel syndrome risk in, 96: 136, 157
  caucasian, reflex sympathetic dystrophy in, 96: 357
Word
  processing with and without mouse use, variation in upper limb posture and movement during, 96: 265
Work
  disability and work-related upper extremity disorders, 97: 262
  of piano virtuosity, 97: 341; 96: 333
  -related Dupuytren's contracture, 97: 305
  -related upper extremity disorders and work disability, 97: 262
  -relatedness of self-reported carpal tunnel syndrome, in U.S. workers, 96: 265
  repetitive movements at, relation to upper limb soft tissue disorders, 96: 258
  return to, after open vs. endoscopic carpal tunnel release, 97: 113
  survivability and cumulative trauma disorders, 97: 261
Workers
  automobile assembly line
    characteristics of forearm-hand exposure in relation to symptoms among, 97: 272

self-reported physical exposure and
musculoskeletal symptoms of
forearm-hand among, 97: 328
carpal malalignment after intra-articular
fractures of distal radius in,
96: 220
carpal tunnel syndrome in,
self-reported, prevalence and
work-relatedness of, in U.S.,
96: 265
compensation
recipients with carpal tunnel
syndrome, validity of self-reported
health measures, 97: 127
status, effect on carpal tunnel surgery
outcomes, 97: 125
Washington State, outcome of carpal
tunnel surgery in, 95: 233
industry (see Industry, workers)
meat processing plant, psychomotor
capacity and wrist tenosynovitis in,
95: 252
metal, prognosis of occupational hand
dermatitis in, 97: 340
office, medical screening for upper
extremity cumulative trauma
disorders in, 95: 244
performing repetitive tasks, detecting
cumulative trauma disorders in,
96: 265
Workplace
surveillance for carpal tunnel syndrome,
95: 248
hand diagrams in, 96: 138
Wound
bite, infected clench-fist human, in area
of metacarpophalangeal joints,
treatment of, 97: 54
bullet, causing penetrating brachial
artery injuries, 96: 345
complications after AO/ASIF wrist
arthrodesis, 96: 194
drainage for palmar space infections,
96: 308
gunshot, low-velocity, of brachial
plexus, 96: 121
knife, causing penetrating brachial
artery injuries, 96: 345
Wrist
(See also Carpal)
approach to, dorsal, triradiate incision
for, 97: 149
arthrodesis (see Arthrodesis, wrist)
arthrography (see Arthrography, wrist)
arthroplasty (see Arthroplasty, wrist)
arthroscopy (see Arthroscopy, wrist)
arthrotomy in evaluation of chronic
wrist pain, 95: 161

cartilage of, articular, wear patterns of,
96: 3
cinearthrography, triple-injection, vs.
arthroscopy, 97: 193
collapse, scapholunate advanced
motion-preserving procedures for,
97: 186
scaphoidectomy and capitolunate
arthrodesis for, 97: 192
contralateral, normal, as reference for
x-ray film measurements of
pathologic wrist, 97: 151
denervation of, Wilhelm's technique,
95: 174
deviation, effect on grip and pinch
strength, 96: 194
disk of, articular, healing of (in dog),
95: 209
extensor orthoses, commercial, 96: 338
flexion-extension after Kapandji
procedure for posttraumatic distal
radioulnar joint problems, 95: 204
fracture, articular, carpal tunnel
pressure in, 96: 217
ganglia (see Ganglia, wrist)
gymnast's
in athletes, adolescent, 96: 225
in females, 96: 223
injuries
acute, epidemiology of, 95: 164
carpal instability after, arthroscopy in
diagnosis of, 95: 159
Galeazzi-equivalent, in children,
95: 61
intercarpal ligamentous, arthroscopic
categorization of, 95: 157
neuropathy after, acute median,
95: 109
instability series, increased yield with
clinical-radiologic screening criteria,
96: 190
joint
innervation, anatomic study of,
95: 174
movement, full range, carpal bone
kinematics and ligament
lengthening during, 95: 170
prosthesis, Meuli cementless, first
experience with, 95: 273
kinematics
during pitching, 97: 157
in tennis players performing
backhand stroke, 96: 334
ligament(s)
carpal (see Carpal, ligament)
defects, symmetric, in contralateral
asymptomatic wrists, wrist
arthrography for, 97: 191

extrinsic, in pathomechanics of ulnar
    translation instability, 96: 1
injuries, partial scapholunate and
    lunotriquetral, arthroscopic
    management of, 97: 170
integrity, wrist arthrography for, in
    young asymptomatic adults,
    97: 190
palmar, clinical relevance of, 96: 177
scapholunate interosseous, MR
    appearances, 96: 205
median nerve lesion at, benign and
    minor, value of special motor and
    sensory tests for diagnosis, 97: 147
motors, biomechanical design and
    application to tendon transfers,
    97: 8
muscle specialization, effect of tendon
    biomechanical properties on, 97: 9
normal, force and pressure transmission
    through, 96: 370
osteoarthritis, asymptomatic
    scapholunate advanced collapse in,
    95: 184
pain (see Pain, wrist)
position
    carpal tunnel pressure and, lowest,
        97: 130
    effect on extensor mechanism after
        disruption separation, 96: 112
prosthesis implant, Meuli III, correctly
    implanted, 96: 288
reflex sympathetic dystrophy,
    microvascular response patterns
    associated with, 95: 27
rheumatoid arthritis of (see Rheumatoid
    arthritis, wrist)
splint (see Splint, wrist)
squareness and median nerve
    impairment, 97: 134
stress situations of, dynamic, topology
    of carpal tunnel during, 96: 23
surgery
    early corrective, in arthrogryposis
        multiplex congenita, 95: 290
    radius bone graft in, distal anterior,
        97: 59
tendon biomechanical properties
    enhance wrist muscle specialization,
    97: 9

tenodesis, secondary, after brachial
    plexus injuries, 96: 251
tenosynovitis
    de Quervain's, MRI in, 97: 265
    psychomotor capacity and, 95: 251
    rheumatoid factor and HLA antigens
        in, 97: 293
ulnar artery repair at, microvascular,
    laser Doppler imaging of finger
    skin blood flow after, 96: 364
ulnar neurovascular bundle at, in
    endoscopic carpal tunnel release,
    95: 148
uninjured, scaphoid shift in, 96: 182
x-rays, digitalized conventional, monitor
    findings of, 96: 38
Writer's cramp
    botulinum toxin in, 95: 308, 309
    tonic vibration reflex and muscle
        afferent block in, 97: 334
WUSPI
    reliability and validity of, 97: 337
Wynn-Perry test
    of hand sensation, 95: 34

X

X-ray (see Radiography)
Xylocaine (see Lidocaine)

Z

Zaidemberg, Carlos
    vascularized graft, anatomical basis of,
        97: 17
Zancolli
    -lasso procedure for hand function
        restoration in spinal cord injury,
        97: 245
    procedure, secondary, after brachial
        plexus injuries, 96: 251
    sesamoid arthrodesis technique,
        modified, for hyperextension of
        thumb metacarpophalangeal joint,
        96: 53
Z-plasty
    for thumb polydactyly, long-term
        results, 97: 319

Author Index

A

Abdullah AF, 128
Abrahamsson S-O, 372
Adani R, 346
Adkins R, 263
Adler L, 375
Akin S, 83
Alemzadeh S, 151
Allampallam K, 140
Allen PE, 154
Altchek DW, 30
Amadio PC, 120, 124
Amarante MTJ, 374
Amiel D, 372
Amis AA, 238
Andersen M, 355
Angel MF, 369
Angrigiani C, 81
Anthony JP, 348
Aoki M, 371
Applegate EB, 337
Ark JW, 3
Asante DK, 34
Ashford RF, 263
Ateshian GA, 3
Atkins RM, 154
Aufranc S, 60

B

Babovic S, 369
Badillet G, 68
Bain GI, 12, 216
Bakhach J, 78
Ballard JL, 134
Barbieri CH, 149
Baruchin AM, 75
Bass RL, 193
Baylis W, 111
Bechtold LL, 89
Behrman MJ, 22
Belkoff SM, 164
Bell-Krotoski JA, 1
Beredjiklian P, 375
Berger AR, 132
Berger RA, 158
Betz RR, 246
Blair WF, 193
Bloom T, 130
Blyth MJG, 34
Bombardier C, 255
Bos KE, 91
Bose KK, 140
Bradbury ET, 345
Brånemark P-I, 62
Braun RM, 85

Bray PW, 26
Breen CJ, 137
Britz GW, 139
Brogmus G, 260
Brown RA, 364
Brown RE, 294
Brunelli GA, 167
Brunelli GR, 167
Brushart TM, 361
Buchbinder R, 255
Büchler U, 39, 43
Buford WL, 6
Bundoc R, 318
Burkholder TJ, 8
Busa R, 346
Butkevich AT, 54
Byström S, 328

C

Cabrera M, 345
Callahan LF, 294
Campbell JP, 26
Capone RA Jr, 289
Caso J, 324
Castagnetti C, 346
Cautilli DA, 224
Chadaev AP, 54
Chakraborty J, 140
Chan WS, 322
Cheng JC, 318
Cherniack MG, 133
Chevaleraud E, 35
Chiu H-Y, 343
Choi KY, 322
Choi S-J, 366
Chotigavanich C, 105
Clayton ML, 236
Cobb TK, 124
Cobby M, 29
Cole WG, 321
Constantinescu MA, 374
Cooke KS, 275
Cornil C, 302
Court-Brown CM, 201
Crain GM, 111
Culp RW, 264
Culver JE, 169
Cuono CB, 188
Curtis KA, 337

D

Dauwe D, 21
Davis S, 231
Dawson J, 60

Decroix J, 70
de Doncker P, 70
Degnan GG, 22
Dell PC, 214, 320
de Smet L, 21
Ditto EW III, 128
Doherty W, 47
Doi K, 103, 106
Domangue B, 22
Doré C, 364, 365
Dumontier C, 196
Dzwierzynski WW, 95

E

Eaton RG, 183
Edwards D, 125
Eggli S, 176
Eglseder WA Jr, 164
Eisenhauer MA, 175
Ejeskär A, 250
Elder KW, 152
Endo T, 71
Erickson S, 95
Esling F, 178
Esser RD, 231
Evanoff B, 191

F

Fagan R, 48
Falco NA, 299
Feldberg L, 323
Fellinger M, 206
Ferenc CC, 214
Ferlic DC, 236
Fernandez DL, 176
Feuerstein M, 262
Field LD, 30
Firoozbakhsh K, 47
Fischer M, 222
Fischer T, 229
Fischer TJ, 114
Fjeldsgaard K, 200
Fogleman M, 260
Foliart DE, 287
Fontaneda JM, 324
Fortems Y, 21, 141
Fortino MD, 155
Fossel KK, 122
Foucher G, 267, 302
Fransson-Hall C, 328
Freeland AE, 204
Froimson AI, 53
Fuchs HA, 294
Fusi S, 188

Fuss FK, 14

G

Garcia-Elias M, 160
Gawkrodger DJ, 340
Gazarian A, 78
Geissler WB, 204
Gelberman RH, 163, 280, 281, 372
Gilula LA, 191
Gingrass MK, 294
Giurintano DJ, 1, 6
Glajchen N, 265
Glicenstein J, 35, 316
Glickel SZ, 275
Glowacki KA, 137
Goel V, 255
Gonzalez J, 324
Gonzalez MH, 45
Gordon DA, 40
Gordon L, 130
Goutallier D, 196
Graf P, 67
Grechenig W, 206
Greenwald D, 10
Greenwald DP, 374
Grilli D, 81
Gröner R, 67
Groth GN, 89
Gu Yu-dong, 104
Guero S, 316
Guo J-h, 179
Gupta A, 43

H

Haasbeek JF, 321
Haddad R, 316
Hagen AD, 337
Hajducka C, 201
Hall RF Jr, 45
Hall S, 365
Hallock GG, 118
Hamanaka I, 115
Hanel DP, 207
Hannafin JA, 270
Harii K, 366
Harris GD, 114
Haws MJ, 363
Hayashi H, 5
Haynor DR, 139
Healey JH, 297
Hernández C, 171
Herskovitz S, 132
Hewison J, 345
Higgs PE, 125
Himmelstein JS, 262

Höglund M, 28
Hollister A, 6
Holmberg J, 285
Hooper G, 301
Hopf C, 268
Höri W, 67
Hotchkiss RN, 233
Hove LM, 200
Hubbard PP, 193
Huene D, 248
Hung L, 318
Hurtado P, 171
Huuskonen M, 293

I

Ide J, 367
Igram CM, 45
Ihara K, 103
Ilstrup DM, 120
Ishii S, 319
Ishikawa J-I, 223

J

Jacobsen MB, 113
James MA, 315
Janssen A, 323
Jeng O-J, 24
Jobe CM, 239
Johanson ME, 252
Johnson JA, 12
Jonsson K, 237
Judkins A, 277
Jukhtin VI, 54
Jupiter JB, 198

K

Kadiyala RK, 280
Kaji R, 334
Kanaya F, 317
Kanje M, 362
Karacalar A, 83
Kashiwagi D, 234
Katayama M, 334
Kato S, 234
Katz JN, 122, 127, 163
Kawaguchi Y, 123
Kay SPJ, 345
Keith MW, 245
Kerboull L, 283
Kiefhaber TR, 186
Kihara H, 210, 220
Kilbom Å, 328
Kilgore KL, 245
Kinninmonth AWG, 34
Kirschenbaum D, 190

Kitay GS, 97
Klinenberg E, 136
Klug MS, 40
Kneeland JB, 97
Kollias SC, 172
Kour A-K, 335
Kozin SH, 50
Krause JO, 51
Kreder HJ, 207
Küllmer K, 268
Kuntz C, 139
Kuwata N, 106
Kwon B, 280

L

Labosky DA, 56
Laitung G, 353
Lam TP, 322
Lamoreux LW, 252
Landrieu KW, 22
Landsman JC, 53
Lantieri LA, 283
Lanzetta M, 267
Lawrence T, 141
Lawson GM, 301
Leatherwood DF, 124
Lederman RJ, 330
Lee GW, 355
Lee J-W, 343
Lee KSL, 353
Lee M-J, 366
Leijnse JNAL, 7
Leit ME, 217
Lenoble E, 196, 302
Leow E-L, 335
Le Viet D, 99
Le Viet DT, 283
Levin LS, 348
Lewis FM, 340
Lieber RL, 9
Lins RE, 281
Linscheid RL, 180
Lintner S, 229
Lipton RB, 132
Liss GM, 305
Livesey JP, 282
Ljung P, 237
Loren GJ, 8, 9
Lundborg G, 62, 285, 362
Lutz DA, 118

M

Ma M-K, 104
MacDermid JC, 216
Mahaisavariya B, 105
Mahoney JL, 26

Maki S, 58
Malczewski MC, 363
Malmivaara A, 293
Manchester RA, 331
Manske PR, 51, 59, 315, 371
Marczyk SC, 94
Martin DS, 125
Martin MA, 171
Mass D, 11
Mathur V, 361
Matloub HS, 95
Matthews JP, 279
May EJ, 108
Mazzer N, 149
McCarroll HR Jr, 315
McKee M, 207
McKee MD, 218
McKeown L, 281
McQueen MM, 201
Melhorn JM, 258, 261
Mikkelsen S, 355
Miller CD, 239
Miller JG, 353
Minami A, 223
Minami M, 234
Minguella J, 345
Mirly HL, 51, 59
Moalli D, 133
Mobbs P, 141
Moneim MS, 47
Morgan JP, 40
Morgan WJ, 157
Morwessel RM, 270
Mulcahey MJ, 246
Muren C, 28
Murphy DG, 175
Murray PM, 187

N

Nagano A, 143
Nagelburg S, 263
Nagle DJ, 114
Nahlieli O, 75
Naidu SH, 375
Nakajima Y, 31
Nakamichi K, 131
Nakamura R, 162
Nakayama Y, 71
Nalebuff EA, 302
Nanchahal J, 290
Nancollas MP, 126
Neill-Cage DJ, 85
Newport ML, 93
Nguyen J, 248
Nomoto Y, 123
Nonnenmacher J, 194

Norris SH, 282

O

Oepkes CT, 91
Ogino T, 319
Ohira S, 123
Okutsu I, 115
Özcan M, 83

P

Page RE, 282
Palmer AK, 208, 210
Pappas AM, 157
Parentis M, 277
Park S, 331
Pasque CB, 146
Patterson RM, 152
Peckham PH, 245
Peimer CA, 126
Pellegrini VD Jr, 277
Pereira BP, 335
Petersen R, 355
Peterson CA II, 58
Phillips C, 11
Piérard GE, 70
Pincus T, 294
Poehling GG, 170
Pollack GR, 93
Potter HG, 270
Povlsen B, 349
Powe J, 175
Pruitt DL, 371
Pugh DMW, 216
Punnett L, 127

Q

Quenzer DE, 180

R

Rader CP, 198
Radwin RG, 24
Ragot JM, 35
Rahme H, 113
Rao SB, 169
Raphael JS, 94, 264
Räuber C, 198
Ray TD, 320
Rayan GM, 146, 304
Rechnic M, 85
Rehm KE, 198
Reider B, 332
Rempel D, 136
Ress AM, 369
Rettig AC, 172

Ribe M, 160
Richards RR, 218
Riley MW, 134
Ring D, 198
Riordan DC, 1
Rispler D, 10
Ritter EF, 348
Roach KE, 337
Rodriguez J, 160
Rompe JD, 268
Rosenwasser MP, 3
Rosén B, 62
Rothwell JC, 334
Roulot E, 99
Rousselin B, 99
Rubin DA, 97
Ruby LK, 214
Ruch DS, 170
Ruf S, 43
Rydholm U, 237
Ryu J, 48

S

Sachar K, 137
Saffar P, 173
Sagerman SD, 208
Saint Cast Y, 78
Sakai K, 103, 106
Salomon GD, 183
Salter DM, 301
Samuelson M, 332
Sanders DW, 12
Savoie FH, 204
Savornin C, 178
Sayag J, 68
Scheker LR, 80
Schuind F, 151
Schulz LA, 157
Schweitzer M, 265
Scott JR, 29
Seibert FJ, 206
Seitz WH Jr, 53
Sennwald G, 222
Sennwald GR, 182
Seradge H, 144
Shah M, 340
Sheth DS, 297
Shibata K, 143
Shieh S-J, 343
Shitara T, 31
Shoemaker SD, 8
Short WH, 155, 220
Shumway S, 10
Siebert J, 81
Sieler S, 190
Silfverskiöld KL, 108
Silverstein MD, 120

Simmons B, 117
Simmons BP, 122, 127
Singson RD, 275
Skinner SR, 252
Skjeie R, 200
Smith BT, 246
Smith DK, 187
Smith GR, 233
So Y, 136
Sobel M, 297
Sollerman C, 250
Solonick D, 190
Songcharoen P, 105
Sood R, 361
Sotereanos DG, 217
Sposato RC, 134
Srinivasan VB, 279
Stallenberg B, 151
Stanek EJ III, 262
Stern PJ, 186
Stock SR, 305
Stokes HM, 22
Suenaga N, 223
Sundine M, 80
Svoboda SJ, 164
Sykes PJ, 290
Szerzinski JM, 59

T

Taavao T, 231
Tachibana S, 131
Taggart I, 29
Takahata S, 319
Takei TR, 302

Tanabe T, 115
Tanoue M, 367
Taras JS, 22, 94, 264
Tessler RH, 320
Tokimura H, 143
Tomasek J, 304
Tordai P, 28
Trail IA, 180
Tsai T-M, 73

U

Ufenast H, 182
Upton J, 299
Urban M, 323

V

van Alphen JC, 91
Van Heest A, 117
Vickery CW, 154
Viegas SF, 152
Viikari-Juntura E, 293
Viscolli C, 133
Vizethum F, 75

W

Waggy CA, 56
Wagner TF, 14
Wajima Z, 31
Wang W-Z, 111
Warwick L, 144
Waters P, 117
Watson HK, 188

Weeks PM, 355
Wehbé MA, 224
Wei F-C, 77
Weiss A-PC, 42
Weiss D, 332
Weiss ND, 130
Werner FW, 155, 210, 220
Wheeler DR, 126
Whitworth IH, 364, 365
Williams CD, 93
Williams RL, 290
Wintman BI, 163
Wolber PH, 128
Wood MB, 58, 337
Wood VE, 248
Wright MH, 239
Wright TW, 337
Wyrick JD, 186
Wyrsch B, 60

Y

Yamaga M, 367
Yelin E, 327
Yim KK, 77
Yin YM, 191
Yoshimura M, 76
Young VL, 89
Yuen JC, 73

Z

Zafiropoulos G, 238
Zagula M, 68
Zamboni WA, 363
Zogby RG, 208
Zook EG, 294